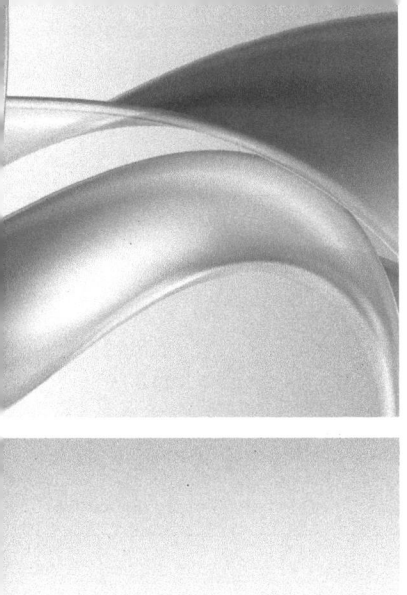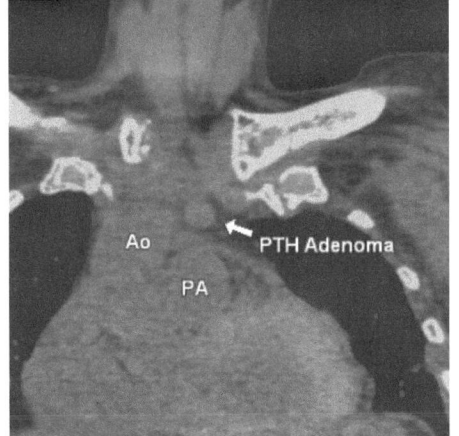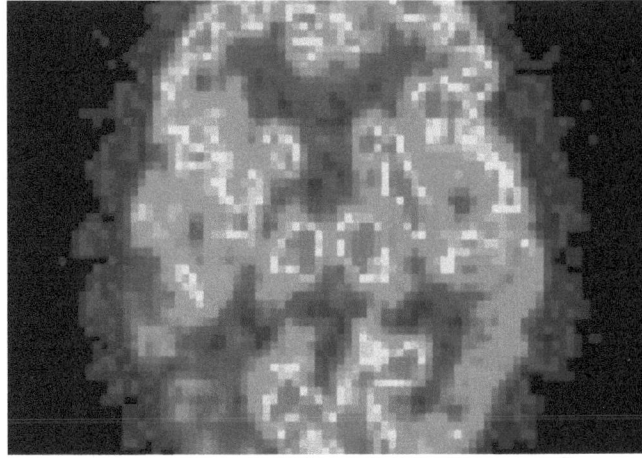

Nuclear Medicine INSTRUMENTATION

JENNIFER PREKEGES, MS, CNMT
Bellevue College
Bellevue, WA

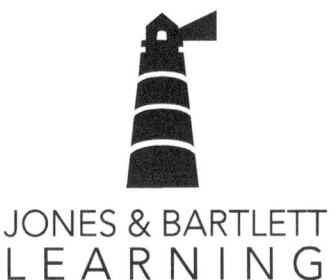

JONES & BARTLETT
LEARNING

World Headquarters
Jones & Bartlett Learning
25 Mall Road
Burlington, MA 01803
978-443-5000
info@jblearning.com
www.jblearning.com

Jones & Bartlett Learning books and products are available through most bookstores and online booksellers. To contact Jones & Bartlett Learning directly, call 800-832-0034, fax 978-443-8000, or visit our website, www.jblearning.com.

Substantial discounts on bulk quantities of Jones & Bartlett Learning publications are available to corporations, professional associations, and other qualified organizations. For details and specific discount information, contact the special sales department at Jones & Bartlett Learning via the above contact information or send an email to specialsales@jblearning.com.

Copyright © 2013 by Jones & Bartlett Learning, LLC, an Ascend Learning Company

All rights reserved. No part of the material protected by this copyright may be reproduced or utilized in any form, electronic or mechanical, including photocopying, recording, or by any information storage and retrieval system, without written permission from the copyright owner.

Nuclear Medicine Instrumentation, Second Edition is an independent publication and has not been authorized, sponsored, or otherwise approved by the owners of the trademarks or service marks referenced in this product.

Some images in this book feature models. These models do not necessarily endorse, represent, or participate in the activities represented in the images.

Production Credits
Publisher: William Brottmiller
Executive Editor: Cathy L. Esperti
Managing Editor: Maro Gartside
Associate Editor: Teresa Reilly
Editorial Assistant: Kayla Dos Santos
Director of Production: Amy Rose
Production Editor: Joanna Lundeen
Marketing Manager: Grace Richards
Manufacturing and Inventory Control Supervisor: Amy Bacus
Composition: Laserwords Private Limited, Chennai, India
Cover Design: Kristin E. Parker
Cover Images: Left to right, top to bottom are as follows:
    Swirl: © Christophe Rolland/ShutterStock, Inc.; Scan: Courtesy of Jennifer Prekeges;
    Bone Scan: Courtesy of Jennifer Prekeges; Brain: © Lawrence Berkeley National Library/Photodisc/Thinkstock;
    Bone Scan: Courtesy of Jennifer Prekeges (same as above); Swirl: © Jiri Vaclavek/ShutterStock, Inc.
Printing and Binding: Gasch Printing
Cover Printing: Gasch Printing

To order this product, use ISBN: 978-1-4496-5288-3

Library of Congress Cataloging-in-Publication Data
Prekeges, Jennifer.
  Nuclear medicine instrumentation / Jennifer Prekeges. — 2nd ed.
    p. ; cm.
  Includes bibliographical references and index.
  ISBN 978-1-4496-4537-3 (pbk.) — ISBN 1-4496-4537-2 (pbk.)
  I. Title.
  [DNLM: 1. Nuclear Medicine—instrumentation. 2. Positron-Emission Tomography—methods.
3. Radioisotopes—diagnostic use. 4. Tomography, Emission-Computed, Single-Photon—methods. WN 440]
  616.07'548—dc23
                                                        2012013953

6048

Printed in the United States of America
23 22   10 9 8 7 6

BRIEF CONTENTS

PART 1	Small Instruments	1
CHAPTER 1	Gas-Filled Detectors	3
CHAPTER 2	Scintillation Detectors	17
CHAPTER 3	Semiconductor Detectors	29
CHAPTER 4	Factors Relating to Radiation Measurement	39
PART 2	Gamma Camera	53
CHAPTER 5	The Gamma Camera	55
CHAPTER 6	Image Digitization and Display	71
CHAPTER 7	Collimators	83
CHAPTER 8	Image Characteristics and Performance Measures in Planar Imaging	95
CHAPTER 9	Departmental Quality Assurance and Quality Control of Gamma Cameras	111
PART 3	Single-Photon Emission Computed Tomography (SPECT)	129
CHAPTER 10	Single-Photon Emission Computed Tomography (SPECT)	131
CHAPTER 11	Image Characteristics and Effect of Acquisition Parameters in SPECT Imaging	151
CHAPTER 12	Improving SPECT Images	163
CHAPTER 13	Quality Control and Artifacts in SPECT	179
PART 4	Positron Emission Tomography (PET)	195
CHAPTER 14	Principles of Positron Emission Tomography (PET)	197
CHAPTER 15	PET Instrumentation	209
CHAPTER 16	Image Characteristics, Performance Measures, and Quantitation in PET	227
CHAPTER 17	Quality Control and Artifacts in PET	243
CHAPTER 18	Computed Tomography and Its Application to Nuclear Medicine	253
CHAPTER 19	Magnetic Resonance Imaging and Its Application to Nuclear Medicine	277
APPENDIX A	Atomic Structure and Interactions of High-Energy Radiation	297
APPENDIX B	Basic Electronics and Devices	305

APPENDIX C	Film and Film Processing	323
APPENDIX D	Computer Fundamentals and Systems	329
APPENDIX E	Collimator Mathematics	339
APPENDIX F	Laboratory Accreditation	347

CONTENTS

Preface xiii
Acknowledgments xv
About the Author xvii
Reviewers xix
Contributors xxi
List of Abbreviations xxiii

PART 1	**Small Instruments** 1	
CHAPTER 1	**Gas-Filled Detectors** 3	
	Learning Outcomes 3	
	Introduction 3	
	Basic Operation 3	
	Dose Calibrator 6	
	Ionization Survey Meter 8	
	Geiger–Müller Survey Meter 9	
	Quality Control 11	
	Limitations of Gas-Filled Detectors 15	
	Summary 16	
CHAPTER 2	**Scintillation Detectors** 17	
	Learning Outcomes 17	
	Introduction 17	
	Basic Principles of Scintillation 17	
	Associated Electronics 21	
	Calibration 23	
	Scintillation Detector Applications 24	
	Peak Broadening and Energy Resolution 26	
	Quality Control 27	
	Summary 27	
CHAPTER 3	**Semiconductor Detectors** 29	
	Learning Outcomes 29	
	Introduction 29	
	Properties of Semiconductors 29	

Operation 32

Uses of Semiconductor Detectors in Nuclear Medicine 33

Performance Measures 34

Quality Control and Care 35

Summary 36

CHAPTER 4   **Factors Relating to Radiation Measurement** **39**

Learning Outcomes 39

Introduction 39

Background 39

Nuclear Counting Statistics 40

Dead Time 44

Energy Spectra 44

Baseline Shift and Pulse Pileup 47

Detection Efficiency 48

Summary 51

PART 2   **Gamma Camera** **53**

CHAPTER 5   **The Gamma Camera** **55**

Learning Outcomes 55

Introduction 55

Historical Background 56

Basic Concepts of Anger's Camera 56

Anger Gamma Camera Components 60

Modern Gamma Cameras 61

Uniformity Corrections and Autotuning 62

General Guidelines for the Use and Care of a Gamma Camera 66

Non-Anger Gamma Cameras 68

Summary 70

CHAPTER 6   **Image Digitization and Display** **71**

Learning Outcomes 71

Introduction 71

Analog Images 71

Digital Images and Image Matrices 72

Acquisition of Digital Images 76

Digital Image Display 77

Limitations of Image Display 80

Summary 81

CHAPTER 7	**Collimators** **83**
	Learning Outcomes 83
	Introduction 83
	Manufacturing Collimators 84
	Collimator Concepts 84
	Design Parameters 85
	Parallel-Hole Collimators 88
	Pinhole Collimator 89
	Other Types of Collimators 92
	Summary 93
CHAPTER 8	**Image Characteristics and Performance Measures in Planar Imaging** **95**
	Learning Outcomes 95
	Introduction 95
	Characteristics of Planar Images 95
	Contrast 98
	Uniformity and Sensitivity 99
	Spatial Resolution 101
	Effects of Acquisition Parameters 106
	Summary 108
CHAPTER 9	**Departmental Quality Assurance and Quality Control of Gamma Cameras** **111**
	Learning Outcomes 111
	Introduction 111
	Quality Assurance 111
	Routine Quality Control Testing for Planar Gamma Cameras 112
	Nonroutine Quality Control Tests 119
	Camera Purchase and Acceptance Testing 122
	Troubleshooting Gamma Cameras 122
	Summary 125
PART 3	**Single-Photon Emission Computed Tomography (SPECT)** **129**
CHAPTER 10	**Single-Photon Emission Computed Tomography (SPECT)** **131**
	Learning Outcomes 131
	Introduction 131
	Development of Computed Tomography Techniques 132
	Overview of the SPECT Process 132
	Analytic Reconstruction 134
	Iterative Reconstruction 142

Image Display..144
Summary..149

CHAPTER 11 Image Characteristics and Effect of Acquisition Parameters in SPECT Imaging..151

Learning Outcomes...151
Introduction..151
Image Characteristics in SPECT..151
Performance Measures in SPECT...154
Effect of Acquisition Parameters..155
Improving Image Quality after Acquisition.....................................159
Summary...161

CHAPTER 12 Improving SPECT Images..163

Learning Outcomes...163
Introduction..163
Attenuation and Scatter...164
Chang Attenuation Correction..166
Patient-Specific Attenuation Maps...166
Compensation for Scatter, Resolution Loss, and Noise..........................172
Implementation..174
Clinical Benefits...177
Summary...178

CHAPTER 13 Quality Control and Artifacts in SPECT..................................179

Learning Outcomes...179
Introduction..179
Acceptance Testing..180
SPECT Quality Control...180
Tomographic Measures of SPECT Performance.....................................187
SPECT Artifacts...190
Summary...194

PART 4 Positron Emission Tomography (PET)..195

CHAPTER 14 Principles of Positron Emission Tomography (PET)........................197

Learning Outcomes...197
Introduction..197
A Brief History of PET..198
Physics of Positron Emitters and Annihilation Photons.........................199

Scintillation Crystals for Annihilation Photon Detection 200

Data Collection 201

Types of Events in PET. 203

Correction for Attenuation 204

Time-of-Flight PET. 205

Quantitative Abilities 206

Summary 207

CHAPTER 15 PET Instrumentation 209

Learning Outcomes 209

Introduction. 209

Overview of PET Tomograph Composition 210

Overview of Acquisition, Reconstruction, and Image Display 210

Detector Blocks 215

Energy Discrimination 216

Coincidences and Random Events 217

Transmission Sources and Geometries 218

Corrections. 220

Acquisition Options 223

Summary 226

CHAPTER 16 Image Characteristics, Performance Measures, and Quantitation in PET. 227

Learning Outcomes 227

Introduction. 227

Image Characteristics in PET 227

Performance Measures in PET 231

Operator-Determined Parameters in PET 235

Factors Affecting Performance Measures. 235

Standardized Uptake Value. 238

Summary 240

CHAPTER 17 Quality Control and Artifacts in PET. 243

Learning Outcomes 243

Introduction. 243

Acceptance Testing. 243

Routine Quality Control. 244

Infrequent Quality Control Tests 246

Artifacts in PET 249

Summary 251

CHAPTER 18	Computed Tomography and Its Application to Nuclear Medicine	253
	Learning Outcomes	253
	Introduction	253
	Basics of X-Ray and CT	254
	Practical Aspects of CT Acquisition, Reconstruction, and Display	257
	Image Quality in CT	264
	Radiation Dosimetry	265
	SPECT/CT Systems	267
	PET/CT Tomographs	268
	Technical Issues in PET/CT	269
	Regulatory Issues	273
	Summary	274

CHAPTER 19	Magnetic Resonance Imaging and Its Application to Nuclear Medicine	277
	Learning Outcomes	277
	Introduction	277
	Electromagnetism and Its Effect on Hydrogen Atoms	278
	Tissue Disturbance and Differentiation	281
	The Pulse Sequence	283
	Forming the Magnetic Resonance Image	284
	MRI Instrumentation	288
	Tissue Characteristics and Image Appearance	290
	Safety Issues	291
	PET/MRI	293
	Summary	295

APPENDIX A	Atomic Structure and Interactions of High-Energy Radiation	297
	Learning Outcomes	297
	Introduction	297
	Atomic Structure	298
	Interactions of Charged Particles	298
	Interactions of Photons	300
	Consequences of Radiation Interactions	301
	Summary	303

APPENDIX B	Basic Electronics and Devices	305
	Learning Outcomes	305
	Introduction	305
	Behavior of Electric Charges	305

	Molecular Bonding	307
	Electric Circuits	308
	RC Circuits	310
	Transistors and Logic Circuits	312
	Electrical Components of Radiation Detectors	316
	Image Display Devices	318
	Summary	321

APPENDIX C Film and Film Processing 323

Learning Outcomes 323
Introduction 323
Film Composition 323
Film Exposure 324
Film Developing 324
Film Densitometry 326
Summary 327

APPENDIX D Computer Fundamentals and Systems 329

Learning Outcomes 329
Introduction 329
Analog vs Digital 329
Computer Fundamentals 330
Computer Architecture 333
Computer Networks 335
Radiology-Specific Computer Systems 337
Summary 338

APPENDIX E Collimator Mathematics 339

Learning Outcomes 339
Introduction 339
Flat-Field Collimator 339
Multihole Collimator 340
Pinhole Collimator 344
Summary 346

APPENDIX F Laboratory Accreditation 347

Learning Objectives 347
Introduction 347
Accrediting Organizations 348
The Accreditation Process 348

Study Protocols and Patient Care Policies 349
Tips for Successful Accreditation 350
Summary 350

Glossary 351

Index 361

PREFACE

As a first-time author, I have a tremendous sense of satisfaction to be asked to prepare a second edition. Many thanks to my fellow nuclear medicine technology program directors who were willing to give a brand-new textbook a try. I am delighted to have the opportunity to correct mistakes, concepts, clarify and bring various topics to a more current state of affairs. I am also quite pleased to have two contributing authors for this edition. Michael Teters and Fady Kassem are medical physicists with wide experience in radiology and a deep understanding of nuclear medicine instrumentation. Both have been of great assistance to me in the process of preparing the Second Edition. Fady in particular contributed the initial draft of the chapter on magnetic resonance imaging, for which I am very grateful.

I have made major changes in a number of chapters and have added two new chapters. I would like to call your attention to these:

- Chapter 2—there is a new concept map elucidating the operation of a scintillation detector, a better description of calibration, and clarification of energy resolution (the property being measured) vs FWHM (the mechanism by which it is measured).
- Chapter 5—the section on non-Anger cameras was rewritten to address planar devices only, with descriptions of non-Anger SPECT systems in Chapter 12.
- Chapter 12—this chapter was updated to include recent improvements, a section on noise regularization, and more information on implementation and clinical benefits. Both software methods of incorporating improvements and non-Anger 3D imaging systems are discussed.
- Chapter 15—photos of a PET tomograph taken apart are included so that the reader can see crystals, septa, electronics, and a rod source. The description of direct and cross-planes is expanded. There is decreased emphasis on 2D vs 3D imaging, and new sections on dynamic and gated imaging and organ-specific PET systems are included.
- Chapter 16—the section on the SUV is rewritten to reflect its increasing importance, and a new section on the benefits of time-of-flight PET is included.
- Chapter 19—this is a completely new chapter on MRI, written as the first PET/MRI scanners are coming into clinical use. It aims to provide a modest rather than in-depth level of understanding of MRI as well as the technological challenges and clinical benefits of combining MRI with PET imaging.
- Appendix A—this has been extensively rewritten to emphasize the consequences of radiation interactions.
- Appendix F—this is a new appendix on laboratory accreditation; references to the requirements of accrediting agencies are also sprinkled throughout the text as appropriate.

How to Use this Text

- **Parts:** The text is broken into four parts that, for the most part, can be comprehended separately, without reference to the others. The only exception is that an understanding of Part II (Gamma Cameras) is assumed in Part III (Single-Photon Emission Computed Tomography).
- **Key terms:** Important words and phrases are italicized when they are introduced. These terms are defined in the new glossary found at the end of the book.
- **Abbreviations:** All abbreviations are spelled out at their first mention in each chapter. A comprehensive list of abbreviations and scientific units are provided in the front matter and a general list is printed inside the back cover as a helpful reference.
- **Sample calculations:** These are included to illustrate the mathematical application of the referenced equations throughout the text.
- **Appendices:** The appendices provide a deeper level of understanding for those who are interested in greater insight on specific topics.
- **References:** I have cited resources used in writing and updating this edition. They may or may not be helpful in expanding learning.
- **Additional resources:** I have compiled a list of additional resources to provide readers with helpful books and articles that will aide in further learning.

ACKNOWLEDGMENTS

When I was in graduate school, I wrote a paper on the environmental effects of the practice of nuclear medicine. In the paper, I referred a number of times to nuclear medicine *technologists*. The professor, a nuclear engineer, crossed out every occurrence of that word and wrote the word *technician* in its place. When I asked why he did that, he replied that "technologist" implied an understanding of the technology. I was quite insulted by that and vowed that my students would have a good understanding of the technology that underlies nuclear medicine. So, my first (somewhat backhanded) acknowledgment is to Dr. Maurice Robkin for providing the impetus for me to write this textbook.

As is true of many books, this work reflects my own understanding, which has been shaped by many other people, a few of whom I would therefore like to acknowledge. Dr. Paul Brown taught me nuclear medicine and has always been a role model. Barbara Ratliff, CNMT, taught the instrumentation course in my training program for many years, and the chapters on gamma cameras and SPECT imaging were originally based on her lecture notes. I have benefitted from a number of continuing-education sessions at national nuclear medicine meetings and the insights of those who truly are experts in the field. Drs. Mike Yester and Tom Lewellen, and Robert Hobbs, MS, provided initial reviews of different sections of the first edition. Tony Knight read through the entire manuscript of the first edition several times.

For this second edition, I would like to express my deep gratitude to Fady Kassem and Michael Teters for assisting me with this edition; their advice, guidance, and clarification on the finer points of medical physics were invaluable. Fady provided the first draft of the chapter on MRI, and tirelessly reviewed my additions and edits. Several people who I consider giants in the field of nuclear medicine, including Dr. F. David Rollo, Dr. Michael Phelps, and Dr. Thomas Budinger, allowed me to use figures that they had created. I am grateful to my publisher, Jones & Bartlett Learning, my production editor Amy Rose, and my art editor Joanna Lundeen. Some of the work was done by people I did not have the pleasure of meeting, but the copyeditor and proofreader provided several rounds of careful reading and editing (and certainly got an education in nuclear medicine instrumentation while doing so).

I would especially like to acknowledge my fellow nuclear medicine educators. I appreciate those who let me know about errors in the first edition and made suggestions for improvements. I am grateful to those who have given me encouragement, especially those who have indicated that their ability to teach this subject has been enhanced by the textbook. My goal in writing this text was to address a significant deficit in our available resources, and your praise has given me the assurance that I have indeed met that goal.

My students continue to give me inspiration, as I see their understanding of the field reach higher and higher levels. Every year, through their struggles, I gain new insights. My coworkers at Virginia Mason Medical Center, and more recently at Bellevue College, have been supportive and encouraging. Finally and most importantly, I thank my husband, Peter, and my daughter, Krysta, for their patience through the many, many hours spent preparing the first and then the second edition. Publication of this text has been a labor of love for my profession, but it has been possible only because of the love and support of my family.

ABOUT THE AUTHOR

Jennifer Prekeges, MS, CNMT, graduated from the nuclear medicine technology program at the Veterans Administration Medical Center in Portland, Oregon, in 1980. Prior to attending that program, she received a bachelor of arts degree in biology and chemistry from Whitman College in Walla Walla, Washington. Jennifer worked as a nuclear medicine technologist for 20 years in the Seattle, Washington, area, and has been involved in nuclear medicine education since about 1983. She started the nuclear medicine technology program at Bellevue College in 1989, after receiving a master of science degree in radiological sciences from the University of Washington. She simultaneously directed the program and worked as a staff technologist at Virginia Mason Medical Center for the first 14 years of its existence, moving to a full-time position at Bellevue College in 2003. In addition to her work as an educator, Jennifer has served as a director and secretary of the Nuclear Medicine Technology Certification Board (1997–2005), reviewer for the *Journal of Nuclear Medicine Technology* (1995–present), member of the Academic Affairs committee of the Society of Nuclear Medicine Technologist Section (1995–1997 and 1998–1999), and copresident of the Pacific Northwest Chapter, Society of Nuclear Medicine Technologist Section (1999–2000). She has authored eight journal articles and one book chapter in addition to this text. In her spare time, she enjoys reading, birdwatching, cross-stitching, and Sudoku puzzles.

REVIEWERS

Mark H. Crosthwaite, Med, CNMT
Program Director and Associate Professor
Department of Radiation Sciences
Virginia Commonwealth University

HM1 Edward R. Eck, BS, RT(R)(CT)(QM), CNMT
Program Director
Nuclear Medicine Technology School
Naval School of Health Sciences

LaRay A. Fox, CNMT, MEd
Program Director
School of Nuclear Medicine
Delaware Technical and Community College
Christiana Care Health System

Germaine C. Frosolone, CNMT, ARRT(N)
Professor, Clinical Coordinator
Nuclear Medicine Technology Program
Gateway Community College

Beata I. Gebuza, BS, CNMT, NCT
Assistant Professor, Program Director
Nuclear Medicine Technology Program
Gateway Community College

Robert F. George, PhD, CNMT, RT(N)
Program Director
Nuclear Medicine Imaging
Wheeling Jesuit University

Joseph Hawkins, MSEd, CNMT
Program Director
Nuclear Medicine Technology
Florida Hospital College of Health Sciences

Glen Heggie, RTNM, BE, ME, EdD, FCAMRT
Clinical Associate Professor, Chair
Cardiopulmonary and Diagnostic Sciences
University of Missouri

Mary E. Klug, CNMT
Instructor, Program Director
Nuclear Medicine Technology
Moraine Park Technical College

Sheila MacEachron, MS, CNMT
Program Director
Nuclear Medicine Technology
Ferris State University

Gregory Passmore, PhD, CNMT
Associate Professor
Department of Biomedical and Radiological Technologies
Medical College of Georgia

Ryan Smith, MBA, CNMT
Clinical Coordinator, Nuclear Medicine Institute
Instructor of Nuclear Medicine
The University of Findlay

David Stout, PhD
Associate Adjunct Professor
Department of Molecular and Medical Pharmacology
UCLA Crump Institute for Molecular Imaging

Lori Kloman Williamson, CNMT
Clinical Coordinator, Nuclear Medicine Institute
Instructor of Nuclear Medicine
The University of Findlay

CONTRIBUTORS

Fady Kassem, MS
Medical Physicist
MRPS Inc.
Long Beach, CA

Michael Teters, MS
Program Director
Nuclear Medicine Technology
Assistant Professor
Medical Imaging Sciences
University of Medicine and Dentistry of New Jersey
Scotch Plains, NJ

LIST OF ABBREVIATIONS

General Scientific Abbreviations

g = gram
m = meter
cm = 0.01 meter; cm^2 = square centimeter, cm^3 = cubic centimeter
ml = milliliter
in = inch
sec = second
hr = hour
° = degrees of a circle
°C, °F = degrees on the Celsius (centigrade) or Fahrenheit temperature scales
Hz = Hertz (cycles/sec)
V = volts
eV = electron volt
kVp = kilovolt peak
ΔV = electrical potential difference between two charged objects
A = ampere
C = capacitance or Coulomb
cts = counts
cps = counts/second
cpm = counts/minute
dpm = disintegrations per minute
dps = disintegrations per second
Ci = Curie
Bq = Becquerel
ppm = parts per million
R = Roentgen
rem = Roentgen-equivalent man
s.d. = standard deviation
σ = standard deviation based on Poisson estimation
Sv = Sievert
τ = time constant (e.g., in a RC circuit)
T = tesla
μ_ℓ = linear attenuation coefficient
μ_m = mass attenuation coefficient
1D = one-dimensional
2D = two-dimensional
3D = three-dimensional
4D = four-dimensional

Standard order-of-magnitude abbreviations:

G = giga = $\times 10^9$
M = mega = $\times 10^6$
k = kilo = $\times 10^3$
m = milli = $\times 10^{-3}$
μ = micro = $\times 10^{-6}$
n = nano = $\times 10^{-9}$
p = pico = $\times 10^{-12}$

Greek Letters

Uppercase	Lowercase	Name
A	α	alpha
B	β	beta
Γ	γ	gamma
Δ	δ	delta
E	ϵ	epsilon
Z	ζ	zeta
H	η	eta
Θ	θ	theta
I	ι	iota
K	κ	kappa
Λ	λ	lambda
M	μ	mu
N	ν	nu
Ξ	ξ	xi
O	o	omicron
Π	π	pi
P	ρ	rho
Σ	σ	sigma
T	τ	tau
Υ	υ	upsilon
Φ	ϕ	phi
X	χ	chi
Ψ	ψ	psi
Ω	ω	omega

Other Abbreviations

AAPM = American Association of Physicists in Medicine
AC = attenuation correction
ACF = attenuation correction factor
ACR = American College of Radiology
ADC = analog-to-digital converter
ALU = arithmetic-logic unit
AOR = axis of rotation
ARRT = American Registry of Radiologic Technologists
BGO = bismuth germanate

CFOV = central field of view
CNR = contrast–noise ratio
COR = center of rotation
CPU = central processing unit
CR = capacitor-resistor (circuit)
CRT = cathode ray tube
CSF = cerebrospinal fluid
CT = computed tomography
CTDI = CT dose index
CTW = coincidence timing window
CV = coefficient of variation
CZT = cadmium–zinc–tellurium
DAS = data acquisition system
DCA = decimal counting assembly
DICOM = Digital Imaging and Communications in Medicine
DLP = dose-length product
E = emission image
ECG = electrocardiogram
EM = expectation maximization
FBP = filtered backprojection
FDA = (United States) Food and Drug Administration
FDG = F-18 fluorodeoxyglucose
FID = free induction decay
fMRI = functional MRI
FORE = Fourier rebinning
FOV = field of view
FT = Fourier transform
FWHM = full-width at half-maximum
FWTM = full-width at tenth-maximum
GI = gastrointestinal
GSO = gadolinium oxyorthosilicate
GUI = graphical user interface
HIS = hospital information system
HU = Hounsfield units
IAC = Intersocietal Accreditation Commission
ICANL = Intersocietal Commission on Accreditation of Nuclear Laboratories
IEC = International Electrotechnical Commission
IMRT = intensity-modulated radiation therapy
IV = intravenous
JCAHO = Joint Commission on Accreditation of Healthcare Organizations
LAN = local-area network
LCD = liquid crystal display
LEAP = low-energy all-purpose
LED = light-emitting diode
LLD = lower-level discriminator
LOR = line of response
LSF = line-spread function
LSO = lutetium oxyorthosilicate
LUT = look-up table
LYSO = lutetium yttrium oxyorthosilicate
MAP = maximum a posteriori
MCA = multichannel analyzer
MIP = maximum intensity projection
MIPPA = Medicare Improvements for Patients and Providers Act
ML = maximum likelihood
MLEM = maximum-likelihood expectation maximization
MPI = myocardial perfusion imaging
MR, MRI = magnetic resonance imaging
MTF = modulation transfer function
MWSR = multiple window spatial registration
NaI (Tl) = thallium-activated sodium iodide scintillation crystal
NECR = noise-equivalent count rate
NEMA = National Electrical Manufacturers Association
NEX = number of excitations
NIST = National Institute of Standards and Testing
NMR = nuclear magnetic resonance
NR = noise regularization
NSA = number of signal averages
OS = operating system
OSEM = ordered-subsets expectation maximization
PACS = picture archiving and communications system
PET = positron emission tomography
PHA = pulse-height analyzer
PLES = parallel-line equal-spacing
PMT = photomultiplier tube
PP = pulse programmer
PROM = programmable read-only memory
PSF = point-spread function
PSPMT = position-sensitive photomultiplier tube
PVE = partial volume effect
q, Q = electrical charge
QC = quality control
R_{coll} = collimator resolution
R_{int} = intrinsic resolution
R_{system} = system resolution
RAM = random access memory
RC = resistor-capacitor (circuit)
RF = radio frequency
RIS = radiology information system
ROM = read-only memory
RR = resolution recovery
rSF = residual scatter fraction
SC = scatter compensation
SCA = single-channel analyzer
SI = Systeme International
SMPTE = Society of Motion Picture and Television Engineers
SNM = Society of Nuclear Medicine
SNMTS = Society of Nuclear Medicine Technologist Section
SNR = signal-to-noise ratio
SPECT = single-photon emission computed tomography
SUV = standardized uptake value
T = transmission image
TBAC = transmission-based attenuation correction
TE = time to echo
TJC = The Joint Commission
TOF = time of flight
TR = time to repetition
UBP = unfiltered backprojection
UFOV = useful field of view
ULD = upper-level discriminator
UV = ultraviolet
VDT = video display terminal
WAN = wide-area network

PART I

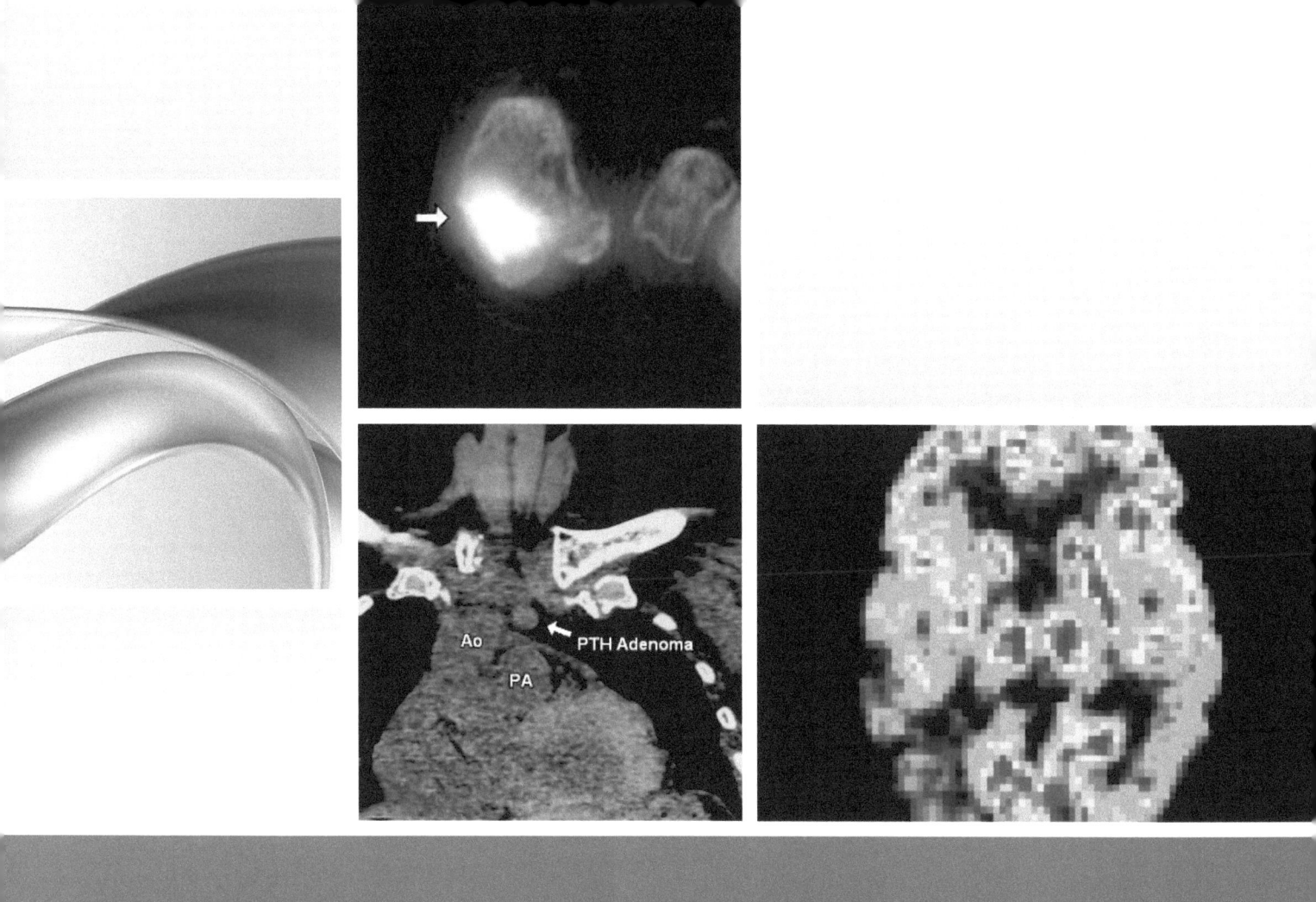

Small Instruments

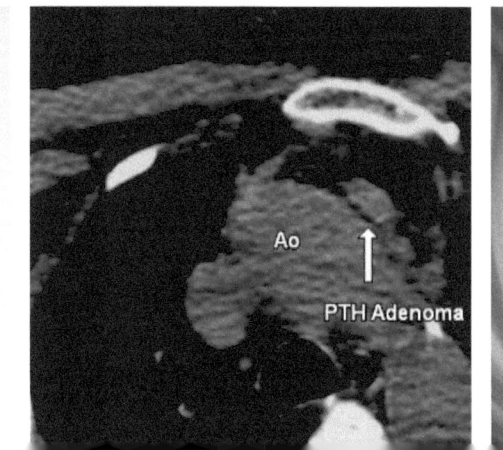

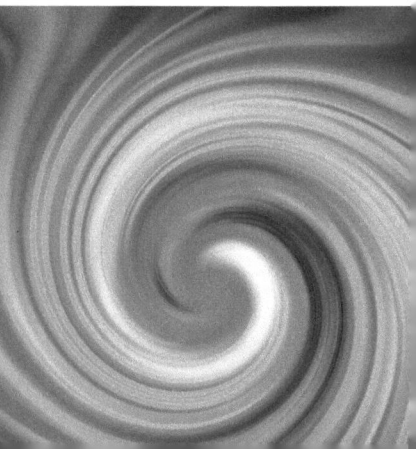

CHAPTER 1 Gas-Filled Detectors

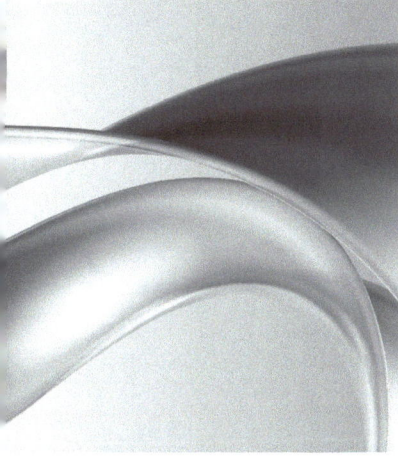
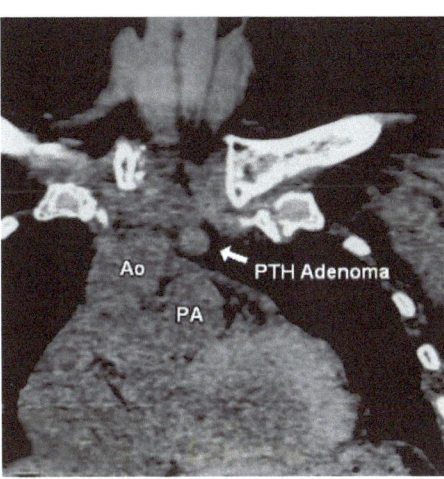
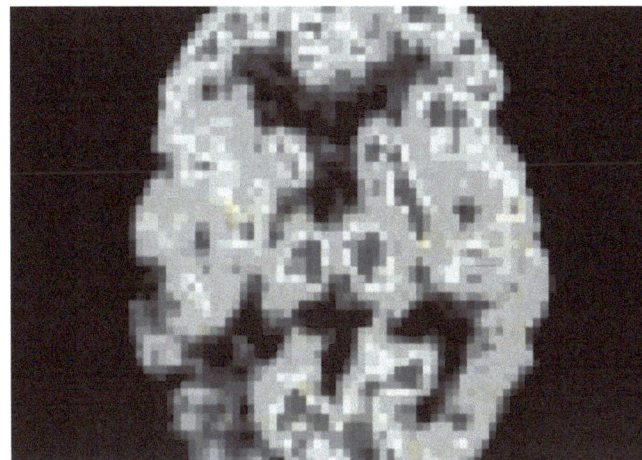

Learning Outcomes

1. Diagram a gas-filled detector and describe how it detects radiation.
2. Draw the voltage response curve for gas-filled detectors and describe each region.
3. Distinguish between current mode and pulse mode, and discuss the consequences of each in common gas-filled detectors.
4. Describe the proper use of a dose calibrator, including the importance of the isotope selector buttons.
5. Distinguish between an ionization survey meter and a Geiger counter, in regard to their operation and appropriate use.
6. Outline the process of radiation detection in a Geiger counter, including the time constant and the need for recovery of the gas chamber.
7. List the recommended quality control tests for gas-filled detectors and their frequencies.
8. Discuss the limitations of gas-filled detectors.

Introduction

Radiation interacts with atoms and molecules, resulting in ionization, which creates ion pairs. An *ion pair* consists of a free electron and the remaining ionized atom or molecule, now positively charged. Each ion pair requires a finite amount of radiation energy, so the number of electrons created is related to the amount of radiation or radioactivity present. These electrons can be caused to move by the application of an electrical field. Thus, the most direct way to detect ionizing radiation is to use electronic equipment to measure the number of electrons created by radiation interactions. The simplest radiation detectors that operate on this principle are called gas-filled detectors, because the ion pairs are created in a chamber filled with gas. Within this class of radiation detectors, we discuss dose calibrators, ionization survey meters, and Geiger counters. Several other gas-filled detectors make useful radiation detectors, but those discussed here are those in common use in nuclear medicine.

Basic Operation

A simple model with only two essential parts—a chamber filled with a gas (hence the term *gas-filled detector*) and a basic electric circuit—is used to illustrate the operation of these instruments (**Figure 1-1**). The structure of the chamber allows it to function as a capacitor; the reader is referred to Appendix B for more information about the electronics of radiation detection instruments. The chamber consists of a positively charged central wire (the *anode*) surrounded by a negatively charged metal tube (the *cathode*). The anode and cathode are separated by a gas and are connected to an external power source. The power source keeps the anode and cathode charged with

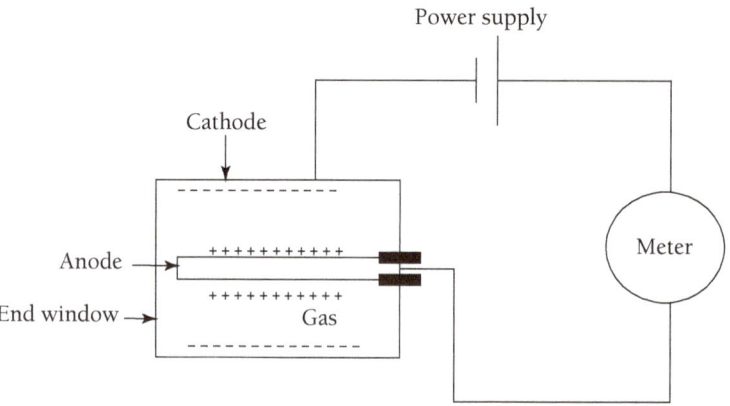

Figure 1-1 Block diagram of a gas-filled detector. The cathode usually forms the outside of the detector, and the anode is an internal plate or wire. The detector has a power source that keeps the cathode and anode charged with negative and positive charge, respectively. The anode and cathode thus form a capacitor, as described in Appendix B. The meter measures either voltage or current, depending on the particulars of the detector design.

as much positive and negative charge, respectively, as their size and the power source's voltage allow. The meter measures the flow of electricity that occurs as a result of neutralization of charge at the anode and cathode.

In the absence of radiation interactions, the gas between the anode and cathode acts as an insulator, and there is no movement of electrical charge. When radiation (gamma rays, x-rays, or charged particles with energy greater than 10 electron volts [eV]) passes through the gas, it ionizes one or more gas molecules, producing free electrons and positive ions. (A brief review of atomic structure and radiation interactions is found in Appendix A.) The average amount of energy required to cause an ionization depends on the type of gas used in the chamber, but is generally between 20 and 45 eV per ion pair. The free electrons and positive ions drift toward the anode and cathode, respectively. Electrons move much faster than the positive ions they leave behind, so we can discuss the collection of electrons at the anode, ignoring for the moment the positive ions created by the radiation interactions. As they move, both electrons and positive ions undergo ionization and excitation interactions with other gas molecules, producing many low-energy *tertiary electrons*. Electrons that reach the anode neutralize some of the positive charge, thus causing electricity to flow through the connecting circuitry to restore the capacitor to its original state. We can measure this neutralization as either current (current mode) or voltage (pulse mode), as discussed in a later section.

The number of electrons measured will depend on several factors, including the number of charged particles and/or photons being measured (i.e., the strength of the radiation source or field); the energy of the radiation; the geometric configuration of the detector; the composition of the gas in the chamber; and the volume, pressure, and temperature of the gas. But a major determinant is the applied voltage between the anode and cathode. Because the electrical potential difference between the anode and cathode provides the driving force behind the movement of the electrons, its magnitude determines how many electrons reach the anode and cathode and what happens to them along the way. For now, let us leave aside the effects of energy, geometry, and gas composition and look at the effect of changing the voltage between the anode and cathode.

Voltage Response Curve

The applied voltage between the anode and cathode is the most important determinant of how many electrons are measured. **Figure 1-2** shows a typical voltage response curve. Its shape can be understood by looking at what is happening in each of the six regions.

Recombination Region

If the applied voltage is quite low, the electrons are moving so slowly that some recombine with other ionized gas molecules and do not reach the anode and cathode, resulting in an incomplete collection of ions. In this region, as the applied voltage is increased, more electrons reach the anode and the measured signal gets larger. There are no usable detectors that operate in this region of the voltage response curve.

Ionization Region (Saturation Region)

As the applied voltage is increased, the system reaches a point at which all electrons are being collected, with no recombination. The *saturation voltage* is a voltage sufficient for this condition of saturation to be reached. There is a

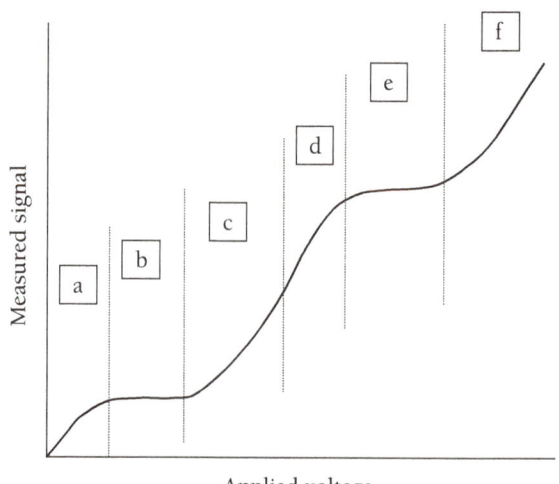

Figure 1-2 Voltage response curve for a gas-filled detector. The regions are (a) recombination, (b) ionization, (c) proportional, (d) limited proportional, (e) Geiger–Müller, and (f) continuous discharge. The shape of the curve is explained in the text.

wide range over which the response is flat, such that even if the voltage fluctuates, the same number of electrons will be collected. The magnitude of the signal is thus proportional to the rate at which photons or charged particles are interacting in the detector. The dose calibrator and ionization survey meter operate in this region.

Proportional Region

If we increase the applied voltage above the saturation voltage, the tertiary electrons are accelerated. They may gain enough kinetic energy to exceed the 10-eV threshold, meaning that they will cause additional secondary ionizations through collisions with other gas molecules. This produces a cascade of electrons called a *Townsend avalanche*. An increase in the applied voltage above the saturation voltage thus produces a signal that is larger than, but still proportional to, the number of ion pairs produced by the radiation (a phenomenon known as *gas amplification*). Gas-filled detectors that operate in this region, called *proportional counters*, are primarily used to detect and distinguish between alpha and beta particles and to identify radionuclides based on these decay products. Proportional counters are quite useful in many physics applications but are not commonly employed in nuclear medicine.

Region of Limited Proportionality

It is in this region that we must begin to consider the fate of the positive ions created by the interaction of radiation with gas molecules. These ions are much larger than electrons and hence drift slowly toward the cathode. In this voltage range, each interaction produces a cloud of positive ions that takes a finite amount of time to disperse. The electric field experienced by the electrons is momentarily decreased, because they are being pulled in two directions—toward the anode and toward the clouds of positive ions. This causes a decrease in the amount of gas amplification. Thus the voltage response curve no longer changes linearly with increasing voltage. This region is not useful for radiation detection.

Geiger–Müller Region

At very high voltages, the gas amplification effect is maximized, so that each electron created produces many ionizations as it races toward the anode. In addition, the moving electrons raise many other gas molecules to excited states via collision interactions, from which they may deexcite by emission of ultraviolet (UV) photons. These UV photons can interact with other gas molecules via photoelectric interactions, producing more free electrons, which in turn are accelerated toward the anode and cause more ionizations and excitations. Thus, each radiation event produces a large avalanche of ions called a *Geiger discharge* throughout the chamber (**Figure 1-3**). The circuit in this case produces a large electrical pulse in response to each radiation event, regardless of the applied voltage (within the Geiger–Müller range) or the energy of the radiation. The pulse size is essentially the same for all radiation events, no matter the type of radiation or the amount of energy transfer. The Geiger counter, a commonly used radiation detector, operates in this region.

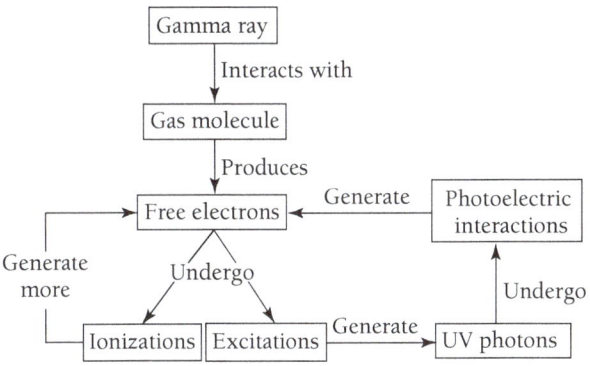

Figure 1-3 Concept map illustrating the Geiger discharge. Each electron created in the chamber interacts with gas molecules via ionization interactions (which create more electrons, the left-hand branch in the diagram) or excitation (which produces UV photons that may be energetic enough to cause more ionizations, the right-hand branch in the diagram). This cycle recurs many, many times. Thus, in a gas-filled detector operating in the Geiger–Müller region, each detected gamma ray creates a large electrical signal.

Continuous Discharge Region

An increase in the voltage above the Geiger–Müller voltage range causes spontaneous ionizations in the detector in the absence of radiation. There are no useful radiation detectors here; operation of a radiation detector in the continuous discharge region can result in permanent damage to the detector.

Current vs Pulse Mode

The electrons that are created in the gas chamber are collected at the anode. The number of electrons collected is correlated to the amount of radioactivity or the strength of the radiation field. This measurement is accomplished in one of two ways. *Current mode* measures the number of electrons per second required to keep the anode and cathode charged. Detectors that operate in current mode are connected to a power supply that constantly strives to keep the anode and cathode charged to their fullest capacity. As electrons produced by radiation interactions neutralize some of the charge on the capacitor, electrons flow from the power source to restore the charge; this electron flow constitutes the measured current. The measurement is therefore based on the time-averaged number of ionizations occurring per second. Current-mode detectors generally operate at high-voltage values that place them in the ionization region.

Because it is an average, an instrument operated in current mode will reach a steady reading over time, as long as the source strength and source-detector distance remain the same. When the radiation level is changing, the reading from a current-mode detector will change based on its averaging time. Some systems allow for the averaging time to take on different values; others do not. Current mode requires a relatively large amount of radiation (many events per second) to produce a precise reading, and even then it generates current in the picoampere (1 pA = 10^{-12} ampere [A]) range. At low levels of radiation, current-mode detectors are subject to statistical fluctuations and interference from leakage currents (movement of electrons through the circuitry in the absence of radiation).

In *pulse mode*, the electrons created by each radiation interaction are treated as a group, and the pulse they create is measured as a single entity. The size of the pulse (either its height or the area under the signal-vs-time function, integrated over time) represents the total charge deposited in the detector by a single radiation interaction. Restoring the electrical potential between anode and cathode still requires an electric current, as in the current-mode detector, but in practice it is easier to measure voltage changes than current changes. Therefore, an RC circuit (a resistor and a capacitor in parallel) is introduced into the circuitry of most pulse-mode detectors, to convert current to voltage (see Appendix B for more details). This also allows the shaping of the pulse, which is necessary for pulse separation and counting. The detector thus reports the number of pulses registered per second, which in turn depends on the amount of radioactivity or the strength of the radiation field.

The underlying assumption of pulse mode is that radiation interactions are separated by enough time that the system can register each one individually. Pulse-mode operation therefore requires a lower rate of radiation interactions in the detector than current mode does. As the interaction rate increases, the readings obtained from a pulse-mode detector will become less accurate, primarily due to dead time. In addition, instruments operating in pulse mode will demonstrate more of the variability characteristic of low-level radiation detection, such that the reading will tend to bounce around, depending on the source intensity and the particular settings used.

Two of the radiation detection instruments discussed in this chapter, the dose calibrator and the ionization survey meter, operate in current mode. The third, the Geiger counter, operates in pulse mode. Most other nuclear medicine equipment, including semiconductor detectors, scintillation detectors, and all forms of imaging systems, also operate in pulse mode. These instruments differ from gas-filled detectors in that the amplitude of each pulse represents the energy deposited in the detector by an individual gamma ray. The ability to determine energy gives these detectors an edge over gas-filled detectors for applications in which energy discrimination is needed.

Dose Calibrator

A *dose calibrator* is used to measure the activity of radionuclide samples. It is calibrated in units of Curies (Ci) and/or Becquerels (Bq). It is truly a workhorse of nuclear medicine, because most departments use a dose calibrator to check every radiopharmaceutical dose that is received or dispensed. A good understanding of how a dose calibrator works, and what it can and cannot do, is therefore vital to the proper care of patients.

Design Features

The basic design of a dose calibrator is shown in **Figure 1-4**, and **Figure 1-5** shows a commercially available model. It operates in the ionization region of the voltage response graph, meaning that all of the primary electrons created in the chamber of the dose calibrator reach the anode, without gas amplification. A dose calibrator is a current-mode instrument: the number of electrons reaching the anode per second is integrated over time, so that it reaches a steady reading over a second or two.

The anode and cathode are found inside the chamber of the dose calibrator. The voltage supply is about 150 volts (V). Typically, the chamber contains either air or argon gas under high pressure (12 or more atmospheres [atm]), which increases the likelihood of gamma ray interactions with the gas. A *dipper* (a gravy-ladle-shaped device fabricated out of Plexiglas®) is used to lower the source container into the cylindrical space that is surrounded by the gas chamber. The outside of the chamber is shielded by a lead cylinder both to prevent external radiation sources from contributing to the measurement and to shield the surrounding area from the

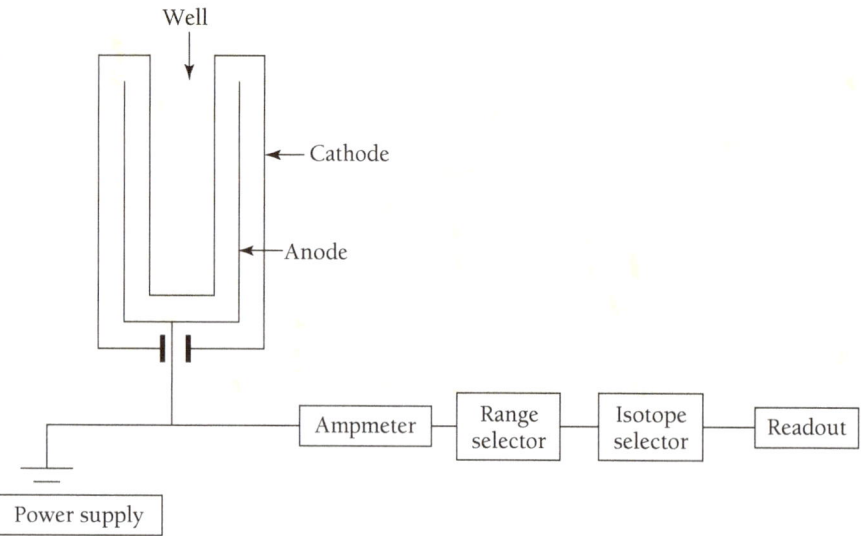

Figure 1-4 Block diagram of a dose calibrator. In addition to the components shown, most dose calibrators sold today have a microprocessor unit that does decay mathematics, saving the user from many calculations. The dose calibrator may also be tied to a computer for tracking of dosage administrations, quality control data entry, and so on.

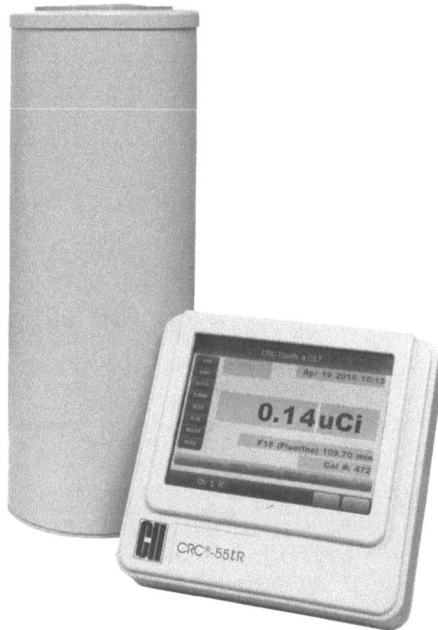

Figure 1-5 A commercial dose calibrator. One can see the shield of the ionization chamber with the dipper handle at the top, as well as the electronic readout module. Photo courtesy of Capintec, Inc.

source being measured. This shield causes some gamma rays to backscatter into the gas chamber, increasing the ionization current when it is present compared to when it is absent. The dose calibrator is calibrated with its shield, and readings are accurate only if it remains in place.

Isotope Selector Buttons

The current that is produced by a radioactive source in the dose calibrator is proportional to both the amount of radioactivity (the desired information) and the energy of the photons, which is dependent on the radionuclide being measured. The dose calibrator by itself cannot distinguish between photons of different energies, and therefore it cannot discriminate between different radionuclides. The operator must do this job using *isotope selector buttons*, which multiply the measured current by a current→activity conversion factor that is specific for each radionuclide. The values of these conversion factors are determined during the initial calibration of the dose calibrator. In older, electromechanical dose calibrators, the values were hardwired into the electronics of the dose calibrator (usually through incorporation of resistors), whereas in newer microprocessor-driven machines they are programmed into the readout as multiplication factors. In either case, it is important to recognize that the dose calibrator will not give an accurate measurement if an incorrect isotope selector button is chosen.

At the factory, a calibration curve is determined using a series of long-lived radionuclide sources, whose activities are traceable to standards at the National Institute of Standards and Testing (NIST) and are thus known exactly. The calibration curve is in turn used to determine conversion factors for the short-lived radionuclides used in nuclear medicine. It is these values that are programmed into the isotope selector buttons. A manual mode allows the user to enter conversion factors not available as preset buttons; the manufacturer usually supplies a table of conversion factor values for a wide variety of radionuclides in addition to those with preset buttons. Once established, the conversion factor for a given isotope selector button is applied to the current measured when a radioactive source is placed in the well.

Sample Calculation 1-1 Isotope-Specific Conversion Factors

The following conversion factors apply to a specific dose calibrator:

$$\text{Tc-99m} : \frac{0.5 \text{ pA}}{\text{mCi}}.$$

$$\text{I-131} : \frac{0.2 \text{ pA}}{\text{mCi}}.$$

A syringe containing a radionuclide is put into the dose calibrator. It generates a current of 2 pA. Calculate the activity if the Tc-99m button is chosen and if the I-131 button is chosen.

$$\text{Tc-99m}: \quad \frac{2 \text{ pA}}{0.5 \text{ pA/mCi}} = 4 \text{ mCi}.$$

$$\text{I-131}: \quad \frac{2 \text{ pA}}{0.2 \text{ pA/mCi}} = 10 \text{ mCi}.$$

The dose calibrator cannot tell which value is correct. It will faithfully give a value for the activity of a sample, based on whichever isotope selector button is engaged. It is incumbent on the operator to make sure that the correct button is chosen.

Operation

The use of a dose calibrator is quite elementary: with the correct isotope selector button depressed, one puts a vial or syringe of radioactive material into the dipper, which is lowered into the well. The number of ionizations created in the gas chamber per second is measured and converted by the isotope selector button to a readout in Ci or Bq. Dose calibrators can measure quantities down to about 20 μCi (740 kBq) to within ±5% (1); below this level, they are less accurate and may take a longer time to reach a steady value. A sodium iodide scintillation detector should be used if accuracy is important at very low activities.

Often nuclear medicine doses are assayed at a different time than they are administered. The dose calibrator reading must then be decay-corrected to the time of administration. Many modern dose calibrators incorporate a clock and calculate radioactive decay internally, thus eliminating the requirement for a separate calculation to determine present activity based on a desired future dosage. These dose calibrators can also keep track of elution vial activities and radiopharmaceutical kit activity concentrations. Many dose calibrator vendors offer computers, printers, and data ports for communication with other devices.

Dose calibrators have an electronic means of setting the background to zero when the source chamber is empty. This process should be engaged at least once per day and preferably several times each day. However, the zero point will be incorrect if there is contamination inside the well. Dose calibrators have a removable plastic liner to protect the inside of the well. If either the liner or the dipper becomes contaminated and the background-setting process is engaged, the machine will rezero to a different level, accounting for the elevated background reading. As the contamination decays, the reading of the empty dose calibrator becomes more and more negative. Dippers and liners should be cleaned if contamination is suspected; it is recommended to have a spare dipper and liner for such occasions.

As was stated previously, dose calibrators cannot distinguish between photons of different energies. The operator can, however, estimate the activity of a radionuclide with high-energy gamma rays in the presence of a radionuclide with low-energy gamma rays through the use of a lead vial shield, as is routinely done in measuring the Mo-99 contents of a generator elution. The *moly shield* is a lead vial shield or "pig" of about 0.5 cm thickness. This is plenty of lead to absorb the great majority of Tc-99m gamma rays (140 keV), but about 50% of Mo-99 gamma rays (750–800 keV) pass through the shield and are measured by the dose calibrator. A correction factor is incorporated into the "Moly assay" selector button that accounts for the partial absorption of Mo-99 gamma rays in the moly shield. The correction factor may also include the 12-hour decay factors for Tc-99m and Mo-99, corresponding to the eluate's expiration time. Using the moly shield and the correction factor, µCi (kBq) amounts of Mo-99 can be measured in the presence of Ci (GBq) amounts of Tc-99m.

Dose calibrators are not able to measure the activity of most pure beta-emitting radionuclides directly, because the beta particles cannot penetrate the liner and wall of the chamber to enter the gas space. However, most commercially available dose calibrators have a correction table to allow estimation of the assay of beta-emitting radionuclides based on the Bremsstrahlung radiation emissions they generate. Such readings are still subject to inaccuracies due to the container the radionuclide is in (see the information on geometry testing in Quality Control). One way to accurately assay a pure beta-emitting radiopharmaceutical dosage is as follows (**Table 1-1**): Prior to administration, place the syringe or vial into the dose calibrator, and dial in the conversion factor for the radionuclide. Then manually adjust the conversion factor so that the measured activity matches the activity calculated from the calibration data. (With some radionuclides, the Bremsstrahlung radiation is so weak that the reading cannot be adjusted to the calculated activity. In such a case, adjust the manual setting so that the reading is some fraction [e.g., 10%] of the calculated value.) After drawing or administering the dose,

Table 1-1

Example Measurement of a Pure Beta-Emitting Radionuclide

Sr-89 strontium chloride assay	
Activity based on calibration data	4.11 mCi
Adjust dose calibrator to read calculated activity	4.11 mCi
Draw dose	
Measure vial after drawing dose (add water to restore original volume)	0.23 mCi
Dosage withdrawn from vial	3.88 mCi

remeasure the syringe or vial on the same setting and in the same container. The administered amount is equal to the difference between the two measurements (multiplied by the inverse of the correction fraction if one was needed).

Ionization Survey Meter

These gas-filled detectors are primarily used to measure exposure rates from radiation fields. (The colloquial name for such detectors, "Cutie Pie," derives from the symbols $Qd\pi$, which are included in the mathematical formula for the detector's sensitivity.) They may also be called *ion chambers* or *exposure rate meters*. An example of an ionization survey meter is shown in **Figure 1-6**.

Design Features

Most commercially available ionization survey meters are filled with air and are battery driven (50–500 V), operating in the ionization region and in current mode. A range setting or scale knob allows radiation exposure rates over several orders of magnitude to be measured. Ionization survey meters may read in *rate mode*, the time-averaged radiation exposure rate in milliroentgens per hour (mR/hr), or in *integrate mode*, giving the total accumulated radiation exposure in mR over a period of time. (A *Roentgen* [R] is an

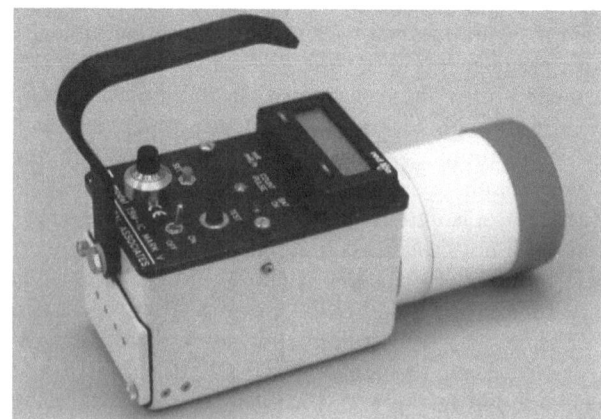

Figure 1-6 Ionization survey meter. Note the single-unit construction, which distinguishes an ionization survey meter from most Geiger counters. Photo courtesy of Biodex Medical Systems, Inc.

amount of radiation that produces 1 electrostatic unit of charge [about 2 billion ion pairs] in 1 cm^3 of air. It is commonly used to describe the strength of a radiation field.)

An ionization survey meter generally has a *thin entrance window* made of a thin layer of mica, mylar, or other low-atomic-number material, that is protected by a sliding or removable shield. If the measurement is to include only photon radiation, the shield is left in place, covering the thin entrance window, so that it absorbs any particulate radiations (i.e., electrons, beta particles, and/or alpha particles) and low-energy photons. If the measurement is to include particulate radiation or low-energy gamma rays, the shield is moved aside to allow these radiation types to cross through the thin entrance window. The readings with and without the shield can be compared to determine the relative amounts of penetrating and nonpenetrating radiation.

Uses

Ionization survey meters are often utilized interchangeably with Geiger counters, but there are important differences that the operator should understand. First, ionization survey meters require a higher radiation flux than do Geiger counters to produce a precise reading. They generally read accurately down to about 1 mR/hr (2). They are therefore applicable to situations such as monitoring radiation levels of patients receiving radionuclides or radioactive implants for therapy, but are not appropriate for detecting radioactive contamination. Second, ionization survey meters have a relatively constant response over a range of gamma ray energies between about 20 and 1,300 keV. They are thus suitable for measuring ambient radiation levels involving mixed photon energies.

Finally, the measured exposure accurately reflects the ionization density in air and can therefore be used as a starting point for some calculations of radiation-absorbed dose for dosimetry purposes. A number called the *work function* estimates the energy required to create one ion pair in the fill gas of the meter. This number can be multiplied by the meter's reading (converted from mR to ion pairs) to calculate the total energy deposited in the gas chamber. This value in turn can be converted to an equivalent value for water (which for radiation absorption purposes is similar to tissue). Using this type of procedure, one can, for example, convert the ionization survey meter "integrate" reading from a nurse's visit with a radioactive patient into an absorbed-dose value for the nurse.

Geiger–Müller Survey Meter

The Geiger–Müller survey meter or Geiger counter is another workhorse of health physics in general and of nuclear medicine departments in particular. It is also one of the oldest radiation detectors, having been invented by Hans Geiger in 1908–1912 and improved by Walther Müller in 1928. It operates in the Geiger–Müller region of the voltage response curve, at 400 to 2,000 V. The electronic signal in a Geiger counter is more complex than in detectors operating in the ionization region and deserves additional explanation.

Operation

In the Geiger–Müller region, each electron produced in an ionization interaction is given a large amount of kinetic energy, so that it causes additional ionizations (a *Townsend avalanche*) and excitations of gas molecules as it is pulled toward the anode. Gas molecules raised to an excited state may produce ultraviolet-wavelength photons, which in turn may be absorbed in photoelectric interactions with other gas molecules, producing additional free electrons. Each of these in turn is also accelerated by the high voltage, generating more Townsend avalanches. The end result is a very large number of ionizations in the chamber called a *Geiger discharge* (Fig. 1-3), producing a billion or more ion pairs (3).

Meanwhile, the positive ions are being pulled toward the cathode, but because they are much larger than electrons, they move relatively slowly. There comes a point at which the anode is completely surrounded by an envelope or "hose" of positively charged gas molecules. Due to the high concentration of positive ions and the effective decrease in the anode's electric field, the electric field felt by free electrons no longer is high enough to cause gas multiplication. New electrons produced at this point (whether between the anode and hose or outside of the hose) will be more likely to recombine with a gas molecule than to cause another ionization. Thus the avalanche finally ends, after producing a large pulse of electricity. A pulse takes about 1 (μsec) to be created and about 50 to 100 μsec to dissipate.

The size of the electrical pulse created by each photon interaction does not vary significantly with either the applied voltage or the energy of the radiation. We will consider each electrical pulse registered by the Geiger counter to be the result of a single gamma ray causing a single ionization in the chamber as it passes through. Geiger counters are thus very sensitive, because a single interaction potentially produces a measurable event. They are very good for detecting small amounts of contamination.

Geiger counters operate in pulse mode. The units of measurement are either contamination units of counts per minute (cpm), or exposure units of mR/hr, or both. In cpm operation, each count represents one Geiger discharge. Calibration for exposure units uses a source with fixed gamma ray energy, so that the Geiger counter reading will change directly with the source strength, at that energy. However, the Geiger counter has significant energy dependence, such that when the source includes gamma rays with a variety of energies, the conversion to mR/hr is not correct for all of the gamma rays. Thus, the exposure reading varies with gamma ray energy, leading to a potential error factor of 2 to 3 (3). In addition, Geiger counters have a low efficiency for gamma rays of only a few percent (3). (Efficiency can be briefly defined as the number of gamma rays detected divided by the number arriving at the detector; see Appendix A for more information.) Its readouts should not, therefore, be used directly to calculate the radiation-absorbed dose. Rather, the Geiger counter is best used as a qualitative or semiquantitative indicator of the presence of radiation. It excels at this task because of its ability to detect small numbers of gamma rays.

Design Features

Geiger–Müller survey meters may operate via direct current from a battery or via alternating current from a wall outlet that is converted internally to direct current. The gas in the chamber is usually helium or argon, and it is often at less than atmospheric pressure, which minimizes the charge differential between anode and cathode that is required to bring about a Geiger discharge. Geiger counters are generally portable and ruggedly built. Some have audible alarms or "chirps" to allow the user to "hear" the radiation level. Like the ionization survey meter, the Geiger counter usually has a range knob or a logarithmic scale, giving it measurement abilities over several orders of magnitude. A low-level electronic discriminator is often included to prevent the detector from registering electrical noise and small-amplitude pulses as radiation events.

The pulse produced by a Geiger counter is quite large (about 10 V), which permits the detector module to be separated from the other electrical components by an insulated wire. The detectors come in a variety of configurations (**Figure 1-7**). A pancake detector (Fig. 1-7a) is designed to detect contamination by virtue of its unidirectional geometry and metal backing that scatters gamma rays back into the active volume. Another common geometry is a cylindrical detector called a G–M tube (Fig. 1-7b), which is used for general radiation detection purposes.

Like ionization survey meters, many Geiger counters have a thin entrance window to allow for measurement of particulate radiation, protected by either a wire screen or a removable cover. With the latter type, the cover must be removed if nonpenetrating radiation is to be counted in addition to penetrating gamma radiation. These end windows are quite fragile and easily broken. A perforated or damaged end window also allows the fill gas to escape, including the quench gas (see the following discussion). In addition, the pressure in the tube increases to the ambient pressure, rendering the unit nonfunctional.

Most Geiger counters read out in a rate meter format, in which the reading is expressed as cpm or mR/hr. The readout reflects the average number of pulses being received at the rate meter each second. As the amount of radiation increases, so will the rate meter output, but how fast it changes depends on the *time constant* τ of the rate meter. This is shown by illustration in **Figure 1-8**. A short time constant causes the Geiger counter reading to change quickly as the radiation field strength changes, but also allows it to bounce around a lot. A long time constant causes the reading to be steadier, but also to change more slowly than the instantaneous radiation field strength. Many instruments allow the operator to vary the time constant. In day-to-day operations, it is important to recognize that a quick response cannot be achieved with a long time constant, while a precise measurement cannot be made with a short time constant.

(a) Geiger counter with pancake detector

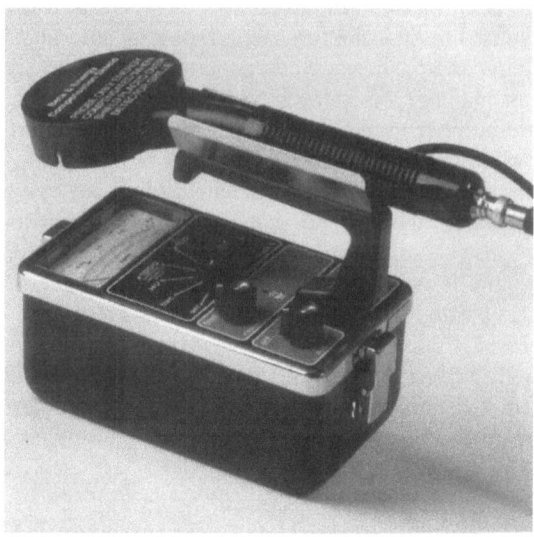

(b) Geiger counter with G–M tube detector

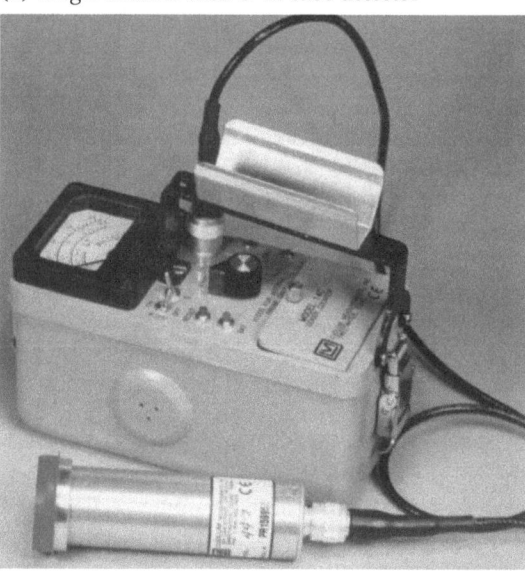

Figure 1-7 Geiger counters. (a) A pancake-type detector, useful for finding contamination. Photo courtesy of Capintec, Inc. (b) A typical Geiger–Müller tube attachment. Photo courtesy of Biodex Medical Systems, Inc.

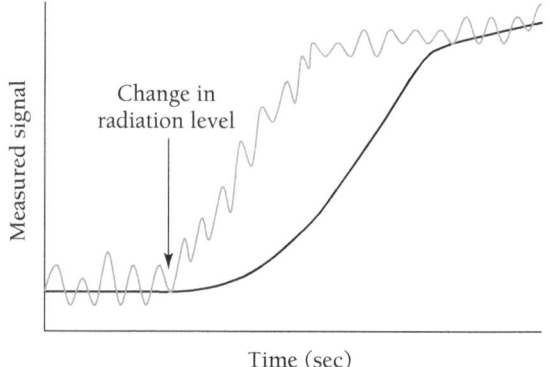

Figure 1-8 Illustration of short vs long time constants. The solid line illustrates a long time constant, while the gray line represents a short time constant.

One problem particular to Geiger counters is the possibility of a continuous avalanche. As electrons recombine with positive ions at the cathode in the final phase of the avalanche, it is possible for one to enter the orbital structure of the positive ion at an excited level and produce a UV photon as it drops down to ground level. If this occurs late in the tube's recovery process, the UV photon could cause a new ionization within the cathode and thus restart the avalanche, leading to either a continuous avalanche or a spurious event. A *quench gas* is added to the chamber at the time of manufacture to prevent this from happening. A quench gas is either an organic or (more likely) a halogen gas that will absorb UV photons without becoming ionized. Because this is taken care of in the manufacturing process, it is not a problem on a day-to-day basis.

Geiger counters are highly reliable instruments, but they tend to suffer from a lack of proper care. A Geiger counter that does not respond to a radioactive source has one of three problems: the battery is dead, the cable wires are broken, or the thin end window is damaged. Broken cable wires can result from dangling the detector while holding the cable. If the response of the Geiger counter to a radiation source is higher than expected, it may be contaminated. Because a Geiger counter may be hard to clean, this may render it unusable until the contamination has decayed to background.

Quality Control

The subject of *quality control* (QC) is a very important one in nuclear medicine. It can be defined as "an established set of ongoing measurements and analyses designed to ensure that the performance of a procedure or instrument is within a predefined acceptable range" (4). If a department does not pay close attention to QC, it cannot be certain that its clinical studies are producing correct results. Hence QC is emphasized in all parts of this text. Even though gas-filled detectors are quite simplistic in their operation, they too must be evaluated on a regular basis (**Table 1-2**).

Ionization Survey Meter and Geiger Counter

The important routine test on these instruments is their functionality for detection of radiation. A daily operations check includes a verification that the battery is working, a reading of background radiation level, and a check on the constancy of the detector's response to a radioactive source. Many ionization detectors have a "battery check" setting and a readout or rate meter output area that indicates whether the battery is supplying voltage in an acceptable range. If such readout is not available, the battery's functionality can be implied by the response to the constancy check. Determination that the background radiation level is in its normal range verifies that the detector has not become contaminated with radioactivity.

The *constancy check* measures a radioactive reference source in a reproducible geometry. The reading should be about the same (constant) from day to day, to within about 10% of an average value. When one of these detectors fails its constancy check, only a few possibilities exist for the source of the problem (**Table 1-3**) and these can easily be checked out.

Ionization survey meters and Geiger counters need to be checked for the accuracy of their output on an annual basis. *Accuracy testing* compares the reading given by the detector to the reading expected from a source with a known amount of radioactivity. In this case, the gamma constant of the reference standard provides the correlation between the activity and exposure rate reading. The *gamma constant* for a given radionuclide gives the radiation field strength (in mR/hr) produced by 1 mCi of that radionuclide at a specified distance (either 1 cm or 1 m). The expected radiation flux in mR/hr can be calculated by multiplying its gamma constant by the reference source's

Table 1-2

Recommended Quality Control Tests for Gas-Filled Detectors

Instrument	Test	Recommended Frequency
Dose calibrator	Constancy	Daily[1,2,3,4]
	Activity linearity	Quarterly[1,2,3,4]
	Accuracy	Annually[1,2,3,4]
	Geometry	At installation and after repair only
Ionization survey meter	Battery functionality	Daily[4]
Geiger–Müller survey meter	Constancy	Daily[4]
	Accuracy/calibration	Annually[4]

Note: All of these tests should be performed after an instrument has been serviced.
[1] Graham LS, ed. *Nuclear Medicine: Self-Study Program II: Instrumentation*. Reston, VA: Society of Nuclear Medicine; 1996:3,5.
[2] Christian PE. Radiation detection. In: Fahey FH, Harkness BA, eds. *Basic Science of Nuclear Medicine* [CD-ROM]. Reston, VA: Society of Nuclear Medicine; 2001.
[3] Klingensmith WC, Eshima D, Goddard J. *Nuclear Medicine Procedure Manual 2003–05*. Englewood, CO: Wick; 2003:20-1-20-4.
[4] Zanzonico P. Routine quality control of clinical nuclear medicine instrumentation: a brief review. *J Nucl Med*. 2008;49:1114–1131.

activity and dividing by the square of the distance between the source and the detector. There must be nothing but air between the source and the detector, and the distance should be great enough that the reference source looks like a point source.

Accuracy determination is usually performed annually by a commercial calibration laboratory, health physics consulting firm, or nuclear medicine product vendor. Each of the instrument's scale or range settings must be checked to verify accuracy. A Geiger counter or ionization survey meter is considered out of compliance if its accuracy reading is not within ±10% of the expected value. A *calibration process* is then employed, which involves adjusting the detector's output to bring it back into compliance. A detector that demonstrates 10 to 20% error can be used if a correction chart is supplied (5). Appropriate documentation and a sticker indicating the date of accuracy testing and/or calibration are supplied by the testing company.

Dose Calibrator

Dose calibrators are very reliable instruments that rarely have problems. They can remain stable to within ±0.1% over several years (3). However, because they are critical to the work of a nuclear medicine department, their operation must be checked daily. In addition, several quality control measures need to be done on a quarterly or annual basis, and all should be repeated after any repair. Table 1-2 lists the tests required for the dose calibrator.

A dose calibrator must be checked annually for accuracy using a reference standard whose activity is traceable to NIST. The procedure for accuracy testing (6) requires three separate measurements of the reference standard, which are averaged and compared to the known activity of the standard. This is repeated with two or three different radionuclides with different gamma ray energies. A dose calibrator is considered accurate if its reading is within ±5% of the reference standard activity (6).

The essential daily quality control test of a dose calibrator is a constancy reading of the activity of a long-lived source (usually Cs-137, although some users employ two or three radionuclides of varying energies). This test can be considered an accuracy evaluation only if the source is NIST-traceable. The constancy test verifies the proper operation of a dose calibrator on a given day, and it must therefore be performed every day that the dose calibrator is used, before its first clinical measurement. An error of ±10% (measured activity vs calibration data) or less is considered acceptable (6). It is also common practice to check the reading of the constancy source with each of the isotope selector buttons. In older electromechanical (as opposed to digital) dose calibrators, this step verifies that the electrical and mechanical components are providing correct outputs. For newer microprocessor-driven models, the numbers will not change unless the microprocessor is reprogrammed. At the time of the constancy check, the dose calibrator should also be checked for contamination and zeroed, and the voltage of the power supply noted.

One of the drawbacks of a constancy measurement is that it evaluates the operation of a dose calibrator at only one activity level. To know whether the dose calibrator is appropriately measuring at a variety of activity levels, a quality control test called activity linearity must be performed. *Linearity* refers to the ability of an instrument to measure variable quantities in a linear fashion. *Activity linearity* is defined as the ability of a dose calibrator to measure, in a proportional manner, sources with activities spanning several orders of magnitude. This test can be done in one of two ways. One is to measure a short-lived source such as Tc-99m at several time points over 2 to 3 days, plotting the measured activity vs time on semilogarithmic graph paper. The points should plot out linearly and match a Tc-99m decay plot. Consistent and accurate timing is necessary for this test; an error of 10 minutes (min) can give an apparent 2% linearity error (6).

Table 1-3

Troubleshooting Gas-Filled Detectors

Instrument	Problem	Possible Causes
Dose calibrator	Higher than expected constancy reading	• Contamination of dipper and/or liner
	Negative background reading or lower than expected constancy reading	• System zeroing engaged with contamination present; contamination has now decayed
Ionization survey meter, Geiger counter	Higher than expected constancy reading	• Contamination • Incorrect measuring distance or reference standard
	Lower than expected constancy reading	• Incorrect measuring distance or reference standard • Shielding material between standard and detector
	No reading on constancy check	• Dead battery • Broken cable (Geiger counter) • Thin end window integrity broken
Geiger counter	Reading decreases as distance decreases	• Dead time is affecting reading

Sample Calculation 1-2   Activity Linearity Based on Decay

A dose calibrator is tested for activity linearity over 3 days, using a Tc-99m source, with the following results:

Day	Time	Activity
1	0800	96.4 mCi
1	1400	48.6 mCi
2	0800	6.08 mCi
2	1400	3.02 mCi
3	0800	0.381 mCi
3	1400	0.160 mCi

Plot these results on semilogarithmic graph paper to determine the linearity response of the detector. Decay-correct all other results to 0800 on day 2 to determine the variability relative to that value.

The graph looks very linear except for the last data point.

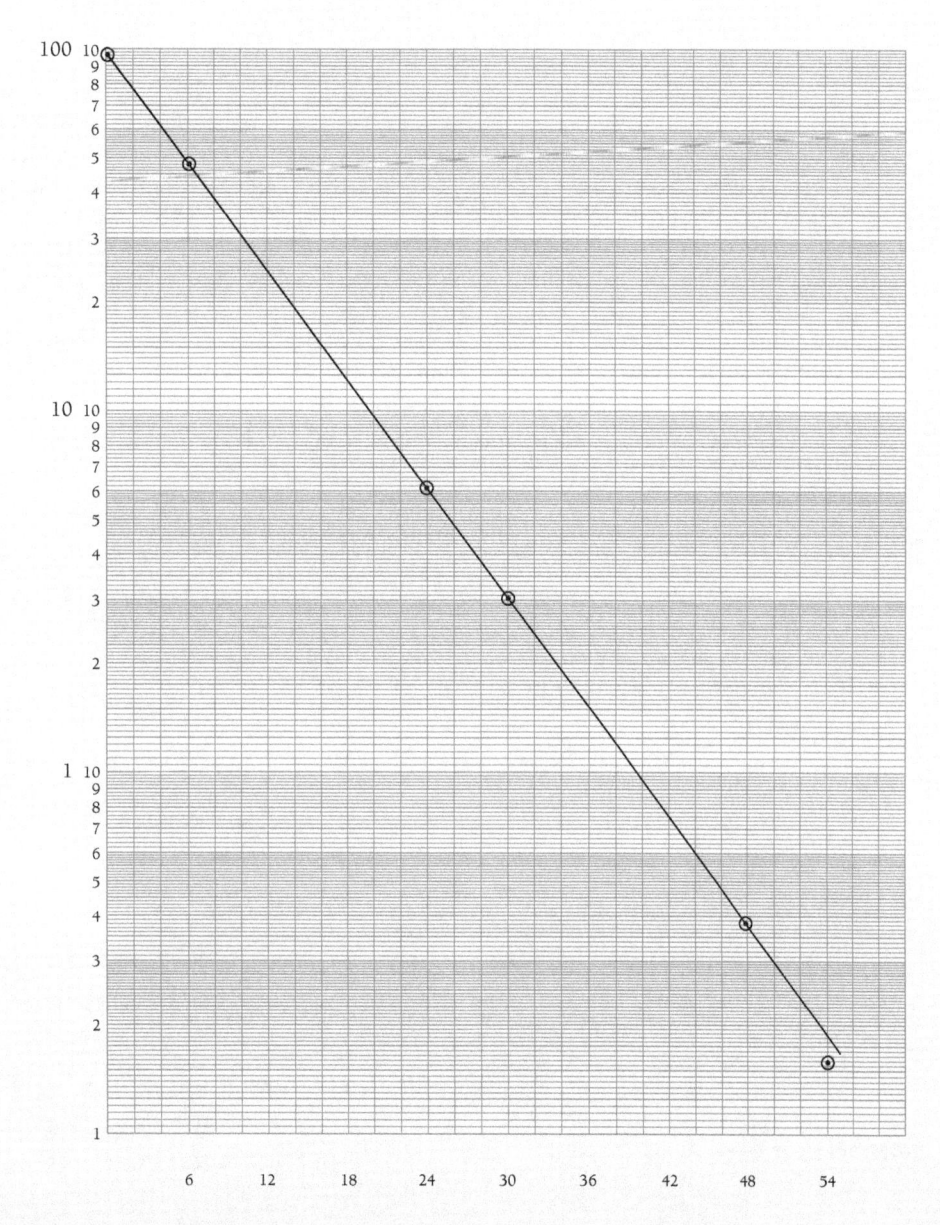

The decay-correction calculation assumes that decay is happening according to the half-life of Tc-99m, and it allows us to evaluate whether the dose calibrator is reflecting that accurately, at the high and low ends of the activity relative to the middle (where the dose calibrator is most likely to give a good measurement).

Continues

Simply apply the decay equation to each value:

$$\text{Activity (day 1, 0800): } 96.4 \text{ mCi} \left(e^{-\left(\frac{0.693}{6.02 \text{ hr}}\right)(24 \text{ hr})} \right)$$
$$= 6.08 \text{ mCi}.$$

$$\text{Activity (day 1, 1400): } 48.6 \text{ mCi} \left(e^{-\left(\frac{0.693}{6.02 \text{ hr}}\right)(18 \text{ hr})} \right)$$
$$= 6.12 \text{ mCi}.$$

$$\text{Activity (day 2, 1400): } 3.02 \text{ mCi} \left(e^{-\left(\frac{0.693}{6.02 \text{ hr}}\right)(-6 \text{ hr})} \right)$$
$$= 6.02 \text{ mCi}.$$

$$\text{Activity (day 3, 0800): } 0.381 \text{ mCi} \left(e^{-\left(\frac{0.693}{6.02 \text{ hr}}\right)(-24 \text{ hr})} \right)$$
$$= 6.04 \text{ mCi}.$$

$$\text{Activity (day 3, 1400): } 0.160 \text{ mCi} \left(e^{-\left(\frac{0.693}{6.02 \text{ hr}}\right)(-30 \text{ hr})} \right)$$
$$= 5.05 \text{ mCi}.$$

Note that the time becomes negative in the last three calculations in order to decay-correct backward in time. This dose calibrator demonstrates good activity linearity, with a range of values of 0.10 mCi or 1.6% around the nominal value of 6.08 mCi, down to the last value, which is only 83% of what the decay equation predicts.

An alternative method for evaluating activity linearity is to use a set of commercially available lead sleeves and a single high-activity source. The source is put into each of the sleeves, and the measured activity is compared to that expected based on the known amount of attenuation by the sleeve. After each reading is corrected by the known attenuation factor for each sleeve, the corrected values are averaged, and the percent error of each measurement relative to the average is obtained. The "sleeve method" for testing activity linearity is accomplished in a much shorter time frame than the decay method described above.

Activity linearity should be checked quarterly over a range of activities from the maximum activity dispensed down to 30 μCi (1.1 MBq). Percent error is calculated as (observed ÷ predicted × 100%). When the decay method is used, calculate the predicted amount of Tc-99m at each measurement time based on a reading between 1 and 50 mCi, because the dose calibrator is least likely to have measurement errors in this range. When the sleeve method is used, a long-lived source of known activity is used, and a table of predicted values is easily generated. **Figure 1-9** shows two examples of dose calibrators exhibiting nonlinearity, for different reasons. If the dose calibrator proves to have nonlinearity greater than ±10% in any activity range, it should be serviced (6).

Sample Calculation 1-3 Activity Linearity Using the Sleeve Method

The following readings are obtained on a Cs-137 source measured in a dose calibrator, using a set of lead attenuating sleeves. The four sleeves are combined to create a total of seven attenuation levels; the attenuation factors and the respective readings are given.

Attenuation Factor of Sleeve	Source Reading
1.000	214.0 mCi
3.379	62.9 mCi
5.088	42.1 mCi
17.694	12.15 mCi
41.368	5.22 mCi
139.226	1.56 mCi
206.937	1.04 mCi
696.105	0.31 mCi

Does this dose calibrator exhibit good activity linearity?
Multiply each reading by its corresponding attenuation factor.
Corrected readings:

$$214.0 \text{ mCi} \times 1.000 = 214.0 \text{ mCi}.$$
$$62.9 \text{ mCi} \times 3.379 = 212.5 \text{ mCi}.$$
$$42.1 \text{ mCi} \times 5.088 = 214.2 \text{ mCi}.$$
$$12.15 \text{ mCi} \times 17.694 = 215.0 \text{ mCi}.$$
$$5.22 \text{ mCi} \times 41.368 = 215.9 \text{ mCi}.$$
$$1.56 \text{ mCi} \times 139.226 = 217.2 \text{ mCi}.$$
$$1.04 \text{ mCi} \times 206.937 = 215.2 \text{ mCi}.$$
$$0.31 \text{ mCi} \times 696.105 = 215.8 \text{ mCi}.$$

Choose 12.15 mCi as a reading unlikely to be affected by any problems, and use its corrected value as the 100% value for this test. Express all other corrected readings as a percentage of this value:

$$214.0 \text{ mCi} = 99.5\% \text{ of } 215.0 \text{ mCi}.$$
$$212.5 \text{ mCi} = 98.8\% \text{ of } 215.0 \text{ mCi}.$$
$$214.2 \text{ mCi} = 99.6\% \text{ of } 215.0 \text{ mCi}.$$
$$215.9 \text{ mCi} = 100.4\% \text{ of } 215.0 \text{ mCi}.$$
$$217.2 \text{ mCi} = 101.0\% \text{ of } 215.0 \text{ mCi}.$$
$$215.2 \text{ mCi} = 100.1\% \text{ of } 215.0 \text{ mCi}.$$
$$215.8 \text{ mCi} = 100.4\% \text{ of } 215.0 \text{ mCi}.$$

The dose calibrator exhibits good activity linearity, because the largest deviation is 1.2% from the 100% value. If the percent values were greater than 10%, the dose calibrator would require servicing.

(a) Activity nonlinearity due to saturation of capacitor

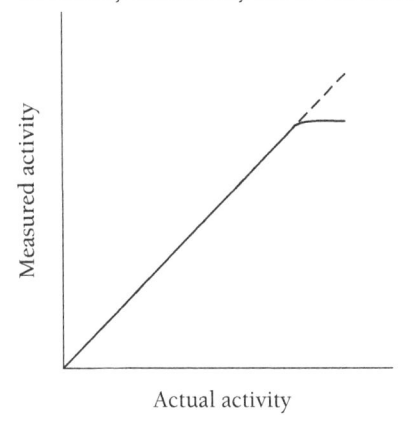

(b) Activity nonlinearity due to recombination

— Measured
--- Extrapolated

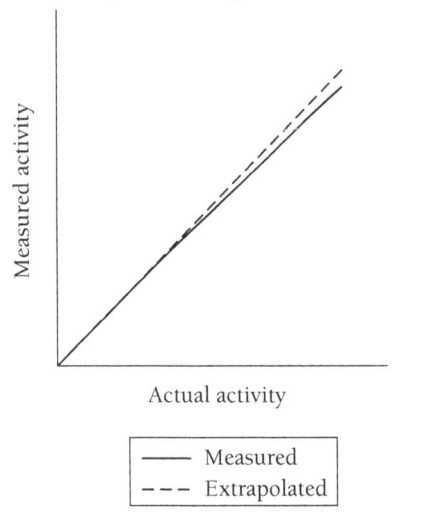

Figure 1-9 Graphs demonstrating poor activity linearity. (a) Activity nonlinearity due to saturation of capacitor. The measured activity line is flat at high activities, indicating that the chamber has exceeded the dose calibrator's ability to neutralize the large number of ion pairs being created. (b) Activity nonlinearity due to recombination. This graph, in contrast, shows a dose calibrator in which recombination is occurring at high activity levels, as indicated by a gradual separation between the measured and extrapolated lines as activity increases.

Finally, a dose calibrator may respond differently to different source containers, especially with certain kinds of radionuclides. When radionuclides that emit beta particles or low-energy gamma rays are measured, the dose calibrator's response is subject to inaccuracies, specifically when the radionuclide is contained in a glass vial vs a plastic syringe. These differences are evaluated by the manufacturer prior to installation of the dose calibrator and are collectively termed *geometry factors*. *Geometry testing* involves the measurement of a variety of radioactive sources in different geometric and volumetric configurations. A common procedure involves incremental additions of water to a radioactive solution, with a dose calibrator measurement after each addition (6). The procedure is performed with 3-ml syringes and 30-ml glass vials, both of which are commonly encountered in nuclear medicine practice. Care must be taken not to lose any radioactivity in the process, or the results will be invalidated. Again, the limit for geometry variation is ±10%; if this value is exceeded, mathematical corrections should be made to compensate.

While it is the manufacturer's responsibility to evaluate geometry issues, it is the user's responsibility to take geometric considerations into account when measuring a specific radionuclide. The particular radionuclides subject to geometric inaccuracies are generally listed in a chart that accompanies the dose calibrator. Geometry measurements need only be performed at installation and repair, so they should be kept on file for the life of the dose calibrator (6).

Limitations of Gas-Filled Detectors

Gas-filled detectors have several characteristics that make them quite useful in the detection of radiation. It is relatively easy to measure electric signals over several orders of magnitude, allowing these detectors to operate over a wide range of radiation intensity. They generally demonstrate excellent linearity of response (i.e., the measured value reported by the detector changes in direct relation to the strength of the radiation field). In addition, the unsophisticated design and simple electronics of these detectors combine to make them highly reliable instruments. But they have important drawbacks when compared to other categories of radiation detectors.

Efficiency for High-Energy Photons

Because the active volume of a gas-filled detector is a gas, these detectors have low efficiency for interaction with high-energy photons. In fact, most of the ionization events registered in a gas-filled detector result not from photon interactions in the gas itself, but rather from interactions in the detector walls, from which energetic secondary electrons escape into the gas chamber (3). The user of any gas-filled detector should be aware that many energetic photons do not interact in either the gas volume or the detector wall and are therefore not being detected. In addition, the relatively few ionizations produced in a gas-filled detector per radiation interaction (as compared to other types of detectors) prevent determination of the energy of that interaction.

Detection of Particulate Radiation

The measurement of charged particles with gas-filled chambers is problematic. Charged particles (alpha particles, beta particles, and electrons) interact via the electrical or Coulomb force. Because the Coulomb force operates over a distance, charged particles are constantly interacting, even in the low density of a gas-filled chamber. This fact makes an accurate measurement of their intensity in any of the gas-filled detectors discussed in this chapter imprecise, for two reasons. First, the walls of the chamber enclosing the gas volume may absorb the charged particles partially or completely, in which case the measurement may represent secondary electrons and/or secondary photons.

Second, if charged particles do get into the chamber (as they do in detectors that have a thin entrance window or open window), the measured ionization rate can have more than one meaning. Imagine two radioactive sources, each emitting only beta particles but with different beta particle energies, interacting in a radiation detector. The higher-energy beta particles, because they are traveling faster, interact with fewer molecules in the time they are inside the chamber. The slower, low-energy beta particles, on the other hand, have time to interact with more gas molecules as they travel through the chamber. In this situation, we cannot tell whether there are a few low-energy beta particles or a lot of high-energy beta particles—both situations can create similar numbers of ionizations in the gas. Gas-filled detectors can measure Bremsstrahlung radiation; this is commonly done with dose calibrators, albeit with necessary corrections (see previous discussion). But the operator should be aware of the potential for error when beta particles are the only radiation emissions.

Dead Time

This problem is encountered with Geiger counters and other detectors operating in pulse mode. *Dead time*, in the general sense, is the minimum time separation required in order that two radiation events be correctly recorded as two separate pulses. In a Geiger counter, this is determined by the time required for the positive ions surrounding the anode to dissipate. If a new radiation event occurs in the chamber before dissipation is complete, the electrical pulse produced will be smaller than usual and may not be detected by the pulse-counting electronics. The maximum observed count rate is limited to about 4,000 to 8,000 counts per second (cps) (corresponding to a true count rate of about 6,000 to 15,000 cps). Further, because the dead time is paralyzable, trying to count at rates above this maximum will lead to a decreasing count rate. A Geiger counter may register a very low count rate in the presence of a significant radiation field.

Summary

The small instruments discussed in this chapter are used daily in the nuclear medicine department. The operation of the department as a whole depends in a significant way on these simple but highly useful radiation detectors. Starting from the detection of the ionizations created by the interactions of gamma rays in air, they produce the measures of radiation field strength and activity needed by those who work with radiation. These instruments are rugged and reliable and will function properly for years if treated with a measure of care.

One must keep in mind, however, that while gas-filled detectors are relatively simple to operate, the user must be thoroughly knowledgeable of their strengths, weaknesses, and potential pitfalls. The use of an ionization survey meter to do contamination surveys or a Geiger counter with a pancake probe to monitor a radionuclide therapy patient would be likely to yield erroneous but apparently valid results. A dose calibrator reading may seem perfectly reasonable, even though the wrong isotope selector button has been chosen. An adequate understanding of the construction and operation of these instruments can prevent errors such as these.

References

1. Graham LS, ed. *Nuclear Medicine: Self-Study Program II: Instrumentation*. Reston, VA: Society of Nuclear Medicine; 1996:3,5.
2. Cherry SR, Sorenson JA, Phelps ME. *Physics in Nuclear Medicine*. 3rd ed. Philadelphia, PA: Saunders; 2003:91.
3. Knoll GF. *Radiation Detection and Measurement*. 3rd ed. New York, NY: John Wiley and Sons; 2000:146, 201, 212, 213, 215.
4. Christian PE. Radiation detection. In: Fahey FH, Harkness BA, eds. *Basic Science of Nuclear Medicine* [CD-ROM]. Reston, VA: Society of Nuclear Medicine; 2001.
5. Klingensmith WC, Eshima D, Goddard J. *Nuclear Medicine Procedure Manual 2003–05*. Englewood, CO: Wick; 2003:20-1–20-4.
6. Zanzonico P. Routine quality control of clinical nuclear medicine instrumentation: a brief review. *J Nucl Med*. 2008;49:1114–1131.

Additional Resources

Graham LS, ed. *Nuclear Medicine: Self-Study Program II: Instrumentation*. Reston, VA: Society of Nuclear Medicine; 1996:1–5.
Henkin RE, Boles MA, Dillehay GL, et al., eds. *Nuclear Medicine*. St. Louis, MO: Mosby-Year Book; 1996:Chapter 5.
Klingensmith WC, Eshima D, Goddard J. *Nuclear Medicine Procedure Manual 2003–05*, Englewood, CO: Wick; 2003:20-1–20-4.
Knoll GF. *Radiation Detection and Measurement*. 3rd ed. New York, NY: John Wiley and Sons; 2000:Chapters 5, 7.
Ramberg-Laskaris KL. Quality control in the radiopharmacy. *J Nucl Med Technol*. 1984;12:33–36.
Zanzonico P. Routine quality control of clinical nuclear medicine instrumentation: a brief review. *J Nucl Med*. 2008;49:1114–1131.

CHAPTER 2 Scintillation Detectors

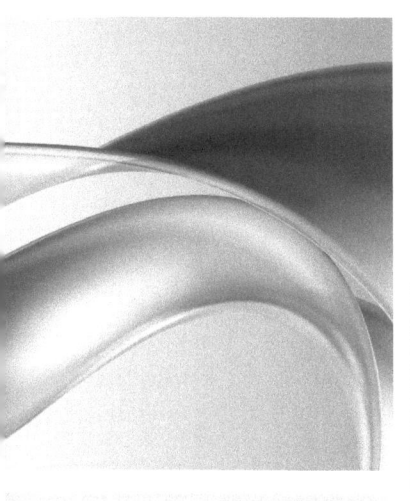

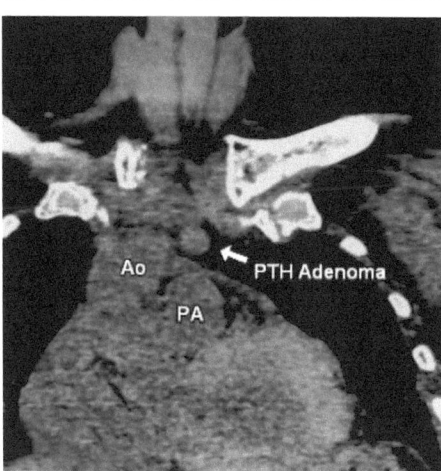

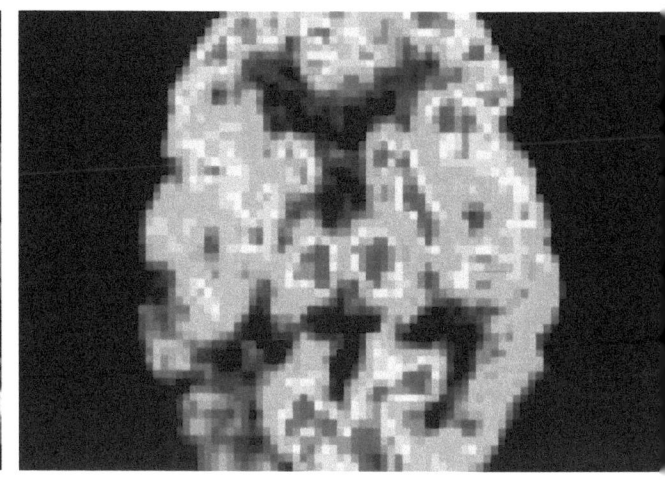

Learning Outcomes

1. Identify the essential steps of radiation detection using a scintillation detector.
2. Describe the delocalized bonding structure of thallium-activated sodium iodide, the emission of scintillation photons in response to absorption of a gamma ray, and the relationship between gamma ray energy and scintillation light emission.
3. Identify the parts of a photomultiplier tube, and state the function of each.
4. List additional electronic components needed for a scintillation detector and the function of each.
5. Distinguish between the output of single-channel and multichannel analyzer scintillation detectors, and discuss counting measurement techniques using well counter and probe configurations.
6. Discuss why and how a scintillation detector is calibrated, for both single-channel and multichannel analyzer types.
7. Outline the causes of peak broadening, the calculation of a percentage energy window and the determination of the percentage energy resolution (including the calculation of the *full width at half-maximum* [FWHM]), and the use of the energy resolution as a quality control test.
8. List recommended quality control tests for scintillation detectors and their frequencies.

Introduction

Scintillation detectors constitute a second major class of radiation detectors used in nuclear medicine. They have significant advantages over gas-filled detectors. Because they are solid rather than gaseous, they have much greater efficiency for interactions with gamma rays compared to gas-filled detectors. This in turn provides a means to measure the energy of a radiation interaction, which allows us to identify radionuclides based on their gamma ray energies, or to distinguish unscattered from scattered gamma rays. Scintillation detectors have wide application in many processes that involve the detection of gamma rays. In nuclear medicine, they are found in thyroid probes, well counters, gamma cameras, and *positron emission tomography* (PET) tomographs. Liquid scintillation counters operate on somewhat similar principles, but are rarely used in clinical nuclear medicine.

Basic Principles of Scintillation

Scintillation is a general term referring to the process of giving off light; it is used both literally and figuratively. More specifically in the sciences, a *scintillator* is any material that can release a photon in the ultraviolet (UV) or visible-light range, when an excited electron in the scintillator returns to its ground state. These *scintillation photons* are detected by a *photomultiplier tube* (PMT) and converted to an electronic signal. Some of the terms used to describe nuclear medicine studies, such as *scintigraphy* and *scintiscans*, derive from this aspect of the detection process.

Scintillator

Many different kinds of materials have the ability to scintillate. Organic materials, particularly conjugated ring compounds, produce scintillation photons in the process of de-excitation of orbital electrons. Scintillators can also be made of glass or of noble gases such as xenon or helium, both of which may be used for detection of particulate radiation. However, all of these scintillators have a low average atomic number, and therefore they are not very efficient for interactions with gamma rays.

The scintillators used in nuclear medicine applications are inorganic crystalline scintillators, often with small amounts of impurities that help them scintillate more efficiently. The process of intentionally introducing an impurity into a pure metal to improve its performance is called *doping*. The most common inorganic scintillator employed in nuclear medicine is thallium-activated sodium iodide, or NaI(Tl). It was developed for use in radiation detection by Robert Hofstadter in 1948. It is used primarily in detectors designed to detect lower-energy gamma rays such as those emitted by Tc-99m. Detectors designed for high-energy photons, such as annihilation photons, are made of scintillators with even higher atomic number and density, such as bismuth germanate, lutetium oxyorthosilicate, and gadolinium oxyorthosilicate.

Scintillation crystals are made to exacting tolerances and require exceptional care in the manufacturing process. The crystal must be optically transparent, without cracks or boundaries that could cause scintillation photons to be reflected. Scintillation crystals are quite fragile, and can fracture under conditions of mechanical stress or rapid temperature change (>5°C or 9°F per hr). Extreme care must be used when working near an exposed crystal. In addition, sodium iodide is *hygroscopic*, meaning that it absorbs moisture from the air. When this happens, the crystal turns yellow and absorbs scintillation photons rather than transmitting them. As a result, scintillation crystals must be hermetically sealed, so that no air or water comes into contact with the crystal.

The most desirable characteristic of sodium iodide is its excellent *scintillation light yield* (number of scintillation photons emitted per eV of radiation energy absorbed), which is higher than that of most other scintillators. This is important because the greater number of scintillation photons leads to greater precision in measuring the energy of the absorbed gamma ray. The scintillation photons produced in sodium iodide range from 325 to 550 nm, primarily in the ultraviolet spectrum but just touching the high end of the visible-light spectrum. This range perfectly matches the response function of the bialkali photomultiplier tube (1), the most common type of PMT used in radiation detection applications.

Another important characteristic of a scintillator is its *decay time*, which indicates how long scintillation photons are released after a radiation interaction. A long decay time means that radiation events will need to be more widely spaced if we desire to count them in pulse mode. The decay time for sodium iodide is relatively long at 230 nsec, which in turn contributes to the detector's overall dead time. As with any material, sodium iodide shows decreased efficiency for interaction as gamma ray energy increases (linear attenuation coefficient μ_ℓ = 2.16/cm at 150 keV vs 0.294/cm at 600 keV).

The Scintillation Process in NaI(Tl)

Thallium-activated sodium iodide is crystalline in physical form, with a small amount of thallium replacing sodium (about 1 in 1,000 atoms) to provide the impurity. It is the delocalized molecular bonding of the crystal that gives it the ability to scintillate (**Figure 2-1**). Delocalized bonding is discussed in greater detail in Appendix B; briefly, the electron orbitals of the sodium and iodine atoms combine to form a valence band and a conduction band of molecular orbitals. The valence band (analogous to the bonding orbital of a covalent bond) is at a lower energy than the conduction band (analogous to the antibonding orbital). The thallium impurities create electron orbitals between the conduction band and the valence band called *activation centers*. In the ground state, the valence band and the ground-state level of each activation center are filled with electrons. The conduction band and the excited energy levels of the activation centers are empty. Thus there is no electron movement in the absence of radiation.

When a gamma ray enters the crystal and undergoes an interaction, it produces one or more secondary electrons with high kinetic energy (see Appendix A). These electrons cause ionizations and excitations as they move, creating many low-energy tertiary electrons. Most of these low-energy electrons lose their energy as heat, but some have the right amount of energy to jump up to the conduction band (Fig. 2-1b, Step *a*). A hole is left in the valence band for each electron excited into the conduction band. The electrons that get into the conduction band are free to move around, but are not allowed to drop directly back into the valence band (this is "forbidden," meaning highly unlikely according to quantum physics). However, the electrons will still seek to find the lowest energy levels available to them, which are the excited-state levels of the activation centers (Fig. 2-1b, Step *b*). Likewise, the holes will allow electrons in the valence band to move, such that eventually the holes will be filled by electrons from activation centers, leaving vacancies in the activation center ground-state orbitals. Quantum mechanics does allow the transition of an electron from the excited state to the ground state in an activation center. The electron drops down and fills the hole, with the release of the excess energy in the form of a scintillation photon (Fig. 2-1b, Step *c*).

Let us consider two important consequences of this process. First, of the energy deposited in the scintillation crystal by the gamma ray, some but by no means all of it is transferred to scintillation photons. (As will be discussed, the detection of radiation by scintillation is an inherently inefficient process. Sodium iodide, with a scintillation efficiency of 13%, is considered a highly efficient scintillator.) From the standpoint of radiation detection, the critical fact is that a *proportionality* exists between the

(a) Band structure of NaI(Tl)

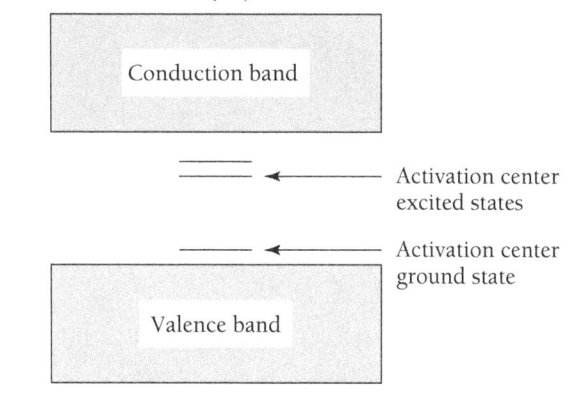

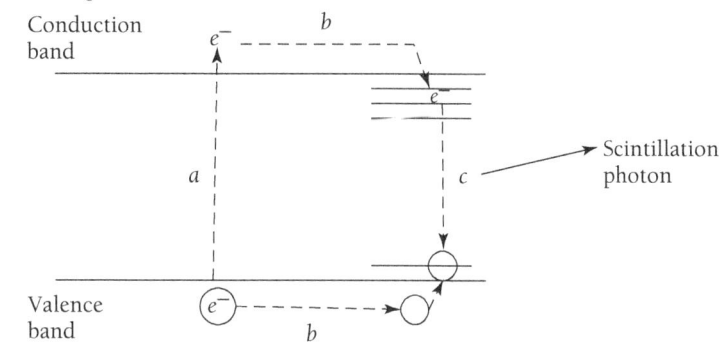

Figure 2-1 Band structure and scintillation process in thallium-activated sodium iodide. The three steps in the scintillation process are as follows (Figure 2-1b): (*a*) some of the free electrons created by a gamma ray interaction have enough energy to jump across the forbidden gap to the conduction band; (*b*) once in the conduction band, these electrons migrate to the activation center excited-state orbitals, and the holes in the valence band to the activation center ground-state orbitals; (*c*) the transition of an electron from an activation center excited-state orbital to an activation center ground-state orbital produces a scintillation photon.

energy that the gamma ray deposits in the crystal and the *number* of scintillation photons produced. A 20-keV gamma ray will produce one-fifth as many scintillation photons as a 100-keV gamma ray. Thus, if we count the scintillation photons, and if we carry this proportionality through the rest of the detection process, we can determine the energy of each gamma ray.

The other important fact is that this all happens very quickly. Because the gamma ray and the secondary electrons it creates are traveling very fast, the process of absorbing the gamma ray's energy takes only a few nanoseconds. The emission of scintillation photons reaches a maximum at about 30 nsec after the gamma ray interaction and declines thereafter with a half-life of about 150 nsec, such that two-thirds of the scintillation light is emitted within 230 nsec. As long as the count rate stays relatively low, the interaction of one gamma ray in the crystal will be completed before the next one occurs. Thus, scintillation detectors generally operate in pulse mode.

Photomultiplier Tube

Having scintillation photons is not enough; we need to convert them to an electronic signal. This is accomplished by a PMT. The thyroid probe and well counter each have one PMT. Gamma cameras have many PMTs, allowing both position and energy to be determined. A diagram of a PMT is shown in **Figure 2-2**. To understand its function, we need to consider each of its parts.

The *photocathode* is closest to the scintillation crystal; it converts scintillation photons to electrons. It is made of a very thin layer of material that is *photoemissive* (i.e., emits electrons when exposed to UV and visible-light photons). Photoemissive materials used in PMTs are most often metal alloys that have extra electrons, usually bialkali antimonide compounds such as K_2CsSb and Na_2KSb. As scintillation photons are released in the scintillation process, some will strike the photocathode and cause it to emit electrons that are released into the vacuum space of the PMT itself. Once the electrons are emitted from the photocathode, the *focusing grid* provides the proper electric field to direct the electrons toward the first dynode. Note that a vacuum must be maintained inside the PMT, so that no electrons are lost due to interaction with any gas molecules. The PMT must also be shielded against stray magnetic fields, as these will alter the trajectory of the electrons (1).

A series of *dynodes* multiply the small number of electrons generated at the photocathode into a measurable electronic signal. They are made of metal alloys (again with an excess of electrons) and are maintained at positive electrical potentials, each one higher than the last. They are curved or positioned so as to direct the emitted electrons toward the next dynode. The absorption of one electron at a dynode causes emission of three to six electrons, depending on the potential difference from dynode to dynode. The electrons released at each dynode are

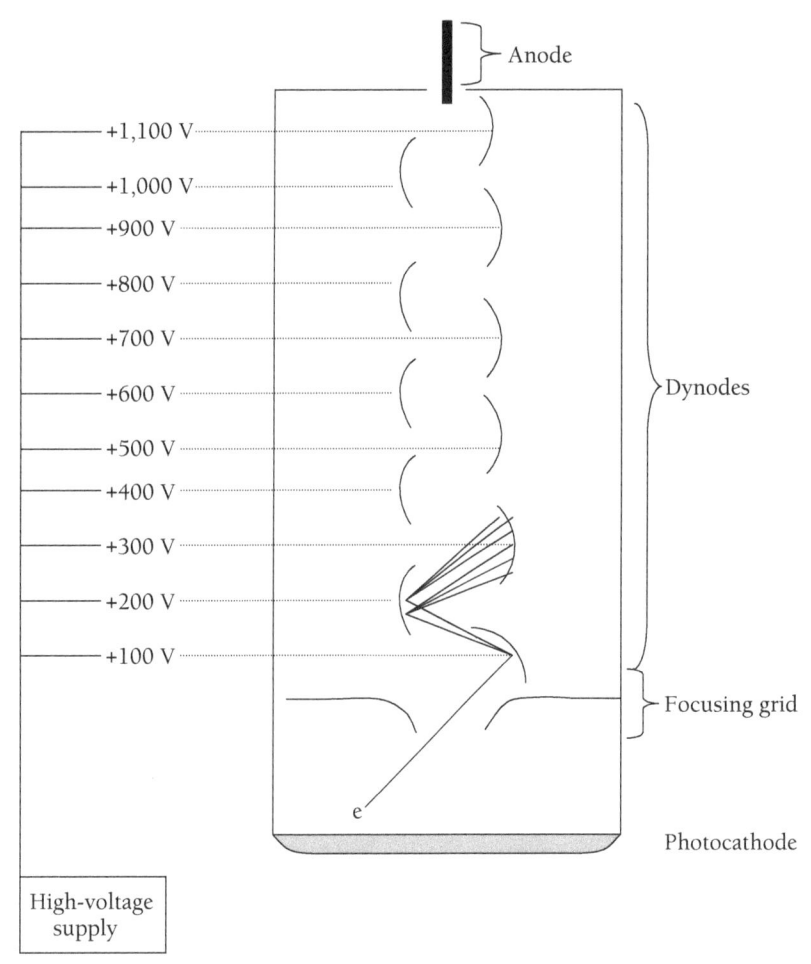

Figure 2-2 Photomultiplier tube. Its basic structure is an evacuated cylinder enclosed in glass, with a photocathode on one end, an anode at the opposite end, and small curved dynodes in between. The electrical potential to the dynodes causes multiplication of the electrical signal created at the photocathode. The passage of an electron through the focusing grid, its interaction with the first dynode, and its multiplication at the second dynode are shown, using a multiplication factor of 3.

accelerated toward the next dynode, again because of the potential difference between dynodes. The process continues for 9 to 12 dynodes, for a total multiplication factor of about 1 million, producing a small but measurable electronic signal. Finally, the *anode* collects all the electrons produced from the final dynode and emits an output voltage signal.

The high-voltage supply of the PMT determines the potential difference between the dynodes and therefore the final size of the PMT output pulse. A typical scintillation detector has a high voltage of 1,000 volts (V) or more, with 100-V increments between dynodes. The exact setting of the high voltage is determined each day using the calibration procedure discussed later in this chapter. Scintillation detectors are very sensitive to changes in the high voltage; a 1% change in the high voltage results in a 10% change in the pulse size (measured at the anode). The high-voltage supply must therefore be steady and well regulated.

To recapitulate the process of radiation detection in a scintillation detector (**Figure 2-3**): A gamma ray interacts in the scintillation crystal to bump electrons into the conduction band, which produce scintillation photons as they transition back to the ground state. The scintillation photons in turn cause the emission of a few electrons at the photocathode of the PMT. These few electrons are converted to a measurable electronic signal at the PMT's anode. The height of the pulse generated in the PMT is therefore proportional to the energy absorbed in the scintillator from the gamma ray interaction. Note, however, that three conversions between energy (photons) and mass (electrons) are required. With each conversion step, there is some inefficiency and therefore a loss of energy. Consider the process for Tc-99m and Cs-137 (**Table 2-1**). The number of information carriers (the scintillation photons or electrons in each step) decreases with each conversion between mass and energy, a fact that has important implications.

Looking at Table 2-1, we can see that the number of information carriers decreases as the process moves toward the photocathode, and then increases as the dynodes multiply the signal beyond the photocathode. However, the number of information carriers is approximate, not exact, and is subject to statistical variation. The point of greatest statistical variation is found at the point in the process where the number of information carriers is the lowest, namely, the release of electrons from the photocathode. As a result, the measured output (the pulse height) is not

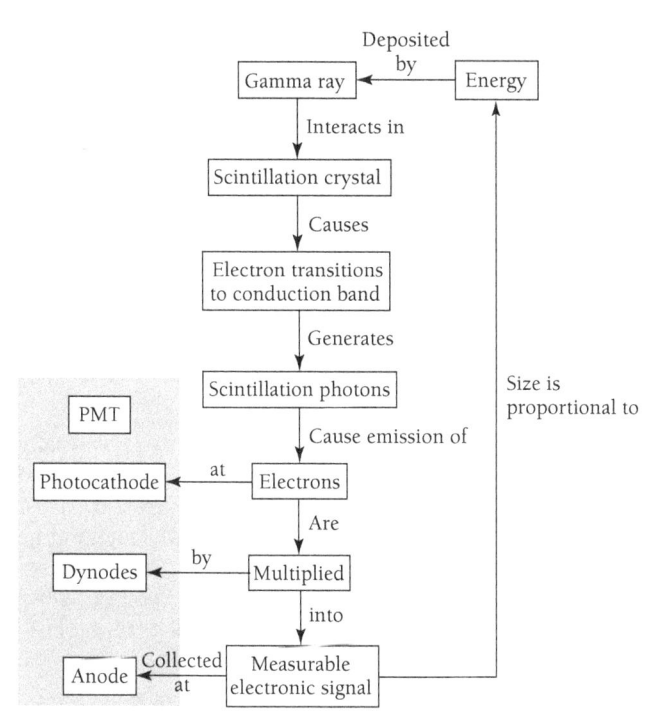

Figure 2-3 Concept map of the scintillation detection process. Note the linearity of the diagram; this indicates that the process will happen in the same way for each gamma ray. The key advantage of the scintillation detector over gas-filled detectors is the connecting line between the size of the electronic signal and the energy that the gamma ray has deposited in the scintillation crystal.

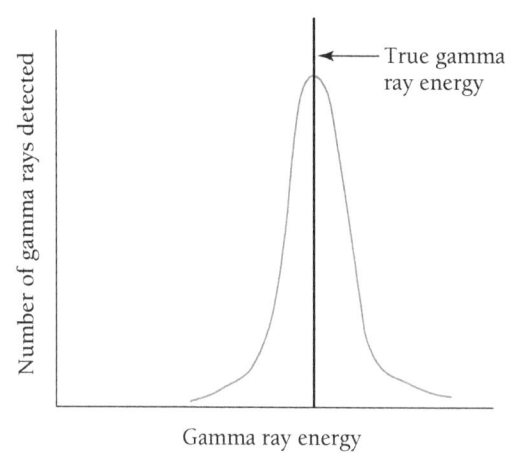

Figure 2-4 Peak broadening as seen with scintillation detectors. The straight line is what would be seen with a detector that translated gamma ray energy into an electronic signal with no statistical variability; the Gaussian curve is seen with scintillation detectors because of the statistical variation that occurs in the detection process.

always exactly proportional to the energy of the photon creating the signal, but has random fluctuations from one gamma ray to the next. For the total absorption of a Tc-99m gamma ray, we do not measure a single pulse height corresponding to exactly 140 keV. Instead, we get a distribution of pulse heights with a Gaussian shape, centered at 140 keV (**Figure 2-4**). This *peak broadening* prevents the separate detection of gamma rays with closely spaced energies. It has important implications for the use of scintillation detectors in nuclear medicine, as will be discussed.

Associated Electronics

Figure 2-5 shows the scintillation crystal and PMT in a block diagram of a scintillation detector. The scintillation crystal sits inside an aluminum "can," which has its inner surface coated with a reflective layer to reflect scintillation photons back into the crystal. The back end of the crystal may be optically coupled to a light pipe made of quartz or Lucite, which is in turn coupled to the PMT. The light pipe acts as a guide for the scintillation photons, internally reflecting wide-angle scintillation photons toward the photocathode. Optical coupling grease (usually some kind of silicon grease) reduces the loss of scintillation photons by preventing reflection at the scintillation crystal/light pipe and light pipe/photocathode interfaces (or the crystal/photocathode interface, in systems without a light pipe). If the coupling grease degrades, the number of scintillation photons reaching the PMT is greatly diminished.

Table 2-1

Scintillation Detector Efficiency

Site in Detector	Conversion Factor	Information Carriers for Tc-99m	Information Carriers for Cs-137
		140 keV photon	662 keV photon
Scintillation crystal	Scintillation efficiency = 12%	16.8 keV converted to scintillation photons	79 keV converted to scintillation photons
Scintillation photons	Each scintillation photon has energy of 3 eV	5,600 scintillation photons	26,480 scintillation photons
PMT at front of photocathode	75% absorption at photocathode	4,200 scintillation photons absorbed	19,860 scintillation photons absorbed
PMT after photocathode	Photocathode efficiency = 20%	840 electrons emitted into PMT space	3,972 electrons emitted into PMT space
Dynodes	Multiplication factor = 10^8	84 trillion electrons	400 trillion electrons

Adapted from: Knoll GF. *Radiation Detection and Measurement*. 3rd ed. New York, NY: Wiley & Sons; 2000:330.

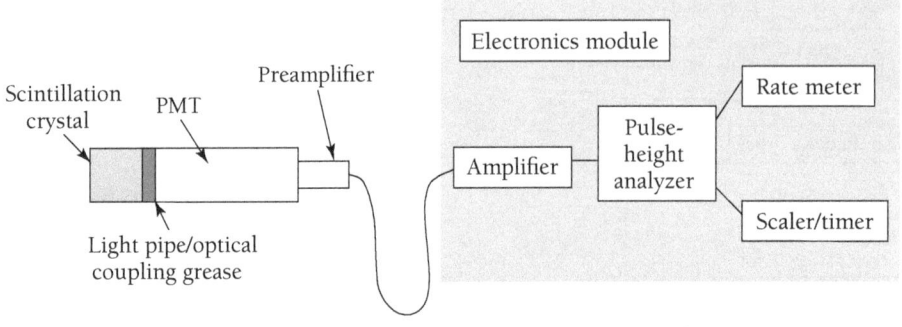

Figure 2-5 Block diagram of a scintillation detector. The detector/PMT assembly is usually separated from the electronics module by a cable.

Signal Amplification

While measurable, the signal output of the PMT anode is still very small. A *preamplifier* (attached directly to the PMT, to minimize signal distortion) boosts the strength of the PMT output signal to allow its passage through the remaining detector electronics. To facilitate complete charge collection, the preamplifier is adjusted to have a long decay time, resulting in a pulse with a long tail, requiring about 50–100 (μsec) to return to baseline. An *amplifier* (housed in an accompanying electronic module) then amplifies the preamplifier output signal by a variable amount. Multiplication factors in amplifiers are typically between 1 and 100 and are adjusted via the coarse and fine gain controls or the energy multiplication knob on the electronics module. The amplifier also shapes the pulse and shortens it to provide a series of discrete pulses that are easier to analyze (see Appendix B for further details).

Determination of Energy Acceptability

Next, the *pulse height analyzer* (PHA) determines the amplitude of the pulse, which correlates with the gamma ray's energy. There are two types of PHAs: the single-channel analyzer (SCA) and the multichannel analyzer (MCA). An SCA consists of a lower-level discriminator (LLD), an upper-level discriminator (ULD), and an anticoincidence logic circuit. The values of the LLD and the ULD are set by the operator and are related to the energy of the photons being measured, as discussed in the following section on calibration. Each pulse in turn is compared to the LLD and the ULD, and pulses with amplitude greater than the LLD but less than the ULD, as detected by the anticoincidence circuit, produce PHA output pulses. (The electronic operation of the PHA is used as an example of a logic circuit in Appendix B.) All output pulses from the PHA are the same size and are sent on to the scaler and the rate meter. The SCA thus essentially extracts the gamma ray energy information from the voltage signal and, based on that energy, either accepts or rejects each pulse. Its output therefore is a string of logic (yes/no or 1/0) pulses that can be counted, but that contain no additional information about the gamma rays they represent beyond the fact that those gamma rays fell within the preset energy range.

Energy Spectrum

The chief drawback of an SCA is that it rejects radiation events that do not fall between the LLD and the ULD, thus preventing us from visualizing a large amount of potentially useful information. An MCA shows all radiation events on an energy graph or *pulse height spectrum* (**Figure 2-6**). Most MCAs work by digitizing the PMT output and assigning the event to one of a series of predefined bins or channels based on the signal's size. We can think of an MCA as consisting of a series of PHAs, each representing a small portion of the energy spectrum. Each gamma ray is recorded as a 1 in one PHA and a 0 in all of the other PHAs.

In the pulse height spectrum of Figure 2-6, each column or bin on the *X*-axis represents a specific narrow range of pulse heights (note that height is represented on the *X*-axis), which in turn represents event energy. The *Y*-axis represents the number of events with energy in that range. The spectrum has several identifiable peaks. The rightmost peak in the figure corresponds to events in which the entire gamma ray energy is registered in the scintillation crystal. This peak is called the *photopeak*, because it corresponds to gamma rays that have undergone photoelectric absorption in the scintillation crystal. Counts to the left of the photopeak represent gamma rays that did not deposit all of their energy in the scintillation crystal. Most have undergone a Compton interaction and are considered "scattered" photons.

The photopeak is used for the calibration procedure described in a following section and for most counting applications. An energy range encompassing the photopeak, shown as the shaded area, contains "acceptable" events that fall within the energy window and hence generate a PHA output pulse. The limits of the shaded area thus correspond

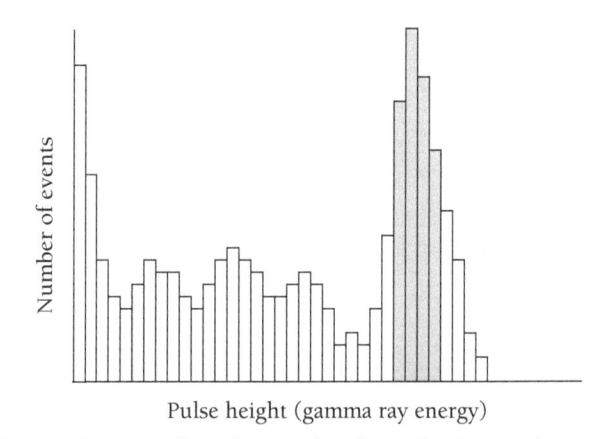

Figure 2-6 Output of a multichannel analyzer. The size or pulse height of each event is plotted on the *X*-axis, and the number of events at each pulse height provides the *Y*-axis value. The shaded bars of the histogram are those within the chosen energy range.

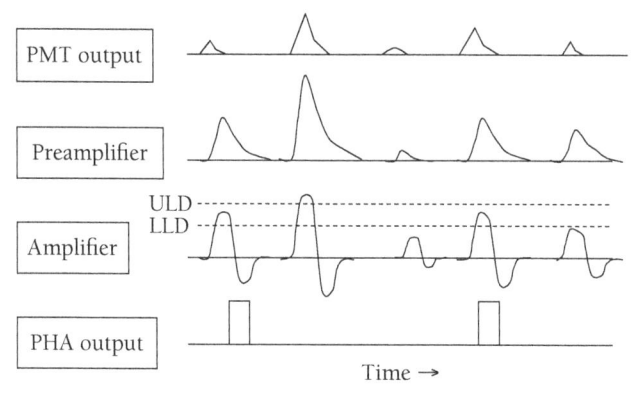

Figure 2-7 Pulse shapes in a scintillation detector. The amplifier line shows the LLD and the ULD levels superimposed on the amplifier output pulses. The PHA output line shows the logic pulses generated when the amplified pulse height falls between the ULD and the LLD. Sizes not to scale; the PMT output signals are much smaller than the preamplifier signals, which in turn are much smaller than the amplifier signals.

to the LLD and the ULD of the SCA. Similar energy spectrum information can be obtained from an SCA, by manually changing the LLD and the ULD to determine the counts at each energy interval and then plotting the spectrum by hand.

Tracking Counts

The last two devices in the block diagram are the scaler/timer and the rate meter. The *scaler/timer* records accepted PHA output pulses during a specified time interval. (The term *scaler* stems from the days when digital registers could not go very high, requiring a scaling circuit to divide the incoming pulse rate by a fixed factor [for example, 100 or 1,000] so that the register could record all the pulses.) A *rate meter* determines the average current produced by the PHA output pulses, which drives a meter calibrated in average counting rate.

Pulse Shapes

Let us consider the block diagram from the standpoint of the pulse shapes at each point in the process (**Figure 2-7**). The PMT output is a very small pulse. The preamplifier, in matching the PMT output pulse to the impedance of the detector electronics, widens it considerably, to about 2 to 5 μsec. The amplifier amplifies and shapes the pulse to make it narrower, usually with a negative overshoot. The PHA output line shows that the PHA only creates an output pulse for input pulses of acceptable height. All of the PHA output pulses are the same height. This sequence works well when the count rate is relatively low, but creates problems called *baseline shift* and *pulse pileup* when counting rates are high.

Calibration

The goal of calibration in a scintillation detector is to define the relationship between the size of the pulse outputs from the PMT and the gamma ray energy. According to an operations manual of one commercially available MCA-type scintillation detector, calibration involves "knowing the energy equivalence of each channel" (2). Recall that the high voltage to the PMT dynodes can be varied by the operator, allowing the pulse size to take on any value. Calibration is needed to correlate pulse size to the energy of the gamma rays being detected. One cannot completely evaluate the energy of a radionuclide sample until this correlation is established. Calibration is accomplished by setting the threshold and window to some desired value and then adjusting the high voltage so that the PMT output pulses are counted within that window.

This section may seem superfluous to some, as most modern scintillation detector systems operate on a "push-button" basis, and many are self-calibrating. However, the author firmly believes that technologists should understand the operation of the machines they work with. The text therefore discusses the energy window determination and calibration of both SCAs and MCAs.

Single-Channel Analyzer

Older scintillation detector systems have two knobs located on the electronics module labeled "threshold" and "window." In relation to our prior discussion, the threshold corresponds to the LLD. The window sits on top of the threshold, so that the value of the ULD is equal to the threshold plus the window. *Calibration* refers to the correlation of these knobs or settings with gamma ray energy in keV. This is typically done with Cs-137, which has a long (30-year) half-life and emits 662-keV gamma rays. The essence of calibration, for single-PMT systems, is to adjust the high voltage so that the photopeak sits in the middle of the window. Once calibrated, the high voltage is locked in, and the threshold and window are changed as needed for clinical measurements.

The threshold and window knobs on an SCA are typically potentiometers with 1,000 distinct settings. It would be highly advantageous to calibrate the detector so that each possible setting on the potentiometer is equal to 1 keV. We first must set the threshold and window to appropriate calibration values. For Cs-137, if a 3% (20-keV) window centered on the 662-keV photopeak is desired, we would set the threshold knob to 652 and the window knob to 20. Once properly calibrated, this would provide a convenient one-to-one correlation between the potentiometer settings and the gamma ray energy.

After the threshold and window are set, the next step is to adjust the high voltage so that the 662-keV photons actually register in the SCA window we have set (**Figure 2-8**). To start from scratch, the voltage is turned down to a low level and the Cs-137 source placed in (or in front of) the detector. Then the high voltage is slowly increased, causing the height (or voltage) of each pulse to get larger (recall that pulse height is plotted along the X-axis of the pulse height spectrum). When the count rate in the window reaches a maximum, the bell-shaped curve is centered on the window, and 662 on the detector dial is equivalent to 662 keV of photon energy. (Note that if we continue to increase the high voltage beyond the maximum, the number of counts will drop but will not reach zero, because scattered photons will be registered in the window. Thus, always start with the high voltage below its expected value.)

Multichannel Analyzer

An MCA is easier to calibrate than an SCA because we can see the whole range of gamma ray energies. We need only

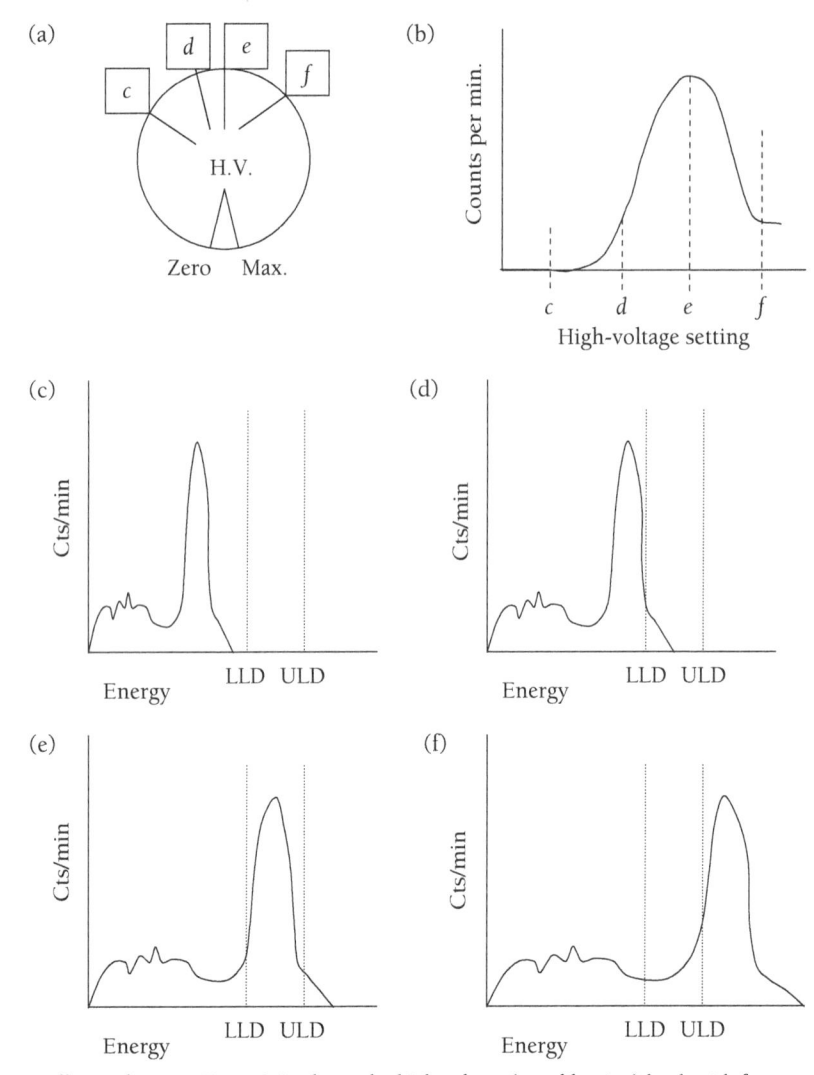

Figure 2-8 Calibration of a scintillation detector. Figure 2-8a shows the high-voltage (or calibration) knob with four settings corresponding to the four energy spectra in Figures 2-8c to Figure 2-8f. Figure 2-8b shows the detector count rate at each knob setting, with the letters corresponding to the pulse height spectra shown in Figures 2-8c to 2-8f. The operator-determined LLD and ULD are shown superimposed on the energy spectra. As the high voltage is increased, the sizes of all pulses increase, and the energy spectrum is "stretched out" along the X-axis. The detector is correctly calibrated in Figure 2-8e, when the number of counts registered in the LLD-ULD window reaches a maximum. In Figure 2-8f, the high voltage has increased the pulse size beyond the center of the window; note that the measured count value does not decrease all the way to zero. Adapted from: Christian P. Radiation detection. In Fahey FH, Harkness BA, eds. *Basic Science of Nuclear Medicine* [CD-ROM]. Reston, VA: Society of Nuclear Medicine, 2001. Reprinted with permission from the Society of Nuclear Medicine.

tweak the high-voltage knob until the highest point of the photopeak corresponds to a specified bin. However, MCAs often don't have a scale that is easily correlated to photon energy in a one-to-one fashion. They may require a conversion factor (e.g., channel 150 = 662 keV) to determine the energy of any other channel.

Energy Linearity

An important quality of a scintillation detector is its ability to measure high- vs low-energy gamma rays in a proportional manner, a concept called *energy linearity* (compare this definition to activity linearity). If a detector properly calibrated with Cs-137 demonstrates good energy linearity, it is able to register any other gamma ray energy at the proper pulse height setting. For example, if SCA knobs are calibrated such that a window centered on 662 corresponds to 662 keV, then a window centered on 140 should register maximum counts with a Tc-99m source. In essence, what we have done by calibration is to set our scale, and the detector's energy linearity characteristics determine how well that scale applies throughout the energy range of interest (**Figure 2-9**). In fact, sodium iodide and other alkali halide scintillators do demonstrate some nonlinearity, mainly at the low end of the energy scale, below about 200 keV (1). For most nuclear medicine applications, this nonlinearity will be small, but its presence should be recognized and measured at least occasionally (3).

Scintillation Detector Applications

Operation

Once the scintillation detector has been calibrated, it is typically used to make a timed measurement of a radioactive

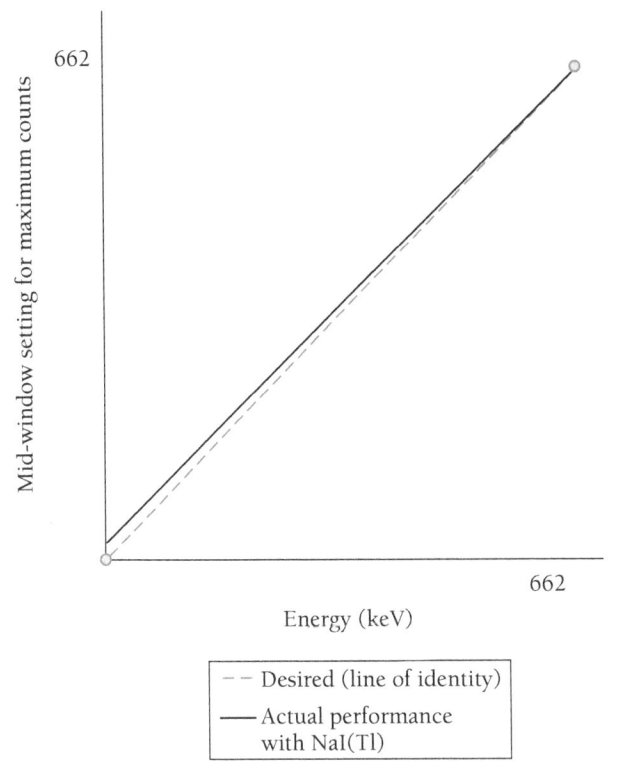

Figure 2-9 Graph illustrating energy linearity. The calibration point at (662, 662) is determined by the calibration procedure, and energy linearity assumes a straight line between this point and (0, 0). It is up to the operator to determine whether a specific scintillation detector is linear with respect to energy; that is, if the detector actually behaves as indicated by the dashed line between 0 and 662 keV.

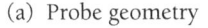

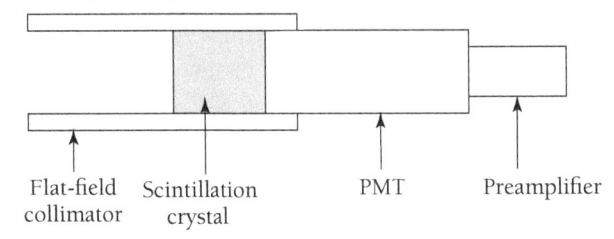

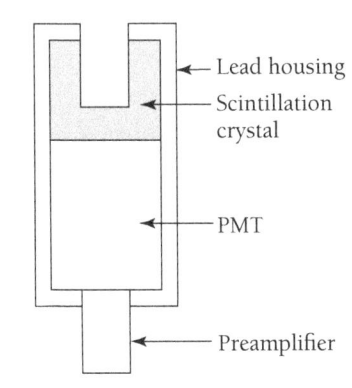

Figure 2-10 Two common scintillation detector configurations. In the organ probe, the scintillation crystal is a right cylinder with a diameter of about 2 in. and a height of 2 in. The well detector has a 4- to 5-in-diameter crystal that is 3 in high, with a ¾-in diameter well cut into the cylinder.

source. The output is a number of counts, each count representing a gamma ray whose total energy deposition in the scintillation crystal fits within the PHA window. A typical measurement has hundreds or thousands of counts, for a typical counting time of 0.5 to 10 minutes (min).

A single measurement thus produces a single value for the amount of radioactivity present in the source. This value is generally expressed in a rate format of *counts per minute* (cpm). A repeat measurement of the same source in the same geometry will usually produce a different value, due to the statistical nature of radioactive decay. We can use this inherent variability to our advantage. In clinical situations, a measurement may be repeated to verify that the procedure was performed correctly. If the two readings are similar, they might then be averaged to generate the final result. Two readings that are significantly different should prompt the operator to consider whether the procedure was done correctly.

Configurations

Scintillation detectors with a single PMT are made in two specific configurations: the probe configuration and the well configuration. These are diagrammed in **Figure 2-10**, with common dimensions given. The probe configuration is designed for external counting of radioactivity in organs such as the thyroid gland. A cylindrical crystal is optically coupled to a single PMT, which is shielded from magnetic fields with a mu-metal housing. A wide-bore lead collimator called a *flat-field collimator* is used to shield the scintillation crystal from stray gamma rays and protect it from mechanical damage. This geometric arrangement allows the probe to accurately measure a small amount of radioactivity, while still being directional enough to give meaningful measurements of individual organs. Appendix E on collimator mathematics discusses the calculation of organ-detector distances when using a flat-field collimator. The operator should bear in mind the possibility that the probe could be detecting radiation coming from sources other than the patient; for example, a radioactive patient in the next room, or a source left unshielded and in the probe's "line of sight." Alternative causes for an unexpectedly high value should be explored.

Most commercially available thyroid probes include a positioning rod, so that patients can be positioned at a reproducible distance from the scintillation crystal. These rods can be made from a variety of materials. One manufacturer uses graphite and states, "Up to 10% attenuation can occur if the rod obstructs the field of view of the capsule from the crystal surface" (3). Good practice requires that the rod be moved out of the field of view after positioning is verified.

The well arrangement is designed to measure samples of radioactive materials in test tubes. The well is formed out of the middle of a cylindrical scintillation crystal, and the PMT is attached to the opposite end of the crystal. This allows for excellent detection efficiency, because a radioactive source in the well is almost completely surrounded by the scintillation crystal, so that more than 90% of emitted photons are absorbed. Well counters work excellently for small sample volumes with low activity (less than about 1 μCi [37 kBq]).

Commercially available scintillation detectors used in nuclear medicine often come as a set, with a probe and a well counter and a single electronics module. While this is a cost-effective arrangement, it requires the user to be aware of several facts. First and most obviously, one must be sure that the correct detector is selected. Second, because they are two separate scintillation detectors, each one must be calibrated separately before use. Finally, due to their differences in geometric efficiency, one should not expect that measurement of the same source will produce similar results with each detector. While all of these facts may be obvious to the experienced user, they have been known to trip up even the best technologists.

Peak Broadening and Energy Resolution

Sources of Peak Broadening

Recall that the gamma rays from a given nuclear transition are always monoenergetic. For example, all Tc-99m gamma-2 photons are emitted from the nucleus with energy of exactly 140.5 keV. However, the detector registers the photons as having slightly different signals and hence slightly different energies. The actual spectrum seen with a sodium iodide detector, instead of consisting of a sharp line at 140.5 keV, shows a broad peak. *Peak broadening* occurs because the gamma ray energy is not reproduced exactly in the detector electronics. The reasons for peak broadening include statistical variations in electron production at the crystal, nonuniformity of photocathode and/or PMT sensitivity, statistical variations in electron production at the photocathode, statistical variations in dynode multiplication, energy nonlinearity, electrical noise, and high-voltage fluctuations. As can be seen in Table 2-1, it is at the photocathode that the number of information carriers reaches its lowest value, and thus the statistical variation in the number of electrons produced at the photocathode causes the majority of the peak broadening seen with sodium iodide.

Percentage Energy Window

We deal with peak broadening in nuclear medicine by setting the detector to look at a range of energies around the photopeak. Because we are generally using a single radionuclide with a photopeak that is adequately separated from the other peaks in the energy spectrum, we can set up an *energy window* to include most of the photopeak and exclude everything else. Window widths are specified as a percentage of the photopeak energy. A narrow window (2–5%) should be used for calibration and a wider window (15–20%) for imaging and other measurements. Some scintillation detectors have a "Window In/Out" toggle. When the toggle is "out," all events above the LLD are counted. This is used when counting wipe test swabs for radioactive contamination.

Sample Calculation 2-1 Calculation of a Percentage Energy Window

Calculate a 20% window centered on the 140-keV photopeak of Tc-99m.

Twenty percent of 140 keV is 28 keV. In order to center the photopeak on 140 keV, we need to put $28 \div 2 = 14$ keV on each side of 140 keV (we could also call this a ±10% window). Thus,

Threshold (LLD) = $140 - 14 = 126$ keV

Window = 28 keV

Upper level discriminator = $140 + 14 = 154$ keV.

Energy Resolution

Peak broadening is also used as a performance measure for scintillation detectors. *Energy resolution* evaluates how well a given detector distinguishes between gamma rays of closely spaced energies. (Note: A very important concept in imaging is *spatial resolution*, the ability of an imaging device to separate objects close together in space. Throughout this text, energy resolution will be specifically identified and "resolution" [without further qualification] will refer to spatial resolution.) We can quantify the energy resolution by calculating the percentage energy resolution, which measures the width of the photopeak relative to the photopeak energy. This is done as follows (**Figure 2-11**):

- Obtain an energy spectrum using Cs-137.
- Measure the height of the photopeak in counts.
- Find the line on the *Y*-axis corresponding to one-half of the peak's height.
- Measure the full width of the peak in keV at this height. This is the *full width at half-maximum* (FWHM).
- Divide the width by the photopeak energy and express as a percentage.

$$\text{FWHM} = \frac{B - A}{E_\gamma} \times 100\% \qquad (2\text{-}1)$$

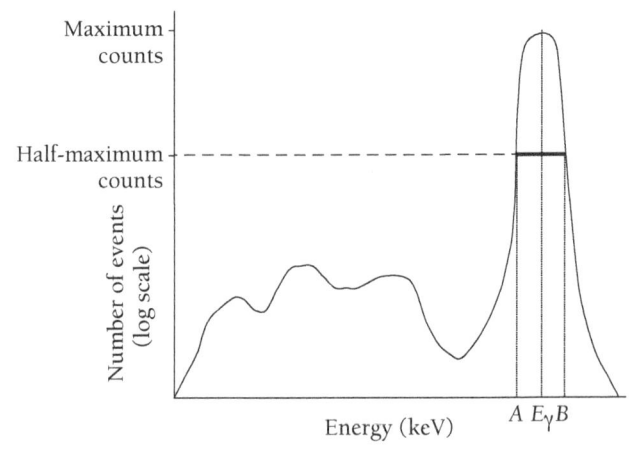

Figure 2-11 Determination of the FWHM of a scintillation detector. Note that *A*, *B*, and E_γ must all be in like units (either keV or channel number on a multichannel analzyer).

The energy resolution can be tracked over time to detect changes in detector performance. A significant change in energy resolution should prompt a service call.

Sample Calculation 2-2 Full Width at Half-Maximum

On an MCA, the photopeak for Cs-137 is found in channel number 380, and the half-height channels are numbers 365 and 396. Calculate the FWHM and energy resolution.

We can work in either energy units (keV) or channel numbers, but not both in the same calculation. To put everything into keV, convert the half-height channels to keV using the conversion factor 662 keV = 380 channels.

$$\text{Channel } 365 \times \frac{662 \text{ keV}}{\text{channel } 380} = 636 \text{ keV}$$

$$\text{Channel } 396 \times \frac{662 \text{ keV}}{\text{channel } 380} = 690 \text{ keV}$$

Using Equation 2-1, we calculate:

$$\text{Energy resolution} = \frac{690 \text{ keV} - 636 \text{ keV}}{662 \text{ keV}} \times 100\%$$
$$= 8.16\%.$$

Or we can do the entire calculation in channel units:

$$\text{Energy resolution} = \frac{\text{channel } 396 - \text{channel } 365}{\text{channel } 380} \times 100\% = 8.16\%.$$

Variation of Energy Resolution with Gamma Ray Energy

Peak broadening is primarily due to the statistical variations in the number of electrons created at the photocathode, and higher-energy gamma rays create more electrons at the photocathode than do lower-energy gamma rays (Table 2-1). Therefore, the energy resolution of a given detector will be larger for lower-energy photopeaks than for higher-energy photopeaks. Sodium iodide scintillation detectors have energy resolution in the range of 6 to 8% FWHM for Cs-137, and 10 to 12% for Tc-99m (4). Because of this variability, Cs-137 is always used to compare energy resolution between detectors.

Quality Control

Daily Tests

A scintillation detector should be calibrated each day it is used (3). This ensures that the high voltage is multiplying the gamma ray signal by an amount that is appropriately related to the settings of the detector. The high-voltage setting

Table 2-2

Recommended Quality Control Tests for Well Counters and Thyroid Probes

Test	Recommended Frequency
Calibration (peaking)	Daily[1,2]
Constancy/sensitivity	Daily[1,2]
Energy resolution	Quarterly/annually[1,2]
Chi-square test	Monthly/quarterly[1,2]
Detector efficiency	Annually[1]

[1]Hall A. A review of the Captus® 3000 thyroid uptake module. Capintec. Fall 2006 newsletter.
[2]Graham LS, ed. *Nuclear Medicine: Self-Study Program II: Instrumentation*. Reston, VA: Society of Nuclear Medicine; 1996:8–9.

should be nearly constant from day to day; a fluctuating value may indicate an unstable high-voltage supply, while a gradual change may signal a loss of optical coupling or hermetic seal.

As a part of the calibration procedure, a sensitivity or *constancy* measurement is made. When a long-lived source such as Cs-137 is used, the cpm should be about the same from day to day (assuming that the energy window and the geometric arrangement of the source and the detector are the same). A change of 10% or more indicates a significant high-voltage fluctuation or other malfunction (5). Calibration and constancy checks will detect most of the common errors associated with scintillation detectors. A background measurement, also done on a daily basis, will ensure that there are no extraneous sources of radioactivity or contamination of the detector.

Infrequent Tests

The energy resolution should be checked at least quarterly; an increasing value indicates a problem with electronic noise, decoupling of the crystal and the PMT, yellowing of the crystal, or a cracked crystal (6). With an MCA, the FWHM is easily checked in conjunction with daily calibration. The measured energy resolution should be less than 10%, using Cs-137 as the source (5). Another quality control measure that should be checked quarterly is the *chi-square test*, a measurement of the statistical variability of the detector. Finally, a detector that is being used to determine absolute radioactivity in μCi or kBq must have an efficiency factor determination at least annually. The efficiency factor correlates the measured count rate to the absolute activity, using a radioactive source of known activity strength. **Table 2-2** summarizes these tests, and **Table 2-3** provides some suggestions for troubleshooting.

Summary

A scintillation detector provides us with more information than a gas-filled detector, because it has the ability to determine the energy of the interacting gamma ray. The resulting ability to perform energy discrimination improves the quality of the information available, be it in identifying different radionuclides or discriminating between unscattered and scattered gamma rays. This energy discrimination

Table 2-3
Troubleshooting Scintillation Detectors

Problem	Possible Causes
Lower than expected constancy reading	• Incorrect high-voltage setting/incorrectly calibrated instrument • Incorrect threshold and/or window setting • Incorrect source-detector geometry (farther away than usual) • Toggle switch pointing to the other detector
Higher than expected constancy reading	• Extraneous radiation source in detector's active volume • Incorrect source-detector geometry (closer than usual) • Contamination of detector or housing
Widening FWHM	• Decoupling of the PMT from the scintillation crystal[1] • Crystal damage

[1]Knoll GF. *Radiation Detection and Measurement.* 3rd ed. New York, NY: John Wiley & Sons; 2000:331.

depends on the proportionality of the information carriers through the scintillation crystal, the PMT, and subsequent electronics, and we can correlate it to an energy scale in keV using the calibration procedures described.

The development of the sodium iodide scintillation detector was an important milestone for nuclear medicine as well as for high-energy physics. Thyroid probes and well counters are important clinical tools, and the technologist must understand the underlying principles as well as their operation. Otherwise, incorrect numeric values and therefore incorrect clinical diagnoses may result.

References

1. Knoll GF. *Radiation Detection and Measurement.* 3rd ed. New York, NY: Wiley & Sons; 2000:233, 234, 286–287, 330, 331.
2. Atom Lab 950 Operator Manual, Biodex Medical Systems, 1/6/99, p. 21.
3. Hall A. A review of the Captus® 3000 thyroid uptake module. Capintec. Fall 2006 newsletter.
4. Cherry SR, Sorenson JA, Phelps ME. *Physics in Nuclear Medicine.* 3rd ed. Philadelphia, PA: Saunders; 2003:159.
5. Graham LS, ed. *Nuclear Medicine: Self-Study Program II: Instrumentation.* Reston, VA: Society of Nuclear Medicine; 1996:8–9.
6. Henkin RE, Boles MA, Dillehay GL, et al., eds. *Nuclear Medicine.* St. Louis, MO: Mosby-Year Book; 1996:82.

Additional Resources

Cherry SR, Sorenson JA, Phelps ME. *Physics in Nuclear Medicine.* 3rd ed. Philadelphia, PA: Saunders; 2003: Chapter 7.
Graham LS, ed. *Nuclear Medicine: Self-Study Program II: Instrumentation.* Reston, VA: Society of Nuclear Medicine; 1996:5–9.
Henkin RE, Boles MA, Dillehay GL, et al., eds. *Nuclear Medicine.* St. Louis, MO: Mosby-Year Book; 1996: Chapter 6.
Knoll GF. *Radiation Detection and Measurement.* 3rd ed. New York, NY: John Wiley & Sons; 2000: Chapters 8, 9.
Nuclear Regulatory Commission. Publication NUREG-1556, Vol. 9, Program-specific guidance about medical use licenses. Available at: www.nrc.gov/reading-rm/doc-collections/nuregs/staff/sr1556/v9/. Accessed February 20, 2009.
Wells P. *Practical Mathematics for Nuclear Medicine.* Reston, VA: Society of Nuclear Medicine; 2000: Chapter 4.

CHAPTER 3 Semiconductor Detectors

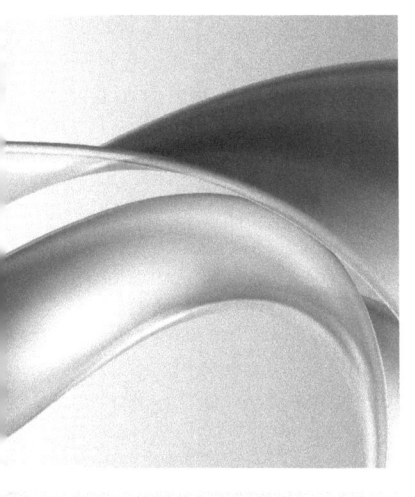

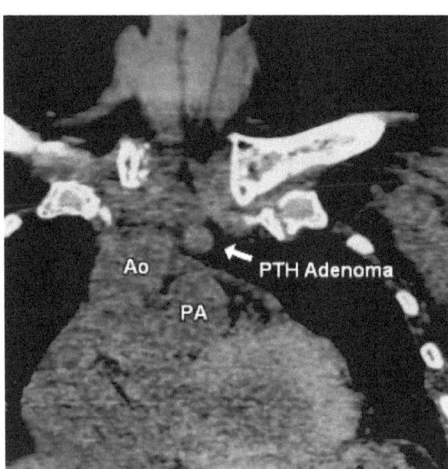

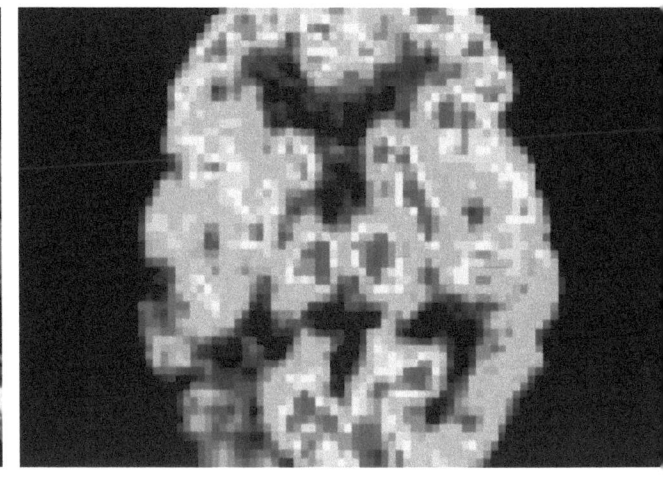

Learning Outcomes

1. Describe the molecular orbital structure of *n*-type and *p*-type semiconductors and what happens when the two are brought together.
2. Explain the operation of a semiconductor radiation detector, including the reverse bias and the depletion layer, as well as the additional features needed for use as an intraoperative probe.
3. Outline the use of an intraoperative probe in sentinel lymph node and parathyroid adenoma localization procedures.
4. Discuss performance measures, quality control testing, and care of intraoperative probes.
5. Contrast the energy spectrum produced by a semiconductor detector with that of a scintillation detector, and discuss the importance of this difference.

Introduction

Sodium iodide is sufficient for many uses in nuclear medicine, but it has two specific disadvantages that limit its application as a small-diameter radiation probe. First, the size and flexibility of a scintillation detector are limited by the need for a photomultiplier tube (PMT). Second, scintillators, while quite acceptable for most nuclear medicine applications, have relatively poor energy resolution compared to other energy-sensitive radiation detectors, primarily due to the multiplicity of inefficient conversion steps and consequent statistical fluctuations (1). These difficulties are overcome in a different type of detector: the semiconductor detector.

The *semiconductor radiation detector* is an ionization detector, essentially a solid analog of the gas-filled detector. Electrons created by radiation interactions are collected directly, rather than requiring multiple intermediate steps as in a scintillation detector, resulting in excellent energy resolution. This in turn allows for better separation of photopeak events from Compton scatter events. No photomultiplier tube is needed, so the detector can be made to quite small dimensions. Semiconductor detectors have found application in the operating room, where they are used to locate lymph nodes, parathyroid glands, and tumors that have been made radioactive by prior injection of a radiopharmaceutical. Cameras using semiconductor detectors have also been produced, and several are commercially available.

Properties of Semiconductors

Band Structure

Recall the delocalized band structure of a metal or crystal: valence and conduction bands are separated by a forbidden gap (see Appendix B for more details). In the ground state, the valence band contains electrons and the conduction band is empty. In a particular class of materials called semiconductors, the forbidden gap is only 1 to 3 eV. At very low temperatures, electrons are restricted to the valence band, and the material behaves as an insulator. At higher temperatures, however, the thermal energy possessed by electrons is enough to allow a small number to overcome the forbidden gap, enabling the semiconductor to conduct electricity. The width of the band gap determines the exact temperature at which a given material becomes a semiconductor. Materials found in group IV of the periodic table of the elements, such as silicon and germanium, possess semiconductor properties.

To be able to function as a radiation detector, a semiconductor needs to have either extra electrons or extra electron holes (or both) to act as information carriers. The molecular situations that create these "extras" are illustrated in **Figure 3-1**. We will use silicon (found in group IV of the periodic table) as the "classic" semiconductor, even though commercial semiconductor radiation detectors are more often made from other materials. Figure 3-1a shows pure silicon, in which all the outer-shell electrons are used to complete the crystal lattice bonding structure. If we add an impurity such as phosphorus (group V of the periodic table), as shown in Figure 3-1b, it will contribute an extra electron that is not needed in the crystal lattice, creating a defect in the crystal structure. This electron therefore is only loosely held to the crystal lattice, and consequently it has an energy level (called the *donor level*) just below the level of the conduction band. The extra electron in the donor-level electron orbital is mobile and can be caused to move into the conduction band by the application of an electric field. This is referred to as an *n-type semiconductor*, and the extra electron is called a *conduction electron*.

If we add a trivalent impurity such as boron (which is from group III of the periodic table and has one fewer outer-shell electron than silicon), an acceptor energy level is similarly created just above the valence band (Fig. 3-1c). Under normal conditions, electrons with thermal energy will occupy acceptor-level electron sites, each leaving an empty orbital in the valence band that is referred to as a *hole*. These holes allow electrons to move within the valence band and thus conduct electricity just as well as the extra electrons in Figure 3-1b. In a sense, the holes act as positively charged electrons, because they appear to move toward the cathode. Semiconductors with this type of impurity are known as *p-type semiconductors*.

Radiation Detection

Semiconductor radiation detectors are usually made so that one side has an *n*-type impurity (excess electrons) and the other side a *p*-type impurity (excess holes), as shown in **Figure 3-2**. At the junction between the two types of materials, the conduction electrons and holes combine, leaving behind impurities with positive charge on the *n*

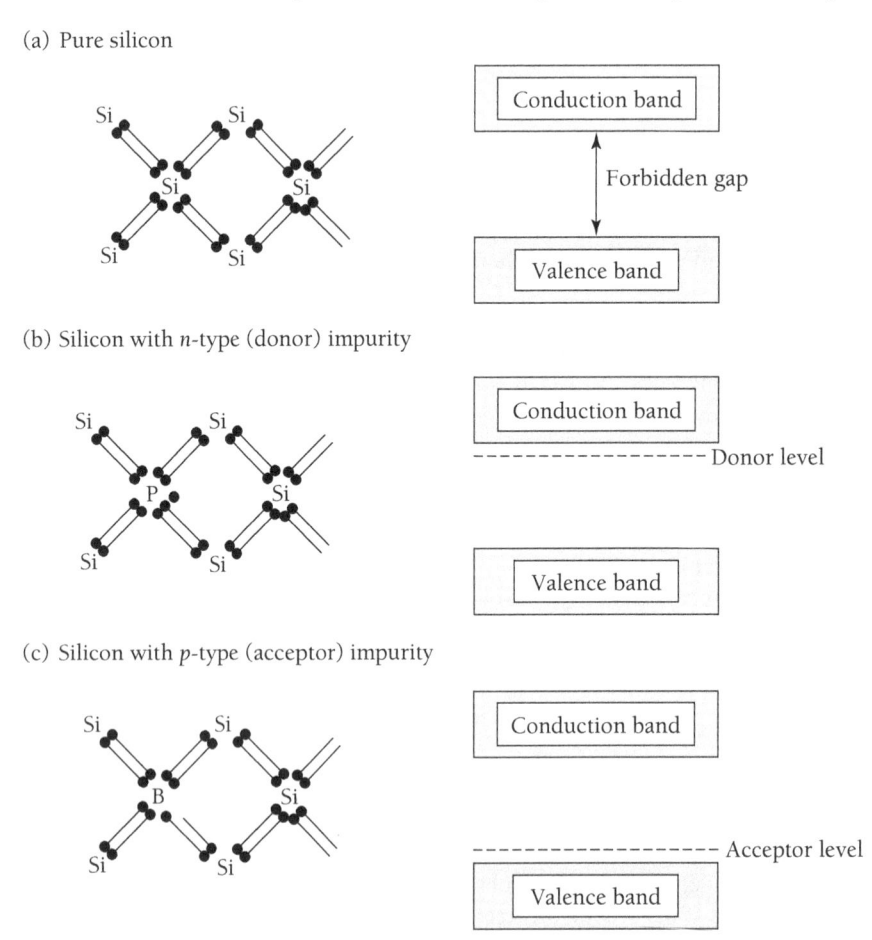

Figure 3-1 Electronic configurations and energy diagrams of pure silicon and silicon with donor and acceptor impurities. Each dot represents an electron and each line a molecular bond. Pure silicon is shown in Figure 3-1a. The addition of a donor impurity such as phosphorus adds an extra electron, creating an *n*-type semiconductor (Fig. 3-1b). The addition of an acceptor impurity such as boron leaves a hole in the electron orbital structure, creating a *p*-type semiconductor (Fig. 3-1c).

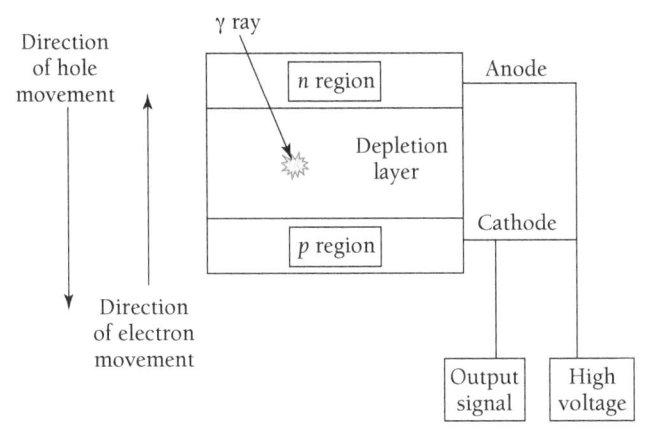

Figure 3-2 Use of a semiconductor block as a radiation detector. The n region and p region may be created by adding impurities or may be intrinsic to the semiconductor itself. The high voltage must be applied in a reverse bias, so that the anode is connected to the n region and the cathode to the p region. When radiation interacts in the depletion layer, the reverse bias draws the electrons and holes out of the depletion layer, as shown by the arrows on the left.

side of the junction and impurities with negative charge on the p side of the junction (both sides having been electrically neutral before being brought together). The combining of conduction electrons and holes means that there are no free charge carriers in this region, a situation that is maintained by the electric field created by the positive and negative charges. This region is called the *depletion layer*. If an electrical potential is applied so that the anode is at the n side and the cathode at the p side (a situation called *reverse bias*), they will attract the electrons and holes, respectively, increasing the size of the depletion layer. (If the anode and cathode are switched, a situation called *forward bias*, electricity will flow freely in the absence of radiation.) The electrical potential maintains the depletion layer, just as in a gas-filled detector it maintains the electrical field between the anode and cathode. The depletion layer thus becomes, in essence, a solid-state ionization chamber.

When a gamma ray interacts in the depletion layer, it creates a number of electron-hole pairs, which are drawn toward the anode (electrons) and cathode (holes). The electric circuit then works to restore the system to its original state, causing current to flow. The time required for the collection of electron-hole pairs is very short (about 10 nsec, which is much faster than a gas-filled ionization chamber), and so each gamma ray interaction can be considered as an individual event (i.e., pulse-mode operation). Further, the number of electron-hole pairs created is proportional to the amount of energy deposited by the gamma rays in the depletion layer, so the energy of each interaction can be determined (given proper calibration).

Semiconductor Radiation Detector Characteristics

Classic semiconductor detectors made from silicon or germanium are unsuitable for most nuclear medicine applications for two reasons: their atomic numbers are too low to provide adequate attenuation for interaction with gamma rays, and they may need to be cooled by liquid nitrogen in order to demonstrate semiconductor behavior. Most semiconductor detectors sold as intraoperative probes for gamma ray detection are made from cadmium, zinc, and tellurium, with varying proportions of ZnTe added to CdTe. The letters CZT are used as a common abbreviation. Relative to Figure 3-1, Cd and Zn act as electron acceptors and Te acts as the electron donor. These materials have atomic numbers similar to that of sodium iodide (48, 52, and 30, respectively) and a high density of around 6 g/cm^3 (compared to 3.67 g/cm^3 for NaI), giving them good efficiency for gamma rays. Conversion of radiation energy to ion pairs in these detectors requires much less energy than in sodium iodide or gas-filled detectors (**Table 3-1**), resulting in superior energy resolution (1.8–2.5% FWHM for 662 keV, compared to 6–8% for NaI). (Another material, HgI$_2$, has an even higher atomic number, higher density, and better energy resolution, but it is not easy to work with and has no current application in commercial intraoperative probes.) Compared to silicon and germanium, the larger forbidden gap of CZT at 1.5 to 2.1 eV allows these materials to be functional as radiation detectors at room temperature. Energy resolution is poorer than with silicon or germanium, mainly because the composition of the cadmium-based alloy is difficult to control; this is not a significant problem for intraoperative probes, which are mainly used for detection and not spectroscopy.

Cadmium-based semiconductor detectors are generally made only a few mm thick. They are therefore best suited to detection of low-energy gamma rays, up to about 200 keV. This is quite sufficient for use with Tc-99m, which is the primary radionuclide in clinical use currently. There is increasing interest in the intraoperative detection of radiopharmaceuticals labeled with I-131 and In-111, which would require either a thicker detector or a different detector material to efficiently interact with the higher-energy gamma rays of these two radionuclides. Probe manufacturers are starting to offer detectors with multiple materials, either within a single probe or as interchangeable probes. Some of these designs combine a semiconductor probe (for lower-energy gamma rays) with a scintillation detector (to facilitate detection of higher-energy gamma rays).

A problem that arises with semiconductor radiation detectors is *charge trapping*, which occurs when electrons

Table 3-1

Comparison of Energy Conversion Factors for Detector Types

Energy needed to create an ion pair:	Semiconductor detector	3–5 eV
	Gas-filled detector	25–35 eV
Incident energy needed to produce a scintillation photon:	Scintillation detector	30 eV

Adapted from: Knoll GF. *Radiation Detection and Measurement*. 3rd ed. New York, NY: John Wiley & Sons; 2000:130, 353, 483.

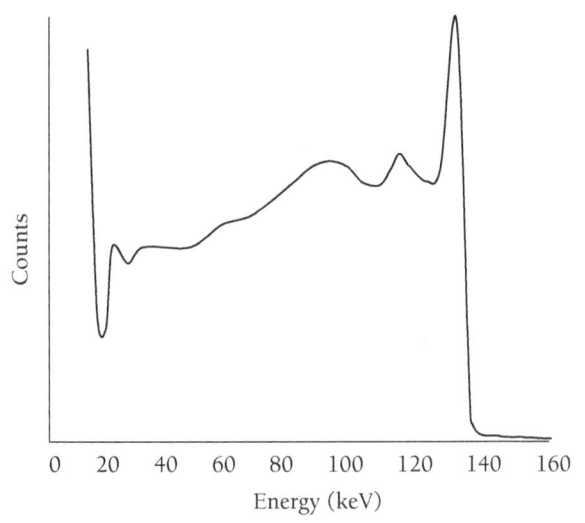

Figure 3-3 Energy spectrum of Tc-99m acquired with a CZT semiconductor detector. The broad plateau of counts below 120 keV is caused primarily by charge trapping.

and/or holes find deep traps within the orbital band structure. These traps are electron orbitals at energy levels in the middle of the forbidden gap, the result of impurities that have been incorporated into the crystal lattice of the semiconductor. An electron or hole that is "caught in a trap" is eventually released, but it may be delayed so that it does not contribute to the signal of the gamma ray that generated it. The end result is an asymmetric widening of the photopeak with a broad tail on its low side, corresponding to measured energies that are less than the true energy of the gamma ray. **Figure 3-3** shows an energy spectrum illustrating this phenomenon. The result of charge trapping is that the statistical uncertainty in pulse heights is increased, degrading both energy resolution and sensitivity (2).

Operation

Electronics

The block diagram of a semiconductor detector looks much like that of a scintillation detector (**Figure 3-4**). An applied voltage of 10 to 500 V is required for the collection of electrons. This bias voltage acts in some ways as a low-level energy threshold, in that small numbers of electrons and holes will not generate a large enough signal to register in the preamplifier. The electric current that results from a radiation interaction is integrated into a voltage pulse that is small, on the order of millivolts, so a preamplifier must increase the signal size significantly without adding noise or increasing the pulse width. Preamplifier performance must therefore be more carefully matched to the detector and its energy resolution characteristics than is required for scintillation detectors. The signal from the preamplifier is further amplified and shaped by an amplifier and then sent to a *pulse height analyzer* (PHA), as with a scintillation detector. Most commercially available models do not have an energy spectrum display, so the pulse height analyzer operates as a single-channel analyzer.

For use as an intraoperative probe, the detector should have several additional electronic features. An audible count rate tone, called a *howler*, allows the operator to watch the probe location and hear the count rate. Either the frequency or the pitch changes with the measured count rate. Electronic background suppression (often called a *squelch feature*) should also be available, so that only count rates above a preset threshold are considered significant. Autoranging of the rate meter allows the system to seamlessly switch to the correct rate meter range. **Figure 3-5** shows two commercially available intraoperative probes and the accompanying electronics module.

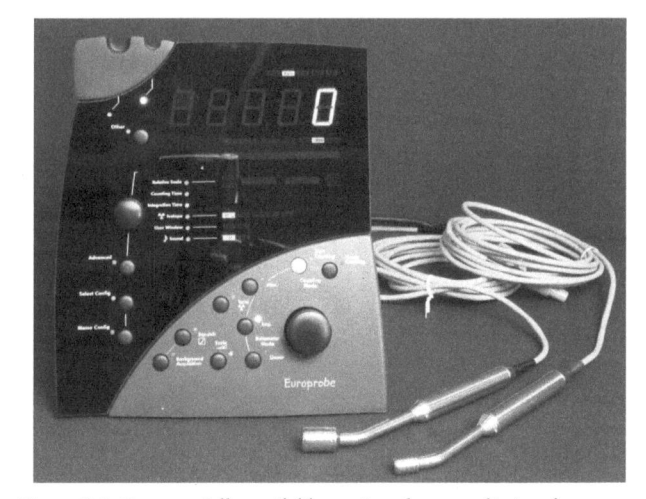

Figure 3-5 Commercially available semiconductor radiation detector. Two intraoperative probe units are shown next to the electronics module. The width of most intraoperative probes is only 1 to 2 cm (2). Photo courtesy of Capintec, Inc.

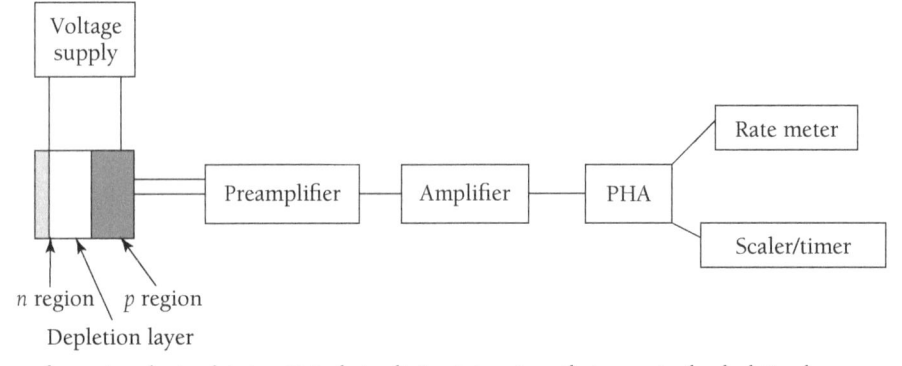

Figure 3-4 Block diagram of a semiconductor detector. Note that radiation interactions that occur in the depletion layer are registered, whereas the *p* and *n* regions are "dead" to radiation detection. The instrument is typically oriented so that the radiation field is beyond the *n* region.

Chapter 3: Semiconductor Detectors

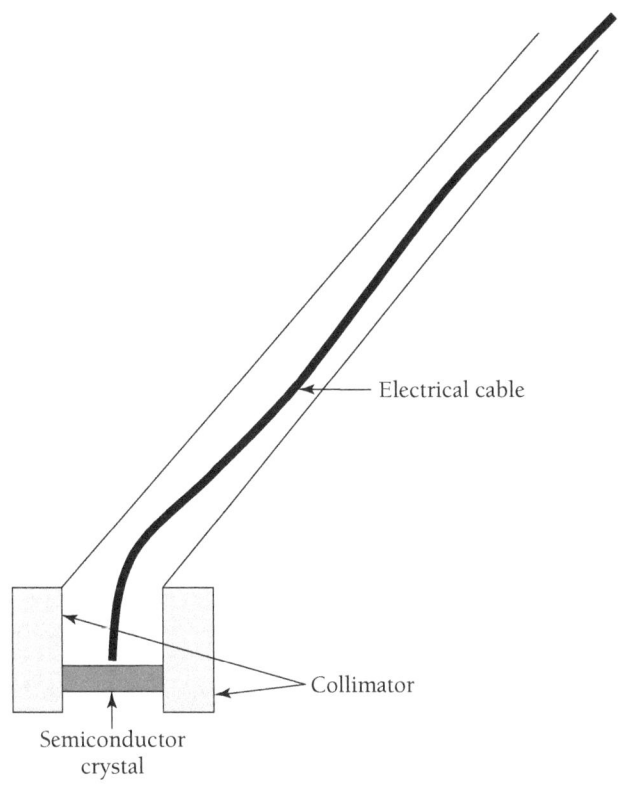

Figure 3-6 Cross section of the functional end of an intraoperative radiation detector. The collimator provides a directional component to the measurement of radiation.

Collimation and Shielding

To be useful as an intraoperative probe, a semiconductor detector must be shielded from radiation coming from directions other than the forward direction. At the same time, however, the probe will perform best if it can get as close as possible to the tissue being localized. The collimator used for semiconductor detectors has a single bore, similar to the flat-field collimator used for probe-type scintillation detectors (**Figure 3-6**), but extending only a very short distance beyond the front surface of the detector. It may be detachable or may be incorporated into the detector housing. Shielding for intraoperative probes has been fashioned from tungsten, gold, and platinum/iridium as well as lead. The operator should be aware of the possibility that characteristic x-rays from the shielding may contaminate the energy window of the desired radionuclide. Shielding and collimation are major determinants of a probe's spatial resolution.

Uses of Semiconductor Detectors in Nuclear Medicine

The demonstrated efficacy of sentinel node localization using radiopharmaceuticals has led to the commercial development of semiconductor probes for intraoperative use. This in turn has stimulated exploration of new potential uses of these devices as well as an increasing connection between the surgery department and the nuclear medicine department. The major advantage of semiconductor detectors for use in surgery is their efficiency, given their small size. For most surgical uses, the detector is used to pinpoint a small volume of radioactive tissue, so it is important to have a small, maneuverable detector. Because the nuclear medicine technologist may not be familiar with the detector's clinical applications, several of these uses are detailed here.

Sentinel Lymph Node Localization

The most common current use of intraoperative probes is for the detection of sentinel lymph nodes of patients with various kinds of cancer. The sentinel lymph node is the node that drains the region of the primary tumor. Filtered Tc-99m sulfur colloid (or another colloidal radiopharmaceutical) is injected at or around the tumor site, and uptake in a lymph node some distance away is identified. In this situation, there is radiopharmaceutical localization only at the injection site and the lymph node, so there is little, if any, background. It is generally considered good practice to image the biodistribution of the radiopharmaceutical with a gamma camera prior to the surgical procedure, especially when the nodal basin draining the primary tumor is in question (3). A mark on the patient's skin indicating the node's approximate location saves operating room time (and potential trauma to the patient). In the operating room, a blue dye (isosulfan blue) may be injected to give a color marking to the sentinel lymph node. The dye is injected around the primary lesion, in approximately the same location(s) as the radiopharmaceutical was injected, and about 20 minutes is allowed for its transit into the lymph nodes.

To use the intraoperative probe, the count rate in a designated reference area is measured to determine background. Then the probe (contained in a sterile sheath) is used to manually scan the marked area, zeroing in on the area with the highest count rate. A location is considered as having increased radionuclide uptake if its count rate is at least 1.5 to 2 times that of the reference area, depending on the situation. The counting time per location depends on the target-to-background ratio, but should be slow enough that no significant activity is missed; 10 to 30 seconds per location is common. The detector head is often angled, for both ergonomic ease and improved eye–hand coordination. It is essential that the operator be aware of the orientation of the head relative to other possible sources of activity, because the detector will register any activity within its field of view, whether the source of that activity is close or deep to the detector's location. Activity in a hot, deep lesion will be recorded similarly to that of a small lesion close to the detector head.

When an area of increased activity is isolated, the surgeon uses a small incision to remove the lymph node. On incision, if the dye has been administered, the surgeon looks for a lymph node that is both blue and radioactive; in practice, nodes that are either blue or radioactive are removed. The node is excised, and its count rate is checked with the probe ex vivo, where its counts are often 10 or more times the background. The probe is reinserted into the incision site to check for additional radioactive lymph nodes. All excised nodes are then sent to the pathology laboratory to look for evidence of metastasis. This determines the remainder of the surgical procedure: a wide lymphatic dissection if metastatic cells are found or closure of the incision and resection of the primary tumor if no evidence of metastasis is seen.

Parathyroid Adenoma Localization

The demonstration of Tc-99m sestamibi uptake in parathyroid adenomas allows the surgeon to use the intraoperative probe in parathyroidectomy procedures as well. The patient is injected with the radiopharmaceutical prior to his or her arrival in surgery. The time required for preoperative tasks and anesthesia induction allows for adequate uptake of the radiopharmaceutical as well as washout from the thyroid gland and other tissues. The intraoperative probe is used to identify the adenoma, allowing for a minimally invasive surgery that in many cases can be done on an outpatient basis. The surgeon needs to bear in mind that there is significant uptake of sestamibi in the myocardium, and to not confuse that activity with the adenoma itself. Parathyroid imaging prior to surgery is recommended to rule out an ectopic location of the adenoma (4).

Tumor Localization

Intraoperative probes are also being suggested for localization of tumors seen with other radiopharmaceuticals, such as monoclonal antibodies and labeled peptides. This is radically different from the sentinel lymph node situation: the tumor takes up a very small amount of the injected dose; the radiopharmaceutical is widely distributed in the body, so there is more background activity than in sentinel node procedures; and the count rate at a given location depends not only on increased activity in the lesion of interest but also on the total activity in the body within the detector's field of view. The small increase in count rate in the area of a tumor may be difficult to detect. The use of I-125 as the radionuclide in this situation is helpful, because its low-energy gamma rays do not penetrate very far in tissue, but I-125 is not easily imaged with gamma cameras. It would be more desirable to be able to detect such isotopes as In-111 that, when labeled to pentetreotide or a monoclonal antibody, for example, demonstrate increased uptake in tumors and metastases. But these studies generally have poor target-to-background ratios, due to both the wide biodistribution of the radiopharmaceutical in the body and the penetrating gamma rays emitted by In-111.

Tumor localization involving In-111 and other high-energy gamma-emitting radionuclides requires reconsideration of both the detector type and the shielding material. Systems have been devised that include both a semiconductor probe for low-energy radionuclides and a scintillation probe for higher-energy radionuclides, the latter using either fiber optics to separate the scintillation crystal from the PMT or a photodiode in place of the PMT, thus decreasing the probe's bulk. Similarly, a dual-detector probe utilizing two plastic scintillators has been developed to detect beta particles in the presence of gamma rays (5). Particulate radiation is stopped in the first scintillator, whereas photon radiation passes through and interacts in the second.

Performance Measures

As with any radiation detection instrument, we need to consider whether the instrument is performing as expected. The specific measures of performance vary with the instrument in question. For semiconductor detectors in use as intraoperative probes, the most important performance tests measure sensitivity and energy resolution. Spatial resolution is of less importance but nonetheless should be considered.

Sensitivity

Sensitivity or *efficiency* is the detected count rate per unit activity. High sensitivity is desirable to improve the detectability of small lesions. For intraoperative probes, sensitivity depends on the intrinsic detector material, probe dimensions, and the geometry of the detector, collimator, and radiation source. Sensitivity also depends to some extent on lesion depth and on the energy emitted by the radionuclide being detected. Sensitivity can be improved through the use of a wider energy window, but this results in acceptance of more scattered photons and consequently a decrease in spatial resolution.

Energy Resolution

The main advantage of a semiconductor detector in applied physics is that the energy resolution is greatly improved compared to that of sodium iodide, because the electrons created in a semiconductor do not need to undergo multiple mass–energy conversions, as is required in a scintillation detector. As Table 3-1 shows, the energy required to create an ion pair in a semiconductor is only 3 to 5 eV, compared to 30 eV to create a scintillation photon in sodium iodide. This large difference between sodium iodide and a semiconductor means that we get many more information carriers per radiation event, resulting in much improved energy resolution (5–10% with CZT) (3). Peak broadening in a semiconductor detector is a function of the applied voltage rather than the gamma ray energy.v

---

Sample Calculation 3-1 Number of Information Carriers

For a 140-keV gamma ray, estimate the number of information carriers created in a gas-filled detector, a scintillation detector, and a semiconductor detector. Assume in each case that all of the gamma ray's energy is used to create information carriers.

Using the values in Table 3-1, we find the following:
Gas-filled detector:

$$140 \text{ keV} \times \frac{1 \text{ ion pair}}{25-35 \text{ eV}} \times \frac{1,000 \text{ eV}}{\text{keV}}$$

$$\cong 4,000-5,600 \text{ ion pairs}.$$

Scintillation detector:

$$140 \text{ keV} \times \frac{1 \text{ scintillation photon}}{30 \text{ eV}} \times \frac{1{,}000 \text{ eV}}{\text{keV}}$$
$$\cong 4{,}700 \text{ scintillation photons.}$$

Semiconductor detector:

$$140 \text{ keV} \times \frac{1 \text{ ion pairs}}{3-5 \text{ eV}} \times \frac{1{,}000 \text{ eV}}{\text{keV}}$$
$$\cong 28{,}000 - 47{,}000 \text{ ion pairs.}$$

Hence, the use of a semiconductor detector increases the number of information carriers in the radiation detection process by a factor of about 10 compared to gas-filled and scintillation detectors.

Figure 3-7 shows two energy spectra of a sample containing both Ag-108m and Ag-110m, one with sodium iodide and one with a lithium-drifted germanium (Ge[Li]) semiconductor. Notice how the few broad peaks seen with sodium iodide become many narrow peaks on Ge(Li), thus allowing identification of both isotopes. Semiconductors such as CZT do not have energy resolution as good as that of Ge(Li), but are superior to that of sodium iodide.

In nuclear medicine applications, energy resolution is important because it determines the ability of the detector to reject scattered photons. The need for good energy resolution depends on the particulars of the radiopharmaceutical biodistribution. It is less critical for lymph node detection, where the only sources of radioactivity are the injection site and the lymph node, and more critical for radio-guided tumor excision, where there is considerable body background. Given the possibilities for this technique, a probe with good energy resolution is always warranted.

Spatial Resolution

Spatial resolution, in the context of an intraoperative probe, is the ability to determine the location of a radioactive source. It is a function of detector size and collimation. It decreases rapidly with distance, especially if a scattering medium such as tissue lies between the detector and the radiation source. The operator must always remember that the probe "sees" a solid column of tissue that extends through the entire patient, and detected activity may be coming from anywhere within that column. Spatial resolution and sensitivity are inversely related for a given detector: any change that improves sensitivity will degrade resolution, and vice versa.

Quality Control and Care

Routine Testing

Semiconductor detectors should be calibrated quarterly or semiannually. Calibration requires tweaking of the amplifier gain to ensure that the preset energy window actually correlates with the gamma ray photopeak energy (just as for scintillation detectors). Unfortunately, most intraoperative probes do not come equipped with a multichannel analyzer display that would make this an easy procedure. Given that the energy window cannot be checked visually, a check of count rate constancy with a long-lived source should be performed daily to verify proper operation. Cobalt-57 is recommended for constancy testing, because its photon energies are close to that of Tc-99m. This is the best single method for determining whether the probe's performance has changed. A visual inspection and battery check should also be performed daily (6). Before every procedure, the user should ideally verify the energy window setting relative to the radionuclide being used; this is especially important when the probe is to be used with multiple radionuclides.

The National Electrical Manufacturers Association (NEMA) has identified a number of quality control tests that may be performed on an intraoperative probe (6). These include measurement of sensitivity in the air and in a scattering medium; energy, spatial, and angular resolution; volume sensitivity; and count rate capabilities, along with several other tests. The probe's performance should be tested annually to ensure that the probe continues to function optimally. Table 3-2 lists suggested quality control procedures and their frequencies. Table 3-3 addresses troubleshooting for these instruments.

Table 3-2

Recommended Quality Control Tests for Semiconductor Probes

Test	Recommended Frequency
Battery check	Daily[1]
Background determination	Daily[1]
Constancy check	Daily[1]
Calibration	Quarterly or semiannually

[1]Adapted from: Zanzonico P. Routine quality control of clinical nuclear medicine instrumentation: a brief review. *J Nucl Med.* 2008;49: 1114–1131.

Table 3-3

Troubleshooting Intraoperative Probes

Problem	Possible Causes
Lower than expected constancy reading	• Energy window not correctly centered on photopeak • Calibration not correct • Incorrect source-detector geometry (farther away than usual)
Higher than expected constancy reading	• Contamination • Extraneous radiation source in detector's line of sight

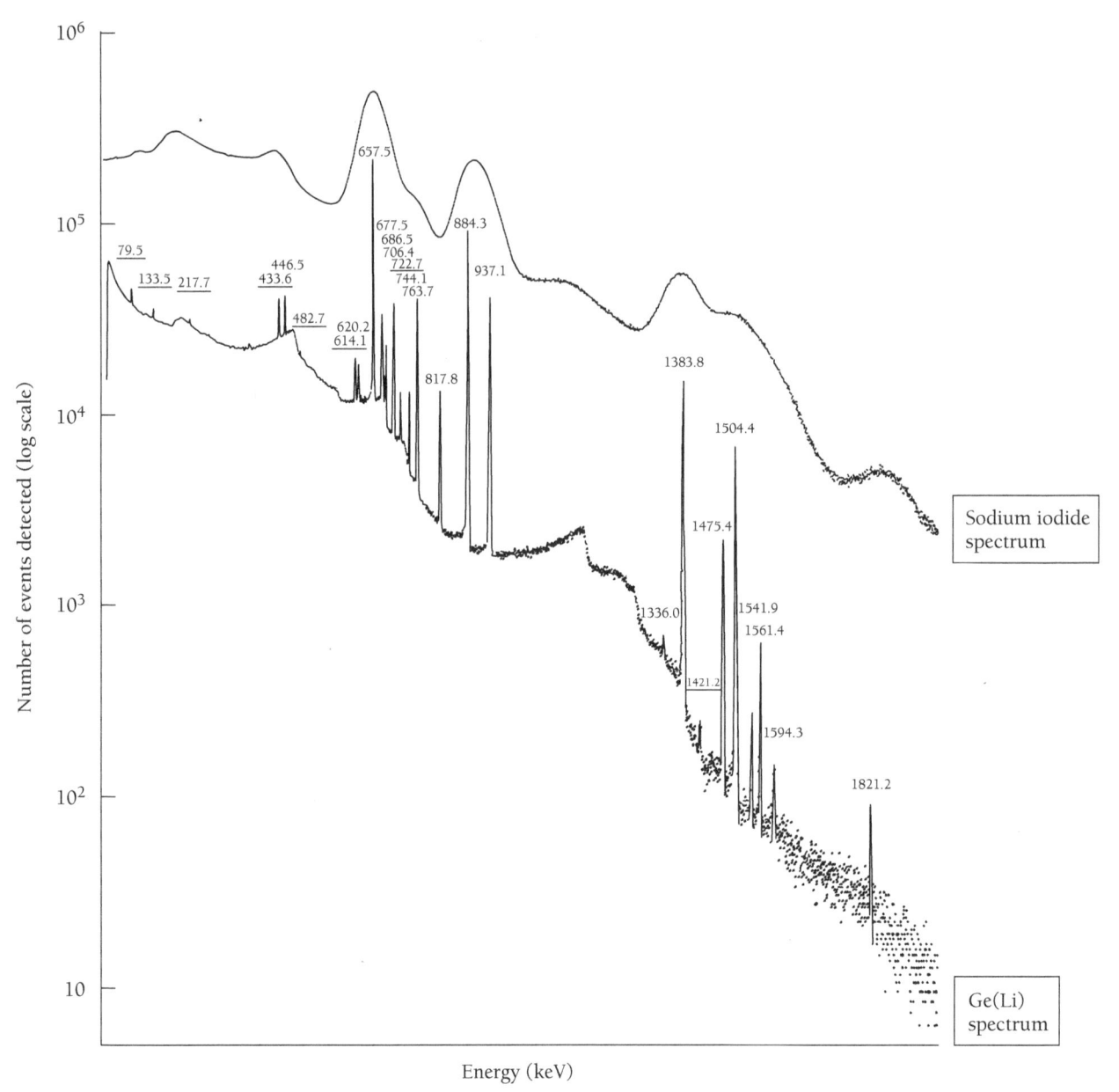

Figure 3-7 Energy spectrum of a combined sample of Ag-108m and Ag-110m. The upper spectrum was obtained using a sodium iodide scintillation detector, the lower spectrum using a lithium-drifted germanium (Ge[Li]) semiconductor detector. From: Knoll GF. *Radiation Detection and Measurement*. 3rd ed. New York, NY: John Wiley & Sons; 2000: 416. Reprinted with permission of John Wiley & Sons, Inc.

Handling

Semiconductor detectors are subject to many of the same concerns as scintillation detectors. They are susceptible to mechanical damage and must be handled with care. Cables and connections should also be treated gently. Rapid temperature changes should be avoided, as should organic solvents, oils, and abrasive or corrosive materials. Manufacturer's instructions regarding sterilization, including maximum temperature, and storage conditions should be followed carefully.

Sterility and electrical safety are of paramount importance in the operative suite. Intraoperative probes should be tested for electrical safety at least annually. Some probes are susceptible to radiofrequency interference from the signals generated by electrocautery equipment, so the two should not be used at the same time. The probe should be either sterilized with ethylene oxide or enclosed in a sterile sheath.

Summary

Semiconductor detectors have some clear advantages over scintillation detectors, and they are in many ways ideally suited for radioactivity detection in the intraoperative setting, at least with low-energy radionuclides, given their high efficiency relative to their size. While nuclear medicine technologists do not operate the probes in most institutions, they should know how the probes work and how their use is complementary to nuclear medicine imaging. However, it is clear that semiconductors will not replace scintillators for most applications in nuclear medicine. We consider semiconductors again when we disuss gamma cameras, as some imaging instruments have been built using semiconductor detector technology.

References

1. Knoll GF. *Radiation Detection and Measurement*. 3rd ed. New York, NY: John Wiley & Sons; 2000:130, 353, 483.
2. Heller S, Zanzonico P. Nuclear probes and intraoperative gamma cameras. *Semin Nucl Med.* 2011;41:166–181.
3. Alazraki N, Glass EC, Castronovo F, Valdés RA, Podoloff D. Society of Nuclear Medicine Procedure Guideline for Lymphoscintigraphy and the Use of Intraoperative Gamma Probe for Sentinel Lymph Node Localization in Melanoma of Intermediate Thickness. Version 1.0. Available at: http://interactive.snm.org/docs/pg_ch24_0403.pdf. Accessed August 5, 2011.
4. Mariani G, Gulec SA, Rubello D, et al. Preoperative localization and radioguided parathyroid surgery. *J Nucl Med.* 2003;44:1443–1458.
5. Daghighian F, Mazziotta JC, Hoffman EJ, et al. Intraoperative beta probe: a device for detecting tissue labeled with positron or electron emitting isotopes during surgery. *Med Phys.* 1994;21:153–157.
6. National Electrical Manufacturers Association. *Performance Measurements and Quality Control Guidelines for Non-Imaging Intraoperative Gamma Probes*. Publication NU 3-2004. Rosslyn, VA: Author.

Additional Resources

Barber HB, Woolfenden JM. Semiconductor detectors in nuclear medicine: progress and prospects. In: Henkin RE, Boles MA, Dillehay GL, et al., eds. *Nuclear Medicine*. St. Louis, MO: Mosby-Year Book; 1996:168–184.

Halkar RK, Aarscold JN. Intraoperative probes. *J Nucl Med Technol.* 1999;27:188–193.

Heller S, Zanzonico P. Nuclear probes and intraoperative gamma cameras. *Semin Nucl Med.* 2011;41:166–181.

Knoll GF. *Radiation Detection and Measurement*. 3rd ed. New York, NY: John Wiley & Sons; 2000:Chapters 11, 13.

National Electrical Manufacturers Association Publication NU 3-2004. *Performance Measurements and Quality Control Guidelines for Non-Imaging Intraoperative Gamma Probes*. 1300 North 17th Street, Suite 1847, Rosslyn, VA 22209.

Wang CH, Willis DL, Loveland WD. *Radiotracer Methodology in the Biological, Environmental, and Physical Sciences*. Englewood Cliffs, NJ: Prentice-Hall; 1975:Chapters 4, 8.

Woolfenden JM, Barber HB. Design and use of radiation detector probes for intraoperative tumor detection using tumor-seeking radionuclides. In: Freeman LM, ed. *Nuclear Medicine Annual 1990*. New York, NY: Raven Press; 1990:151–173.

Zanzonico P. Routine quality control of clinical nuclear medicine instrumentation: a brief review. *J Nucl Med.* 2008;49:1114–1131.

Zanzonico P, Heller S. The intraoperative gamma probe: basic principles and choices available. *Semin Nucl Med.* 2000;30:33–48.

CHAPTER 4

Factors Relating to Radiation Measurement

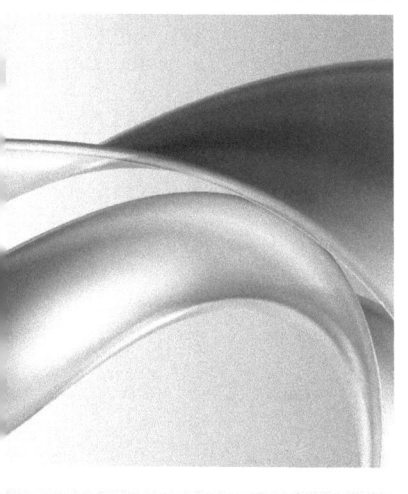

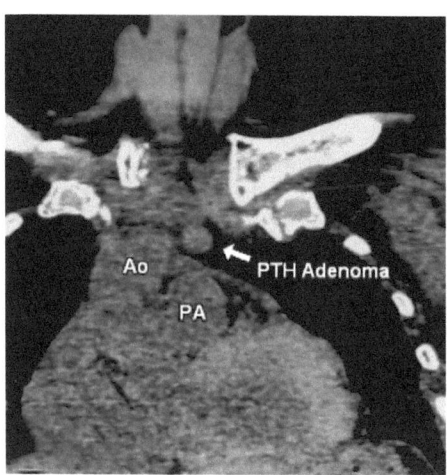

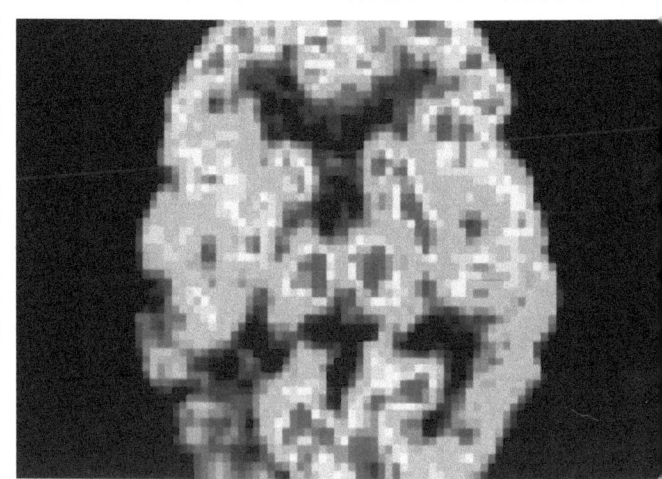

Learning Outcomes

1. State the sources of background in a (nonimaging) counting measurement, and discuss how it is handled.
2. Briefly describe the principles of nuclear counting statistics and their application to counting measurements, including Levy–Jennings plots and chi-square tests.
3. Given a counting measurement, calculate the standard deviation and the coefficient of variation; given sample and background counting measurements, calculate the net count rate and its standard deviation.
4. Define dead time, differentiate between paralyzable and nonparalyzable dead time, and discuss the importance of dead time in radiation measurements.
5. Given the photopeak energy of a radionuclide, calculate the energies of
   a. The Compton edge
   b. The iodine escape peak
   c. The backscatter peak
6. Explain the origin of the following peaks seen in radionuclide energy spectra:
   a. Characteristic x-rays
   b. Lead x-rays
   c. Coincidence and sum peaks
7. Use a variety of scenarios to illustrate the concept of detection efficiency.
8. Discuss the need for and determination of an efficiency factor.

Introduction

In the measurement of a radioactive source or radiation field, a number of factors affect the exact value obtained. It is very important that the technologist understand these factors and their influence on radiation detection tasks. All come into play in imaging as well as counting applications, but they are much more critical to a counting measurement because there is no image to rely on. This chapter discusses these factors in relation to the small instruments covered in Chapters 1–3, and we refer to these same concepts as needed in subsequent chapters.

This chapter has two distinct parts. The first covers topics that apply to all pulse-mode radiation detection instruments, including background, nuclear counting statistics, and dead time. The second part discusses issues specifically related to energy-sensitive detectors. A large part of the second section is devoted to energy spectra. In both parts the emphasis is on concepts rather than formulas.

Background

In any radiation detection situation, background will be present. *Background* refers to detected counts that do not come from the source being measured. It is determined by making a measurement with no source present. In a counting measurement, background counts result from cosmic radiation, from naturally occurring radionuclides found in the walls of the room, from extraneous sources of radiation in the area of the detector, and even from spurious electronic signals within the detector itself. (We discuss other kinds of background that arise in imaging situations in later chapters.) Ideally, whenever a counting measurement is made, background should be measured and subtracted to obtain a net count value. But as a practical matter, if its count rate is less than 1% of the source count rate, background can safely be ignored (1).

Nuclear Counting Statistics

Noise is an unavoidable complication in radiation detection measurements. *Noise* is defined as "any undesired fluctuation that appears superimposed on a signal source" (2). It arises from many sources, including the random nature of radioactive decay, variations in energy transfer within a detector, fluctuations occurring within a detector and its electrical components, and background radiation. Depending on the situation and the context, the term noise may refer to any or all of these sources; in particular, when nuclear counting statistics are discussed, noise specifically references the randomness of radioactive decay. The way to account for this variability is through the use of statistics.

Statistics with Multiple Measurements

When we make several measurements of a sample containing radioactivity using a scintillation detector, we get a different value for each measurement. If we make a number of measurements (and do so instantaneously, so that no appreciable radioactive decay occurs), we could determine the average or *mean value* M of the group of measurements

$$M = \frac{\sum_i^n N_i}{n} \qquad (4\text{-}1)$$

where N_i represents each individual measurement, n represents the total number of measurements, and M is the mean value for the set of measurements.

We could also plot a *frequency distribution* (a graph of measured value vs number of times that value was obtained in the set of measurements). The frequency distribution for a set of 30 measurements of an I-131 source is shown in **Figure 4-1a**. The width of the frequency distribution characterizes the spread of the values obtained, and it can be described by the *standard deviation s*:

$$s = \sqrt{\frac{\sum_i (N_i - M)^2}{n-1}}. \qquad (4\text{-}2)$$

The standard deviation is a measure of the *precision* of the data set (the range of measured values). With many, many measurements, the frequency distribution would become a smooth curve (Fig. 4-1b).

Poisson Statistical Model

We can approximate this information by taking only a single measurement of the radioactive sample. We are allowed to do so because radioactive decay obeys the *Poisson* statistical model. Chapter 3 of Reference 2 gives the entire mathematical derivation of the Poisson model. We will move directly to the major predictions of the model: (1) a single measurement can be used to predict the frequency distribution that we would produce if we took many, many measurements of the sample; and (2) the width of the frequency distribution (its standard deviation σ) can be estimated as the square root of the value of that single measurement. Mathematically,

$$\sigma \cong \sqrt{N} \qquad (4\text{-}3)$$

where N is the value of the single measurement we have made.

The first prediction, stated more fully, says that the frequency distribution of all possible measurements for the sample will fall into a Gaussian or normal curve (Fig. 4-1b) as long as the individual values of each measurement are greater than about 20 counts (cts). This frequency distribution has a width that is fixed relative to the standard deviation:

- Of all possible measurements, 68.3% are within 1 standard deviation of the mean (the peak of the curve).
- Of all possible measurements, 95.4% are within 2 standard deviations of the mean.
- Of all possible measurements, 99.7% are within 3 standard deviations of the mean.

So by taking a single measurement of our sample and applying the second prediction of the Poisson statistical model, we can predict the shape and width of the frequency distribution that would result from taking many measurements of that sample.

The single measurement N, in providing an estimate of the width of the frequency distribution, also provides us with an estimate of the mean value M of the frequency distribution. Because the single value N that we have is one of the many measurements that make up the frequency distribution, we can turn the above statements around to relate M to N:

- The mean value of the sample has a 68.3% likelihood of being within 1 standard deviation ($1\sqrt{N}$) of our single measurement N.
- The mean value of the sample has a 95.4% chance of being within $2\sqrt{N}$ of the single measurement N.
- The mean value of the sample has a 99.7% chance of being within $3\sqrt{N}$ of our single measurement.

Another way to state the first bullet is that we are 68.3% confident that M is within 1 standard deviation of N (and hence ±1 standard deviation is known as the 68.3% *confidence interval*). Similarly, ±2 standard deviations represents a 95.4% confidence interval, and ±3 standard deviations a 99.7% confidence interval. Thus the application of

(a) Frequency distribution of 30 measurements

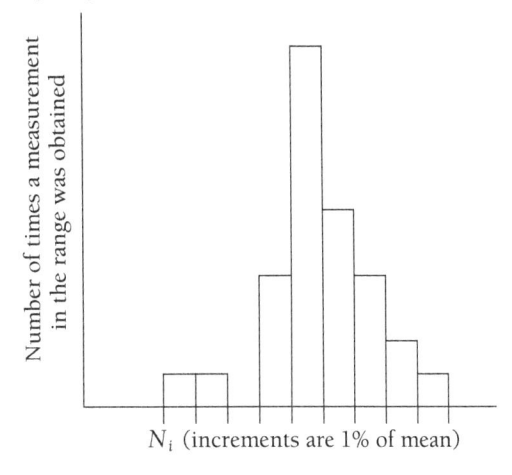

N_i (increments are 1% of mean)

(b) Gaussian frequency distribution

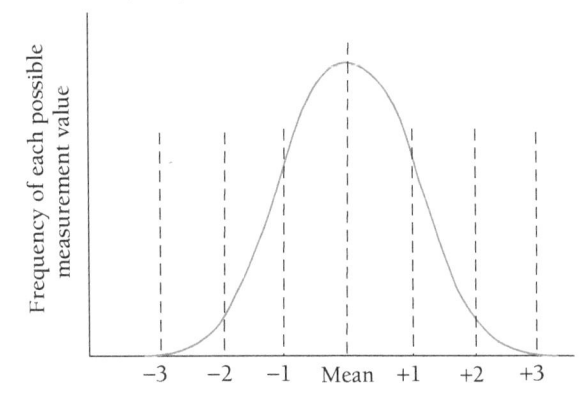

Figure 4-1 Frequency distributions of counting measurements. Figure 4-1a shows an actual frequency distribution of 30 measurements of a radioactive source. The X-axis is demarcated in intervals of 1% of the mean value; the height of each bar indicates the number of measurements in that 1% range. The smooth curve in Figure 4-1b is the frequency distribution of an infinite set of measurements of a radioactive sample. Because radioactive decay obeys Poisson statistics, the curve has a Gaussian shape, and its proportions are well-known. All possible measurements are represented in the area under the curve. Given the curve's known proportions, we can take a single measurement and know its likelihood relative to the mean value of the infinite set of measurements.

the Poisson model allows us to make a single measurement of a radioactive sample and relate it to the mean value for that sample.

One consequence of Equation 4-3 is that as N gets larger, σ (the standard deviation) increases much more slowly. Thus the frequency distribution shown in Figure 4-1b gets narrower as N gets larger. In a counting measurement, the goal is to obtain a result that has good statistical precision or reproducibility. This is characterized by a number called the *coefficient of variation* (CV):

$$\text{CV} = \frac{\sqrt{N}}{N} \times 100\% = \frac{100\%}{\sqrt{N}}. \qquad (4\text{-}4)$$

The CV allows the comparison of standard deviations for measurements with different N values.

The CV is a measure of the *statistical precision* or reproducibility of N. To have a CV less than ±1% (a goal for many counting measurements), a single measurement needs to contain at least 10,000 cts (based on Equation 4-4, if $1/\sqrt{N} = 0.01$, then N = 10,000). This level of statistical precision is sometimes taken as a desirable end point in situations involving in vitro sample counting.

Sample Calculation 4-1   Statistical Analysis of a Single Counting Measurement

A scintillation detector generates a counting measurement of 15,765 cts. What is the standard deviation of this measurement? What is the coefficient of variation? What does this mean in practical terms?

According to Equations 4-3 and 4-4,

$$\sigma = \sqrt{15{,}765 \text{ cts}} = 126 \text{ cts}$$

$$\text{CV} = \frac{126 \text{ cts}}{15{,}765 \text{ cts}} \times 100\% = 0.8\%.$$

What this means is that while the single measurement of 15,765 cts may not be the best value for this radioactive sample, the best value is likely within 1 standard deviation of this value. We express this by quoting the measurement as 15,765 ± 126 cts. The CV tells us that the variability of this measurement is less than ±1%, which is our goal in terms of statistical precision.

Nuclear Counting Statistics

Rules for Combining Standard Deviations

The application of the Poisson model to nuclear counting statistics has one very important restriction: Equation 4-3 can only be used if N represents the number of counts recorded in a counting measurement. N cannot be a count rate or a net count value or any other derived quantity. The practice for generating the standard deviation of a derived quantity is to apply Equation 4-3 to the actual count value to determine its standard deviation, and then to use this number to derive the needed standard deviation. The rules for generating these derived values and two common examples of their use are discussed in this section.

It is always possible to increase the time of a measurement in order to reach a CV of 1%, because the CV can be expressed as a count rate:

$$CV = \frac{\sqrt{N}}{t} \times 100\%. \qquad (4\text{-}5)$$

If the measurement time is increased, the count rate stays the same, but the precision improves (CV gets smaller) as the value of N increases. In patient measurement situations, however, it is often not practical to take a measurement of 10,000 cts. In these cases, the technologist must take extra care to ensure that the measurement reflects the clinical situation accurately. For example, a thyroid uptake protocol may be designed to reach statistical precision in euthyroid and hyperthyroid states. In the hypothyroid patient, however, a statistically precise measurement of 10,000 cts might require a measurement of 10 minutes or longer. Rather than requiring the patient to sit through that 10-min measurement, a shorter and less precise measurement may be taken. It is then incumbent on the technologist to ensure that the technical aspects of this measurement are exactly correct (e.g., that the probe is properly calibrated and is on the "probe" and not the "well" setting).

Often it is necessary to add or subtract two counting measurements; a common example is subtraction of background from a sample measurement. It follows that the standard deviations of the two measurements must both

Sample Calculation 4-2 Adding and Subtracting Counting Measurements

A capsule containing I-131 for a thyroid capsule is counted for 2 min, and background for 1 min, with the following results:

Capsule = 25,294 cts

Background = 108 cts.

Calculate the net count rate and its standard deviation.
First we need to express both values as counts per minute (cpm):

Capsule = 12,647 cpm

Background = 108 cpm.

The net count rate is then

Capsule − background = 12,647 − 108 = 12,539 cpm

To calculate the standard deviation, we need the standard deviations of the capsule and background measurements. To use the Poisson rule in Equation 4-3, we must use the actual counting measurements to determine each standard deviation:

$$\sigma_{\text{capsule}} = \frac{\sqrt{25,294\ \text{cts}}}{2\ \text{min}} = \frac{159\ \text{cts}}{2\ \text{min}} = 80\ \text{cpm}.$$

The standard deviation of the background measurement is

$$\sigma_{\text{bkg}} = \frac{\sqrt{108\ \text{cts}}}{1\ \text{min}} = 10\ \text{cpm}.$$

The standard deviation of the net count rate is then

$$\sigma_{\text{net}} = \sqrt{(80\ \text{cpm})^2 + (10\ \text{cpm})^2} = 80.6\ \text{cpm}.$$

We would express the count rate as $12{,}539 \pm 81$ cpm. Note that the standard deviations *add* in quadrature, even though the operation combining the two measurements is a subtraction operation.

---

be included in the standard deviation of the sum or difference. The rule in this situation is that the standard deviations *add in quadrature*:

$$\sigma_3 = \sqrt{\sigma_1^2 + \sigma_2^2} \qquad (4\text{-}6)$$

where σ_1 and σ_2 are the standard deviations of the two measurements being combined and σ_3 is the standard deviation of the sum or difference.

Thus, the presence of a significant background reading changes not only the value of the counting measurement, as noted previously, but also the statistical certainty of that measurement. We can, however, reach a similar conclusion about the statistical question to what we did when we considered the effect of background on the counting measurement, namely, that when background is small in comparison to the sample measurement, its effect on the standard deviation can be ignored. That is, the resulting value for σ_3 in Equation 4-6 is dominated by the larger of the two terms σ_1 and σ_2. If background is 1% of the sample counting measurement or less, it will not have a significant effect on the combined standard deviation (1).

Statistical Testing

Statistics are useful in several quality control procedures. A *Levy–Jennings plot* can be used to follow the performance of a detector over time. Multiple measurements of a particular quality control parameter are made, and the mean value and standard deviation are determined using

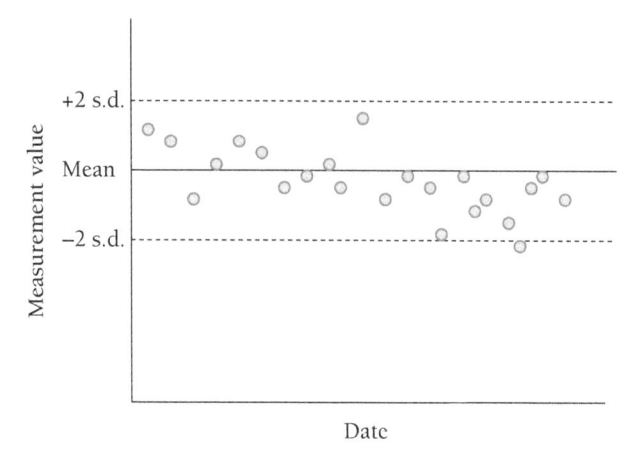

Figure 4-2 A Levy–Jennings plot. The plot is prepared by determining the mean and standard deviation of a group of measurements, made with the same instrument and parameters as the quality control measure in question. If the measurement is of a radioactive source, the lines should be sloped to account for decay. Each day, the value of the daily measurement is plotted on the graph. If the data follow a Poisson frequency distribution, 95% of the daily measurements should fall between the two dashed lines. But we also see changes over time. In the plot shown, it is clear that the measurements are decreasing over time, even though 21 of the 22 points are within ±2 standard deviation limits. In Appendix C, Figure C-5b shows several Levy–Jennings plots.

Equations 4-1 and 4-2; these values are used to create the graph shown in **Figure 4-2**, with an X-axis of time (usually days). If the detector's performance follows Poisson statistics, 95% of all possible measurements should fall between the lines. Measurements of the same parameter are then plotted on the graph, allowing trends to be spotted easily.

The *chi-square test* compares the measured variability of a group of measurements to the Poisson-predicted variability. The test is performed by taking a series of n measurements with a radiation detector such as a well counter or thyroid probe. The mean (M) and standard deviation (s) of the data set are calculated as in Equations 4-1 and 4-2. In addition, a number called the *chi-square statistic* (χ^2) is determined:

$$\chi^2 = \frac{1}{M}\sum_{i=1}^{n}(n_i - M)^2 = \frac{n-1}{M}s^2. \quad (4\text{-}7)$$

Remember that the Poisson-derived standard deviation σ is equal to the square root of an individual counting measurement. This equation therefore compares the experimentally determined standard deviation (s^2) to that predicted by the Poisson distribution ($\sigma^2 \approx M$). The quantity ($n - 1$) is called the *statistical degrees of freedom*, and if s^2 and M are similar, then the value of the χ^2 statistic should be numerically close to the degrees of freedom.

The value obtained in a chi-square calculation is compared to a chi-square table (**Table 4-1**), which shows the probability of obtaining a given value for χ^2 by chance. The calculated χ^2 statistic (Eq. 4-7) is located on the line of the table corresponding to either the number of measurements (n) or the number of degrees of freedom ($n - 1$). Most likely the calculated χ^2 statistic will be between two of the tabulated values. The probabilities (the p values) at the top of those two columns are then recorded.

What do these probabilities tell us? A "perfect" fit between the experimental distribution of measured values and the Poisson-predicted distribution would give a probability of 0.5. The p values that indicate possible equipment problems are at the low and high ends of the probability scale. A χ^2 test that produces a p value less than 0.1 indicates that the data set had a larger variability than expected by statistics alone. A p value greater than 0.9 indicates less variability than expected. Either result should cause the operator to question the function of the detector.

Sample Calculation 4-3   Chi-Square Test

A scintillation detector is tested for statistical precision using the chi-square test. Twenty measurements of a radioactive source are made, and application of Equations 4-1 and 4-2 reveals a mean of 96,643 and a standard deviation of 450 cts. Calculate the chi-square statistic and use Table 4-1 to determine the p value for this test.

From Equation 4-7, we get

$$\chi^2 = \frac{(20-1)(450\text{ cts})^2}{96{,}643\text{ cts}} = 39.81.$$

Use the n = 20 line of Table 4-1 to find the p values that are close to this: p = 0.05 has a chi-square statistic of 30.14.

The calculated chi-square statistic is larger than that for p = 0.05, so the p value for the chi-square test performed must be smaller than 0.05. This indicates that the variability among the 20 measurements is larger than would be predicted by Poisson statistics.

Table 4-1

Chi-Square Statistic Probabilities

Number of Measurements (n)	Degrees of Freedom ($n - 1$)	p = 0.05	p = 0.10	p = 0.5	p = 0.90	p = 0.95
10	9	16.92	14.68	9.34	4.17	3.82
20	19	30.14	27.20	18.34	11.65	10.12
25	24	33.20	36.42	23.34	15.66	13.85

The χ^2 test is not particularly good at identifying problems, in that a detector with significant malfunction may still produce an acceptable p value. But the test does provide a means of analyzing the output of the detector in relation to the expected statistical variability. An acceptable χ^2 test result gives the operator confidence that the detector has good statistical precision.

Dead Time

Dead time is the minimum time separation of two radiation events required to detect them as two distinct events. It is essentially the processing time per event. In a detection system with multiple components, dead time is usually determined by the slowest component. Both energy-sensitive and energy-insensitive detectors may have dead time. For example, in a Geiger counter, the dead time is determined by how long it takes for the detector to recover from the Geiger discharge. In a scintillation detector, the dead time is determined by the decay time of the signal in the crystal and/or the time required for the tail on the amplifier signal to return to baseline. The effect of dead time in either case is that some events are lost because they occur too soon after the preceding event, and therefore the count value we measure is not the true count value, but somewhat less than that.

We need to distinguish between two different ways in which dead time can affect the measured count value. A *nonparalyzable* system is one in which an event occurring during the dead time is simply ignored, with no effect on subsequently occurring events. In a *paralyzable* system, each event (recorded or not) introduces a dead time, creating an extendable period of detector paralysis. The two models are illustrated in **Figure 4-3**. If we graph the observed count rate vs the true count rate (**Figure 4-4**), we see that in the nonparalyzable system, the observed count rate approaches a maximum value. In the paralyzable system, the observed count rate reaches a maximum, then decreases as additional events extend the dead time and paralyze the system. In this case, a measured count rate could correspond to either of two different true count rates.

The dead time of a detector can be determined experimentally (2,3), and once the dead time is known, the maximum observable count rate can be determined. From

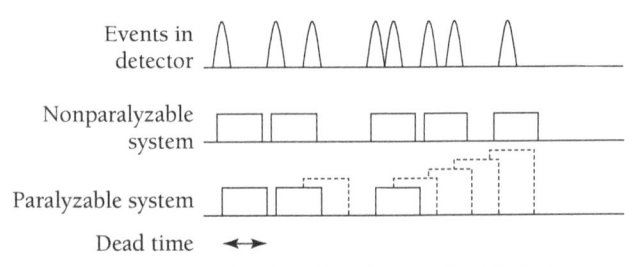

Figure 4-3 Illustration of paralyzable and nonparalyzable dead time. Eight events occur in the detector in this sequence. The nonparalyzable system counts five events and ignores the three events that occur during dead time. The paralyzable system only registers three events, because all events, detected or not, add dead time. The dashed-line rectangles represent the extending system paralysis as additional events incur their own dead time.

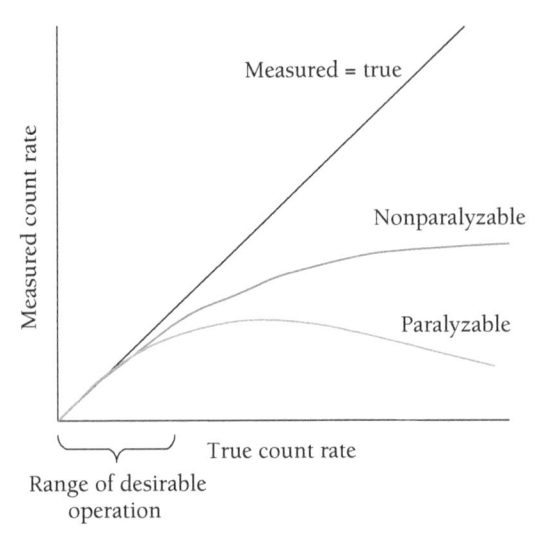

Figure 4-4 Measured count rates in paralyzable and nonparalyzable systems. The line of identity shows where the measured count rate is equal to the true count rate. The nonparalyzable system reaches a maximum measured count rate. The paralyzable system, reaches a maximum and then declines at higher count rates as it becomes paralyzed.

a practical standpoint, the nuclear medicine technologist needs to be aware that radiation detectors can have dead time, ranging from about 2 μsec in a scintillation detector to about 5 μsec in a gamma camera to 50 to 100 μsec in a Geiger counter. One should always be aware that the true count rate may be different from what the detector is reporting, especially at high count rates. Ideally, a detector should be operated only in the range of count rates where the observed count rate is equal to the true count rate (as shown in Fig. 4-4).

Energy Spectra

One of the chief advantages of energy-sensitive detectors such as scintillation and semiconductor detectors is that they allow us not only to detect the presence of radiation, but also to evaluate the energy of detected events. When a radiation detector reaches this level of sophistication, we are presented with new issues beyond those discussed thus far. A particular gamma ray may interact in a way that causes all of its energy to be deposited in the detector, or it may interact in such a way that some of the energy escapes the detector and is not registered. Thus we have to consider a variety of possible interaction scenarios and their results; these are illustrated in **Figure 4-5**. The evaluation of energy spectra obtained using an energy-sensitive detector is called *spectroscopy*.

Energy spectra display the results of interactions of high-energy photons in the material of the radiation detector. An idealized energy spectrum, including several of the peaks described in the following sections, is shown in **Figure 4-6a**. The peaks of this ideal spectrum are sharp and well defined, whereas in real life (Fig. 4-6b) they are broad. This is so because this spectrum was acquired using a sodium iodide detector, in which statistical fluctuations play a large role. Keep in mind that while we identify each peak as a single energy, the actual spectrum shows a broad peak with a sodium iodide scintillation detector and a

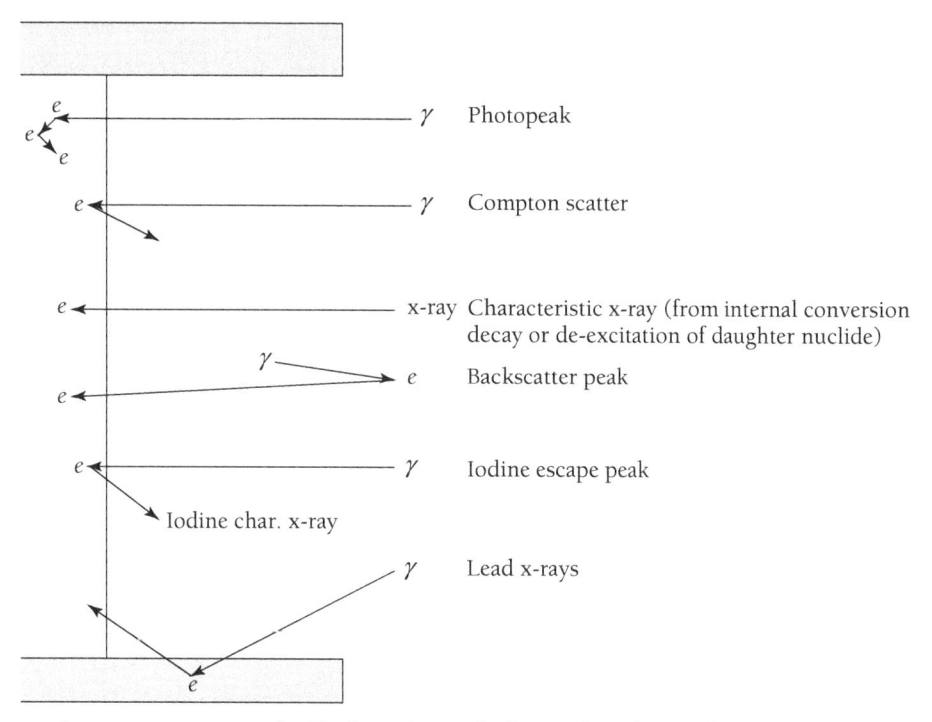

Figure 4-5 Interactions causing energy spectrum peaks. The figure depicts the front surface of a scintillation crystal with a flat-field collimator. Six possible interactions are illustrated; not all will be seen with every radionuclide. Each *e* represents an interaction resulting in the ionization of an atom, and it indicates that the resulting electron's kinetic energy is absorbed in that location. Photons are depicted in the diagram as γ or x-ray; these can escape from the material where the interaction took place.

much narrower peak with a semiconductor detector. We can measure the broadness of the peaks using the full width at half-maximum (FWHM). The presence and significance of various peaks in the energy spectrum depend on the type of radioactive source, its geometry relative to the detector, and other factors described below. In clinical situations, any unexpected peaks should be identified to rule out interfering sources.

Photopeak

The *photopeak* is the peak that corresponds to interactions in which the entire gamma ray energy is absorbed in the scintillation crystal. For most radionuclides, the photopeak is the rightmost peak seen. It represents the total energy of the gamma ray, whereas other peaks in the energy spectrum represent some loss of energy from the detection process and therefore will be to the left of the photopeak. When looking at an energy spectrum, one should first identify the photopeak. Keep in mind, however, that there can be multiple photopeaks for a single radionuclide. For example, In-111 produces two gamma rays for each disintegration, at 173 and 247 keV. Also remember that although we typically use the most frequently emitted gamma ray(s) for our measurements, other gamma ray emissions can show up as small peaks in the energy spectrum. Because the energy of its photopeak(s) is specific to a radionuclide, one of the uses of spectroscopy is to determine the identity of an unknown radionuclide.

Compton Scatter

Now assume that a gamma ray, instead of depositing all of its energy in the crystal, undergoes an initial Compton

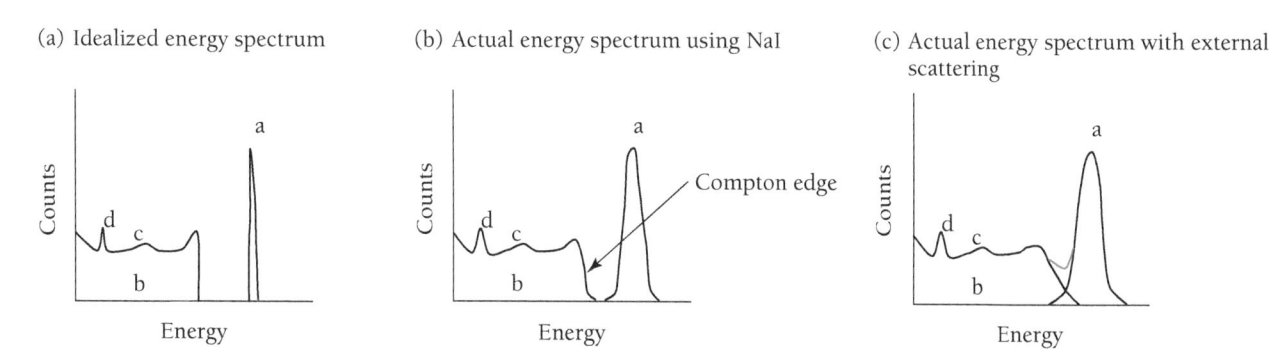

Figure 4-6 Ideal and actual energy spectra. The ideal spectrum has sharp boundaries and narrow peaks, while the actual spectrum has broad peaks and indefinite transitions. The following are identified: (a) photopeak, (b) Compton region, (c) backscatter peak, and (d) lead x-ray and/or other characteristic x-ray peaks. Figure 4-6b shows the spectrum as it is broadened by the finite energy resolution of sodium iodide. Figure 4-6c shows additional events between the Compton and photopeak regions due to multiple and/or external scattering events; the gray line indicates that the total counts in this area are the sum of the Compton and photopeak counts. The Compton edge is defined as the inflection point of the high-energy side of the Compton region.

Energy Spectra   45

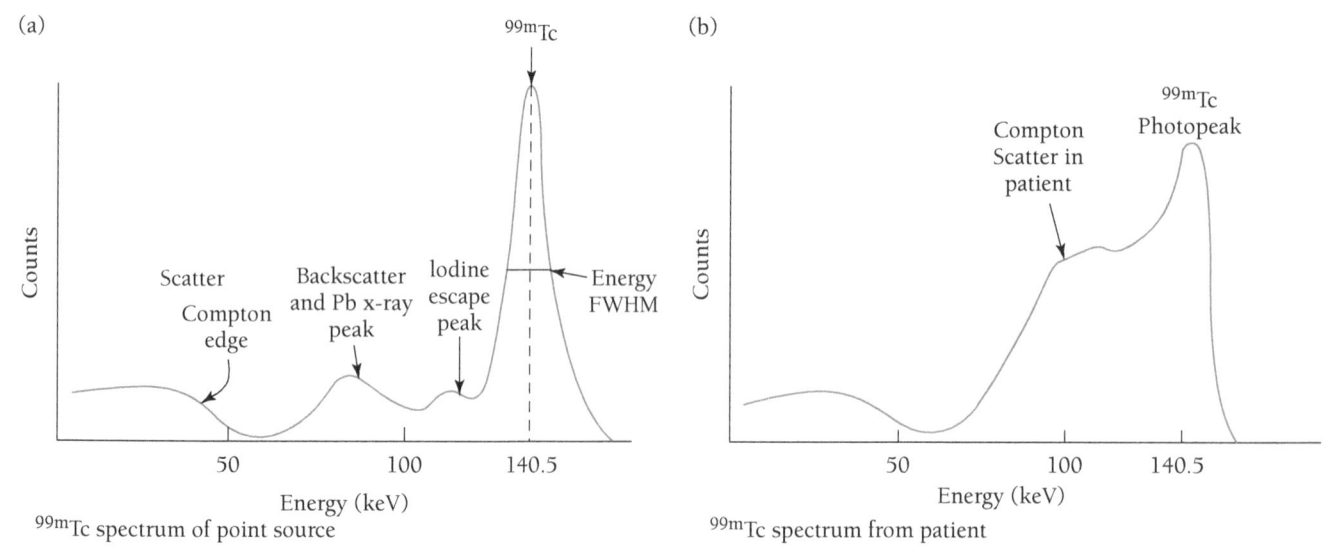

Figure 4-7 Energy spectra showing the location of the Compton edge and the effect of scatter. These spectra are of Tc-99m and were obtained with a gamma camera. The spectrum in Figure 4-7b was generated with a patient as the radiation source; note the greatly increased scatter region and the difficulty in separating the photopeak from the Compton region. Reprinted from: Mettler FA, Guiberteau MJ, eds. *Essentials of Nuclear Medicine Imaging.* 2nd ed. Orlando, FL: Grune & Stratton; 1986:21. Used with permission from Elsevier.

scattering interaction in the detector, following which the scattered gamma ray escapes the crystal. Only the Compton electron (which probably will not escape the crystal, due to its short range) deposits its energy in the crystal. The portion of energy carried out of the crystal by the scattered gamma ray is lost from the pulse, and we measure a lower energy than the photopeak energy. How much lower? Because Compton scattering can occur at any angle, the energy measured has a range of possible values, and therefore a *Compton region* is seen in the energy spectrum. There is an upper limit to the Compton region, because there is an upper limit to how much energy a photon can transfer to a Compton electron. This limit is called the *Compton edge*. The maximum energy a Compton electron can have is given by the Compton scattering equation (Eq. A-3) with $\theta = 180°$ (2):

$$E_{\text{Compton edge}} = E_\gamma - E_{\gamma'} \quad (4\text{-}8)$$

where

$$E_{\gamma'} = \frac{E_\gamma}{1 + (2E_\gamma/511 \text{ keV})} \quad (4\text{-}9)$$

and E_γ and $E_{\gamma'}$ are in keV. On the energy spectrum, the Compton edge is the inflection point of the rightmost downsloping part of the Compton region (Fig. 4-6b). Because a range of Compton scattering angles will cause the scattered photon to leave the crystal, we can see a range of energies from 0 keV up to the Compton edge. If an isotope has multiple photopeaks, each photopeak will have its own Compton edge, although it may be hard to see all of them. Again, these demarcations are not sharp but are smeared out with a sodium iodide detector.

Keep in mind that Compton scattering occurs not only in the detector but also in materials outside of the detector. This is a common occurrence in many nuclear medicine applications. A gamma ray that undergoes a Compton scattering event in a patient may lose only a small amount of energy, so that its energy still falls within or close to the energy window. If such a gamma ray then is absorbed in the detector, its energy may fall between the photopeak and the Compton edge (Fig. 4-6c). Thus the Compton region overlaps the photopeak to an extent that can be significant (**Figure 4-7**). As a general rule, checking the location of the energy window relative to the photopeak (called *calibration* for a probe or well counter and *peaking* for a gamma camera) should not be done with the patient as the radionuclide source.

Characteristic X-Rays

A *characteristic x-ray* is produced when an orbital electron moves from a higher orbital to a lower orbital to fill an inner-shell vacancy (see Appendix A). In the process of radioactive decay, this may occur in two ways: in the original radionuclide itself following an internal conversion decay (the alternative to gamma emission) or from the decay daughter as it deexcites to the ground state. In the first instance, internal conversion ejects a K- or L-shell electron, creating an orbital vacancy that will produce a characteristic x-ray when it is filled. Tc-99m can illustrate this mechanism of characteristic x-ray production; 10% of its decays are by internal conversion, which produce 18- and 20-keV K-shell characteristic x-rays. In the second instance, the decay to the daughter can leave an electron in an excited-state orbital, resulting in a configuration that deexcites with a characteristic x-ray emission. As an example of this source of characteristic x-rays, consider Co-57. It decays by electron capture to Fe-57, which then has an orbital vacancy that produces a 6.4-keV Fe-57 characteristic x-ray. These characteristic x-ray peaks are superimposed on the Compton region.

The photopeak(s), the characteristic x-ray peak(s), and the Compton region are seen in the spectrum of every radionuclide. In addition, other peaks may be seen, depending on the photon energy and the geometry of the detector. These are described next.

Backscatter Peak

The *backscatter peak* occurs when the gamma ray is scattered in the source or surrounding structures (e.g., walls, floors) such that the scattered photon is then absorbed in the scintillation crystal. This is the inverse of the Compton edge situation: now it is the scattered photon rather than the Compton electron that is depositing its energy in the crystal. The energy of the backscatter peak is therefore

$$E_{\text{backscatter peak}} = \frac{E_\gamma}{1 + (2E_\gamma/511 \text{ keV})}. \quad (4\text{-}10)$$

The backscatter peak is broad because backscattered photons may enter the crystal from angles other than 180°. Depending on the geometry and other factors, the backscatter peak may be noticeable, or it may be subsumed by other sources of scattered photons.

Lead X-Rays

Scintillation detectors are generally surrounded with lead to prevent extraneous photons from interacting in the crystal. A gamma ray that is absorbed by a photoelectric interaction with a lead atom will generate a characteristic x-ray, which may then be absorbed in the crystal. A peak would occur at the energy of the lead K-shell characteristic x-rays, which are about 80 to 90 keV (3). The presence of a lead x-ray peak depends on the particular geometry of the detector, but is somewhat more likely to be seen with gamma rays in the 90- to 200-keV range. The K-shell binding energy in lead is 88 keV, so K-shell x-rays will not be seen at gamma ray energies below this level. Any type of shielding material can produce characteristic x-rays, so knowledge of the composition of the detector housing materials may be helpful.

Iodine Escape Peak

In a sodium iodide crystal, an incident or scattered gamma ray most commonly interacts with an iodine atom, via the photoelectric effect. The photoelectron's energy is retained in the crystal, but it is possible for the 28-keV iodine characteristic x-ray to escape the crystal without interacting. The amount of energy deposited in the crystal is then less than the photopeak energy by the amount of the iodine characteristic x-ray:

$$E_{\text{iodine escape peak}} = E_\gamma - 28 \text{ keV}. \quad (4\text{-}11)$$

This is a surface phenomenon. It usually occurs with lower-energy gamma rays (less than 150 keV, for example, Co-57 or Tl-201), because higher-energy gamma rays are more likely to penetrate farther into the crystal before interacting, making the characteristic x-ray's escape less likely.

Coincidence and Sum Peaks

When a radionuclide emits two gamma rays per disintegration, they may interact in the crystal at the exact same time and be detected as one event by the crystal. The energy of such an "event" is the sum of the two gamma ray energies. This peak is more likely seen in well counters, because the detector almost completely surrounds the sample and is more likely to absorb both gamma rays (**Figure 4-8**). We can also have sum peaks of gamma rays with characteristic x-rays and chance (i.e., accidental) coincidences of gamma rays from different disintegrations, with a high-activity sample. The energy peaks are the sum of whatever photons interacted coincidentally in the detector.

Using the above information, the operator of an energy-sensitive detector should be able to predict the general shape of the energy spectrum of any radionuclide. This in turn allows the identification of any unexpected peaks, which may indicate contamination of the radionuclide sample or the detector. Energy spectra are usually best plotted on a semilogarithmic graph, which allows visualization of small peaks that are unimpressive on a linear graph, relative to the much larger height of the photopeak (**Figure 4-9**).

Sample Calculation 4-4 Calculation of Expected Energy Spectrum Peaks

For Hg-203, which has a photopeak energy of 279 keV, calculate the energies of peaks that can be expected on an energy spectrum using a sodium iodide scintillator.

Photopeak = 279 keV

Compton edge (CE) calculation:

$$E_{\text{CE}} = E_\gamma - \left[\frac{E_\gamma}{1 + (2E_\gamma/511 \text{ keV})}\right]$$

$$= 279 - \frac{279}{1 + 1.09} = 279 - 133 = 146 \text{ keV}.$$

Characteristic x-rays = 70–84 keV (from decay data table for Hg-203).

Backscatter peak = $E_\gamma/[1 + (2E_\gamma/511 \text{ keV})]$ = 133 keV.

Lead x-rays = 80–90 keV.

Iodine escape peak = unlikely.

Baseline Shift and Pulse Pileup

The shape of the output pulse created by the amplifier of a radiation detector has consequences that affect radiation measurement. **Figure 4-10a** shows the classic amplifier pulse with its negative undershoot, which is a consequence of the physics of the electronic circuitry (2). However, the negative undershoot causes a problem when

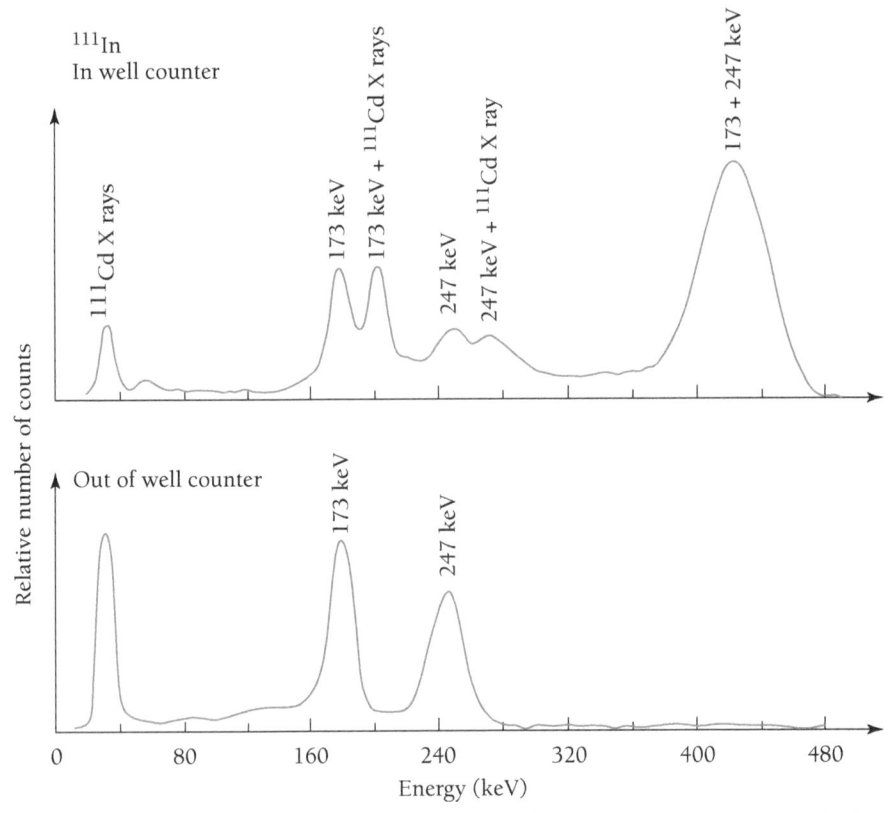

Figure 4-8 Energy spectra for In-111, obtained with the source in the well of the well counter (upper spectrum) and held out of the well (lower spectrum). Three coincidence peaks are identified when the source is within the well counter, at 198, 272, and 420 keV. Note the summed peaks in the upper spectrum that disappear in the lower spectrum, as coincidence events become less likely. Reprinted from: Cherry SP, Sorenson JA, Phelps ME. *Physics in Nuclear Medicine*. 3rd ed. Philadelphia, PA: Saunders; 2003: Fig. 10-7, p. 154. Used with permission from Elsevier.

two pulses occur close together in time. If the next pulse is received before the last pulse has returned to baseline, it will be seen as having a lesser amplitude than it actually does, a situation called *baseline shift* (Fig. 4-10b). If pulses occur even more closely spaced in time, they pile up on one another and are treated as a single event (Fig. 4-10c). This is called *pulse pileup*. Note that in either case, the pulse height analyzer (PHA) incorrectly rejects the pulse it receives, and the measured count rate is lower than the true count rate. On the other hand, two pulses whose sum after pulse pileup puts them into the PHA window will be incorrectly recorded as a "good" event. Baseline shift and pulse pileup become problematic at high count rates, where they must be managed. This is relatively easy to accomplish electronically (2). The better choice, however, is to operate the radiation detector at count rates where baseline shift and pulse pileup are not an issue.

Detection Efficiency

Detection efficiency refers to the ability of a radiation-detecting instrument to convert radiation emissions to useful signals (3). (This is similar to, but more precisely defined than, the term *efficiency* given in Appendix A.) At its most basic level, we can consider detection efficiency to be the ratio of measured events to measurable events, or gamma rays detected vs gamma rays emitted. This is called *absolute efficiency*. However, a number of factors affect its value.

Components of Efficiency

The *efficiency* of a radiation detector is its ability to turn disintegrations into measured counts. The detector's ability to do so depends on a number of factors, including the nature of the detector, the geometry of the detector and the source relative to it, the energy window (in energy-sensitive detectors), and what happens to the photons within the radioactive source. Let us consider these factors by way of some examples.

Detector Composition

Consider a gas-filled detector and a sodium iodide detector. Sodium iodide is better at absorbing gamma rays, so it will register more radiation events from a given source than a gas-filled detector will. Similarly, a sodium iodide crystal will be better at absorbing Tc-99m photons than I-131 photons, because the 140-keV photons of Tc-99m are more likely to undergo a photoelectric interaction than the 364-keV photons of I-131. These differences are due to the inherent properties of the detector material and the gamma rays being detected, and they are collected into a term called *intrinsic efficiency*. In general, materials with higher effective atomic number are better absorbers of gamma rays than those with lower atomic number, because

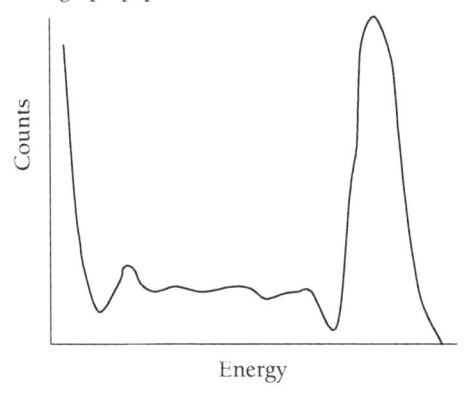

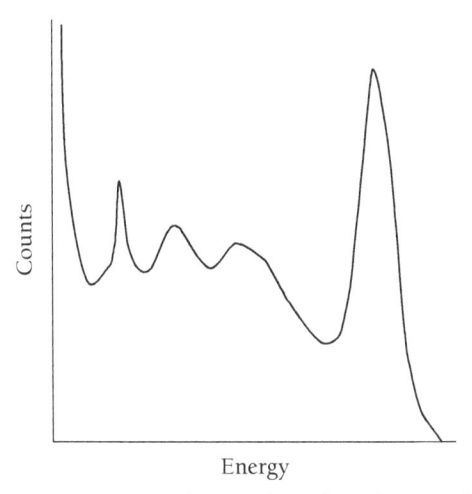

Figure 4-9 Energy spectra using linear and semilogarithmic graph paper. The small peaks found in the Compton region are much more obvious on the semilogarithmic plot, making them easier to recognize.

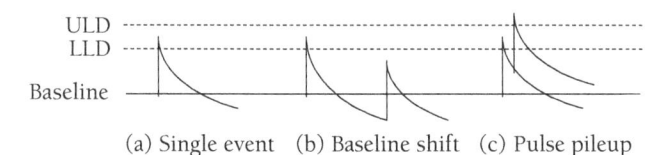

Figure 4-10 Illustration of baseline shift and pulse pileup. The amplifier output pulse typically has a negative overshoot (Fig. 4-10a). In baseline shift (Fig. 4-10b), the next pulse falls in the negative overshoot of the previous pulse. In pulse pileup (Fig. 4-10c), the next event falls on the peak of the previous pulse. In baseline shift, the second pulse is not counted; in pulse pileup, neither is counted. Dashed lines indicate the pulse height analyzer settings, and the solid line indicates the electrical baseline.

the former have higher electron densities. This is particularly important in considering scintillators for 511-keV photons.

Detector Geometry

Next we compare a well counter and a probe, both made of sodium iodide. Given equal-activity sources, the well counter will register more counts than the probe, because a well counter more completely surrounds the radioactive sample (see Fig. 2-10). This is an example of *geometric efficiency*. Geometric efficiency is generally expressed as the fraction or percentage of the total emissions that intersect with the radiation detector in a given source-detector geometry.

As a first estimation, then, detection efficiency is the product of the geometric and intrinsic components, the fraction of emitted photons that reach the detector times the fraction of those reaching the detector that are registered as counts. But the use of an energy-sensitive detector brings additional factors into play.

Energy Window

If the PHA's window size is decreased, the measured count rate in counts per minute by necessity will become smaller, even though the actual activity remains the same. Thus the efficiency decreases as the window width decreases.

Absorption and Scatter

If we have a source within a scattering material and a source not in the scattering material, given the same amount of radioactivity, the source in the scattering material will have more photons absorbed or scattered to a lower energy, so the detector will see fewer photons in the photopeak.

From these examples, it should be apparent that a measurement of a radioactive source or patient depends on many factors. In theory, we could start with a measured count rate, then divide it by a series of modifying factors (all less than 1) based on the above considerations, to determine the actual activity of the source in question. This is not necessary in most clinical situations, however.

In imaging studies, efficiency need be determined only in a relative sense, because areas of abnormal radiopharmaceutical uptake can be identified by comparison to areas of normal uptake. In nonimaging studies, such as measurement of thyroid uptake, a standard is used to compare to the patient value. The standard in these cases is a radionuclide source whose activity can be directly correlated to the amount administered to the patient. In these studies, efficiency is the same for the standard and the clinical measurements (as long as the standard and patient measurements are made with the same instrument, counting parameters, and geometry, and as long as the dead time is not different between the standard and patient measurement). Thus in clinical imaging and nonimaging studies, we do not need an absolute value for detection efficiency to obtain accurate and clinically meaningful information.

Efficiency Factor Determination and Use

Three particular circumstances in nuclear medicine require the actual efficiency of a detector: performing wipe tests to detect removable contamination, checking packages for contamination before opening them, and performing thyroid bioassays. In these cases the required number is in μCi or dpm, but the detector measurement is in cpm. Therefore we need to have an *efficiency factor* of the form cpm/dpm to make this conversion.

To determine the efficiency factor (4), we again need a standard, but we need a more exact definition for this term. A reference standard for an efficiency factor determination is a long-lived calibration source whose absolute activity in dpm is known and which emits gamma rays of approximately the same energy as the isotope of interest. For example, Ba-133 (E_γ = 356 keV) is a common reference standard for a bioassay measurement, which detects thyroid contamination with I-131 (E_γ = 364 keV); for Tc-99m, Co-57 (E_γ = 122 and 137 keV) is often used. By using a reference standard with similar energy to the isotope of interest, the intrinsic efficiency of the detector is kept about the same, and in some situations the same energy window can be used.

The reference standard is put into or in front of the detector in the same geometric orientation as will be used for the sample measurement. The threshold, window, and high voltage are set as they will be for the sample measurement. The standard is counted to determine its cpm, and background is subtracted. Its calibration information is used to calculate the current activity in dpm. The efficiency factor is then the ratio of net cpm to dpm:

$$\text{Efficiency factor} = \frac{\text{net cpm of standard}}{\text{dpm of standard}}. \quad (4\text{-}12)$$

When a thyroid bioassay or contamination wipe (the sample) is measured, its background-subtracted cpm is divided by the efficiency factor to convert the measurement to activity or dpm:

$$\text{dpm (sample)} = \frac{\text{net cpm (sample)}}{\text{efficiency factor}}. \quad (4\text{-}13)$$

We should also account for the differences in emission frequency between the standard and the sample radionuclides:

$$\text{dpm (sample)} = \frac{\text{net cpm (sample)}}{\text{efficiency factor}} \times \frac{\text{gamma rays/disintegration (std)}}{\text{gamma rays/disintegration (sample)}}. \quad (4\text{-}14)$$

For example, Tc-99m emits 140-keV gamma rays in 89.1% of its disintegrations, whereas Co-57 emits either 122- or 136-keV gamma rays in 96% of its disintegrations. A measurement of Tc-99m dpm using an efficiency factor determined with Co-57 needs to be corrected by a factor of 0.96/0.891. If Ba-133 is used as a long-lived standard for I-131 efficiency the correction factor is 0.621(Ba-133)/0.812(I-131) (5). These long-lived radionuclides may be sold as "mock standards." For example, a mixture of Ba-133 and Cs-137 may be called "mock I-131," and its activity may be quoted as "equivalent activity of I-131," in which case the disintegrations ratio is already taken into account.

Sample Calculation 4-5 Efficiency Factor

A thyroid bioassay is to be performed, and the standard for the bioassay is Ba-133, which has an activity of 1.05 µCi today. The following data are obtained:

$$\text{cpm}_{std} = 3{,}479 \text{ cts}$$

$$\text{cpm}_{bkg} = 95 \text{ cts}$$

$$\text{cpm}_{thyroid} = 585 \text{ cts}.$$

First, we need to calculate the dpm of the Ba-133 sample:

$$(1.05\,\mu\text{Ci})\left(\frac{37\text{ kBq}}{\mu\text{Ci}}\right) = 39 \text{ kBq}$$

$$\text{dpm}_{std} = (39 \text{ kBq})\left(\frac{1{,}000 \text{ disintegrations}}{\text{sec} - \text{kBq}}\right)\left(\frac{60 \text{ sec}}{\text{min}}\right)$$

$$= 2.34 \times 10^6 \text{ dpm}.$$

Next, determine the net count rates of the standard and the thyroid measurement:

$$\text{Net std cpm} = 3{,}479 - 95 = 3{,}384 \text{ cpm}.$$

$$\text{Net thyroid cpm} = 585 - 95 = 490 \text{ cpm}.$$

From the net standard cpm and its calculated dpm, we can determine the efficiency factor for measurements made as indicated here:

$$\text{Efficiency factor} = \frac{3{,}384 \text{ cpm}}{2.34 \times 10^6 \text{ dpm}} = 0.00145.$$

We could express this as 0.145%, but to use it in Equation 4-13 we need to keep it in its decimal form. We convert the net count rate of the thyroid measurement to dpm, by dividing by the efficiency factor:

$$\text{dpm}_{thyroid} = \frac{490 \text{ cts}}{0.00145} = 337{,}931 \text{ dpm} \cong 338{,}000 \text{ dpm}.$$

Finally, convert from dpm to µCi:

$$\frac{338{,}000 \text{ disintegrations}}{\text{min}} \times \frac{1 \text{ min}}{60 \text{ sec}} \times \frac{\text{sec}\cdot\text{kBq}}{1{,}000 \text{ disintegrations}} = 5.6 \text{ kBq or } 0.15\,\mu\text{Ci}.$$

In this calculation, we did not take the branching ratio of Ba-133 compared to I-131 into account (see Sample Calculation 4-6).

Note that the efficiency factor is good only for measurements made under exactly the same conditions as when the efficiency factor was determined. If anything changes, a new efficiency factor must be determined. Good practice standards require that the efficiency factor be determined at least annually (6).

Sample Calculation 4-6   Efficiency Factors with Branching Ratios

Complete Sample Calulation 4-5 by incorporating the branching ratios of the two radionuclides involved. The branching ratios are

- Ba-133, γ_8: 0.621 gamma ray emitted per transition
- I-131, γ_{14}: 0.812 gamma ray emitted per transition

Using Equation 4-14, we get

$$\mathrm{dpm}_{\text{thyroid}} = \left(\frac{490 \text{ cpm}}{0.00145}\right)\left(\frac{0.621}{0.812}\right)$$
$$= 258{,}442 \text{ dpm} \approx 258{,}000 \text{ dpm}$$

$$\frac{258{,}000 \text{ disintegrations}}{\text{min}} \times \frac{1 \text{ min}}{60 \text{ sec}} \times \frac{\text{sec} \cdot \text{kBq}}{1{,}000 \text{ disintegrations}} = 4.3 \text{ kBq or } 0.12 \text{ }\mu\text{Ci}.$$

Summary

We often assume that radiation detectors measure exactly what we put in front of them. The point of this chapter is that measurements of radioactive samples are subject to many variables beyond the actual fact of the amount of radioactivity present. When these variables come into play, we no longer have a one-to-one relationship between the counts measured and the amount of radioactivity present. It is important that the technologist know about these factors and recognize when they are affecting a measurement, to ensure that an accurate measurement is obtained.

References

1. Lombardi MH. *Radiation Safety in Nuclear Medicine*. Boca Raton, FL: CRC Press; 1999:59.
2. Knoll GF. *Radiation Detection and Measurement*. 3rd ed. New York, NY: John Wiley & Sons; 2000:121–123, 310, 596, 629, 632–636.
3. Cherry SR, Sorenson JA, Phelps ME. *Physics in Nuclear Medicine*. 3rd ed. Philadelphia, PA: Saunders; 2003:152, 165, 181–182.
4. Wells P. *Practical Mathematics for Nuclear Medicine*. Reston, VA: Society of Nuclear Medicine; 2000:138.
5. Weber DA, Eckerman KF, Dillman LT, Ryman JC. *MIRD: Radionuclide Data and Decay Schemes*. New York, NY: Society of Nuclear Medicine; 1989:229, 271.
6. Zanzonico P. Routine quality control of clinical nuclear medicine instrumentation: a brief review. *J Nucl Med*. 2008;49:1114–1131.

Additional Resources

Cherry SR, Sorenson JA, Phelps ME. *Physics in Nuclear Medicine*. 3rd ed. Philadelphia, PA: Saunders; 2003:Chapters 9–12.

Knoll GF. *Radiation Detection and Measurement*. 3rd ed. New York, NY: John Wiley & Sons; 2000:Chapters 3, 4, 10, 11.

Wells P. *Practical Mathematics for Nuclear Medicine*. Reston, VA: Society of Nuclear Medicine; 2000:Chapter 4.

PART II

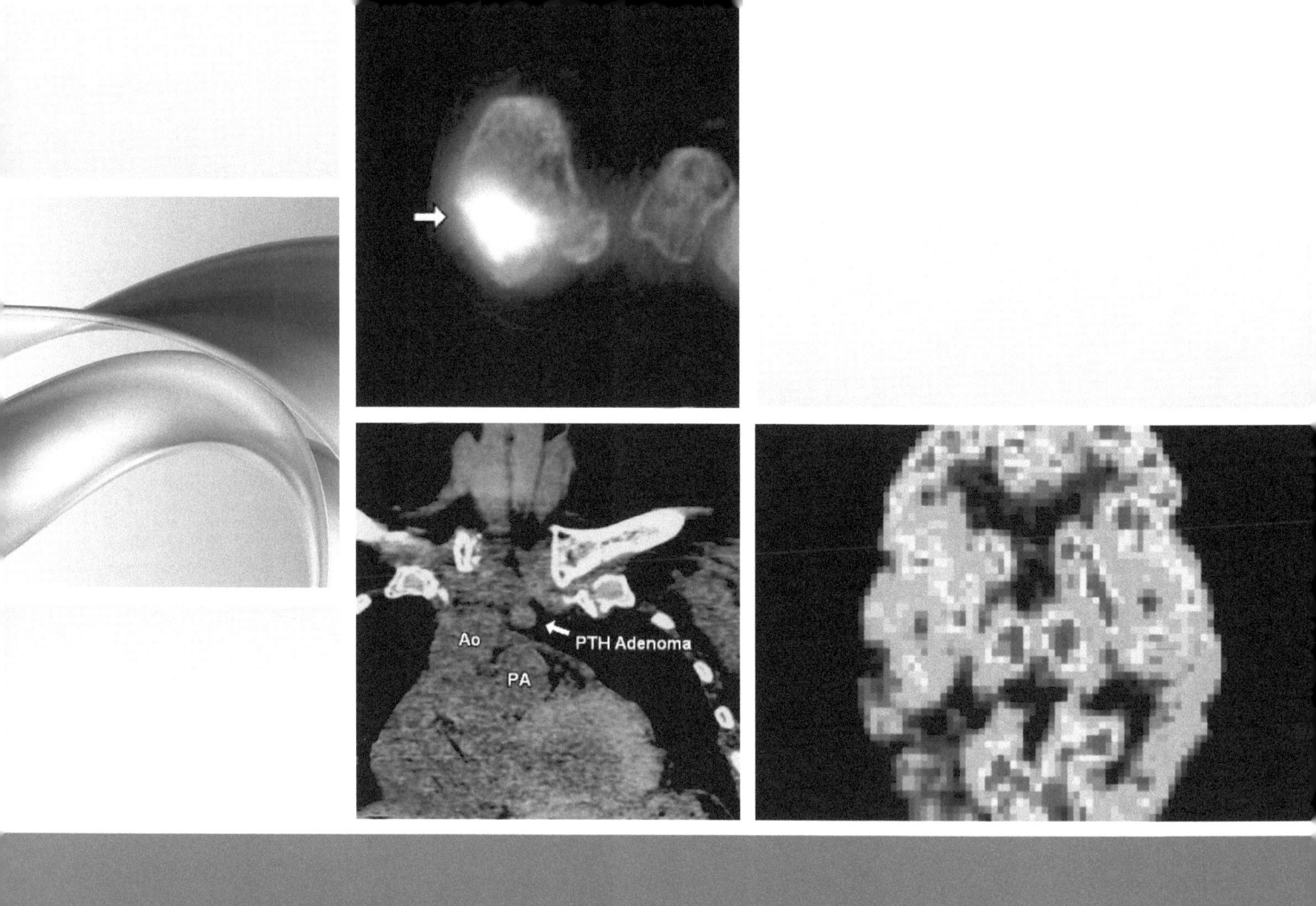

Gamma Camera

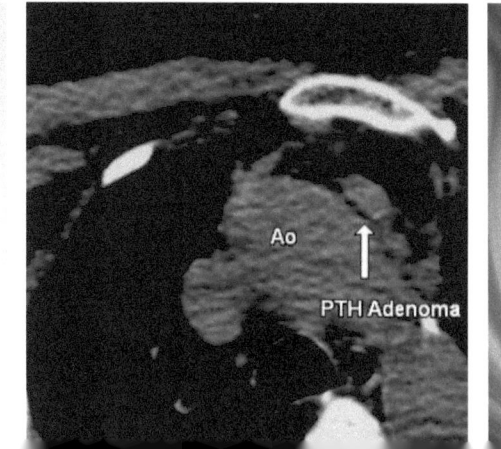

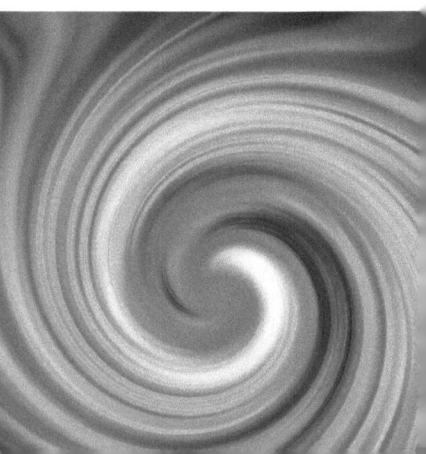

CHAPTER 5: The Gamma Camera

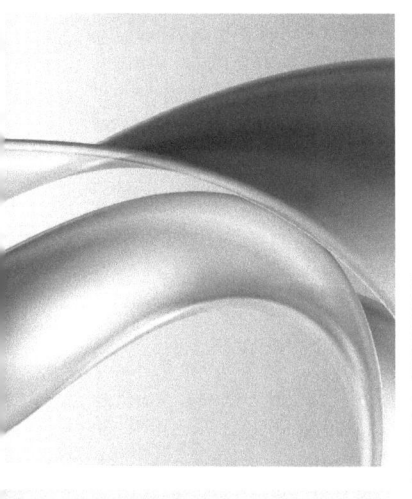

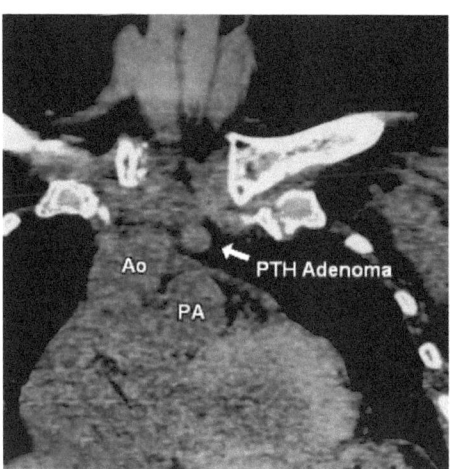

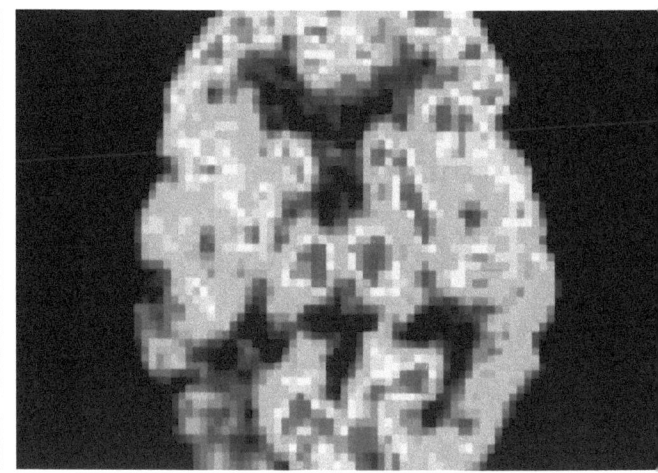

Learning Outcomes

1. Define *uniformity*, *spatial resolution*, and *sensitivity* as these terms apply to gamma cameras.
2. Describe the basic concepts behind Anger's gamma camera, including its positioning logic, the need for energy normalization of the event position, and the requirement for a collimator.
3. Outline the improvements made over the years to Anger's camera design.
4. Discuss the need and the methods used for energy, linearity, and uniformity correction as well as the concomitant need for autotuning of photomultiplier tubes.
5. Describe the use of a gamma camera, including
   a. Patient positioning
   b. Operation and imaging modes
   c. Care
6. Briefly characterize planar gamma cameras not using Anger's positioning logic.

Introduction

The instruments we have discussed so far (Geiger counters, dose calibrators, and scintillation detectors) were well developed by the mid-1950s, but they were not sufficient in themselves to justify the existence of the specialty of nuclear medicine. A device was needed that could create images of gamma rays, allowing the visualization of the distribution of a radiopharmaceutical in the body. This chapter examines the essential operation of the *gamma camera* (also called the *scintillation camera*) invented by Hal Anger, which is the most important instrument that most nuclear medicine professionals work with. We consider briefly the rectilinear scanner (the forerunner of the gamma camera) and the development of the gamma camera. We then look at the operation of Anger's camera as originally designed, discuss improvements that have been incorporated over the last 40 years, and consider guidelines for its use and care. Finally, we examine some newer gamma cameras based on different types of detectors and/or different electronics.

Three terms that describe primary operational characteristics of a gamma camera are:

- *Uniformity*: the ability of a gamma camera to produce a uniform image in response to a uniform source of gamma rays.
- *Sensitivity*: the ability of a gamma camera to use the gamma rays available to it.
- *Resolution*: the ability of a gamma camera to reproduce the details of a nonuniform source of gamma rays (this is spatial resolution, rather than energy resolution).

Uniformity, sensitivity, and resolution are characteristics that depend on the construction of the camera. Uniformity can be improved through the use of electronic manipulations, a topic that is addressed in this chapter. Resolution and sensitivity are highly dependent on the choice of collimator.

Historical Background

Even before the development of nuclear reactors and particle accelerators, which made possible the artificial production of radionuclides, ways to apply the newfound phenomenon of radioactivity to medicine had been discovered. But through the mid-1940s, the only instrument available to measure radioactivity was the Geiger counter. In 1948, Robert Hofstader developed the scintillation detector, using sodium iodide as the radiation-detecting material and a photomultiplier tube (PMT) to convert the resulting scintillation photons into an electronic signal.

The Rectilinear Scanner

In 1949, Benedict Cassen began to work on the idea of coupling a scintillation detector to a mechanical scanning apparatus as a way to record the two-dimensional biodistribution of a radiopharmaceutical in a patient (**Figure 5-1**). The scintillation detector moved back and forth over the patient, registering the count rate at each location. The count rate value in turn controlled the intensity of a light source moving over a film. The generic term *scans* for nuclear medicine images derives from this imaging technique.

The need to physically move the scanner necessitated long imaging times, ranging from 10 to 60 minutes. Moreover, the extended time required to obtain a single image meant that this technology was not adaptable to dynamic studies, thus precluding many studies of organ function. Despite these drawbacks, rectilinear scanning was used for more than 20 years, reaching its peak in 1973 (1). It demonstrated the potential of radionuclide imaging and therefore was an important starting point for the field of nuclear medicine.

Development of the Anger Gamma Camera

The limitations of the rectilinear scanner prompted the development of the gamma camera by Hal Anger in 1958 (2). (Dr. Anger also developed the well counter in 1950 and the first positron camera based on coincident detection of annihilation photons in 1959 [3].) His key insight was that the location of a gamma ray interaction could be determined by the distribution of scintillation light among many PMTs. The positioning determination in Anger's system went beyond just localization of an event to a specific PMT, which would have been unsatisfactory due to the large size of the PMTs, which were about 3 inches in diameter at that time. Instead, Anger used capacitors to modify the measured signal at each PMT, based on the PMT's position relative to the face of a scintillation crystal (a more complete explanation follows). *Anger positioning logic* (as it has come to be known) is described by one author in this way (1): "determination of the pattern and strength of the voltage signals in the individual tubes [identifies] the positions of the scintillations on the crystal." Using this system, the location of a gamma ray interaction on the camera face could be determined to within about 5 mm. Mapping a radiopharmaceutical distribution in a patient thus became a function of the two-dimensional area of the camera face, rather than the changing location of the detector over the patient. A large scintillation crystal, as wide as a patient, could be utilized to obtain an image over an entire organ, eliminating the need for scanning motion. Further, the energy deposited by the interaction could be determined from the sum of the PMT signals, allowing for energy discrimination and rejection of (some) scattered gamma rays.

However, a large-diameter scintillation crystal would register any gamma ray traveling at any angle. Even a point source of radioactivity would illumine the entire crystal, generating a large circle of radiation interactions. In a complex object such as a patient, areas of low radiopharmaceutical uptake would be "filled in" by gamma rays from other areas traveling at oblique angles, and no definition would be achieved. So between the crystal and the patient, Anger added a *collimator* (essentially a lead sheet with many tiny holes or channels through it). The collimator allows the gamma rays traveling in the "correct" direction (usually perpendicular to the face of the camera) to pass through the holes and interact in the scintillation crystal, and the collimator absorbs those with other trajectories.

Anger's invention debuted in commercial form in 1962, but it was not well received at first. To better visualize details, Anger used a thin (0.25-in) sodium iodide scintillation crystal. Most radiopharmaceuticals available at that time used high-energy radionuclides such as I-131 and Hg-203, for which the thicker scintillation crystal of the rectilinear scanner was better suited. Fortuitously, the introduction of lower-energy radionuclides, and concomitant development of methodologies for radiopharmaceutical chemistry, made Anger's camera a success. Technetium-99m, first discovered in 1938, was made available from molybdenum-99 generators in 1960, and radiopharmaceutical kits using Tc-99m were developed by the late 1960s. The confluence of these two developments paved the way for the success of the field of nuclear medicine.

Basic Concepts of Anger's Camera

Overview

Before getting into the nitty-gritty of how the gamma camera works, we look at the big picture. The big picture has two distinct parts: before the gamma rays reach the scintillation crystal and after they are absorbed. **Figure 5-2** shows a cross section of an object containing a radioactive distribution, being imaged by a gamma camera with a parallel-hole collimator. Gamma rays emitted in the object have a variety of possible fates. They can travel in a direction perpendicular to the camera face, passing through one of the holes in the collimator and interacting (usually via a photoelectric interaction) in the scintillation crystal (path *a* in Fig. 5-2). It is these events that we desire to record, because they most accurately depict the position of the radioactivity in the object.

But a number of other outcomes are also possible. A gamma ray could be traveling at something other than a perpendicular angle to the camera face (such as path *b*),

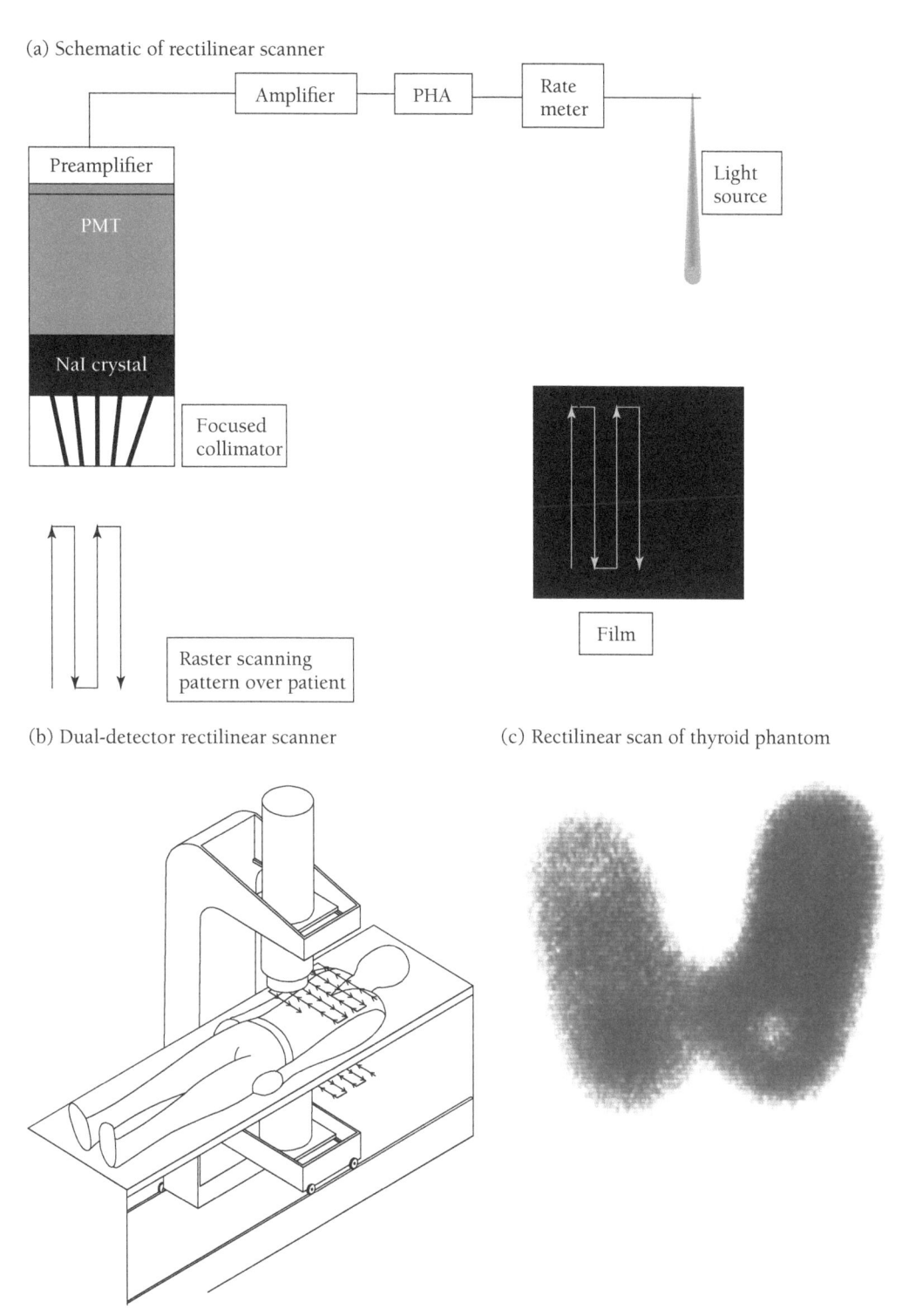

Figure 5-1 Rectilinear scanner. The first nuclear medicine imaging device utilized a single-PMT scintillation detector, similar to a thyroid probe, which scanned back and forth over the patient in a raster pattern. The detector was mechanically linked to a light source, which illuminated a film in proportion to the count rate detected at each location over the patient. The scanner used a thick scintillation crystal (2 in) and a heavy, focused collimator, well suited to absorption of high-energy gamma rays. Figure 5-1b and 5-1c reprinted from: Rollo FD. *Nuclear Medicine Physics, Instrumentation, and Agents*. St. Louis, MO: Mosby-Year Book; 1977. Used with permission of Dr. Rollo.

in which case it is giving incorrect positional information (i.e., the gamma ray's location of interaction in the crystal is different from its point of emission in the object). These events are ideally absorbed by the collimator, to keep them from becoming part of the image. A gamma ray may be scattered within the object, such that its final trajectory takes it through a collimator hole and into the scintillation crystal, but its interaction location does not accurately depict its point of origin in the object (path *c*). We may be able to eliminate some of these scatter events because they have decreased energy relative to the energy window. Finally, a gamma ray may undergo photoelectric

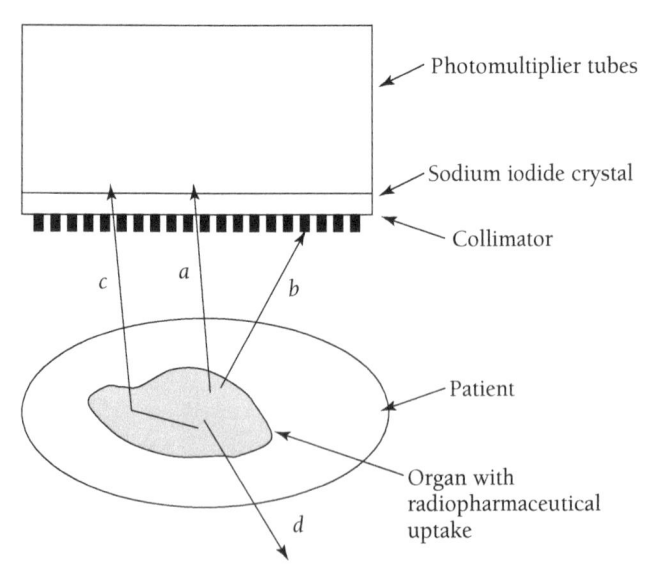

Figure 5-2 Photon paths from patient to collimator. The "front end" of a gamma camera, depicts several paths that gamma rays coming from an object with an internal radiopharmaceutical might take. Path *a* represents a "good" gamma ray that travels more or less perpendicularly into the crystal, passing through the object and a collimator hole without interacting with either. Path *b* shows a gamma ray, traveling in a direction not perpendicular to the crystal face, that is absorbed by the collimator. A gamma ray might be scattered to an angle that allows it to pass through the collimator, but is a "bad" event because its location of interaction in the crystal does not correspond to its location of origin in the object (path *c*). Finally, in path *d*, a gamma ray is emitted in a direction that does not allow it to be registered by the gamma camera.

camera shown in **Figure 5-3**). The gamma rays that successfully traverse the collimator are absorbed in the scintillation crystal. We refer to these absorbed gamma rays as "events." They produce scintillation photons that spread isotropically from the point of interaction. Scintillation light is absorbed by a number of PMTs, each of which converts the light it receives to an electronic signal. The signals from the PMTs are combined to determine the location and energy of the gamma ray's interaction in the scintillation crystal (as explained in the next section). Each event produces three output signals: the X and Y signals indicate the event's location, and the Z signal indicates its energy (based on the linear relationship between gamma ray energy and the total number of scintillation photons produced). If the event's energy is within the designated energy window (i.e., the Z signal meets the requirements of the pulse height analyzer [PHA]), then its X and Y coordinates are passed on to an image-recording device. Each accepted event is considered a "count" and is added to the camera's count register.

Thus, an image acquired with a gamma camera is a collection of counts; the number of counts at different locations is determined by the distribution of radioactivity within the object being imaged. A nuclear medicine image is acquired over time, similar to a time exposure on a photographic camera, in which the shutter of the camera is left open for a long enough period to properly expose the film inside. Stated more generally, the imaging time is extended so that enough counts are registered to produce a readable image. This number depends on the characteristics of the imaging situation and of the organ and/or physiologic process being imaged.

absorption in the object or may be emitted in a direction that does not bring it into contact with the gamma camera (path *d*). These events are not available for imaging.

The second part of the big picture occurs inside the gamma camera (refer to the schematic diagram of a gamma

Anger Positioning Logic

The key to understanding the gamma camera is its method of determining the location of each gamma ray interaction.

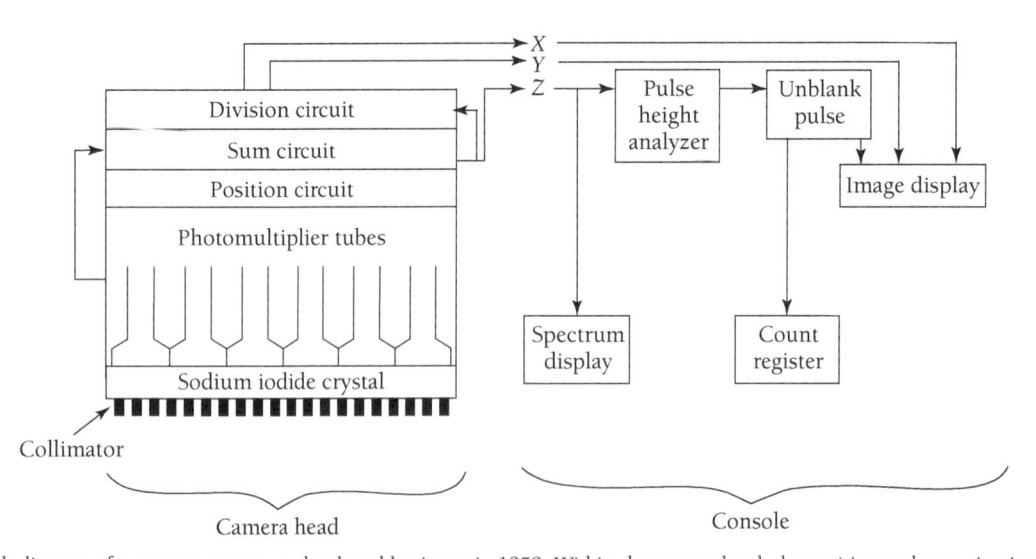

Figure 5-3 Block diagram of a gamma camera, as developed by Anger in 1958. Within the camera head, the position and sum circuits receive input from all PMTs. The sum circuit totals these to create the Z pulse. The position circuits determine the location of each event according to the Anger positioning logic described in the text. The X and Y position signals are normalized to event energy by the division circuit. The console includes the pulse height analyzer, the spectrum display, and the count register; a variety of image display devices may be part of or separate from the console.

Chapter 5: The Gamma Camera

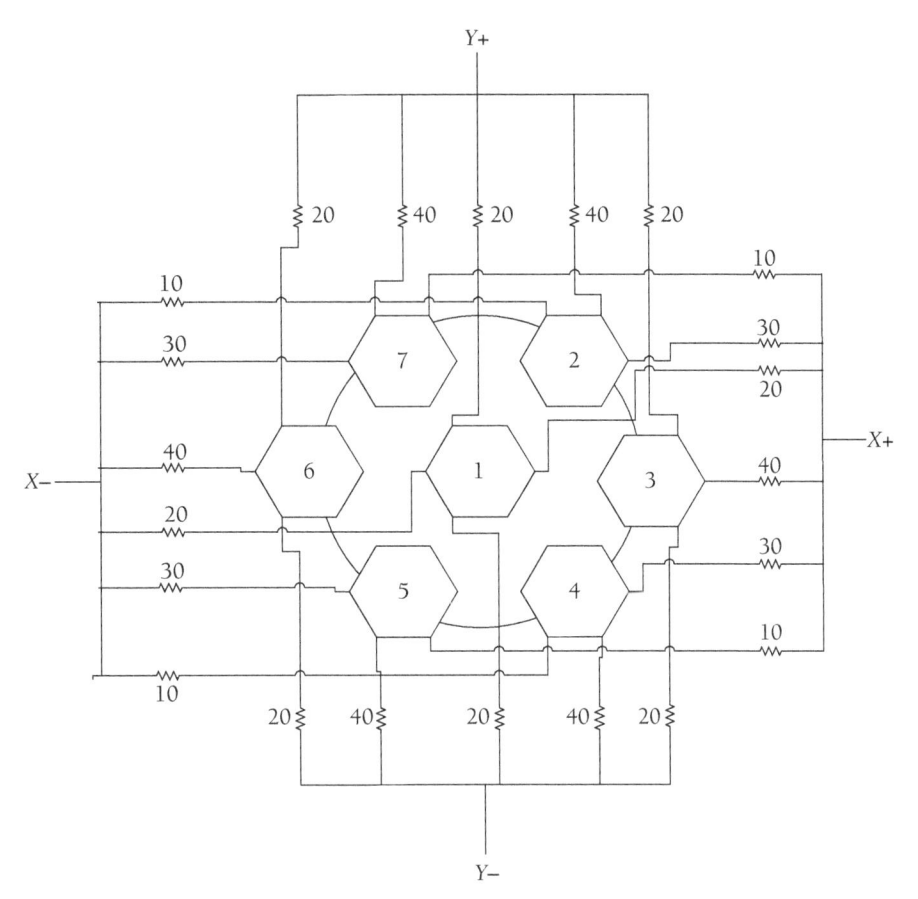

Figure 5-4 Anger's original position circuitry. Anger used a 4-in-diameter scintillation crystal and seven PMTs, connected via Y− (as opposed to Y+) resistors to the four position circuits. The value of each capacitor or resistor is represented here as a weighting factor, which depends on the proximity of a PMT to a given position circuit. For example, PMT 5 contributes significantly to the Y− position circuit and is therefore given a high weighting factor of 40 in that circuit. It contributes very little to the X+ circuit, and so has a weighting factor of only 10 in that circuit.

A diagram of a small seven-PMT gamma camera as originally described by Anger (2) is shown in **Figure 5-4**. The crystal face is given X− and Y− axes that cross at its center; the event location will be determined relative to these axes. There are four *position circuits*, labeled X+, X−, Y+, and Y−. Each PMT is connected to one or more of these circuits. A capacitor located along the wire connecting the PMT to a position circuit acts as a weighting factor for signals from that PMT, relative to its contribution to that position circuit.

The gamma camera operates in pulse mode, treating the scintillation photons from a single event as a unit. Most gamma ray interactions will generate the largest signal in the PMT that sits above the place where the interaction occurred. Surrounding PMTs will see smaller amounts of light. However, the surrounding PMTs that are closest to the interaction will absorb a greater amount of scintillation light. The effect of these secondary signals is to "pull" the point of the interaction to a specific point under the PMT that saw the most scintillation light. Within the gamma camera, the PMT signals, modified by the appropriate weighting factors, are sent to all four position circuits. The X− and Y− outputs are subtracted from the X+ and Y+ outputs, respectively, and the resulting X and Y values indicate the event's location relative to (0, 0) at the center of the *field of view* (FOV). This is illustrated in **Figure 5-5a**.

A couple of important complicating factors need to be considered here. One is that the position signals must be normalized to the total energy of the event. This is accomplished by dividing the X and Y position signals by the Z (total PMT output) signal. If this normalization is not done, two events interacting at the same location, but with different energies, will be mapped to different locations (Fig. 5-5b).

The second complicating factor is what happens at the edge of the scintillation crystal. Gamma rays may scatter off the side of the crystal or the detector housing, such that more are detected near the edge. In addition, position determination by Anger's technique becomes inaccurate as the outer ring of the PMTs is reached, because there are no farther-out PMTs to pull events into their correct positions. Hence many events are incorrectly positioned at or near the edge of the FOV. This phenomenon is called *edge packing*, and up to 50% of all counts may be seen in this area (4). Edge packing is usually masked, either with a lead ring in the collimator or by limiting the displayed FOV electronically to exclude it.

(a) Event located to left of center

PMT	Output	X+	X−	Y+	Y−
1	8	160	160	160	160
2	1	30	10	40	0
3	1	40	0	20	20
4	1	30	10	0	40
5	3	30	90	0	120
6	5	0	200	100	100
7	3	30	90	120	0
Total	22	320	560	440	440

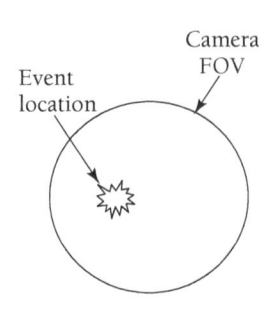

Unnormalized: $X = 320 + (-560) = -240$ $Y = 440 + (-440) = 0$

Normalized: $X = \dfrac{320 + (-560)}{22} = -10.9$ $Y = \dfrac{440 + (-440)}{22} = 0$

(b) Event in same location as event (a) above, but with 10% less energy

PMT	Output	X+	X−	Y+	Y−
1	7.2	144	144	144	144
2	0.9	27	9	36	0
3	0.9	36	0	18	18
4	0.9	27	9	0	36
5	2.7	27	81	0	108
6	4.5	0	180	90	90
7	2.7	27	81	108	0
Total	19.8	288	504	396	396

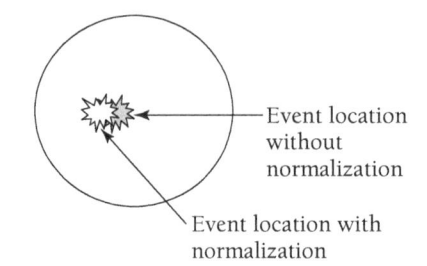

Unnormalized: $X = 288 + (-504) = -216$ $Y = 396 + (-396) = 0$

Normalized: $X = \dfrac{288 + (-504)}{19.8} = -10.9$ $Y = \dfrac{396 + (-396)}{19.8} = 0$

Figure 5-5 Determination of event location. Figure 5-5a illustrates the implementation of Anger positioning logic and is based on the gamma camera diagrammed in Figure 5-4. PMT 1 sees most of the scintillation light generated by the event, but that detected by PMTs 5, 6, and 7 pulls the event location to the left of center. Figure 5-5b demonstrates the need for normalization by event energy. The event in Figure 5-5b is in the exact same location as the event in Figure 5-5a, but has 10% lower energy, as shown by the PMT output signals. If the events are not normalized by dividing by the total of the PMT outputs, the events map to different locations. When normalization to the total of the PMT outputs is carried out, they map to the same location.

Anger Gamma Camera Components

With this overall understanding of the workings of a gamma camera, we can go back and examine each component of the system shown in Figure 5-3. This section covers the elements of gamma cameras as they were constructed through the early 1980s. The next two sections then discuss more recent modifications utilizing digital electronics.

Collimator

The collimator essentially projects the gamma ray distribution onto the scintillation crystal by allowing detection of only those gamma rays that pass through its holes. Gamma rays traveling at undesired angles are (ideally) absorbed by the lead septa between the holes. The angle, diameter, and length of the holes and the thickness of the lead between them determine in large measure both the quality of the images created by the camera and the time required to obtain those images. Collimators can be made to different specifications to maximize either sensitivity or resolution. The three operational characteristics of uniformity, resolution, and sensitivity can be measured either *intrinsically* (without a collimator) or *extrinsically* (with a collimator).

Scintillation Crystal

Sodium iodide is used to this day in gamma cameras due to its excellent scintillation light output and resulting good energy resolution. A scintillation crystal in a modern gamma camera may be circular, rectangular, or square, and its largest dimension may measure up to 20 in. Although gamma cameras are used to image a broad range of gamma ray energies, the thickness of the scintillation crystal (commonly $\frac{3}{8}-\frac{5}{8}$ in) makes them optimally suited for the 100- to 200-keV range. The crystal is *hygroscopic* (absorbs water) and must be hermetically sealed. As with the scintillation detector, the backside of the crystal (opposite the collimator) is optically coupled to the light pipe or the PMTs to prevent reflection of scintillation photons away from the PMT array. Each PMT in Anger's camera has its own preamplifier and amplifier.

Light Pipe and Photomultiplier Tubes

The determination of event location depends on the distribution of scintillation light among several PMTs. But PMTs are not uniformly sensitive to scintillation light. The photoemissive layer of each PMT's photocathode is thickest at the center, making the center more likely to absorb scintillation photons than the periphery. Thus, when PMTs are coupled directly to a scintillation crystal, the outline of each PMT is seen.

Anger incorporated a light pipe (a sheet of optical-quality plastic) into his gamma camera to minimize this effect. The light pipe was machined to refract scintillation photons away from the dead spaces between the PMTs. The areas of the light pipe corresponding to the centers of the PMTs were painted black to absorb some scintillation photons, so as to correct for the increased sensitivity at the PMT centers. High-quality optical coupling grease was used to couple the PMTs to the light pipe. Ultimately, however, the light pipe was a less than satisfactory solution to the problem of the nonlinear PMT response. Further efforts to improve gamma camera performance led to more sophisticated solutions to this problem, which are discussed later in this chapter. These in turn have eliminated the need for a light pipe in most modern cameras.

Position, Sum, and Division Circuits

As discussed previously, the Anger *position circuits* use multiple PMTs and a hardwired capacitor or resistor matrix to locate the position of each gamma ray interaction relative to the X- and Y-axes. The *sum circuit* totals the output signals of all of the PMTs and creates the Z pulse; this represents the energy that the gamma ray deposited in the crystal. The Z pulse is used in several places. First, it is compared to the PHA discriminators to determine whether the event's energy is within the window set by the operator. Second, it is sent to the *division circuit* to normalize the X and Y signals in order to correctly position an event (i.e., the normalization illustrated in Fig. 5-5b). Finally, it is sent to a spectrum display so that the operator may compare the energy spectrum from the radionuclide being imaged to the window(s) set on the PHA.

Pulse Height Analyzer

Like the scintillation detector, the gamma camera uses an energy window to identify the photopeak energy of the radionuclide being imaged. The operator chooses the appropriate percentage window and centers that window on the photopeak visualized on the spectrum display. This in turn determines the settings of the lower- and upper-level discriminators of the PHA. The PHA allows us to eliminate at least some of the events that follow path c in Figure 5-2, because they have lost energy through one or more Compton scattering events. Gamma cameras generally offer three PHA energy windows, allowing for simultaneous acquisition of photons from multiple photopeaks or multiple radionuclides. The PHA output pulse, called the *unblank pulse*, is sent to the count register and to an imaging device and/or computer matrix for inclusion in the final image.

Cathode Ray Tube

Prior to the advent of digital electronics, images were created via a photographic device called a *cathode ray tube* (CRT) (its operation is further described in Appendix B). The CRT receives the X and Y signals from every event and uses them to change the potentials at horizontal and vertical deflector plates. The *unblank pulse* from the PHA turns on (unblanks) an electron source, creating a small burst of electrons in the CRT. The electron burst is focused and accelerated toward the CRT's phosphor screen by accelerating electrodes, and its direction of travel is modified by the potentials at the two deflector plates. On arrival at the phosphor screen, it causes the screen to emit phosphorescent light, which in turn exposes a film, creating a black dot. The final image consists of many dots, whose two-dimensional distribution represents the distribution of the radiopharmaceutical in the object being imaged.

Modern Gamma Cameras

Most modern gamma cameras have two camera heads (**Figure 5-6**); three-headed cameras are available, and a four-headed camera has been produced. Different sizes are available, but the most common size is a rectangle in the neighborhood of 38 × 50 cm (15 × 20 in). Virtually all cameras are capable of longitudinal and/or rotational motion. Utilizing rectangular crystals, software techniques, and head-to-toe scanning, whole-body images can be easily produced. Rotational imaging allows for the creation of tomographic images. These advances have greatly improved both the imaging capabilities and the productivity of nuclear medicine departments.

Digital Image Display and Storage

Since the early 1980s, nuclear medicine images have been digitized. An *image matrix* with many storage locations is created in computer memory prior to image acquisition. Each storage location corresponds to a small portion of the camera's FOV. These small squares are called picture elements, or *pixels*. Every count accepted by the PHA is assigned to a pixel, according to its X and Y values. As the image is acquired, the number of counts assigned to each pixel increases, relative to the activity in the corresponding part of the object. Once acquired and electronically stored, the image is displayed using a color scale to represent the number of counts in each pixel. Choice of the image matrix size is an important one.

Photomultiplier Tubes

PMTs have changed considerably since Anger's invention. They have decreased in diameter from 3 in to about 2 in and are generally made with a square or hexagonal face rather than a round face, which allows for closer packing. Modern gamma cameras have 60 to 120 PMTs. Advances in PMT construction and choice of photoemissive material have increased their efficiency and decreased the amount of background noise produced. Software allows for *thresholding* of PMT response, so that only the PMTs in the

(a) Gamma camera with two heads in 90° orientation

(b) Gamma camera with two heads in 180° orientation

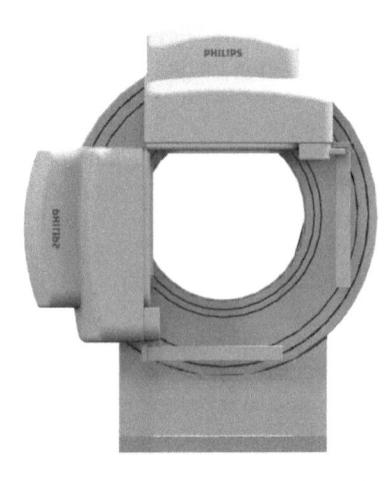

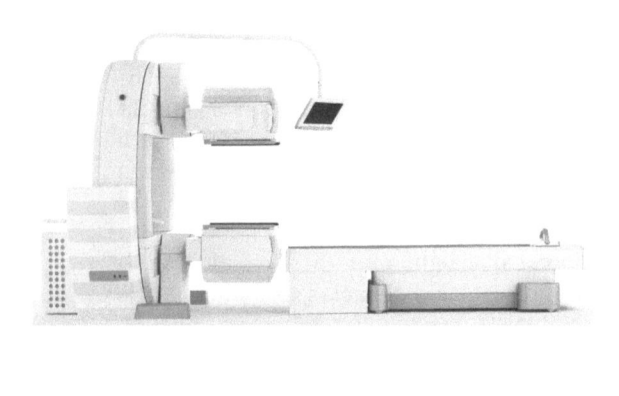

Figure 5-6 Two examples of modern gamma cameras. Both mount two camera heads on a circular gantry, allowing for rotation around the imaging table. The camera in Figure 5-6a shows the two heads in a 90° orientation, which is commonly used for cardiac SPECT imaging. The camera in Figure 5-6b has a computer screen that mirrors some of the information on the acquisition terminal, such as a real-time depiction of counts (i.e., a persistence scope) and a time-elapsed/time-remaining graphic. Both systems allow the imaging table to move in a head-to-toe direction for a whole-body scan. Figure 5-6a courtesy of Philips Healthcare. Figure 5-6b courtesy of Siemens Healthcare.

immediate vicinity of an event are included in the position determination (**Figure 5-7**). Because PMTs that are far from an event produce a signal that is largely noise, thresholding improves the precision of event localization. It also allows for simultaneous detection of multiple events, as only a few PMTs are involved in the detection of any one event.

Electronics

The advent of fast electronic microprocessors has brought about significant changes in the gamma camera. PMT output signals are digitized rather than passing through the resistor matrix as in Anger's design. This allows the sum and position circuits also to be digitized, such that the position of an event can be determined via a software algorithm or a lookup table. The light pipe has been removed in most cameras, and the necessary corrections are made digitally to compensate for the nonuniformity of PMT response. Corrections needed to improve image uniformity (see the following section) are also applied digitally. Digitization of the X and Y signals dovetails nicely with the creation of an image within a computer matrix.

Uniformity Corrections and Autotuning

Uniformity is defined as the ability of a gamma camera to reproduce a uniform radioactive distribution. It can be described as the camera's spatially dependent sensitivity. It is evaluated daily, by exposing the camera to a uniform source of radioactivity in a *flood image*. An ideal flood image has only small variations in count density (cts/cm^2 or cts/pixel) from one area of the image to another. This variation can be quantified; a larger value indicates a less uniform flood.

Causes of Nonuniformity

The ability to produce a uniform distribution of counts in response to a uniform field of gamma rays is not an inherent property of gamma cameras. The most significant cause of nonuniformity is the response differential as one moves from the edge to the center of a PMT (**Figure 5-8**). Because a PMT is less responsive to scintillation photons around the edges of its photocathode surface, events that should be positioned between two PMTs are actually directed toward one or the other. The result is the mispositioning of events, which results in hotter and colder areas on a flood image and nonlinearity of straight-line objects. Another cause of nonuniformity is nonuniform

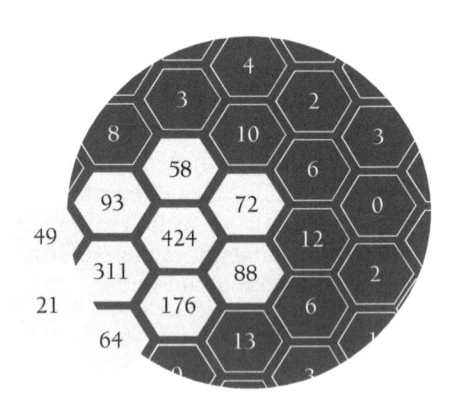

Figure 5-7 Thresholding. Modern electronics allow the gamma camera to limit the PMTs contributing to an event's location by requiring a signal of some minimum size from each PMT. In the diagram, the threshold is 20, so only the light gray PMTs are used to determine the location of the gamma ray interaction. This eliminates the contributions from distant PMTs, which most likely are not generated by the event itself, but rather are manifestations of noise. In addition, thresholding allows the possibility of simultaneous detection of multiple events, as only a few PMTs are required for the position determination of an individual event.

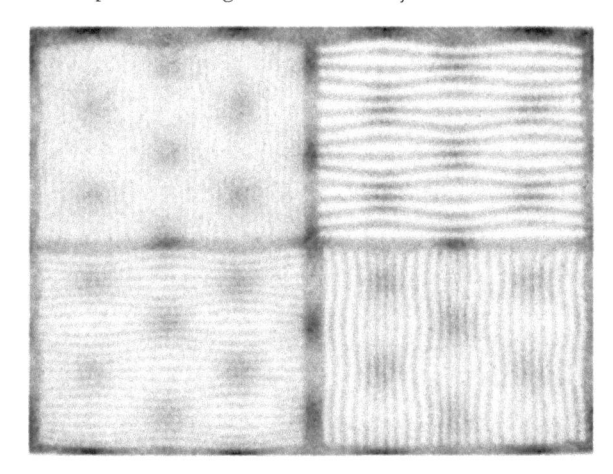

Figure 5-8 Nonuniformity of PMT response. Figure 5-8a shows four locations relative to a single PMT coupled to a large sodium iodide crystal. The expected and actual responses are shown in Figure 5-8b. Based on the equidistant spacing of the four points in Figure 5-8a, Anger positioning logic assumes that the PMT output changes in a linear fashion (the dashed line in Fig. 5-8b). But in fact, the output function has a Gaussian shape, making event localization more difficult to determine, both at the edges and at the center of the PMT. Figure 5-8c shows a bar phantom image with no corrections for the nonuniform response of the PMTs. The nonlinear bars result from events being "pulled" toward the centers of the PMTs (the dark spots). Figures 5-8a and 5-8b adapted from: Madsen M. The scintillation camera. In: *Basic Science of Nuclear Medicine* [CD-ROM]. Reston, VA: Society of Nuclear Medicine; 2001. Used with permission of the Society of Nuclear Medicine. Figure 5-8c courtesy of Group Health Cooperative.

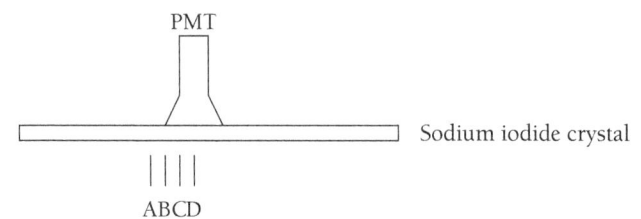

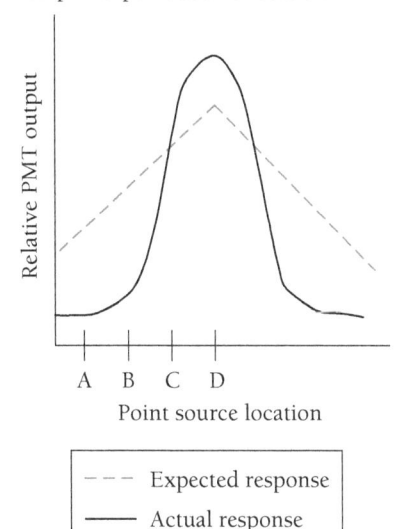

detection efficiency, caused by differences in measured Z pulse size from one point to another. This stems primarily from the nonuniformity of individual PMTs and from variations in the amount of multiplication from one PMT to another.

As Anger's camera design was refined, significant improvements in spatial resolution were made, but these came at the expense of uniformity. The lack of uniform camera response is particularly problematic for SPECT imaging, and so considerable efforts have been made to improve uniformity. These are described in the following sections. The operator should have an in-depth understanding of the layers of correction that are operating in a modern gamma camera.

Uniformity Correction Techniques

In a gamma camera in which no correction for nonuniformity has been applied, the variability in count density from a uniform source can be as much as ±15% of the average, resulting in up to a 30% difference in count density between two points. This can easily be detected by the naked eye, and it must be corrected to do any kind of useful imaging. Historically, the original uniformity correction technique applied to gamma cameras was known as *point-source sensitivity* or *tuning*. It involved adjusting the high voltage to individual PMTs to produce equal count rates across the FOV. Tuning can improve nonuniformity to about ±10% relative to the average. Manual tuning is performed infrequently in modern gamma cameras, because of the large number of PMTs.

Count Skimming or Adding

The advent of fast microprocessor technology in the 1980s initially allowed camera manufacturers to improve uniformity by manipulating count densities, a technique called *count skimming* or *count adding*. In this process, a high-count flood image is analyzed by applying an image matrix to the FOV. The number of counts in each pixel of the matrix is compared to the average across the whole image. These deviations from the average are stored as correction factors for each pixel. Microprocessors then add or subtract counts "on the fly" (as an image is being acquired), according to each pixel's correction factor. For example, if in the flood image a given pixel is too high by 10%, then its microprocessor would "skim off" (i.e., not record) 1 count out of every 10. If a given pixel is too low by 10%, then the microprocessor would double-count every 10th count. Count skimming or adding results in a visually uniform image, with nonuniformity of about ±5%. It does not transfer to gamma rays of different energies, so each different isotope requires a separate correction matrix. Also note that this is a purely cosmetic approach; it does nothing to address the underlying causes of nonuniformity.

Energy and Linearity Corrections

Further advances in microprocessor technology finally allowed manufacturers to deal with the root causes of nonuniformity, namely, the mispositioning and nonuniform detection efficiency noted previously, by storing energy and linearity corrections for each pixel. These correction matrices are determined either at the factory or by field service personnel, and in some cases by the end user. They are applied to images on the fly, even when the image is going directly to film. In completely digital cameras, the corrections can be incorporated into lookup tables that convert measured location and energy to corrected values.

The need for *energy correction* can be demonstrated by a simple illustration. If tuning is done using a point-source sensitivity procedure, the photopeaks at different locations will not be perfectly aligned. But if the energy window used at each location is matched to the photopeak seen at that location, the variation in uniformity over the FOV comes close to what is predicted by Poisson statistics (5). In **Figure 5-9**, the energy spectrum measured at a specific location might be offset by several keV compared to the overall photopeak of the system. Either the PHA window or the local energy spectrum should be shifted to correctly evaluate the energy of events at this location. An event occurring at this location should also have its X and Y position signals normalized by the event energy according to its local energy spectrum, rather than that of the system as a whole. An energy correction matrix is generated that stores the photopeak energy seen by each pixel and applies a ΔZ correction so that the pixel's energy spectrum is aligned with that of the system as a whole. Energy correction circuitry (originally called a *sliding energy window*) therefore more correctly positions each event. It has the added benefit of improving energy resolution (6), allowing the system to eliminate more scatter events. A gamma camera with only energy correction applied still has considerable nonuniformity, but this correction provides the underlying basis for the other corrections.

Event mispositioning, the other main cause of nonuniformity, is caused by the nonlinearity of PMT response (Fig. 5-8). *Linearity correction* information is obtained by imaging micrometrically precise linear phantoms and measuring the amount of displacement needed to produce straight lines in the image (**Figure 5-10**). After acquiring an image of the phantom, a matrix of correction factors is stored for the displacement ΔX that must be added to the X value that is reported by the positioning circuit in order for the line phantom to be exactly reproduced. The phantom is then rotated 90° so that ΔY values can be stored. These ΔX and ΔY correction factor matrices are then further interpolated to create a submatrix of correction factors within each of the original pixels, producing a high-resolution array of correction factors. The displacement corrections must be much more accurate than the gamma camera's X and Y determinations, because any systematic errors will produce visible nonuniformities (7). As an image is acquired, each event is localized to one of these submatrix locations, and the ΔX and ΔY of that

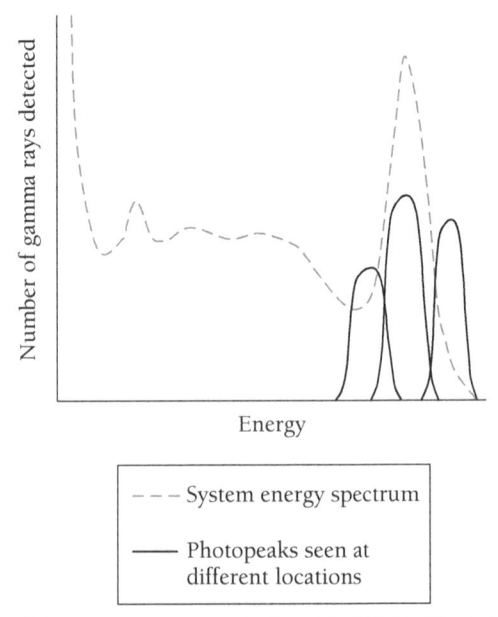

Figure 5-9 Energy spectra as seen by individual PMTs. The dashed line shows the energy spectrum seen by the camera as a whole, the solid lines those photopeaks seen by three PMTs. Because the individual PMTs see the photopeak at slightly different energies, both the energy and the position of events are calculated incorrectly.

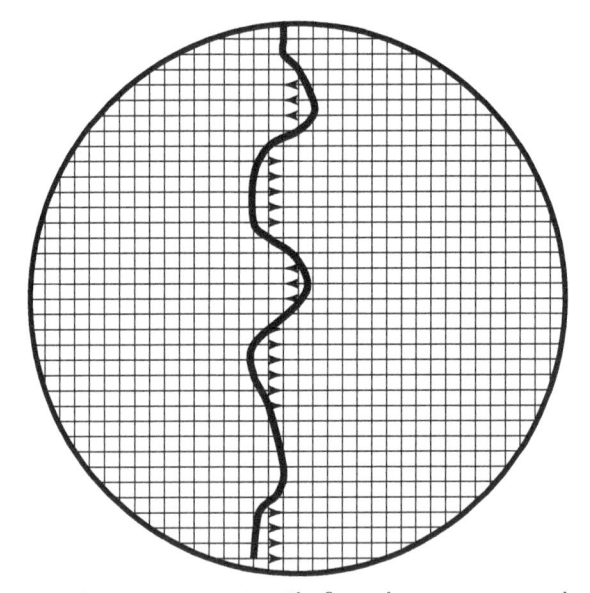

Figure 5-10 Linearity correction. The figure shows an exaggerated example of a linearity phantom applied to a gamma camera without linearity corrections. The arrowheads show some of the displacements necessary to correct for event mispositioning, which would be incorporated into a linearity correction map. Modified from: Simmons G. *The Scintillation Camera*. Reston, VA: Society of Nuclear Medicine; 1988: Fig. 3-4. Used with permission of the Society of Nuclear Medicine.

submatrix location are applied to the event's measured X and Y values.

Energy and linearity corrections greatly improve gamma camera uniformity (**Figure 5-11**) and are used in all modern gamma cameras. Both are applied to images on an event-by-event basis (**Figure 5-12**), resulting in ±3 to 5% nonuniformity. They are stable over time and may be applicable to all imaging conditions and isotopes (depending on the system). Most importantly, this approach leads to a quantitatively correct image, in contrast to count skimming or adding, which by itself only artificially changes the number of counts to get a visually uniform image.

Uniformity Correction Map

Once energy and linearity corrections are in place, the remaining nonuniformity is primarily due to regional variations in sensitivity, for which correction by count skimming or adding is appropriate. Most gamma cameras utilize count skimming or adding techniques in the form of an isotope-specific (and possibly collimator-specific) *uniformity correction map*, to obtain an image with final nonuniformity in the ±1 to 3% range. Uniformity correction maps (also called *sensitivity maps*) are generally acquired on-site, using a high (60–120 million) count acquisition (8). These should be reacquired whenever a gamma camera's measured uniformity deteriorates. Because they are isotope-specific, the operator must remember to change the uniformity correction map when the radionuclide being imaged changes.

Autotuning of Photomultiplier Tubes

Energy and linearity corrections put a greater pressure on the performance of the PMTs, in that the PMTs must be properly tuned and the output of each PMT must be stable if the corrections are to perform properly. Application of energy and linearity corrections assumes that the PMT gains (high-voltage settings) are the same as when those corrections were established. But in fact, PMT gains tend to drift over time, thus potentially invalidating the corrections. As mentioned above, manual tuning is prone to errors with many PMTs, so an automated method is preferred. Modern gamma cameras therefore use some form of *autotuning* to make incremental adjustments of PMT high voltages and preamplifier gains, so that their voltage outputs remain stable and the corrections remain valid. A variety of autotuning methods have been used; a few of the more common ones are discussed here.

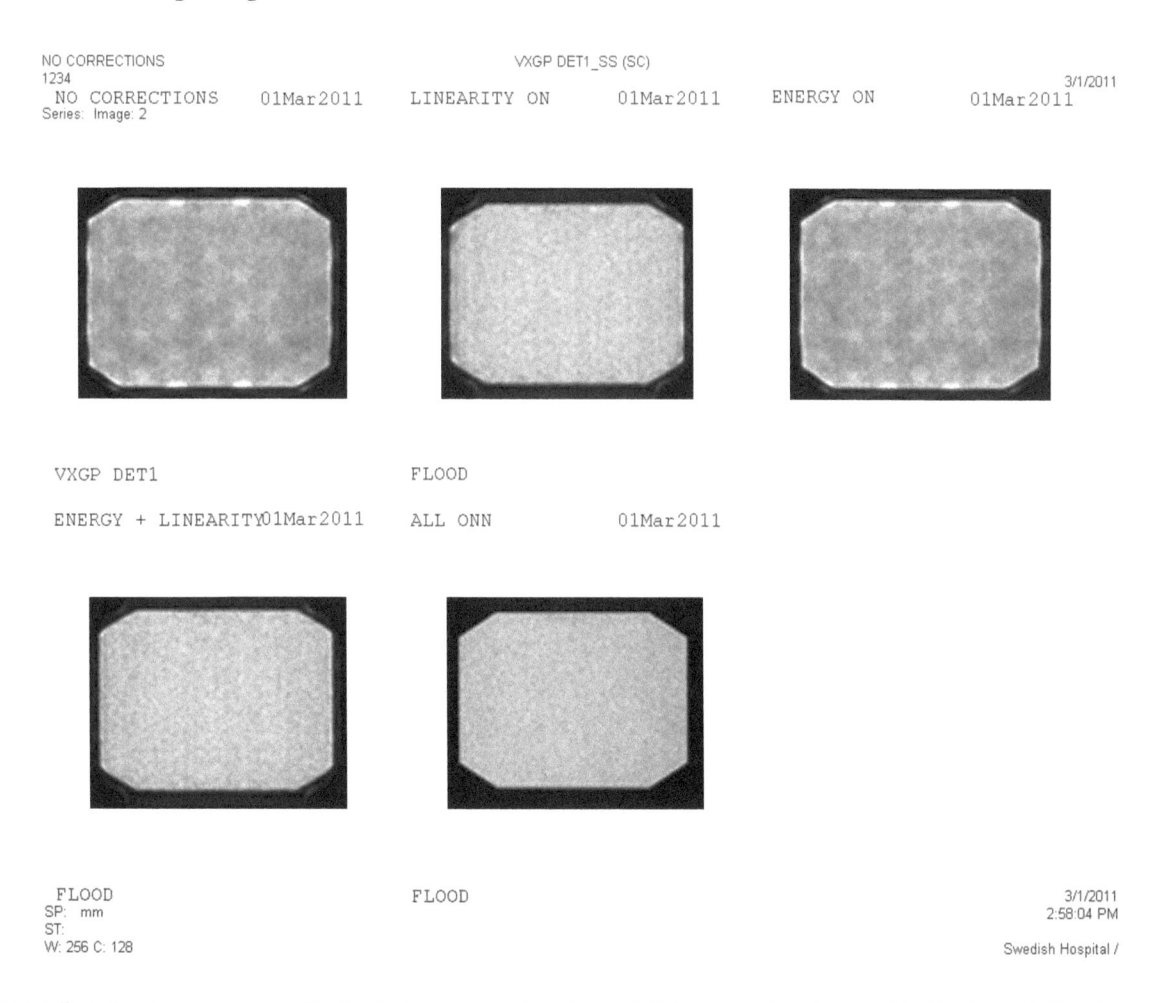

Figure 5-11 Effect of various corrections. The flood with no corrections (upper left) has integral uniformity of 18.2%, that with linearity correction only (upper middle) 7.7%, energy correction only (upper right) 17.8%, energy and linearity (lower left) 6.3%, and all corrections (lower middle) 6.1%. The "all corrections" image includes the uniformity correction map, which includes an electronic edge mask (small areas of activity outside of the flood itself do not appear in the "all on" image). Image courtesy of Swedish Medical Center.

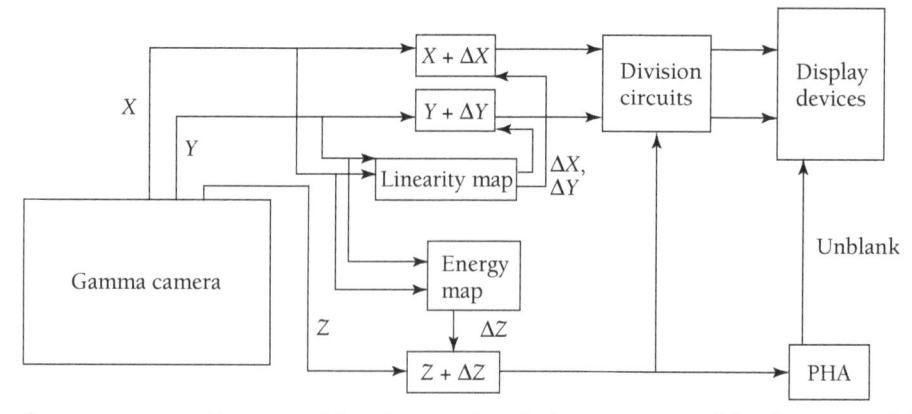

Figure 5-12 Schematic of a gamma camera with energy and linearity corrections. Each event is corrected first for energy and then for location, and the corrected energy is used to normalize the corrected X and Y position signals. Energy correction is accomplished by feeding the X and Y position signals into the energy map, which outputs the position-specific value for ΔZ. The position signals are then sent to the linearity map, where ΔX and ΔY signals are produced. Finally, the position location of the event is determined, using the modified values of $X + \Delta X$, $Y + \Delta Y$, and $Z + \Delta Z$.

Photopeak Monitoring

One technique monitors the photopeak value at each PMT and adjusts the PMT gains relative to a reference value stored during preventive maintenance. This method assumes that PMT drift is a long-term process resulting from the aging of PMTs and their circuits.

Split-Photopeak Monitoring

This approach sets two narrow energy windows on the high side of the photopeak for each PMT. The PMT high voltage is automatically adjusted to keep the number of counts in the two windows at a predetermined ratio. Because this method is dependent on the local count rate, it is applied only to PMTs seeing a significant number of counts; those PMTs not registering that number of counts are assumed not to need gain adjustment at the moment. This method assumes that PMT function is best assessed by its response to a gamma ray flux.

LED Monitoring

Another method uses light-emitting diodes (LEDs), either one in each PMT or a single LED in the detector housing that is seen by all PMTs. The LED produces a flash of light at regular intervals. This light flash generates a large number of photoelectrons within the PMTs, so that an LED event is free of statistical noise and easily distinguishable from gamma ray events. The voltage output for the LED flash from each PMT is compared to a reference value for that PMT, and its gain is adjusted if the difference is larger than a set value. This method is based on the principle that LEDs exhibit greater stability than PMTs and can therefore be used to validate PMT gains.

Most camera manufacturers limit the allowable change in the autotuning procedure to about 3 keV, requiring a service person to adjust PMTs that fall outside of that limit. Fortunately, a poorly adjusted PMT creates a more noticeable nonuniformity with energy and linearity corrections than if no corrections are used, thus prompting a service call. **Figure 5-13** illustrates the multiple layers of correction needed to achieve good uniformity and who or what is responsible for each layer.

General Guidelines for the Use and Care of a Gamma Camera

Physical Construction of a Gamma Camera

It is helpful to recognize how a gamma camera is put together and which functional parts are located in which physical locations. The gamma camera head, which is mounted on a gantry of some kind, contains the scintillation crystal, the PMTs, and the position and energy

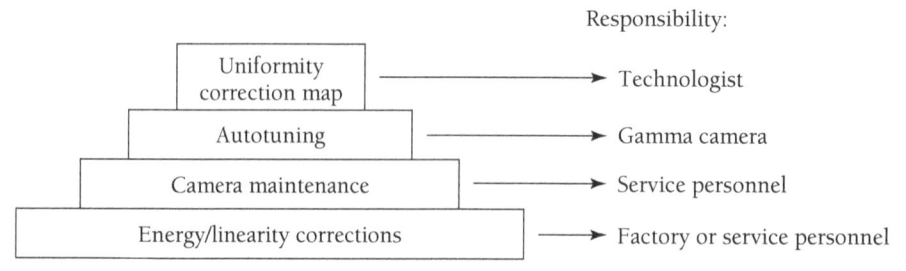

Figure 5-13 Multilayer system for optimal gamma camera performance. The systems necessary to maintain gamma camera performance are shown on the left, with the responsible party indicated at right. The size of each layer indicates its relative importance in improving camera performance. Each of the three upper layers relies on the layers below to provide a foundation, so each party must do its part.

66 Chapter 5: The Gamma Camera

circuitry. The scintillation crystal itself is coated with titanium oxide, a highly reflective material, and is sealed hermetically in a thin aluminum casing. The entire head is in a light-tight housing, usually made of aluminum. Because PMT performance is affected by changes in the earth's magnetic field (e.g., during camera rotation), PMTs may be individually shielded with a mu-metal. The electronics located within the head generate heat, so the housing usually has ventilation fans with openings that should be kept clean and unobstructed. The gamma camera head must have a stable, reliable source of electricity to the PMTs, preamplifiers, and position circuits. The collimator attaches to the housing over the front surface of the crystal, but not resting on it. The mechanisms by which collimators are installed on the camera head are many and varied. The heavy weight of some collimators may require a counterbalance as a part of the gantry.

Emerging from the camera head assembly are the X, Y, and Z signals, which constitute the vital information for the remainder of the system's operation. The PHA, count register, and spectrum display are all located in the camera's control console, which is usually physically separate from the camera head. Computers and image display devices are directly incorporated into modern gamma cameras. It is crucial that the technologist understand the function and interaction of these devices in the particular situation in which he or she works, as they vary from manufacturer to manufacturer and from camera to camera.

Installation Considerations

Gamma cameras require very specific conditions for environment and electric power. Gamma cameras generate heat and operate best when that heat is removed via air circulation. Thus it is recommended that imaging rooms be maintained at about 68 to 70°F, and that air circulation be adequate to keep the temperature at that level throughout the working day. Air filters should be cleaned on a regular schedule, to facilitate air circulation and removal of moisture within the camera head and other components of the system. On the other hand, scintillation crystals can crack if the temperature changes by more than 9°F/hr, so the camera room should not undergo the daily temperature fluctuations brought about by leaving a window open. Stability of the power supply is very important. Power surges can affect any part of the system, so surge protection and/or battery backup is strongly recommended. Most hospitals have emergency electrical generation systems that are tested on a regular basis; gamma cameras may need to have power manually restored after such a test.

The location of a gamma camera relative to other sources of gamma rays should be considered carefully. The ability of a gamma camera to detect gamma rays changes relatively little with distance. It will "see" gamma rays that come from far away as well as those that originate close by. The presence of a nearby patient waiting room or radioactive materials laboratory may lead to image artifacts. This is especially true when 511-keV annihilation photons are present, because these high-energy photons will not be absorbed by a low-energy collimator or by the gamma camera's detector housing. Technologists need to be alert to the possibility of such interference.

Patient Positioning

When a patient is positioned for an image with a gamma camera, two important rules should be followed. First, the collimator should be as close as possible to the patient, even touching the patient in most situations. The theoretical reasons for this rule are covered in Appendix E; at this point, it is sufficient to say that the ability to see detail in the image is degraded as the camera is moved away from the object being imaged. Second, the area of interest should be positioned at or close to the center of the FOV. As one nears the edge of the FOV, edge packing and distortions may degrade image quality.

Patients can be placed in a variety of physical positions relative to the gamma camera head, but the resulting image should always be oriented such that the patient's head is at the top of the image. Some cameras' orientation systems are quite straightforward, using stick figure representations that can be compared to the actual patient position, whereas others utilize reference points on a 360° circle. Some systems have the ability to mirror the orientation; this should be used with great caution and always returned to its unmirrored position.

Imaging Modes

In *static* imaging, a single image is acquired with the camera in one location, after which the camera head or patient position is readjusted prior to starting the next image. Static imaging can be combined with longitudinal motion of the gamma camera to create a *whole-body* image. As the camera head moves, counts are added to the appropriate pixels in a whole-body image matrix. The camera may be stationary at the beginning and end of the acquisition, as it first opens up and then shrinks its FOV, so that all parts of the scan field are imaged for the same length of time. Gamma cameras also have *dynamic* imaging capabilities, in which a series of images are taken sequentially, each for a set length of time. This acquisition mode allows visualization of physiologic processes that change over time, such as blood flow or organ function. The ability to demonstrate organ function through dynamic imaging is a key aspect of nuclear medicine. A third acquisition mode is called *gated* imaging.

For static imaging, the issue of when to terminate image acquisition must be addressed. One commonly used parameter is to acquire a specific number of counts, the value of which is based on the need to produce a statistically adequate image. The exact number needed varies with the situation, but ranges from 100,000 to 1 million or more. The desired number of counts must be balanced against the length of time required to reach that level. The longer the acquisition time, the more likely it is that the patient will move, blurring the image and thus destroying the improvement gained with more counts. Alternatively, one can use time as a stopping condition, based on one's estimate of the counts that can be acquired in that length of time. If two or more images are to be compared, it is often best that they be acquired for the same length of time. Most gamma cameras allow both a time limit and a count value to be set as stopping conditions, so that the camera stops at whichever limit is reached first.

A third approach to stopping conditions is the use of *information density*. The image is acquired for a period of time to reach a specified count density (counts/cm²) in a specified area, according to the equation

$$\text{Imaging time (sec)} = \frac{\left(\text{desired cts/cm}^2\right)\left(\text{area}[\text{cm}^2]\right)}{\text{measured count rate}\left(\text{cts/sec}\right)}.$$

(5-1)

The area in this equation may be the entire FOV, or a small region of interest within a specific part of the body may be identified. This technique is often used to determine an appropriate scanning speed for a whole-body scan. Common information density values in nuclear medicine range from 100 to 3,000 counts per cm². (For comparison purposes, an x-ray has information density of about 1 million events per square *millimeter* [mm²] [9]. This is one major reason that x-rays are more visually appealing than nuclear medicine images.) As the count density increases, the relative noise level decreases, enabling the observer to more easily interpret the image.

Sample Calculation 5-1 Information Density

The desired information density for a planar bone imaging protocol is 2,000 cts/cm² over the spine. A patient is positioned with the gamma camera posterior, and a 20-sec scout image is acquired. A 1-cm² region of interest positioned on the spine in the scout image contains 120 cts. What time should be set for a high-quality image?

The count rate over the spine is 120 cts in 20 sec, or 6 cts/sec. The imaging time is therefore

$$\text{Imaging time} = \frac{\left(2,000 \text{ cts/cm}^2\right)\left(1 \text{ cm}^2\right)}{6 \text{ cts/sec}} = 333 \text{ sec.}$$

All images taken using this information density calculation should have about the same image quality. In the days when images went directly onto film, all images taken for a given information density would use the same filming parameters.

Care of Gamma Cameras

Scintillation crystals are fragile and expensive. The scintillation crystal should therefore always be protected by a collimator except when intrinsic quality control procedures are being performed. For single-head cameras, it is recommended to leave the camera with the collimator facing the floor during long periods of nonuse, such as overnight. For dual- and triple-head systems, follow the manufacturer's instructions for positioning during nonuse periods. Collimators are easily damaged by imaging tables, by objects set on them, and even by using them as a writing surface. They should be treated with as much care as the rest of the gamma camera.

Gamma cameras are subject to issues of aging. The scintillation crystal may become hydrated and yellowed, PMTs may fail, and optical coupling may deteriorate over time. Systems using cathode ray tubes may demonstrate phosphor burn, where an image left on the screen may be seen as a "ghost" even after it is cleared. The most common problem in newer digital systems is malfunction of electronic parts. Service should be performed by properly trained personnel.

Non-Anger Gamma Cameras

Since the mid-1990s, considerable effort has gone into the development of gamma cameras based on designs different from that of the Anger camera. A major motivation for these efforts was the desire to avoid the limitations on sensitivity and spatial resolution imposed by Anger's scheme. In addition, developers have tried to improve the flexibility of patient positioning and decrease the space needs of the camera, often with particular organs in mind. As these new cameras become more common, it will be important for the technologist to understand how they are different from the Anger camera. Planar systems are discussed here and systems designed for tomographic imaging are discussed later. Rather than discuss specific configurations, we will highlight how they differ from the Anger design.

Detector Material

First, most of the new non-Anger devices use detector materials other than sodium iodide. One is CsI(Tl), a scintillator that has higher effective atomic number and higher mass density than NaI(Tl), giving it improved efficiency for absorbing high-energy gamma rays (10). CsI(Tl) releases more scintillation photons per MeV of gamma ray energy, but the scintillation light is a higher wavelength than is optimal for current PMTs, necessitating the use of avalanche photodiodes as the photon transducers (see the following section). The scintillation decay time for CsI(Tl) is much longer than that of NaI(Tl), although this is not usually a problem for single-photon imaging. CsI(Tl) crystals can be grown with a column microstructure, in which each column acts as an optically isolated scintillator (10), which fits very well with the idea of a pixelated detector system (see the following section).

Other manufacturers are utilizing semiconductor materials, namely, cadmium zinc telluride (CZT), in breast imaging devices. Semiconductor radiation detectors eliminate some of the inefficiencies of the scintillation detection process by directly counting electrons produced by gamma ray interactions. Because they count many more electrons per radiation interaction, they consequently have significantly improved energy resolution compared to scintillation detectors (5–10% vs 10–15%). In addition, a 1-mm-thick semiconductor detector has about the same sensitivity for

140-keV photons as a 10-mm-thick scintillation detector (11), a plus when designing a small-field imaging device.

Pixelated Architecture

A second major feature of the non-Anger devices is that they are all pixelated systems, using many small detectors rather than a single large crystal. Pixelated cameras usually identify the individual detector registering a photon interaction rather than the exact (X, Y) location of the interaction as in Anger's design. So smaller detectors mean better resolution, and the detector size in these devices is in the range of 1.5 to 3 mm on each side.

The use of a pixelated system and such small detectors necessitates something other than a standard PMT to convert the basic radiation detection emissions to an electronic signal. One technique is to use a *position-sensitive PMT* (PSPMT). A PSPMT multiplies electrons as a standard PMT does, but maintains spatial separation of the multiplied electron clouds originating at different points on the photocathode. A mesh structure with 16 to 20 stages of multiplication is created by layering many dynodes with guard plates perforated with holes. The anode of a PSPMT is divided into discrete pixels, each with its own connection to the downstream electronics.

A second technique is to replace the PMT with a solid-state device called a *photodiode*. A photodiode converts photons to electrons and then collects those electrons directly—much as the semiconductor radiation detectors do, except that they are registering scintillation photons instead of gamma rays. A photodiode can be modified to accomplish some multiplication of the electronic signal, in which case it is called an *avalanche photodiode*. Both of these devices are discussed in Appendix B.

Collimators

The systems using NaI or CsI scintillation crystals use collimators similar to a regular gamma camera, in that the collimator holes are smaller than the individual crystals and not aligned with them. Slant-hole construction may be utilized to improve the ability to see lesions close to the chest wall and for three-dimensional localization needs such as biopsy. The CZT-based systems, on the other hand, use what is called a *registered collimator*, in which the collimator holes are square and are matched to the geometry of the detector elements. This effectively causes the detector and collimator hole to act as a single radiation detector, such that the collimator resolution determines the system resolution (12). The collimator holes are larger than in a traditional gamma camera collimator, so sensitivity is much higher.

Physical Size

A key advantage of the pixelated architecture is that edge effects are avoided. Because the location of a gamma ray interaction in Anger's design is determined by a group of PMTs, there must always be one ring of PMTs beyond the edge of the FOV. This makes the camera head quite bulky, with several centimeters of "dead space" around the outside. In the pixelated camera, localization to one crystal requires only that crystal's electronics. Most of the commercially available systems have dead space of less than 1 cm around the face of the camera. They generally have imaging FOVs in the range of 15 to 20 cm by 20 to 40 cm.

These cameras can be used for a number of nuclear medicine studies; bone scans of extremities and thyroid scans are two examples. Some are dual-head systems and may allow the two views to be combined into a composite image, creating, for example, a geometric mean of the views from the two camera heads. Depending on the vendor, one may be able to obtain collimators of various grades and even pinhole collimators. These cameras are considerably smaller and less intimidating than a typical Anger camera, and they are being marketed for pediatric and medical office imaging situations. Let us consider breast imaging as one application of these devices.

Breast-Specific Gamma Imaging

We have known since Tc-99m sestamibi came into wide use that it localizes in areas of high metabolic activity, including breast cancers. In fact, the DuPont Company at one point marketed sestamibi separately as Miraluma for breast imaging and Cardiolite for cardiac imaging. However, it is very difficult to get good views of the breast with a traditional gamma camera without having the rest of the thorax and upper abdomen in the FOV. The most common way to obtain breast-only images was to have the patient lay prone on an imaging table that included a breast cutout, so that the breast could hang freely and could be imaged from the lateral aspect. The chief drawback of this imaging configuration was that the breast tissue was several cm from the camera face, significantly degrading resolution.

Pixelated cameras mounted on mammography gantries are now available for nuclear breast imaging (**Figure 5-14**).

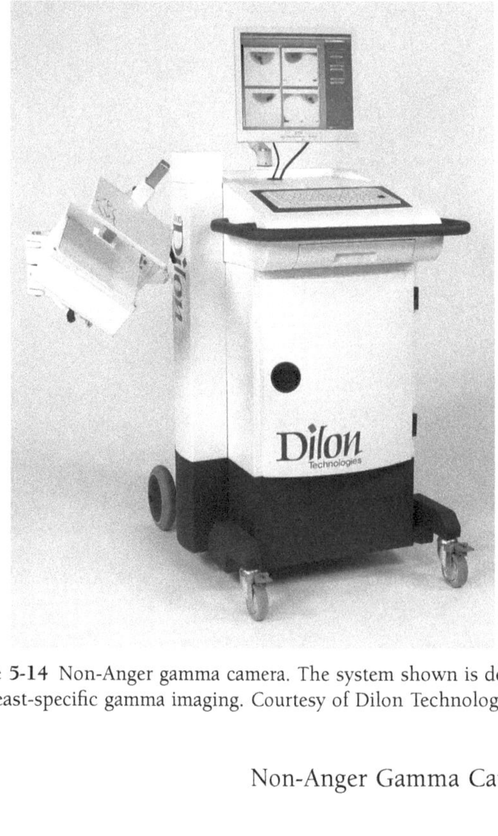

Figure 5-14 Non-Anger gamma camera. The system shown is designed for breast-specific gamma imaging. Courtesy of Dilon Technologies.

Sodium iodide, cesium iodide, and CZT are used as detector materials. The absence of dead space around the FOV allows for positioning of the breast tissue that is similar to standard mammographic views. The breast can be positioned directly on the camera face (light compression is generally used), improving the resolution relative to the prone-dependent position used with the Anger camera. These systems can detect breast lesions of 5 mm or smaller, and because the sestamibi images are directly comparable to the mammographic images, suspicious lesions seen on mammograms can be evaluated as hot (most likely malignant) or not hot (most likely benign). Thus, breast-specific gamma imaging can reduce the number of breast biopsies that turn out to be benign, which without further imaging amounts to as much as two-thirds of all biopsies.

Summary

More than 50 years after their invention, gamma cameras continue to be the most important radiation detecting instruments in almost all nuclear medicine departments. Their operation, while more complex than other radiologic imaging devices, is well understood, such that most technologists can spot problems and address them as they come up. Energy and linearity correction tables, along with other improvements over Anger's original design, have significantly improved image quality. While instruments with different methodologies have been developed to image radionuclide distributions in the human body, to date none have been widely competitive with the gamma camera.

Two basic points about imaging with gamma cameras serve to summarize this chapter. The first point is that imaging in nuclear medicine is essentially a statistical exercise, much like counting with a nonimaging detector. The precision of the information and the quality of the image improve as the total number of counts increases. All nuclear medicine images are time exposures, in that information must be collected for a finite length of time to get enough count statistics for an adequate image.

The second point is that, no matter how long the acquisition time of an image, it will never approach the level of detail of an x-ray, *computed tomography* (CT), or *magnetic resonance imaging* (MRI). The latter are primarily anatomic imaging modalities, and thanks to their excellent information density, they excel at showing the details of anatomy. The gamma camera has inherent limitations that will always cause its images to look "fuzzy" compared to other imaging techniques. Nuclear medicine, in contrast, is a functional imaging modality, and its strength is in the demonstration of organ function. In the arena of physiologic imaging, nuclear medicine has no equal.

References

1. Travin MI. Cardiac cameras. *Semin Nucl Med.* 2011; 41:182–201.
2. Anger HO. Scintillation camera. *Rev Sci Instrumen.* 1958;29:27–33.
3. Tapscott E. First scintillation camera is foundation for modern imaging systems. *J Nucl Med.* 1998;39:15N–27N.
4. Henkin RE, Boles MA, Dillehay GL, et al., eds. *Nuclear Medicine.* St. Louis, MO: Mosby-Year Book; 1996:128.
5. Simmons GH. *The Scintillation Camera.* New York, NY: Society of Nuclear Medicine; 1988:51.
6. Madsen M. The scintillation camera. In: *Basic Science of Nuclear Medicine* [CD-ROM]. Reston, VA: Society of Nuclear Medicine; 2001.
7. Muehllehner G, Colsher JG, Stoub EW. Correction for field nonuniformity in scintillation cameras through removal of spatial distortion. *J Nucl Med.* 1980;21:771–776.
8. Zanzonico P. Routine quality control of clinical nuclear medicine instrumentation: a brief review. *J Nucl Med.* 2008;49:1114–1131.
9. Cherry SR, Sorenson JA, Phelps ME. *Physics in Nuclear Medicine.* 3rd ed. Philadelphia, PA: Saunders; 2003:268.
10. Knoll GF. *Radiation Detection and Measurement.* 3rd ed. New York, NY: John Wiley & Sons; 2000: 235, 238.
11. Heller S, Zanzonico P. Nuclear probes and intraoperative gamma cameras. *Semin Nucl Med.* 2011;41:166–181.
12. Mueller B, O'Connor MK, Blevis I, et al. Evaluation of a small cadmium zinc telluride detector for scintimammography. *J Nucl Med.* 2003;44:602–609.

Additional Resources

Cherry SR, Sorenson JA, Phelps ME. *Physics in Nuclear Medicine.* 3rd ed. Philadelphia, PA: Saunders; 2003:Chapter 13.

Madsen MT. Recent advances in SPECT imaging. *J Nucl Med.* 2007;48:661–673.

CHAPTER 6
Image Digitization and Display

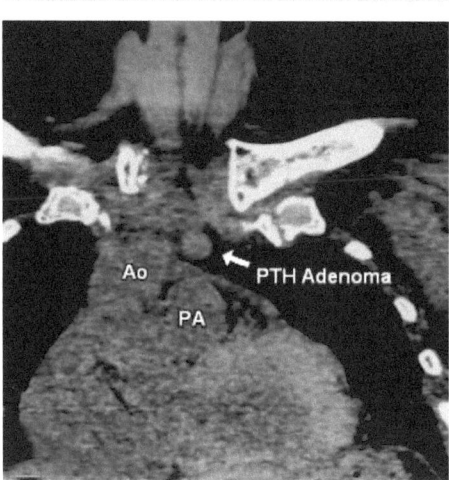

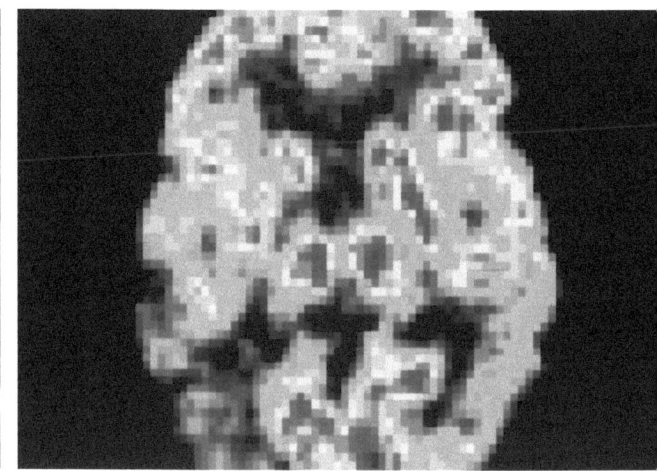

Learning Outcomes

1. Contrast analog and digital images obtained from a gamma camera.
2. Distinguish between a word-mode acquisition and a byte-mode acquisition, and discuss the problems associated with pixel overflow and matrix choice.
3. Identify image matrix choices applicable to nuclear medicine images; determine pixel size, given camera dimensions; and discuss the trade-offs involved in choosing a matrix for a particular situation.
4. Briefly discuss the benefits and limitations of digitally zooming a gamma camera image.
5. Contrast frame-mode and list-mode methods of storing image information, and discuss the need for buffers in frame-mode acquisitions.
6. Explain how count-per-pixel values are converted to pixel intensities on a gray or color scale as well as the purpose of logarithmic and exponential scales relative to a linear scale.
7. Discuss the operation of a screen capture program and its advantages as a storage format.

Introduction

The essential operation of the gamma camera remains much the same as when Anger created it, with one important exception—the manner in which images are displayed. From the early days of 35-mm filmstrips and Polaroid film to multiformatters to the use of computers as add-on devices to their incorporation into the gamma camera itself, this aspect of nuclear medicine imaging has changed more drastically than any other. Whatever photographic or display system is used, it must supply both contrast (i.e., the ability to distinguish between areas of higher and lower counts) and detail (i.e., the ability to show degrees of change between areas of higher vs lower counts). This chapter briefly addresses the concept and creation of an analog image on film and then moves to digitization of nuclear medicine images and the advantages this has brought to the practice of nuclear medicine.

Analog Images

A gamma camera creates the X, Y, and Z signals that carry the essential information of each event interacting in the scintillation crystal. The X and Y signals generated by the Anger positioning logic are analog signals; that is, they can take on any value, to an infinite degree of precision (see Appendix D for further discussion of analog vs digital data). The exact (X, Y) location of each event is different from the (X, Y) location of all other counts in the image. On the other hand, after it goes through the pulse height analyzer (PHA), the Z signal is a digital signal, having only two possible values (on or off). In a cathode ray tube (CRT), these signals turn on (using the digital Z signal) and deflect (via the analog X and Y signals) an electron beam to create a dot on a phosphor screen (see Appendix B for more details). In most early gamma cameras and even into the 1990s, CRTs were used to directly expose a film (the basic concepts of film exposure and development are discussed in Appendix C). The result is an *analog* image, in which many dots, each in its individual location, create a visual display of the two-dimensional distribution of gamma rays interacting in the scintillation crystal. Where there is greater radioactivity in the object, there is a correspondingly greater concentration of dots on the film.

For this process to work successfully, the dots created by the electron beam must be of the right size and sharpness. These qualities are controlled by focus and size or intensity controls on the CRT. If the dots are out of focus, the image will lose its sharpness. If they are too big, the image will be overexposed. If they are too small, the image will be underexposed. These controls are set by the operator, and if they are set incorrectly, in a completely analog system (i.e., one with no digitization process or integrated computer), the entire image must be acquired again.

The analog position information for each count from the Anger position circuit, combined with a CRT to pinpoint that location on a film, creates an aesthetically pleasing image representing the distribution of radioactivity seen by the gamma camera. But once the image is acquired, it can only be evaluated visually—no further manipulation or quantitative analysis can be done. Much greater value can be obtained from nuclear medicine images if we can count the number of gamma rays within a defined region of interest. So while analog images are very pretty, they have significant limitations, and they penalize the technologist who does not pay attention to details. They also penalize the patient if another imaging session is needed.

To get around these limitations, gamma cameras have incorporated computers since the early 1970s. In fact, it is not an overstatement to say that computers have transformed nuclear medicine. Through the mid-1980s, computers were completely separate add-on devices for most gamma cameras. Since the early 1990s, every gamma camera has incorporated at least one and often several computers. Appendix D reviews the fundamental workings of a computer.

Digital Images and Image Matrices

The first thing that a computer requires is a *digital image*. In a digital image, the X and Y values corresponding to the event position are limited to certain discrete values. The conversion process is accomplished by an *analog-to-digital converter* (ADC). The requirement for discrete values leads to a grid-like arrangement called an *image matrix*. Each possible position in the grid is called a picture element, or *pixel*. **Figure 6-1** shows a coarse 16 × 16 image matrix, superimposed on a gamma camera with a circular field of view (FOV).

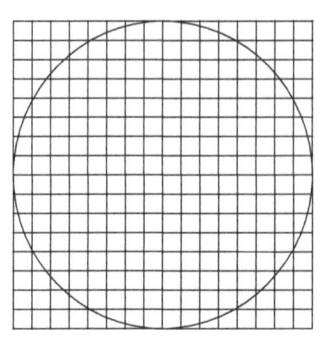

Figure 6-1 Image matrix concept. A 16 × 16 image matrix is applied to the field of view of a circular gamma camera. The corner pixels, which are not needed for the circular FOV, often contain identifying information such as the patient's name and the date the image was acquired.

The analog X and Y signals coming from an event registered by the gamma camera are converted to digital X and Y values that in turn locate the event in one of the pixels of the image matrix; the computer increments the count in that pixel by one. In a completed image, three numbers specify each pixel: its X-coordinate, its Y-coordinate, and the number of counts registered in it. The latter value is correlated to a gray or color scale. The resultant image gives visually much the same information as the analog image, but can be manipulated and analyzed after acquisition and stored on digital media, such as a magnetic tape or optical disk.

Image Matrix Choices

A digital image is characterized by its *matrix dimension*. Matrix dimensions routinely used in nuclear medicine include 64 × 64, 128 × 128, and 256 × 256. **Figure 6-2** shows examples of images acquired using each matrix size. As the matrix dimension increases, the ability to see detail improves: A 64 × 64 matrix is noticeably boxy, whereas a 256 × 256 image is almost as good as an analog image. Nonsquare matrices (for example, 256 × 1,024 for a whole-body scan) are also possible. Pixel size can be estimated by dividing the FOV size by the number of pixels:

$$\text{Pixel size (mm)} = \frac{\text{FOV (mm)}}{\text{matrix dimension}}. \quad (6\text{-}1)$$

For example, a 38-cm diameter camera with a 64 × 64 matrix has pixels that are 38 cm ÷ 64 pixels = ~0.6 cm/pixel (i.e., the pixel's width in the X or Y direction). For a rectangular FOV, divide the longer side of the FOV by the pixel dimension.

Sample Calculation 6-1 Pixel Size Calculation

A gamma camera has a rectangular FOV that is 50 cm × 35 cm. Calculate the pixel dimension for the three image matrix sizes commonly used in nuclear medicine.

Because the FOV is rectangular, we apply the matrix to the longer side of the FOV:

$$64 \times 64 \text{ matrix}: \frac{50 \text{ cm}}{64 \text{ pixels}} = \frac{0.78 \text{ cm}}{\text{pixel}}.$$

$$128 \times 128 \text{ matrix}: \frac{50 \text{ cm}}{128 \text{ pixels}} = \frac{0.39 \text{ cm}}{\text{pixel}}.$$

$$256 \times 256 \text{ matrix}: \frac{50 \text{ cm}}{256 \text{ pixels}} = \frac{0.20 \text{ cm}}{\text{pixel}}.$$

Thus the pixel size in either the X or the Y direction decreases from 0.78 cm in a 64 × 64 matrix to 0.20 cm in a 256 × 256 matrix. Most people would convert these to 7.8, 3.9, and 2.0 mm, or would first convert the 50-cm FOV dimension to 500 mm.

When a nuclear medicine image acquisition is set up on a computer, the computer must locate space in its memory to store that image. The amount of space required depends on both the matrix dimension and the expected maximum number of counts per pixel. Determining the space required for an acquisition was an important issue in the early days of computing, when computer memory was at a premium. Even today, computer storage of nuclear medicine images is not a trivial matter, and hard-disk space can be a problem at times. Computer memory is used more efficiently if we don't reserve a lot of space that isn't needed. So nuclear medicine computers allow the operator to specify "byte mode" or "word mode" for each acquisition. *Byte mode* (often denoted "x8" after the matrix dimension) allows a pixel to accumulate up to 255 counts (cts) (1 byte of information). This amount of memory is not sufficient for many imaging protocols. *Word mode* (denoted "x16") allots 2 bytes to each pixel address, allowing each pixel to accumulate up to 65,535 cts, but requiring twice as much space in memory (See Sample Calculation 6-2 on p. 74).

Pixel Saturation

An important factor to consider when acquiring in byte mode is the issue of pixel saturation. What happens if a pixel reaches 256 counts? The system could (1) stop acquiring in that pixel (the pixel is said to be *saturated*), (2) stop the image acquisition altogether, or (3) roll that pixel back to zero and continue acquiring. The first option loses direct correlation with radioactivity in the patient; the second may produce an image with insufficient total

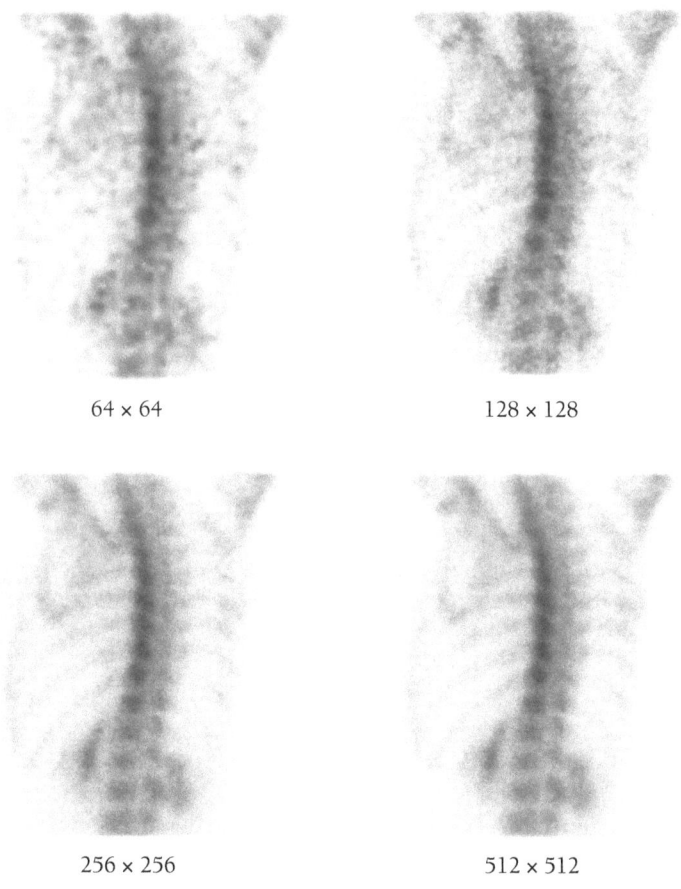

Figure 6-2 Four matrix dimensions commonly used in nuclear medicine. The first three matrices are employed in clinical imaging, and the 512 × 512 matrix is often used for quality control procedures. Image courtesy of Virginia Mason Medical Center.

Digital Images and Image Matrices

Sample Calculation 6-2 Computer Memory Calculations

Calculate the bytes of digital memory needed to store each of the following acquisitions:

a. Five static 256 × 256 word-mode images
b. Dynamic acquisition of twenty-four 2-second (sec) frames of 64 × 64 byte-mode images
c. Dynamic acquisition of sixty 1-sec images followed by one hundred 12-sec images, all in 128 × 128 byte mode

For each image, we need the total number of images times the total number of pixels (assume a square matrix) multiplied by either 1 byte/pixel (byte mode) or 2 bytes/pixel (word mode). Divide by 1,024 to convert to kilobytes (see Appendix D).

a. $5 \text{ images} \times \dfrac{256 \times 256 \text{ pixels}}{\text{image}} \times \dfrac{2 \text{ bytes}}{\text{pixel}}$
$= 655,360 \text{ bytes} = 640 \text{ kbytes.}$

b. $24 \text{ images} \times \dfrac{64 \times 64 \text{ pixels}}{\text{image}} \times \dfrac{1 \text{ byte}}{\text{pixel}}$
$= 98,304 \text{ bytes} = 96 \text{ kbytes.}$

c. $(60 + 100) \text{ images} \times \dfrac{128 \times 128 \text{ pixels}}{\text{image}} \times \dfrac{1 \text{ byte}}{\text{pixel}}$
$= 2,621,440 \text{ bytes} = 2,560 \text{ kbytes}$
$= 2.56 \text{ Mbytes.}$

Sample Calculation 6-3 Relationship between Matrix Size and Statistical Noise

A 50-cm camera with an image matrix of 128 × 128 is used to acquire an image of the spine. Information density in the region of the spine is 1,850 cts/cm². What is the average count density per pixel? If the matrix size is increased to 256 × 256, how does the average count density change? What are the coefficients of variation in each situation?

In the original configuration, the pixels are 3.9 mm or 0.39 cm on a side (see Sample Calculation 6-1; we'll stay in cm because the information density is in cm²). The count density is thus

$$\frac{1{,}850 \text{ cts}}{\text{cm}^2} \times \frac{(0.39 \text{ cm})^2}{\text{pixel}} = \frac{281 \text{ cts}}{\text{pixel}}.$$

With a 256 × 256 matrix, the pixels are 0.2 cm in each direction, and the count density is

$$\frac{1{,}850 \text{ cts}}{\text{cm}^2} \times \frac{(0.20 \text{ cm})^2}{\text{pixel}} = \frac{74 \text{ cts}}{\text{pixel}}.$$

The coefficients of variation, on a per-pixel basis, are therefore (based on Eq. 4-4)

$$128 \times 128 \text{ matrix: CV} = \frac{1}{\sqrt{281 \text{ cts}}} \times 100\% = 6\%.$$

$$256 \times 256 \text{ matrix: CV} = \frac{1}{\sqrt{74 \text{ cts}}} \times 100\% = 12\%.$$

---

counts; and the third option leads to a very confusing image, in which the pixels representing the area of highest activity may be displayed as an area of low counts. An example of pixel saturation can be seen in **Figure 6-3**. Different systems use different pixel overflow rules; some allow the operator to choose from several options. The bottom line is that one must be aware of the possibility that data or image quality might be lost because of pixel overflow in byte mode. Word mode is sufficient for all nuclear medicine studies and is recommended for most acquisitions.

Trade-offs with Image Matrices

At first glance it would appear that a finer matrix would guarantee a higher-quality image, but this is not necessarily true. If the matrix dimension is increased by a factor of 2 (e.g., from 64 × 64 to 128 × 128), the image will have smaller pixels by a factor of 2. But an additional result will be that the counts per pixel will be decreased, on average, by a factor of 4, because a single pixel in the 64 × 64 matrix corresponds to four pixels in the 128 × 128 matrix. Recall that the information contained in the image is really the variation in the number of counts. If the counts are spread out too sparsely, we will lose the effect of that variation and produce a noisy image (**Figure 6-4**).

Image *noise* is the pixel-to-pixel variations in a digital image, which are due to the statistical nature of radioactive decay and detection and to the assignment of counts to specific pixels.

A coarse image matrix (64 × 64, for example) generally solves the problem of noise, but leads to concerns about resolution. The pixels may be large enough that they no longer accurately represent the spatial distribution of the measured counts. Further, a coarse image matrix reduces the ability to define the edge of an organ. A pixel located at the edge of an organ may contain counts from both the organ and the tissue beyond the organ. The computer will therefore average the organ count density and the background count density. (This is the two-dimensional analog of the partial-volume effect.) The eye has a harder time visualizing the edge of the organ, and the counts-per-pixel value is not reflective of the organ count density.

Let us consider how these factors affect the choice of image matrix. One way to think about this is to consider pixel size as it relates to the system's ability to see detail. Ideally, the size of a pixel should be no larger than one-half of the camera's spatial resolution (as measured with a line-spread function). When this condition is met, the image resolution is determined by the system resolution and is

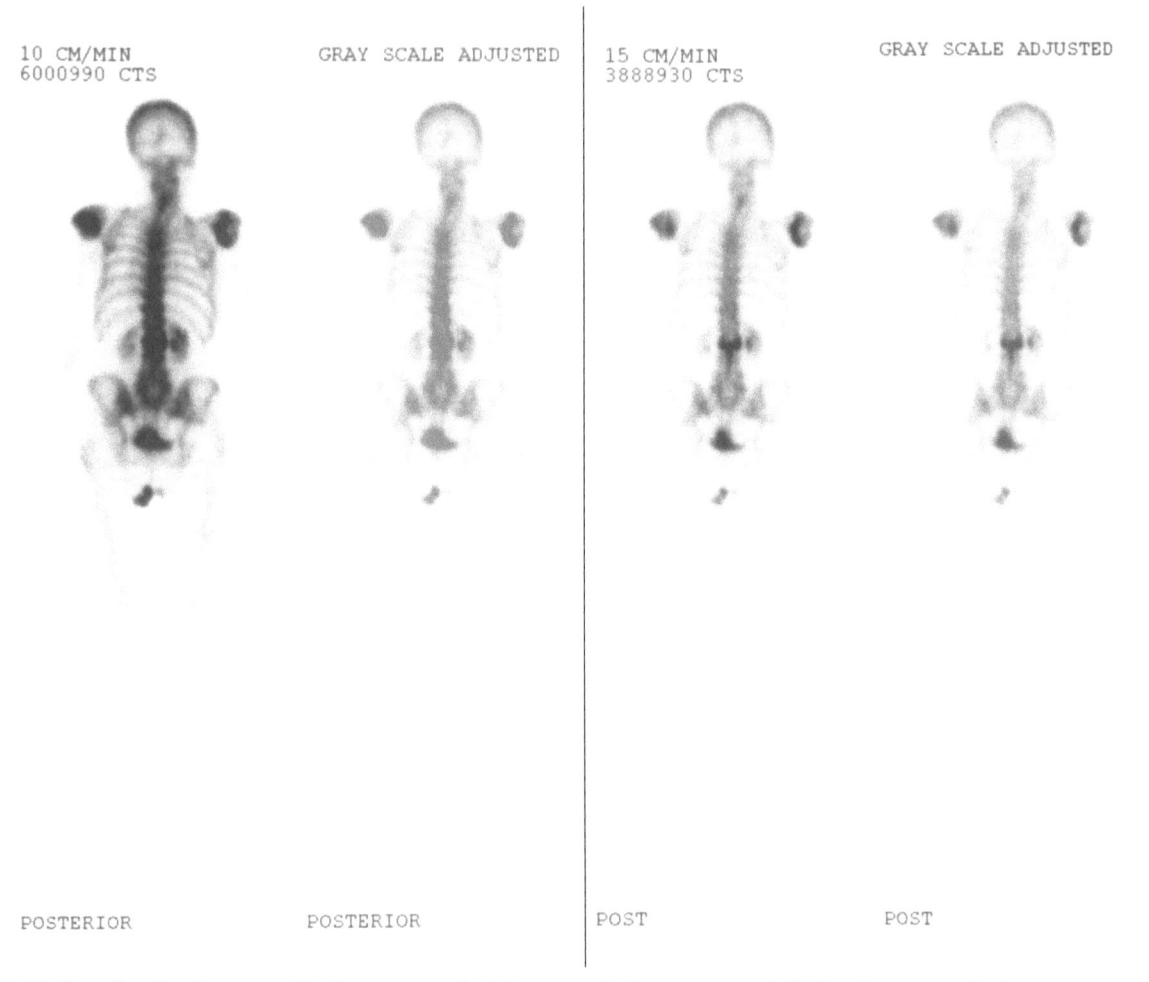

Figure 6-3 Pixel overflow in a bone scan. The bone scan on the left was acquired at a scan speed of 10 cm/min in a mode that stops acquiring counts into any pixel that reaches 256 cts. Note that many pixels are saturated, including most of the vertebral column. Even when the gray scale is adjusted (second image from left), image definition within these saturated regions is lost. The bone scan on the right (also shown in two gray-scale adjustments) is a repeat scan of the same patient, using a scan speed of 15 cm/min. The degree of pixel saturation is greatly reduced, making the abnormality at the L2 vertebra more clearly obvious. Image courtesy of Virginia Mason Medical Center.

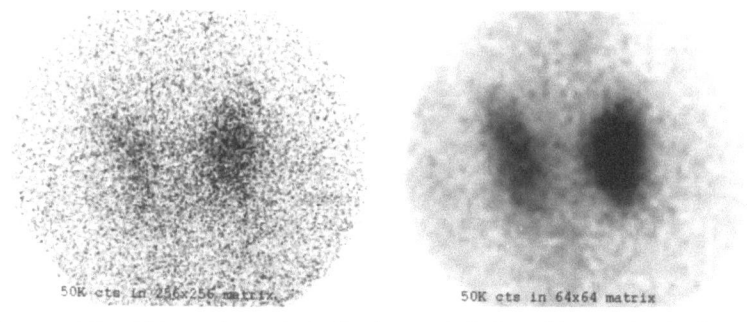

Figure 6-4 Image noise. This low-count thyroid image demonstrates the decreased clarity and increased noise that occur when a matrix dimension too large for the available counts is used. The left-hand image is 50,000 cts acquired into a 256 × 256 image matrix, and the right-hand image shows the same number of counts in a 64 × 64 matrix. Image courtesy of Virginia Mason Medical Center.

not being limited by the pixel size. (This requirement is an application of the sampling theorem.) Applying the sampling theorem to the anatomy of interest, we want the pixels to be no more than one-half as large as the smallest structure we hope to see. However, making the pixel size smaller than one-third the camera's spatial resolution reduces the per-pixel counts and increases the noise level of the image. In practice, therefore, a matrix dimension that generates pixels between one-half and one-third the size of the system resolution is considered the best choice.

Alternatively, given that we have only a few choices for matrix dimension, we can simply consider the best use of each. A 256 × 256 image matrix is warranted when good spatial resolution is needed and plenty of counts are

Digital Images and Image Matrices

Sample Calculation 6-4 Relationship of Pixel Size to Camera Resolution

In the gamma camera described in Sample Calculation 6-1, the system resolution is 9.5 mm. What is the largest pixel dimension that should be used with this system, if we are to take full advantage of the system resolution? How does that compare to the three pixel dimensions calculated in Sample Calculation 6-1?

The sampling theorem says that pixels should be no larger than one-half of the FWHM. For a system resolution of 9.5 mm, the pixels should be no larger than 9.5 ÷ 2 = 4.75 mm.

- The 64 × 64 matrix, with a pixel dimension of 7.8 mm, does not meet the criterion of the sampling theorem.
- The 128 × 128 matrix has pixels that are 3.9 mm on a side, which meets the sampling theorem requirement.
- The 256 × 256 matrix produces 2.0-mm pixels, which are less than one-quarter of the FWHM. These are smaller than warranted and should be used only in high-count situations.

available. An example of this situation is a bone scan: we would like to get good details, especially of vertebrae or extremities, and we can acquire the image for a long period of time. In a gastric emptying study, on the other hand, the stomach is a large organ without many anatomic details. The information of interest in this study is the change in radioactivity in the stomach over time. Further, there is little background activity except for the small intestine inferior to the stomach, so edge effects are not significant. A 64 × 64 image matrix is adequate for this study.

A dynamic renal study is an example of a compromise between two extremes. The kidneys are considerably smaller than the stomach. Each image is acquired for a short time, so counts are not plentiful in any one image. We wish to outline the renal cortex on the functional part of the study, so our pixels must be small enough to identify the cortex separately from the collecting system. And the goal of the study is to obtain quantitative information, so edge effects should be avoided. The choice of a 128 × 128 image matrix provides the best quality images in this situation.

Nuclear medicine computers generally allow for image matrix compression after acquisition. An image acquired in a 256 × 256 matrix can be compressed to 128 × 128 simply by combining each group of four pixels into one. Programs are also available that allow one to increase the matrix dimension of an image by subdividing each pixel into four new pixels, but this is much more problematic. Because the image was acquired with less spatial resolution than the desired image matrix, the program applies a rule of some sort to distribute the counts from each original pixel into the four new pixels. There are several ways to accomplish this, but in the end we have no assurance that the new image accurately reflects the actual count distribution.

Digital Zoom

In analog imaging, one can only increase the size of the organ relative to the FOV through the use of a focused (converging or pinhole) collimator. The creation of a digital image allows for such a change to be made in several ways. First, as has been demonstrated, the use of a larger (finer) matrix dimension produces smaller pixels, increasing resolution. A simplistic way to change the pixel size after acquisition is to apply a zoom factor (sometimes called a *postzoom*) to the image. In this technique, the image is "magnified" by making each pixel bigger. For example, a postzoom factor of 2 applied to a 64 × 64 image might expand the middle 32 × 32 pixels to occupy the full display screen. Each pixel still represents a square of 6 × 6 mm (on a system with a 38-cm FOV), but on the display they are now twice as big.

A more sophisticated approach is to apply the zoom factor to each event *before* assigning it to the image matrix (prezooming). A 64 × 64 acquisition with a zoom factor of 2 puts counts that would have been in the 10th pixel from the origin into the 20th pixel. This produces a 64 × 64 image in which each pixel dimension is one-half of what it was without the zoom factor. Equation 6-2 shows Equation 6-1 modified by the zoom factor:

$$\text{Pixel size (mm)} = \frac{\text{FOV (mm)}}{\text{matrix dimension} \times \text{zoom factor}}.$$

(6-2)

The pixels that were 6 mm on each side in the unzoomed image are now only 3 mm. This approach can easily be adapted to magnify specific parts of the FOV; for example, one can magnify the lower part of the FOV for brain scanning to allow for gamma camera positioning so as to clear the patient's shoulders. The digital nature of the system allows any zoom factor to be used, rather than limiting us to integers or factors of 2.

Does the use of digital zoom really improve the ability to see details? Yes, but only to the level of the gamma camera system. In the above example, an event whose analog location is three-fourths of the way across pixel 19 in the unzoomed image should be found in pixel 39 of the zoomed image. But if the system is only able to place events within an accuracy of 1 cm, that event could end up in any pixel between 37 and 41. So while application of a zoom factor can improve resolution, it can only do so up to the limits of the system resolution.

Acquisition of Digital Images

Frame Mode

The acquisition of nuclear medicine images in a digital format requires allocation of memory locations in the computer system. Most nuclear medicine images are acquired in *frame mode*: an image matrix or frame is created prior to starting the acquisition, and each count is assigned to a pixel in that frame. Typically, the frame is held in an *image buffer* (a short-term memory location) during acquisition. The image is sent to long-term memory only when it is complete. A small but finite amount of time is required to save the frame in the buffer into long-term memory. After the image has been saved to a long-term storage location, all of the buffer's pixel values are reset to zero.

Dynamic images are also acquired in frame mode. But because of the finite time required for saving to disk, a dynamic series of images requires a pair of buffers. Counts are acquired into one buffer, while the other buffer is sending its image to long-term storage and resetting its pixel registers to zero. When it is time to start acquiring the next image in the series, the second buffer is ready to accept data with no loss of time, and the first buffer then transfers its completed image to memory and rezeros its pixel registers.

Gated Frame Mode

Gated images represent a further advance in image capabilities, one that became practical only through the use of computers. In this technique, a repeating physiologic parameter is used as a *gate* to direct the image acquisition. This is most commonly done with cardiac imaging (radionuclide ventriculography and myocardial perfusion imaging), so the cardiac contraction cycle with its repeating R wave (electrocardiographic peak indicating ventricular contraction) will be used to illustrate the technique. The user defines the number of segments or frames into which the cardiac cycle is to be divided. The patient's heart rate is inverted to determine the *R-R interval* (the time between R waves of the electrocardiogram [ECG] in msec/beat), which is then divided by the desired number of frames to determine the time per frame:

$$\frac{\text{time}}{\text{frame}}(\text{msec}) = \frac{\text{min}}{\text{beats}} \times \frac{\text{beat}}{\text{no. of frames}} \times \frac{60 \text{ sec}}{\text{min}} \times \frac{1{,}000 \text{ msec}}{\text{sec}}. \quad (6\text{-}3)$$

Each frame thus corresponds to a small time segment of the contraction-filling (systole–diastole) cycle of the heart.

The computer acquisition process then creates a buffer frameset, which has a number of image buffers equal to the desired number of frames. The R wave of the patient's ECG, acting as the gate, directs the acquisition to start putting counts into buffer frame 1. When buffer frame 1's time is up, the acquisition moves to buffer frame 2, and so on until the last buffer frame's imaging time is complete. Then the computer stops acquiring until the next R wave is detected. Following this process over many heart cycles allows a composite picture of activity relative to the cardiac cycle to be built. If the next R wave arrives early (i.e., a shorter R-R interval than was originally measured), the computer must obey the gate and go back to buffer frame 1. Hence the terminal frame or frames of a gated acquisition often contain fewer counts than the earlier frames.

Abnormal heart contractions may have significantly shorter or longer R-R intervals than usual. We may therefore wish to evaluate the length of each beat before adding it to image memory. To do *beat rejection*, we need a temporary buffer frameset to store data for a single beat and a second buffer frameset to be ready to store the next beat. A beat is accepted or rejected only after its R-R interval is determined. If it is accepted, the data from the first set of buffers are added to a buffer frameset containing the composite data. If a beat is rejected, the pixel registers are all reset to zero so that the buffer frameset can be ready for the next cardiac cycle. Clearly, such complex acquisitions can only occur with the assistance of a computer.

List Mode

The other option besides frame-mode acquisition is the *list-mode* acquisition. In this technique, counts are not assigned to a pixel in an image frame during acquisition. Instead, each count is stored separately as an (X, Y) value. In addition, timing markers and possibly physiologic parameters such as the R wave are stored in sequence. The acquisition speed is limited only by the time needed to store each count or time marker. List-mode acquisition allows the user to wait until after the acquisition to determine the best choice for allocating counts into dynamic frames. List mode requires much more computer memory than frame mode. It is rarely used in clinical nuclear medicine (it is more common in research), but it may find new applicability for dynamic imaging in combined PET/CT imaging of the heart (1).

Digital Image Display

The creation of digital images has three major benefits. First, it allows the operator to adjust the image appearance after acquisition. This saves much time on the part of both the technologist and the patient. Second, regions of interest can be applied to digital images to quantify the radioactivity found in an organ and hence the organ's function. Third, images can be displayed in a variety of gray and color scales, allowing different aspects of the image to be accentuated or deemphasized. It is important to use the various display manipulations in ways that are appropriate to the imaging situation, so that clinically important information is not obscured. Before looking at the use of color scales, however, we consider how to deal with one of the drawbacks of digital images; namely, that they are not as pretty as analog images.

Smoothing

When an analog image is digitized, it loses the "smoothness" that comes with being able to define event locations exactly. As counts are assigned to pixels, some pixels will get extra counts and others will get fewer counts, leading to pixel-to-pixel differences that are due not to variability within the object itself, but rather to the imposition of an image matrix "regimentation" on the image. This variability can make nuclear medicine images hard to interpret. We can decrease it by applying a *smoothing filter*, which generates a new value for each pixel based on a weighted average of that pixel and its neighbors. The 9-point smoothing filter is most commonly used; it is illustrated in **Figure 6-5**.

(a) Nine-pixel area of digitized image

A	B	C
D	E	F
G	H	I

(b) Filter kernel

1	2	1
2	4	2
1	2	1

(c) **Equation to calculate new value for pixel E:**

$$E = \frac{[(4E) + (2)(B + D + F + H) + (1)(A + C + G + I)]}{16}$$

(d) Unsmoothed and smoothed bone scan images of the hands

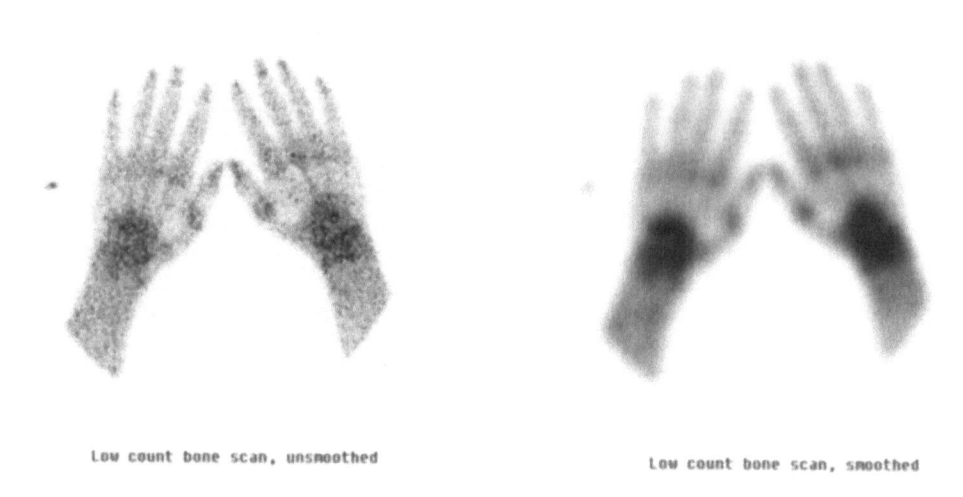

Low count bone scan, unsmoothed

Low count bone scan, smoothed

Figure 6-5 Smoothing. Figure 6-5a represents a small, 3 × 3 pixel region within a digital image with count-per-pixel values denoted as A–I. Figure 6-5b is the filter kernel (the weighting factors applied to each pixel) and the mathematical equation used to calculate the smoothed value for pixel E, based on its original value and the values of its neighbors. The value in the denominator, 16, is the sum of the weighting factors used in the numerator of the kernel. Figure 6-5c shows the effect of smoothing on a low-count bone scan image of the hands. Figure 6-5c image courtesy of Virginia Mason Medical Center.

The filter is applied to each pixel of the original image in succession, and the smoothed pixel values are stored in a new image.

The net result of smoothing is to bring the outlier pixels (those that are high or low compared to their neighbors) back closer to the local norm. This has the desired effect of making the image look less grainy. But it can also be detrimental if the count change from one pixel to the next reflects a real change in the object. For example, a given set of pixels may be aligned with a sharp count boundary in the object, in which case the effect of smoothing would be to decrease the sharpness of this boundary in the image. The ultimate result of repeated smoothing would be a completely flat image.

Gray Scale and Lookup Table

In an analog image, film density reproduces the localization of activity in the object being imaged; more dots mean more blackness (we will assume throughout that we are using a white background or a clear film). In a digital image, counts in a pixel similarly indicate activity in the object; a visual scale is used to show the relative number of counts in each pixel. The most basic visual scale is a *linear gray scale*, in which each number of counts is assigned a specific level of grayness (**Figure 6-6a**), with the gray levels getting darker as counts increase.

A *lookup table* (LUT) assigns a particular shade of gray to a specific count-per-pixel value, wherever that count-per-pixel value is found in the image. The convention in nuclear medicine computer systems is to initially display a set of static images such that within each image, the maximum counts-per-pixel value is set to the highest LUT intensity and 0 cts/pixel to the lowest LUT intensity. (We can say that the images are *normalized* to each other in the display; that is, they are put on a scale relative to the maximum-count pixel in each image.) When a dynamic study is displayed, all images will be normalized to the maximum-count pixel within the entire set. This makes the comparison of images relative to one another meaningful.

A gray scale is the most "true to the eye" of any color scale, in that the human eye registers gray-scale changes in an approximately linear fashion. The number of shades of gray used depends on the system and on parameters set by the user. A scale that uses 8 shades of gray shows distinct thresholds between levels and produces a blocky-looking image.

(a) Linear gray scale

(b) Background subtraction and contrast enhancement

Example lookup table:

Cts/pixel	Grayness
>15	Black
11–15	Dark gray
6–10	Medium gray
1–5	Light gray
0	White

—— Contrast enhancement
—— Background subtraction

(c) Nonlinear gray scales

—— Logarithmic scale
- - - Exponential scale

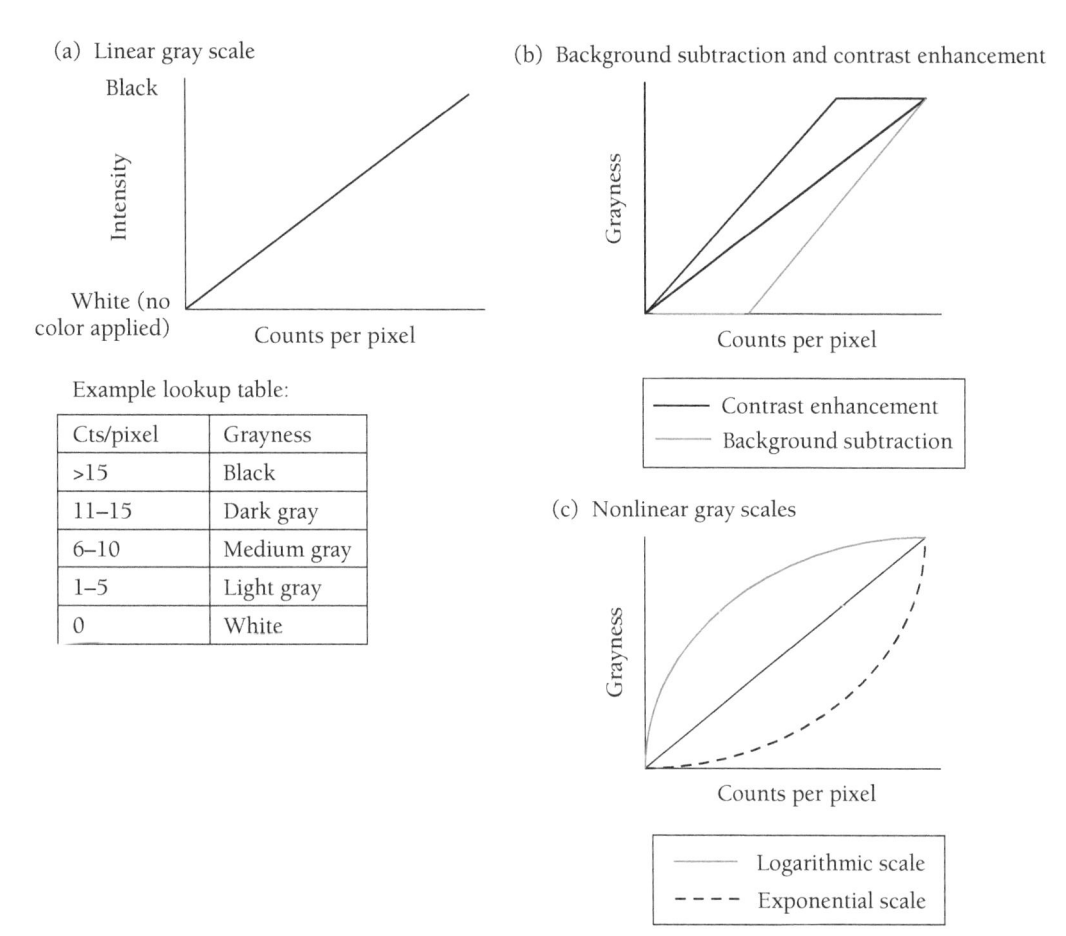

Figure 6-6 Graphical depiction of computer gray scales. These graphs all assume the use of a white background, so that increasing counts per pixel are seen as increasing optical density (grayness). The computer finds the counts-per-pixel value for a given pixel along the X-axis and then assigns the corresponding gray level from the Y-axis. The graph in Figure 6-6a represents a linear scale. The table shows an example of how the graph is translated into five gray levels. Figure 6-6b shows how manipulating the scale increases the contrast (i.e., the slope of the line). Decreasing the count value given maximum intensity is sometimes called *contrast enhancement*, while increasing the count value assigned minimum intensity is sometimes called *background subtraction*. Figure 6-6c shows an exponential and a logarithmic gray scale; these are referred to as "gamma maps" in some systems. Their effect on image appearance is described in the text.

A scale with 64 shades of gray is indistinguishable from completely smooth shading to the human eye, which cannot perceive changes in brightness of less than about 2% (2). The most common configuration is to use an 8-bit LUT, generating 256 gray levels. It is also easy to invert the gray scale, such that the background is black and areas of increased activity are light, similar to an x-ray.

Color Scales

We are not, however, limited to shades of gray. We can assign any colors we desire to the image, using a LUT with three values for each defined step. The three values represent the relative contributions of red, green, and blue needed to produce the desired color. Each of the three primary colors is given an 8-bit LUT, allowing for more than 262,000 different combinations. This greatly increases our ability to perceive details in the image, given that the human eye can discriminate more than 1 million different colors (1). The color LUT values are then applied to the red, green, and blue color phosphors found in video display terminals (VDTs) and liquid-crystal display (LCD) monitors (see Appendix B). These devices can create any color by combining appropriate amounts of the three phosphors. Once the user chooses a color LUT, the computer sends to the video display controller the appropriate intensity values for the three electron guns for each color in a VDT, or to the three subpixels of the LCD.

A variety of color scales have been developed to emphasize specific aspects of nuclear medicine images in specific situations. These are helpful if used as intended, but when applied incorrectly, such scales may cause confusion for the viewer. Many color scales are intrinsically nonlinear, meaning that the human eye responds to the colors of the scale in a different order than their sequence in the scale. For example, the eye is more sensitive to green and yellow light than to blue or red light. When viewing a typical rainbow scale, the eye responds to yellow and green in the middle of the scale out of proportion to the position of these colors on the scale. Some color scales, such as the "hot-body" and "warm-metal" scales, mimic the eye's linear perception of the gray scale, while utilizing our ability to see color.

Discontinuous color scales may make changes in counts per pixel look more significant than they actually are, giving the appearance of a sharp boundary where none exists. Even smoothly varying scales may be interpreted incorrectly if the eye does not assign equal significance to progressive steps of the scale. Color scales are easily misinterpreted by persons not familiar with nuclear medicine images. Standard practice is to include a similarly manipulated color bar along with the image whenever a color other than a linear gray scale is used (3). One should revert to a gray or hot-body scale if there is any doubt about how to best display a particular image.

Image Contrast

We can enhance a digitized image by changing the upper and lower limits of the color scale, a practice called *windowing*. Rather than utilize the entire available counts-per-pixel scale, from zero to the maximum value, we can choose to employ only part of that range. Usually one picks the part of the scale that contains the physiologic or pathologic detail of interest. *Image contrast* is defined mathematically as the change in image intensity per incremental change in counts per pixel (i.e., the slope of the gray-scale map in Fig. 6-6a). Contrast can thus be changed by moving either the top or the bottom of the line or both, as shown in Figure 6-6b. Care must be taken not to obscure important image details when using windowing to increase image contrast.

An example might be instructive here. When the hepatobiliary system is imaged, the gall bladder accumulates a considerable portion of the radiopharmaceutical. Once this has occurred, our interest is not in the gall bladder, but in the small amount of activity that has entered the duodenum. Rather than use the gall bladder's maximum counts per pixel to set the high end of the visual scale, a good technologist "dials down" the image intensity so that any intestinal activity can be visualized. The gall bladder is now completely black, but this is acceptable because the activity of physiologic interest at this point is in the intestines.

Another, gentler way to change image contrast is to use a nonlinear scale (Fig. 6-6c). An *exponential* scale de-emphasizes (suppresses) the low counts in an image; a *logarithmic* scale increases the visibility of low-count structures. Another way to say this is that a logarithmic scale puts the greatest contrast (the steepest slope) in the low-count range, whereas an exponential scale puts the greatest contrast in the high-count range. These scales are sometimes referred to as *gamma curves*. A specific gamma value, usually included in the scale's name, is used to define the scale according to the gamma function equation:

$$\text{Grayness} = (\text{cts/pixel})e^{1/\text{gamma value}}. \quad (6\text{-}4)$$

The gamma value can vary from 0.0 to 10.0. A gamma of 1.0 generates a linear scale; a gamma less than 1, an exponential scale; and a gamma between 1 and 10, a logarithmic scale.

Screen Capture

All computers have *screen capture* programs that store images and other information after they have been formatted for presentation. This allows for the addition of graphs and annotation as well as images of various sizes. Most screen capture programs save the images as the visual scale has been adjusted, translating that scale to a standardized visual scale. Once this has been done, the image can only be adjusted according to the standardized scale. For example, one might capture an image after adjusting to 10 cts/pixel as the lowest intensity, rather than 0 cts/pixel. The captured image cannot be adjusted back to a baseline of 0 cts/pixel; that information was lost when the screen was "captured." One would need to return to the original image to be able to display that information.

Image Display Devices

Once an image is stored in digital format, it can be displayed using a variety of devices, including various computer display monitors and hard-copy devices such as formatters and printers. These devices should be able to reproduce the image in its digital form, without imposing any limitations or distortions. Appendix B discusses the operational details of monitors and printers, and Appendix D covers computers.

Limitations of Image Display

It is important to recognize that the processes by which images are created, displayed, and photographed do not ultimately determine what we are able to see. The ability of a particular observer to see a particular detail depends on many factors, of which the image itself is only one. Two extensive reviews of the issue of visual psychophysics are found in References 2 and 4; a few of the concepts that pertain to nuclear medicine are discussed here.

First, we must realize that an image can be no better than the imaging situation allows it to be. The parameters that are most important to interpretation of nuclear medicine images are count density, contrast, and lesion size. Radiopharmaceutical characteristics and patient physiology may produce a biodistribution that fundamentally lacks contrast and/or detail. The inherent resolution and count limits of gamma cameras may also limit lesion detectability. The finite size of the pixels in a digital image affects the ability to define the edge of an organ or lesion. Image manipulation and display techniques can improve one's ability to detect details, but only to the point at which these other factors become limiting.

Second, image interpretation is not a cut-and-dried exercise of one's observational powers. It is rather a dynamic interplay of visual input with mental "reality maps" that we subconsciously construct in our brains and that are constantly being modified by experience. One's ability to interpret an image depends as much (or more) on one's knowledge and expertise as on the quality of an image. Artifact recognition is one example of how vision and prior knowledge must work together.

An element of visual psychophysics that helps to convey the complexity of the interaction of the brain and eyes is the visualization of edges. Some neurons fire only when a stimulus is turned on or off; when the stimulus is

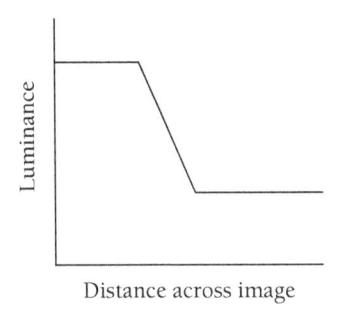

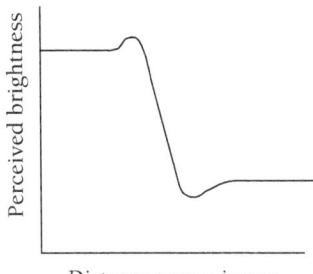

Figure 6-7 Mach bands. The left-hand graph shows the measured luminance of a test pattern. The right-hand graph shows the increased sensitivity that the eye has for a boundary, which aids in edge detection. Extra neurons fire at the boundary, causing an increased neural output signal that is interpreted by the eye as increased luminance. The result is the perception of a narrow band of bright or dark at the point of intersection of two areas with sharply different luminances. Reprinted from: Lotto RB, Williams SM, Purves D. An empirical basis for Mach bands. *Proc Natl Acad Sci USA*. 1999;96:5239–5244. Copyright 1999 National Academy of Sciences, USA.

left in place, these neurons gradually cease firing. When the eye reaches an edge or boundary within an image, the additional firing of these neurons produces an exaggeration of the boundary (**Figure 6-7**). The *Mach band phenomenon*, as it is called, causes us to see narrow bands of light and dark at the transition point of a luminance step. As a result, the level of brightness needed to adequately display an image depends on the presence or absence of sharp boundaries. One of the reasons that nuclear medicine images are perceived as "fuzzy" by many radiologists is that they have fewer sharp edges than other radiologic images. The sharp boundaries encountered in x-rays and other types of radiologic images are enhanced by the Mach band phenomenon.

Human vision responds strongly to objects in motion. Some neurons in the visual cortex are active only when movement is detected, indicating that motion is a fundamental dimension of the visual system. We can use this to our advantage in displaying nuclear medicine images. The display of a beating heart from a myocardial perfusion study conveys more information to the viewer than the polar map that summarizes the wall motion. A rotating three-dimensional reconstruction conveys greater depth perception than a stationary view of the same reconstruction.

Several aspects of visual psychophysics affect nuclear medicine images. Because of their inherent fuzziness, nuclear medicine images generally look worse with magnification. Areas of increased activity are easier to detect than photopenic areas. Nuclear medicine images can be displayed in either a positive (white on a black background) or negative (black on a white background); there are perceptual differences between the two that are not completely understood, and each offers advantages. When images are put onto film, the characteristics of the film play a large role in the ability to visually appreciate image details and count density changes. Finally, the use of view boxes adds a veiling glare of excess light that decreases the eye's sensitivity for the subtle changes that may be significant in nuclear medicine images.

All of these factors play into the interpretation of a nuclear medicine study by a given individual. But we must go even beyond that, to the fact that different individuals will be affected differently by each factor. When nuclear medicine studies are in the development process and when nuclear medicine departments are evaluating their diagnostic quality, two of the parameters considered are intraobserver and interobserver variability. *Intraobserver* refers to the ability of an individual reader to reach the same conclusion about a particular study on two occasions. *Interobserver* refers to the ability of multiple individuals to reach the same conclusion about a study. A nuclear medicine test is useful only if its results can be reported consistently. Good intra- and interobserver results rely in part on agreement on how to display and view images.

Summary

The essence of nuclear medicine is the creation of images that can be viewed on film or on a computer screen. The X, Y, and Z signals emanating from a gamma camera are only the starting point; we take those signals and lay them out in two-dimensional space, in either an analog or a digital fashion. But the work does not end here. Physicians and technologists working in nuclear medicine need to understand how the display systems work and how a given display choice (such as a particular color scale) affects one's perception of the image. They also need to understand how images are perceived by the eye and how the information contained in them is interpreted by the brain.

References

1. Schwaiger M, Ziegler S, Nekolla SG. PET/CT: challenge for nuclear cardiology. *J Nucl Med*. 2005;46:1664–1668.
2. Jaffe CC. Medical imaging, vision, and visual psychophysics. *Med Radiog Photog*. 1984;60:1–48.
3. Wagner HN, Szabo Z, Buchanan JW, eds. *Principles of Nuclear Medicine*. 2nd ed. Philadelphia, PA: WB Saunders; 1995:392.
4. Pizer SM, ter Haar Romeny BM. Fundamental properties of medical image perception. *J Digital Imaging*. 1991;4:1–20.

Additional Resources

Cherry SR, Sorenson JA, Phelps ME. *Physics in Nuclear Medicine*. 3rd ed. Philadelphia, PA: Saunders; 2003:Chapter 19.

Henkin RE, Boles MA, Dillehay GL, et al. *Nuclear Medicine*. St. Louis, MO: Mosby-Year Book; 1996:Chapter 15.

Lee KH. *Computers in Nuclear Medicine: A Practical Approach*. 2nd ed. Reston, VA: Society of Nuclear Medicine; 2005:Chapters 7, 8.

CHAPTER 7 Collimators

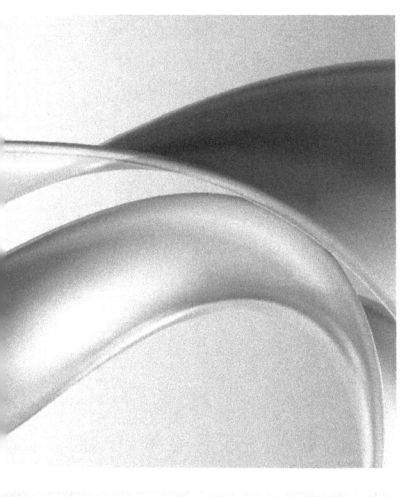

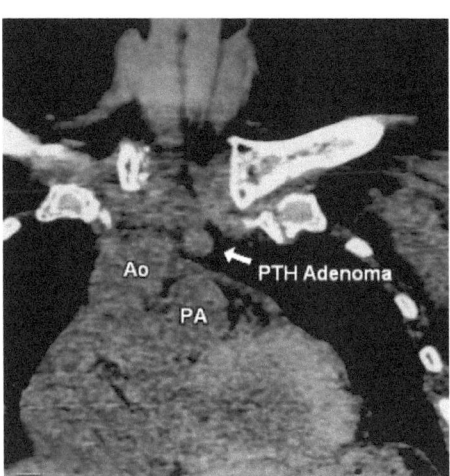

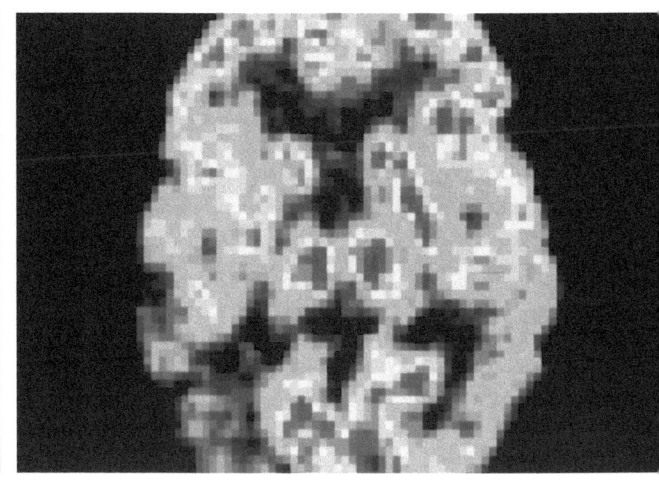

Learning Outcomes

1. Distinguish between the foil and cast methods of collimator manufacture, and discuss the advantages and disadvantages of each.
2. Diagram the geometric, penetration, absorption, and scatter components of a gamma ray source illuminating a collimator, and discuss how each affects resolution and sensitivity.
3. Identify the effect of changing the hole diameter, hole length, and object–collimator distance on collimator resolution, and illustrate with diagrams.
4. Given collimator and intrinsic resolution, calculate the system resolution.
5. Discuss issues related to septal thickness for low-energy vs high-energy radionuclides and how collimators are made to address these issues.
6. State concepts and issues related to the use of a pinhole collimator.
7. Characterize and briefly discuss uses for slant-hole, converging, diverging, cone-beam, and fan-beam collimators.
8. Draw graphs illustrating the changes in resolution, sensitivity, and field-of-view size vs object–collimator distance for parallel-hole and focused collimators.

Introduction

A collimator is an essential part of any gamma camera. In Anger-type cameras, it is a lead sheet with many very small holes, usually parallel, through the thickness of the sheet. Its function is to create a geometric correspondence or mapping between gamma rays emitted in the object and the location of their interaction in the scintillation crystal. Two examples of collimators are shown in **Figure 7-1**. **Figure 7-2** shows the internal structure of a parallel-hole collimator.

Without a collimator, gamma rays from many angles are absorbed in the scintillation crystal, and no useful spatial information is obtained. With a collimator, only the gamma rays that are carrying "good" information (based on their angle relative to the camera) are projected onto the scintillation crystal. This is called *absorptive collimation*, because the collimator eliminates the "bad" (i.e., off-angle) gamma rays by passively absorbing them in the *septa* (the lead between the holes). This arrangement is simultaneously too good and not good enough. It is too good in that more than 99.9% of all gamma rays are absorbed (1). But it is not good enough in that the holes must be of some finite width, so we can't stop all gamma rays that we don't want, namely, those not exactly perpendicular to the crystal face.

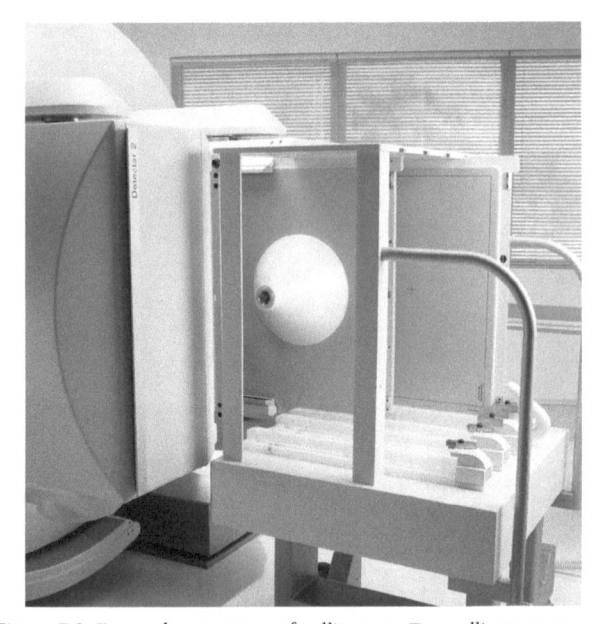

Figure 7-1 External appearance of collimators. Two collimators are shown: a pinhole collimator is in the middle of the photograph, and behind it (to the right of the pinhole collimator) is a parallel-hole collimator. The pinhole collimator is in the process of being installed onto one head of the gamma camera at the left. It is used to magnify small organs such as the thyroid gland. Photo courtesy of Siemens Medical Systems.

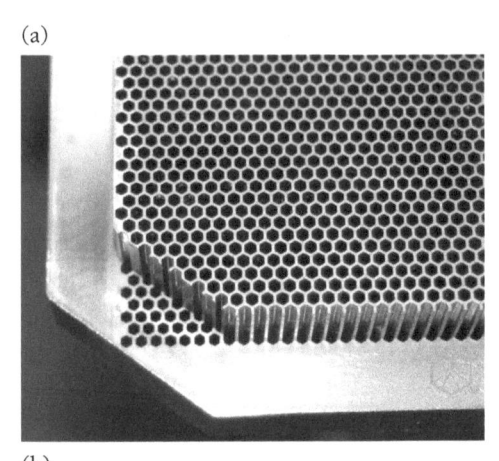

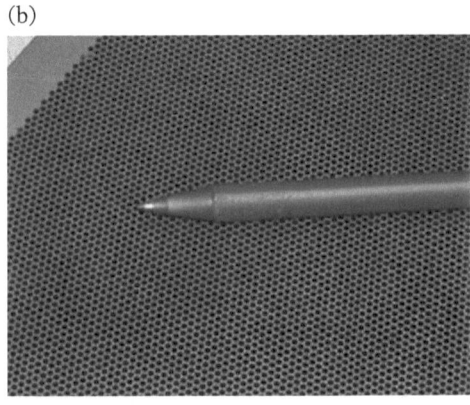

Figure 7-2 Internal construction of a parallel-hole collimator. (a) The holes are most commonly hexagonally shaped, and they have considerable length, as the cut-away shows. (b) The size of the holes is on the order of the tip of a pen. The septa constitute the walls between the holes; their thickness depends on the energy of the radionuclide being used with the collimator. Photos courtesy of Nuclear Fields, Inc.

The collimator therefore constitutes the most significant limitation on gamma camera performance (1), and it is the major determinant of both resolution and sensitivity. These parameters are determined by the collimator's geometric dimensions, specifically the diameter and number of holes it has, and the length and thickness of the septa. We can describe collimators from a mathematical standpoint, and readers interested in such descriptions are referred to Appendix E. However, nuclear medicine technologists are generally not involved in the design of collimators, but rather in choosing collimators for specific imaging situations. This chapter covers the concepts and applications of collimator design as they pertain to clinical imaging situations.

Manufacturing Collimators

Collimators are usually made from lead, because of its high atomic number and density. Tungsten, gold, and depleted uranium have better attenuation properties, but all are more expensive and/or harder to work with than lead (2). Lead is a very soft metal that is difficult to drill. Collimators are easily damaged and must be handled with care. Collimator damage is a major cause of artifacts in nuclear medicine images.

Collimator holes can be round, square, or hexagonal (**Figure 7-3**). Round holes are easy to make and can be packed closely together, but leave dead spaces, resulting in decreased sensitivity. Square holes are also easy to manufacture, but because the length of the hole's diagonal is considerably larger than the length of its sides, resolution varies with the direction of measurement. The most common choice currently is hexagonal close-packed holes, an arrangement that maximizes sensitivity for a given resolution (2).

Collimators can be fashioned using several methods. A *foil* collimator is made from corrugated lead sheets in which the folds are lined up and glued together to create the septa (Figs. 7-3b and 7-3c). Thin lead sheets work well for low-energy radionuclides, especially Tc-99m and Tl-201. *Cast* collimators are made by casting or etching the lead into the desired shape. This method is used to fabricate collimators used with high-energy gamma rays, because thicker septa are required than can be made with lead foils. *Microcast* collimators are also cast from molten lead, but the holes are created using steel pins held in place by two steel plates, and the lead is quick-cooled to reduce shrinkage. These collimators are less easily damaged and generally are more uniform than foil collimators (3), but may be considerably more expensive. A recent innovation in collimator manufacture is the *microlinear* collimator, which uses thin lead foil, but incorporates a slight arc where the foils join to prevent misalignment (Fig. 7-3d). Pinhole collimators are made from a mold.

Collimator Concepts

Figure 7-4 shows the possible outcomes of gamma rays leaving the object and interacting (or not interacting) in

(a) Round

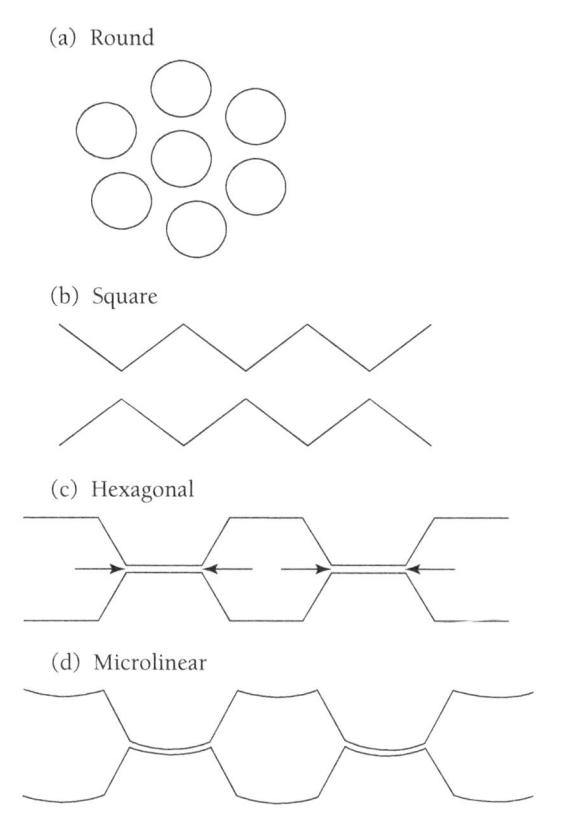

(b) Square

(c) Hexagonal

(d) Microlinear

Figure 7-3 Several possible shapes for collimator holes. The choice of hole geometry is dependent on the method used to construct the collimator. Round holes (Fig. 7-3a) are most often created by a cast methodology. Figures 7-3b, c, and d each show two foils coming together to create the collimator holes. The arrows in Figure 7-3c indicate the space where glue is needed to hold the foils together; mechanical stress can misalign the foils along the arrows. Microlinear construction (Fig. 7-3d) eliminates the need for glue and decreases the likelihood of misalignment. Figures 7-3c and 7-3d reprinted with permission of Nuclear Fields, Inc.

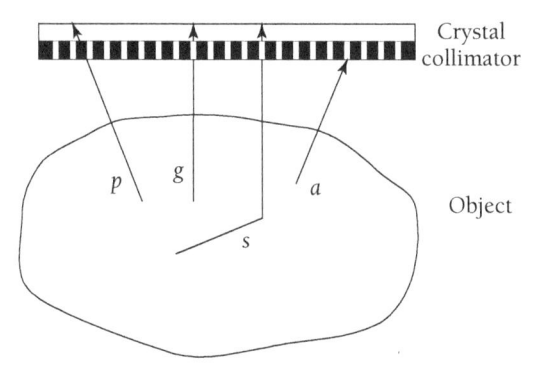

Figure 7-4 Possible outcomes of gamma rays as they interact with a gamma camera collimator; g = geometric component (gamma rays that pass through the collimator holes and interact in the scintillation crystal), p = penetration component (gamma rays that have penetrated one or more septa without being absorbed), s = scatter component (gamma rays that undergo Compton scatter interactions in the object, such that the scattered gamma rays pass through the collimator holes without interacting), and a = absorption component (gamma rays that are absorbed in the collimator septa).

a collimator. (We assume for the moment that all the collimator holes are parallel to one another and perpendicular to the camera face. Collimators that differ in one or both of these assumptions are available and are discussed later in this chapter.) The *geometric* fraction is the fraction of photons that pass through the collimator holes without interacting with the septa, thus entering the crystal in a perpendicular direction. The *absorption* fraction consists of those photons that are absorbed in the lead septa. The *penetration* fraction is the subset of photons that have passed through one or more septa without having an interaction with the lead atoms. Finally, the *scatter* fraction includes photons that pass through the collimator without interacting, but only after they have been scattered in the object (scatter within the collimator itself is generally negligible, at least with low-energy radionuclides).

The geometric and absorption components are thus giving good information: those photons passing through a collimator hole at a 90° angle to the crystal face are accepted (with a small range around 90°, because the holes have a finite diameter), and photons outside this narrow range are eliminated by absorption in the septa. The penetration and scatter components are adding bad information into the image, because in each case photons are emitted in the object at one location, but are absorbed in the scintillation crystal at a different location.

These four fractions can be used to understand how collimator design and radionuclide selection affect resolution and sensitivity. Overall, the geometric fraction is the most important determinant of collimator characteristics. Resolution—the ability to see details—is improved by decreasing the size of the collimator holes (and therefore the geometric fraction). In addition, any change in the collimator design that decreases the penetration fraction will improve resolution. Sensitivity, or the number of photons detected, will be increased by design changes that increase the geometric fraction and decreased by changes that decrease the penetration fraction. Penetration and scatter contribute to background and thus degrade image contrast. In practice, collimators are generally designed to maximize either resolution or sensitivity while keeping the penetration component at an acceptable level. The definition of "an acceptable level" depends on the particulars of a given imaging situation, so a selection of collimators is generally needed.

Design Parameters

Translation of these concepts into a physical collimator is based on relatively simple principles of geometry (Reference 4 is Anger's article describing the mathematics of parallel-hole collimators). The mathematics of resolution and sensitivity relative to the design parameters of a collimator are discussed in Appendix E. While many readers will shudder at the thought of trying to understand the math, it is actually fairly straightforward. This section describes in words and diagrams how the hole diameter, hole length, and septal thickness affect collimator performance. But some may find that the geometric relationships and mathematical formulas shown in Appendix E will make the concepts clearer.

Figure 7-5 illustrates the design parameters of hole diameter and hole length, as well as the effect of object–collimator

(a) Illustration of R_{coll}

(b) Increased hole diameter

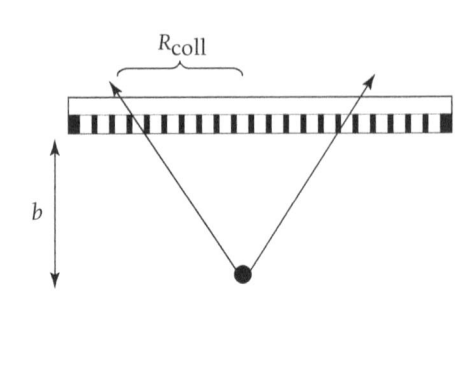

(c) Increased hole length

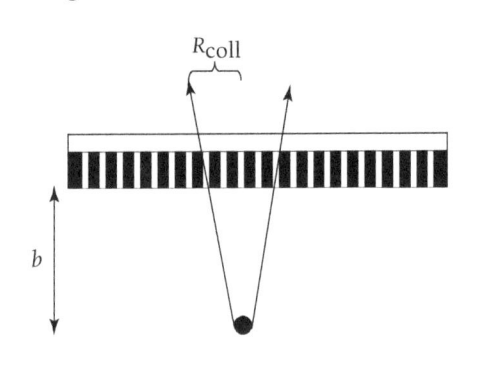

(d) Increased distance

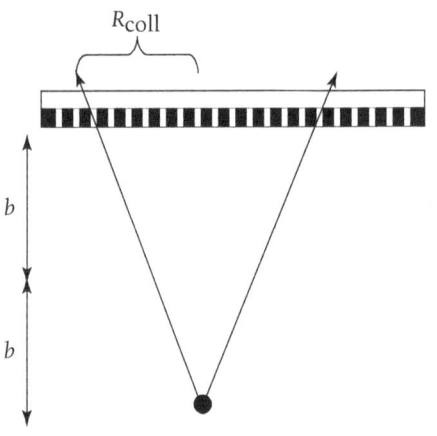

Figure 7-5 Effect of hole diameter, hole length, and object–collimator distance on resolution. In each diagram, the arrows from the point source to the crystal are shown at the maximum angle that does not intercept any lead septa. Figure 7-5a illustrates the concept of R_{coll}. A count profile through the point source is shown above the collimator; R_{coll} is the radius of the circle that the point source projects onto the crystal, taken midway between the outer edge of counts and the center of the circle. A smaller R_{coll} indicates improved resolution. This figure should be used as the basis for comparison for the other figures. In Figure 7-5b, the holes are twice the diameter in Figure 7-5a, and R_{coll} increases (resolution is degraded). Figure 7-5c shows that if the septa are made longer than in Figure 7-5a, R_{coll} decreases (resolution is improved). Finally, as the distance between the point source and the collimator is increased, R_{coll} increases (Fig. 7-5d).

distance. In these diagrams, the collimator resolution R_{coll} is the radius of the circle of gamma rays projected onto the crystal by the collimator, from a point source at some distance from the collimator (Fig. 7-5a). It thus provides a measure of the perceived size of the source at this distance, as shown by the idealized count profile above the collimator. A smaller R_{coll} indicates a collimator with better resolution; a larger R_{coll}, one with worse resolution.

Hole Diameter

The diameter of the holes in a multihole collimator determines both its resolution and its sensitivity. As the hole diameter increases, photons at greater angles pass through the collimator without being absorbed in the septa (Fig. 7-5b). If the hole diameter is made smaller, we restrict the photons passing through the holes to a narrower range of angles. Thus, a collimator with small holes will have better resolution (smaller R_{coll}) and lower sensitivity, whereas a collimator with large holes will have poorer resolution and higher sensitivity. If the hole size increases beyond the camera's intrinsic (uncollimated) resolution, however, the hole pattern itself will be visualized, decreasing the diagnostic utility of the images. This can be seen in extrinsic floods with high-energy collimators, in which hole diameter is increased in order to improve sensitivity (see Parallel-hole Collimators).

Hole Length

The length or *bore* of the collimator holes also affects resolution and sensitivity (Fig. 7-5c). As the holes are made longer, gamma rays that are not quite perpendicular to the collimator are more likely to be absorbed in the septa before they reach the scintillation crystal. Increasing the hole length is a tactic that can improve resolution without sacrificing too much in the way of sensitivity. Long-bore collimators have found application in SPECT imaging, where they are used to maintain resolution at the greater distances required to allow rotation of the camera around the patient.

Distance

The object–collimator distance is the other important factor in collimator resolution (Fig. 7-5d). As this distance is increased, gamma rays are able to pass through a wider area of collimator holes without intercepting the lead septa. Radius R_{coll} is increased, indicating that resolution is degraded. A cardinal rule of planar gamma camera imaging is therefore to bring the collimator as close to the patient as possible. Not doing so counteracts the collimator's design parameters. The use of a high-resolution collimator is pointless if the collimator is not literally touching the object being imaged.

On the other hand, sensitivity remains constant as distance increases for a parallel-hole collimator. This is so because the same number of gamma rays pass through a larger number of holes. Object–collimator distance is thus the one factor that does not involve a trade-off between resolution and sensitivity, and it is the only factor under the direct control of the operator. Optimal gamma camera imaging always requires minimizing the object–collimator distance.

Septal Thickness

The thickness of the lead septa between collimator holes is the major determinant of the penetration component of Figure 7-4. *Septal penetration* is the ability of gamma rays to cross from one hole to another without being absorbed in the septum. We know from nuclear physics that photon absorption is a probabilistic function, and we cannot guarantee that any thickness of lead will stop all gamma rays. We will always have a penetration fraction. But if we get much septal penetration, resolution is degraded and the resulting image is less clear.

The energy of the radionuclide being utilized is therefore the main determinant of septal thickness: a higher-energy isotope requires thicker septa, as can be seen in **Figure 7-6**. Collimators are therefore specified by photon energy; a collimator's stated energy is generally the highest energy that can be effectively imaged with that collimator. **Table 7-1** shows the septal thickness and septal penetration for several collimators designed for different maximum photon energies. **Figure 7-7** shows images of a high-energy source with low-, medium-, and high-energy collimators. When an imaging situation requires a specific but not commonly used isotope, it is possible to have a collimator custom-made, taking septal penetration and the desired resolution into account.

Septal penetration is a significant issue when imaging with high-energy radionuclides. As the photon energy increases, the septal thickness must also increase, or too many of the gamma rays will penetrate the collimator. But if the septa are made thick enough to minimize the penetration fraction, the collimator loses sensitivity and becomes very heavy. So we compromise and use less lead than we need, but we must in turn accept significant septal

Table 7-1

Relationship of Radionuclide Energy, Septal Thickness, and Septal Penetration for Selected Collimators

Energy Rating of Collimator	Septal Thickness	Septal Penetration
140 keV	0.25 mm	< 1%
160 keV	0.3 mm	2%
200 keV	0.5 mm	1%
250 keV	1.0 mm	1%
364 keV	2.2 mm	> 5%

Used with permission of Nuclear Fields USA, 1645 River Road, Suite 5, Des Plaines, IL 60018.

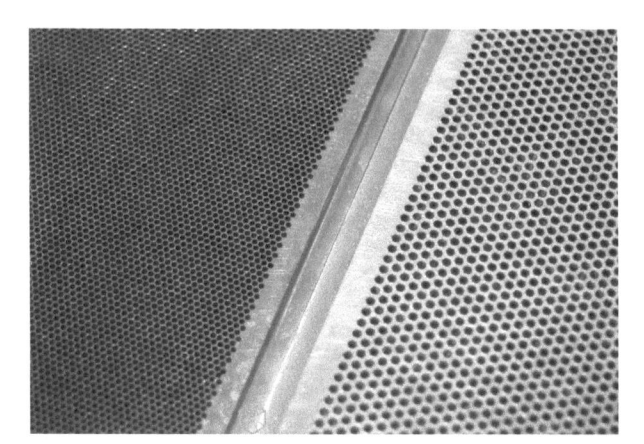

Figure 7-6 Comparison of septal thickness for low- vs medium-energy collimators. The low-energy collimator is on the left and the medium-energy collimator on the right in this photo. When they are placed side by side, the increase in septal thickness needed for increasing gamma ray energy is apparent. Photo courtesy of Nuclear Fields, Inc.

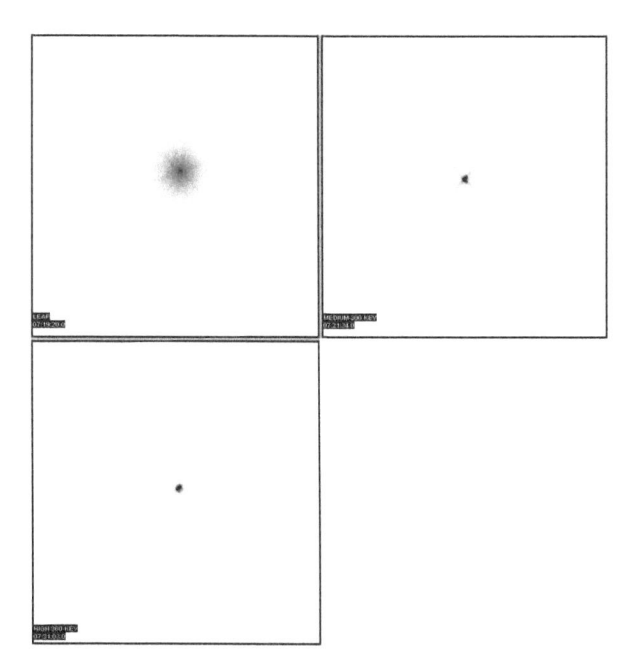

Figure 7-7 Images of a high-energy source with low-, medium-, and high-energy collimators. The source being imaged is an I-131 uptake capsule. The 364-keV gamma rays are not absorbed to any significant extent in the low-energy collimator (upper left), so the image demonstrates a complete lack of definition. The medium-energy (upper right) and high-energy (lower left) collimators stop more of the I-131 gamma rays, but are still hampered by a star artifact. Image courtesy of Virginia Mason Medical Center.

Design Parameters

(a) Square-hole alignment (b) Hexagonal-hole alignment

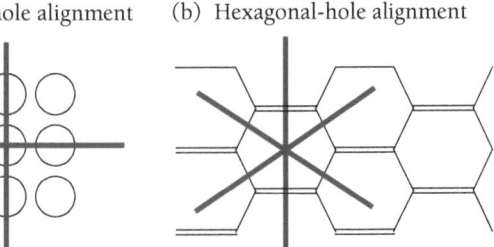

Figure 7-8 Star artifact. The arms of the star are in the direction of the least amount of lead. (a) A four-arm star indicates that the holes are aligned in a square pattern. (b) A six-arm star indicates that the holes are aligned in a hexagonal pattern.

penetration, often in the form of a *star artifact*. Star artifacts can be seen in many situations, but are especially noticeable when a high-energy radionuclide is concentrated in a small volume. The images in Figure 7-7 all illustrate star artifacts. Photons are most likely to penetrate the septa at their thinnest point, which in a collimator is between the centers of the holes. Thus a star artifact illuminates the hole geometry of the collimator (**Figure 7-8**).

System Performance

System resolution (R_{sys}) is determined by both collimator resolution (R_{coll}) and the inherent resolution of the uncollimated camera (called its *intrinsic resolution* and abbreviated R_{int}). (The term *system* in this context refers to the camera as it is used for imaging, with a collimator. We could also refer to it as *extrinsic* resolution.) These are combined according to a root–mean–square type of calculation:

$$R_{sys} = \sqrt{R_{int}^2 + R_{coll}^2} \qquad (7\text{-}1)$$

The value for R_{coll} in this calculation is usually calculated rather than measured, using Equation E-5 (or the appropriate formula for a non-parallel-hole collimator). The larger of the two values in this formula has the greater influence on the value of R_{sys}. When we consider a typical imaging situation with some distance between the collimator and the organ being imaged, it is the collimator resolution that dominates.

Sample Calculation 7-1   System Resolution

Calculate the system resolution for a gamma camera that has an intrinsic resolution of 4.0 mm and collimator resolution of 2.1 mm at the surface and 7.1 mm at 10 cm from the collimator surface.

At the surface: $R_{sys} = \sqrt{(4.0 \text{ mm})^2 + (2.1 \text{ mm})^2} = 4.5 \text{ mm}.$

At 10 cm: $R_{sys} = \sqrt{(4.0 \text{ mm})^2 + (7.1 \text{ mm})^2} = 8.1 \text{ mm}.$

Note that in each case, the larger of the two values dominates the R_{sys} calculation. Note also the large change in system resolution at a distance from the collimator.

Similarly, system sensitivity is determined by intrinsic sensitivity and collimator sensitivity, but in a different fashion. Intrinsic sensitivity is mainly dependent on the thickness of the scintillation crystal. At low gamma ray energies, intrinsic sensitivity approaches unity (i.e., all gamma rays are absorbed in the crystal), and collimator sensitivity determines system sensitivity. At higher gamma ray energies, on the other hand, intrinsic sensitivity drops below 50% (see Fig. 8-4), while collimator sensitivity increases due to septal penetration. While the collimator is still the main determinant of system sensitivity, it may be advantageous to consider nontraditional combinations of cameras and collimators for high-energy radionuclides.

For example, consider the imaging dilemma presented by the thyroid cancer metastatic survey using iodine-131 as sodium iodide. Radiation dosimetry considerations and the (debated) phenomenon of thyroid stunning have led many nuclear medicine practitioners to drop the dosage of I-131 as sodium iodide from 5–10 mCi down to 2 mCi. Most of the radiopharmaceutical clears from the body, so that at the time of imaging, only a small amount remains. Using a standard gamma camera with a $\frac{3}{8}$-inch (in) scintillation crystal and a high-energy collimator, a 10-minute image may yield only 20,000 to 50,000 counts, barely enough for statistical significance. If a camera with a thicker crystal (say, 1 in) is available, its increased intrinsic sensitivity yields many more counts and/or a much decreased imaging time. Even if the only available collimator for this latter camera is designed for medium-energy isotopes, the time savings and increased number of counts may trump the increase in septal penetration and loss of resolution that come with using the medium-energy collimator.

Summary

With this background on collimator parameters and their effect on system performance, we can now discuss the different kinds of collimators used on gamma cameras. Not every department has every variety of collimator. For example, pinhole collimators are often omitted in favor of digital zooming, especially on multihead systems. This saves cost and space, but forfeits the increased resolution that the pinhole collimator offers. Keep in mind also that new advances in gamma camera technology will continue to bring new types of collimators into prominence, so the following examples should not be considered exhaustive.

Parallel-Hole Collimators

Parallel-hole collimators provide a one-to-one mapping between activity in the object being imaged and count density in the image, without magnification or distortion. The great majority of nuclear medicine studies are performed with parallel-hole collimators. If a different kind of collimator is used for a particular situation, it is because a parallel-hole collimator is specifically felt to be inadequate for that situation.

Parallel-hole collimators are often "graded" based on their performance characteristics and the maximum

Table 7-2

Comparison of Design Features, Sensitivity, and Resolution of Low-Energy Collimators

Characteristic	High Sensitivity	General Purpose	High Resolution
Hole diameter	2.5 mm	1.9 mm	1.9 mm
Hole length	30 mm	30 mm	41 mm
Septal thickness	0.3 mm	0.5 mm	0.25 mm
Resolution:			
at surface[1]	2.9 mm	2.2 mm	2.1 mm
10 cm[1]	11.9 mm	9.0 mm	7.1 mm
Sensitivity (cpm/µCi)	800	450	240

[1]These values are calculated from the formulas in Appendix E.
Used with permission of Nuclear Fields USA, 1645 River Road, Suite 5, Des Plaines, IL 60018.

photon energy to be used (**Tables 7-2** and **7-3**). The most common designation system describes a given collimator as high-sensitivity, general-purpose, high-resolution, or ultra-high-resolution. These designations are not hard and fast (5); one rationale for doing collimator calculations such as those described in Appendix E is to verify the manufacturer's quoted values for resolution and sensitivity (2).

Resolution/Sensitivity Choices

High-sensitivity collimators are used only in situations where sensitivity is significantly more important than resolution; for example, in first-pass cardiac studies. When a high-sensitivity collimator is purchased, extrinsic bar phantom studies should be done to determine its resolution (see discussion of Moiré patterns).

The more common choice is between a general-purpose (also called a low-energy all-purpose or LEAP) collimator and a high-resolution collimator. The general-purpose collimator is quite suitable for dynamic and functional imaging where anatomic information is secondary; examples include renal and gastric-emptying studies. A high-resolution collimator should be used when imaging time can be extended and when good anatomic information is required (e.g., bone scan images of the hands or feet). In addition to the improved resolution, a high-resolution collimator improves contrast (6).

Energy Choices

Parallel-hole collimators can be made for a variety of photon energies, but significant compromises must be made as photon energy increases. First, the septa must get much thicker (>2 mm for I-131; see Table 7-3). This limits the area of crystal surface available for photon absorption, thus decreasing sensitivity. But administered activity is often low to begin with, so the hole diameter is increased to make the imaging time more tolerable. The hole length is increased to cut down on septal penetration and to regain some of the resolution lost to the increased hole diameter, but resolution is still degraded compared to low-energy collimators.

While it is possible to make several grades of collimators at each gamma ray energy employed, cost becomes an issue, and most departments purchase one medium-energy (up to 250 keV) and one high-energy (up to 364 keV) general-purpose collimator for each gamma camera. Using a collimator with an energy maximum lower than the gamma ray energy being imaged may result in severe septal penetration, star artifacts, and loss of image detail. This is especially true if a low-energy collimator is used to image gamma rays with energies higher than about 160 keV (see upper-left image of Fig. 7-7).

Pinhole Collimator

The pinhole collimator is a large, hollow lead cone with a single small (3- to 7-mm) hole or aperture at the point of the cone (**Figure 7-9**). It is used to magnify very small organs such as the thyroid gland. It works much like an

Table 7-3

Comparison of Design Features, Sensitivity, and Resolution of Low-, Medium-, and High-Energy Collimators

Characteristic	Low-Energy All-Purpose	Medium-Energy All-Purpose (250 keV)	High-Energy All-Purpose (364 keV)
Hole diameter	1.9 mm	3.0 mm	3.4 mm
Hole length	30 mm	40 mm	45 mm
Septal thickness	0.5 mm	1.0 mm	2.2 mm
Resolution at surface[1]	2.2 mm	3.5 mm	4.0 mm
Resolution at 10 cm[1]	9.0 mm	11.8 mm	13.5 mm
Sensitivity (cpm/µCi)	450	1,000	465

[1]These values are calculated from the formulas in Appendix E.
Used with permission of Nuclear Fields USA, 1645 River Road, Suite 5, Des Plaines, IL 60018.

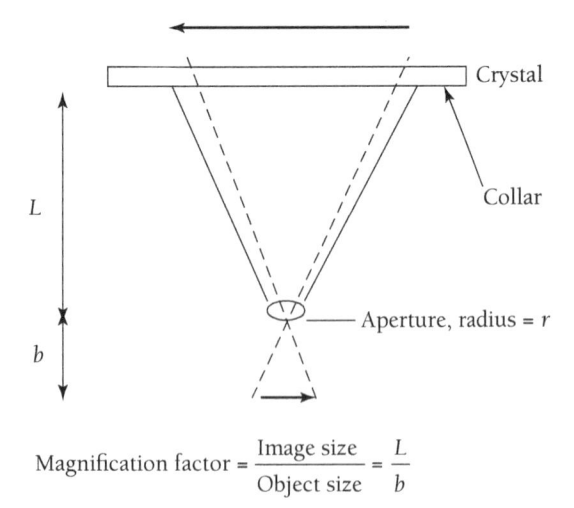

Figure 7-9 Pinhole collimator. The figure shows the inversion of the arrow (the object being imaged) and the magnification factor, which depends on the length of the collimator (L) and the distance between the aperture and the object being imaged (b).

$$\text{Magnification factor} = \frac{\text{Image size}}{\text{Object size}} = \frac{L}{b}$$

old-fashioned box camera, in that it both inverts and magnifies the image. The operator must be aware that the image is inverted relative to normal (parallel-hole) orientation, and she or he may need to physically correct for this inversion, if the system does not do so automatically. The aperture insert is commonly made of tungsten, platinum, or even gold to absorb more high-energy gamma rays; this insert may be interchangeable with other inserts, allowing the operator to vary the aperture size. Using an insert matched to the photon energy will improve resolution (because there will be decreased penetration through the insert) and decrease background from scatter (7).

The distance between the aperture and the organ being imaged affects the resolution, sensitivity, magnification, and field of view (FOV) size. As the object is moved closer to the aperture, the magnification factor increases and resolution improves. But sensitivity decreases, because fewer photons are traveling at angles that allow their passage through the aperture, and the diameter of the FOV decreases as well. Increasing the aperture radius will improve sensitivity and degrade resolution. For small organs such as the thyroid, the pinhole collimator provides the best combination of resolution and sensitivity. It will, however, demonstrate image distortion and loss of counts near the edges of the FOV, because of the three-dimensional nature of the object and the subsequent differential magnification. A well-positioned image of a thyroid gland, for example, should extend across no more than two-thirds to three-fourths of the FOV.

The large end of the cone may be made to occupy only the central part of the FOV, and the remainder of the crystal surface is covered with a lead "collar" (**Figure 7-10a**). The thickness of this collar is kept to a minimum on account of weight considerations, such that it may not absorb many high-energy gamma rays. Figure 7-10b shows a pinhole collimator thyroid image using Tc-99m pertechnetate; note that the edge of the aperture is easily perceived. Figure 7-10c shows an I-123 thyroid image that demonstrates penetration through the collar by the 159-keV photons. This penetration can make it difficult to determine where the edge of the pinhole aperture is. Figure 7-10d demonstrates a

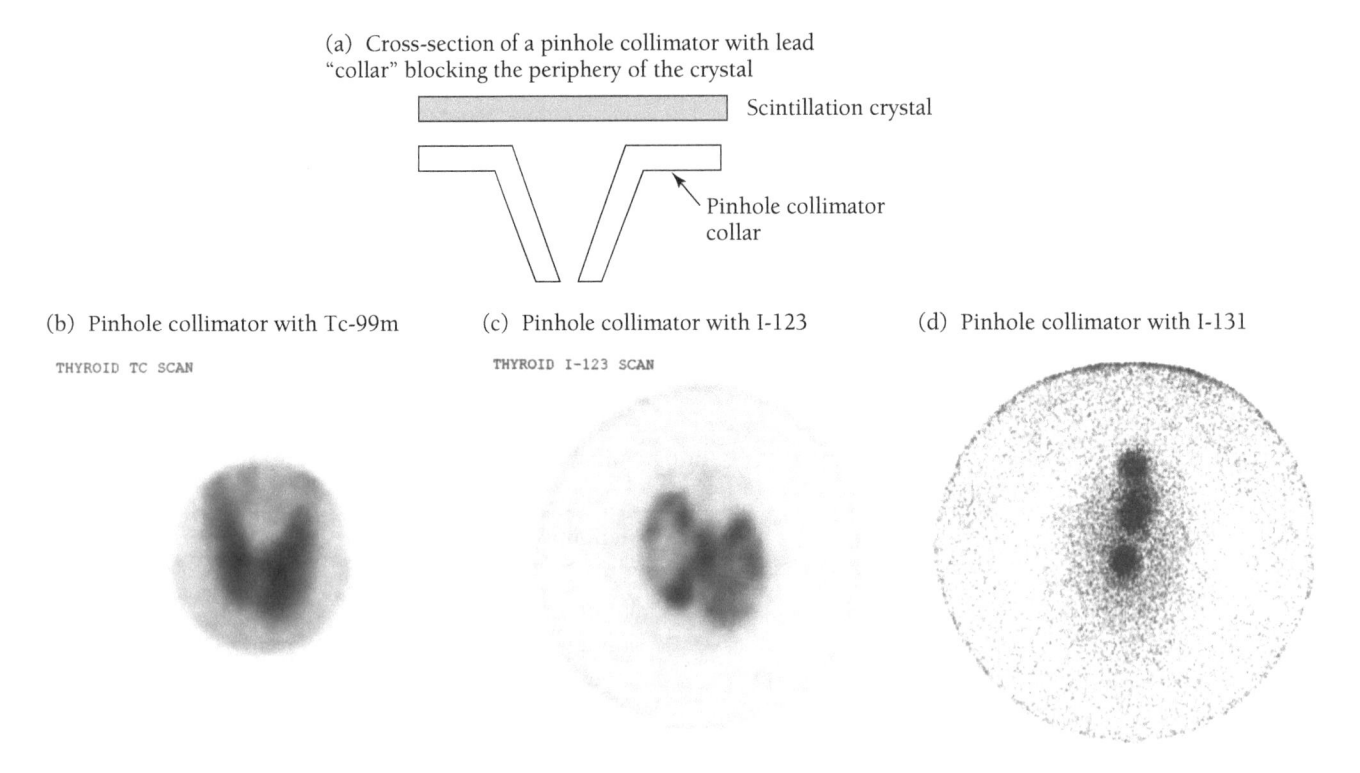

Figure 7-10 Pinhole images of the thyroid, using three different radionuclides. Figure 7-10a shows a cross section illustrating the collimator's construction. With Tc-99m 140-keV gamma rays (Fig. 7-10b), the pinhole collimator's collar blocks most gamma rays that reach it. Using I-123, with its 159-keV gamma rays (Fig. 7-10c), gamma rays are not stopped by the collar and are seen in the image. With I-131 and its 364-keV gamma rays (Fig. 7-10d), gamma rays penetrate the collar and produce edge packing. Figures 7-10b, 7-10c, and 7-10d courtesy of Virginia Mason Medical Center.

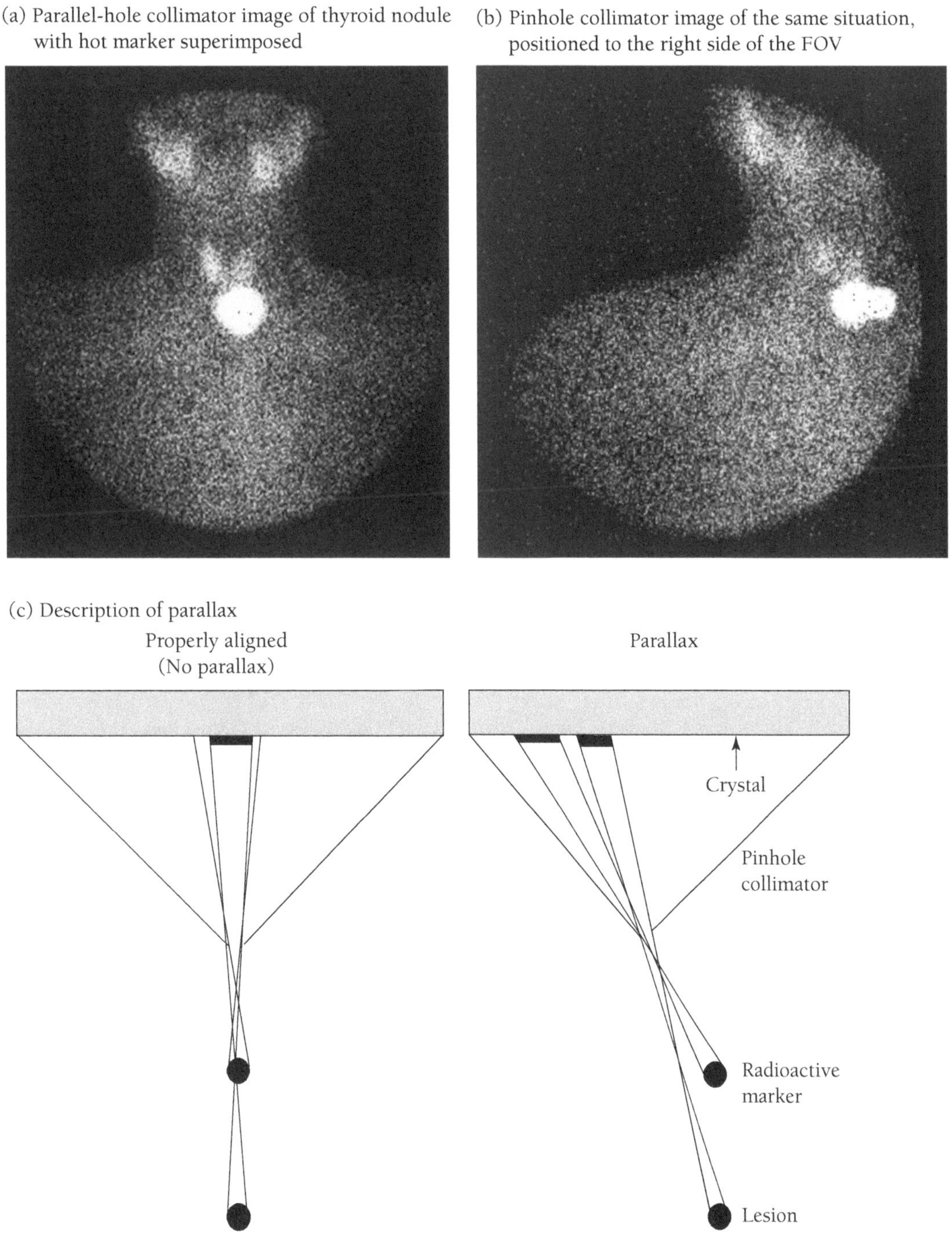

(a) Parallel-hole collimator image of thyroid nodule with hot marker superimposed

(b) Pinhole collimator image of the same situation, positioned to the right side of the FOV

(c) Description of parallax

Properly aligned (No parallax)

Parallax

Crystal

Pinhole collimator

Radioactive marker

Lesion

Figure 7-11 Demonstration of parallax in a pinhole collimator. Figures 7-11a and 7-11b are images of a thyroid gland with an overactive nodule, with a hot marker indicating its palpable location. In the pinhole image (Fig. 7-11b), the nodule and marker are positioned to the right edge of the FOV, causing the marker to project to a different location than the nodule. Figure 7-11c illustrates how the position changes from centered to off-center positioning. Images and diagram courtesy of Dr. David Hillier.

similar situation with I-131. In addition to penetration through the collar, there are extra counts seen at the top of the image, beyond the top of the patient's head. Where are these counts coming from? Recall that the image within the pinhole is inverted, but that the "collar" area is not. Thus the gamma rays seen at the top of the image are emanating from the abdomen and not the skull.

Pinhole collimators are subject to parallax errors (8). *Parallax* is an apparent change in the location of an object due to one's point of observation (**Figure 7-11**). A parallel-hole collimator image of a thyroid gland with a hot nodule and a hot marker is shown in Figure 7-11a. The hot marker directly overlays the nodule, so that the two are indistinguishable. The same situation is imaged with a pinhole collimator in Figure 7-11b; the positioning of the thyroid in this image is to the far right of the FOV. The scintillation crystal "sees" the hot marker at a different location than the hot nodule below it, because the marker is at a different vertical location than the nodule (Fig. 7-11c).

With the increasing popularity of dual-head gamma cameras and electronic zooming capabilities, the pinhole collimator may be facing obsolescence. Some, even many, who read this text will never use a pinhole collimator. But its value for imaging small organs can be demonstrated (9). The Society of Nuclear Medicine (SNM) *Procedure Guideline for Thyroid Imaging* recommends the use of a pinhole collimator (10).

Other Types of Collimators

Collimators can be made with the holes at angles other than 90° to the face of the collimator. Holes can be parallel but at some specific angle, or the holes can be made to come together (converge) or spread apart (diverge) (**Figure 7-12**). Such collimators can be used in a variety of situations; the operator needs to recognize both the strengths and the weaknesses of such collimators.

Slant-Hole Collimators

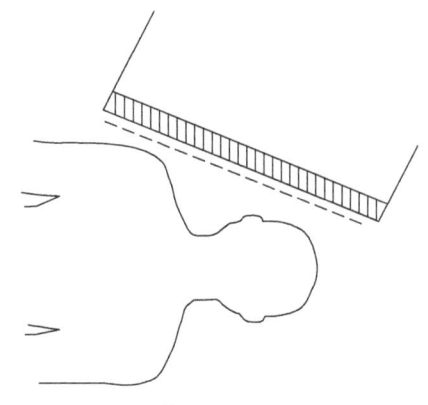

Collimators with holes that are parallel to one another but not perpendicular to the surface of the collimator are called *slant-hole collimators*. They are used to provide a parallel-hole view of a particular organ at a particular angle, while still minimizing the patient–collimator distance. One use of a slant-hole collimator is to provide a fixed angle for equilibrium cardiac gated blood-pool scanning; another is to obtain SPECT images of the brain with the camera close to all parts of the head while avoiding the shoulders (Fig. 7-12a). Because the holes are slanted at a particular angle (a common choice is 30°), the collimator must be positioned at a related angle relative to the patient or the organ of interest. Keep in mind that the plane of equal resolution is still parallel to the camera face, not perpendicular to the angle of the holes, as shown by the dashed line in Figure 7-12a. Parts of the brain farther from this line will have worse resolution than parts of the brain closer to this line.

Converging and Diverging Collimators

In the early days of nuclear medicine, when many cameras had 10-in-diameter fields of view, *diverging collimators* were common. In a diverging collimator, the holes are farther apart on the object side and closer together on the camera side, thus taking a large object and minifying it to fit in the FOV (Fig. 7-12b). If the area of interest is too large for the FOV when the object is close to the camera face, the area can be made smaller by moving the object away from the collimator face.

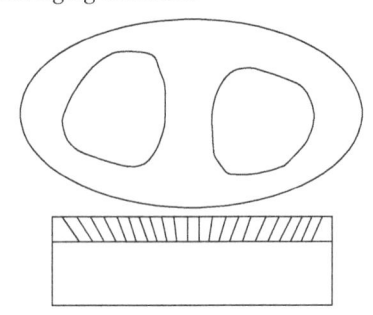

Converging collimators are the opposite of diverging collimators, in that the holes are closer together on the object side and farther apart on the crystal side, so that the image is magnified (Fig. 7-12c). In fact, a converging collimator flipped over becomes a diverging collimator, and collimators with names such as "Divcon" were produced for small-FOV cameras. Converging collimators (now called cone-beam collimators) continue to find

(a) Slant-hole collimator

(b) Diverging collimator

(c) Converging collimator

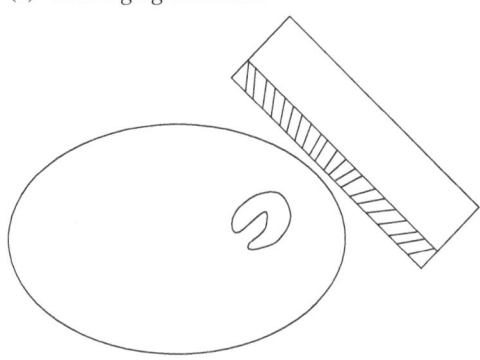

Figure 7-12 Non-parallel-hole collimators. One use of a slant-hole collimator (Figure 7-12a) is to image the brain; the dashed line shows the plane of equal resolution. A diverging collimator is shown in Figure 7-12b, imaging the lungs. Small organs like the heart are often imaged with a converging collimator (Fig. 7-12c).

application in cardiac and pediatric studies, where a large-FOV camera does not adequately magnify the organ of interest.

Figure 7-13 shows how sensitivity, resolution, and FOV change with distance for parallel-hole, diverging, converging, and pinhole collimators. In general, magnification improves resolution and minification degrades it, as can be seen in the graphs for the converging and diverging collimators, respectively. Converging collimators in particular have better resolution than the other nonpinhole collimators, because the distance-dependent resolution loss is balanced by the distance-dependent magnification (11). But because the amount of magnification or minification changes with depth, both converging and

(a) Resolution vs distance

(b) Sensitivity vs distance

(c) Field of view vs distance

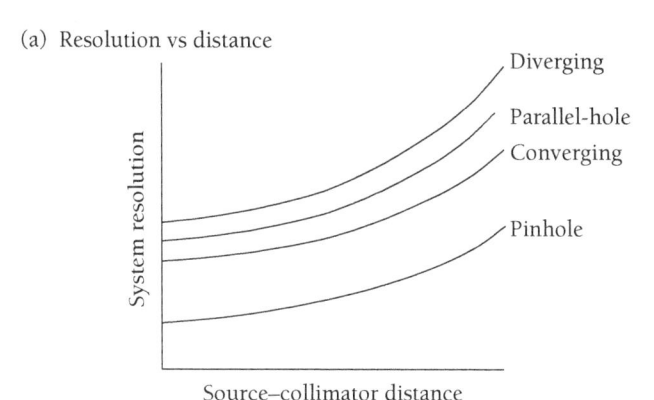

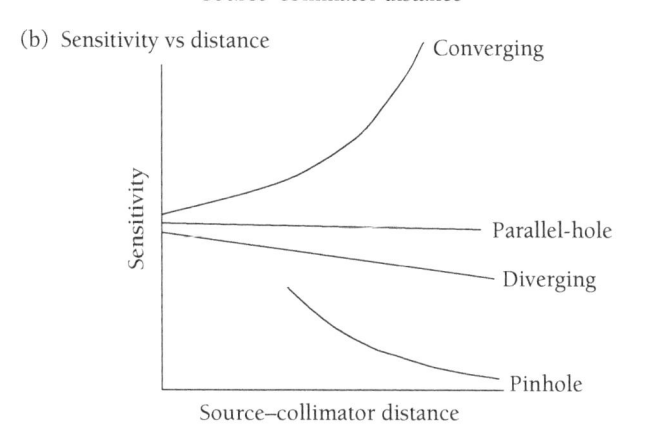

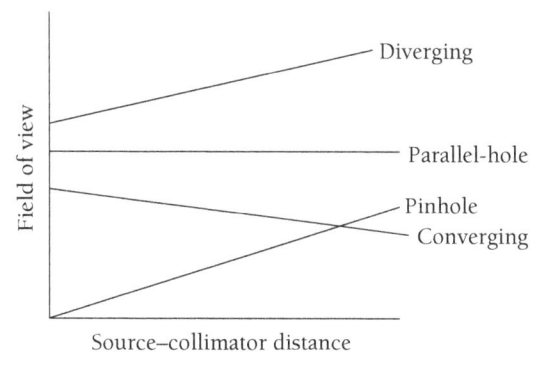

Figure 7-13 Change in resolution, sensitivity, and field-of-view size for four different types of collimators. (a) Resolution vs distance. (b) Sensitivity vs distance. (c) Field of view vs distance.

diverging collimators show image distortion due to the three-dimensional shape of the object being imaged. Note that the resolution of the pinhole collimator is much better than any of the other collimators. The diameter of the FOV is constant with distance for parallel-hole collimators, decreases as distance increases for converging collimators, and increases greatly with distance for the pinhole collimator (although at the expense of magnification and resolution).

Fan-Beam and Cone-Beam Collimators

Collimators can also be made to converge or diverge in only one axis, or in only part of the collimator. In modern gamma cameras, rectangular collimators used for whole-body scanning may have divergent holes near the lateral edges, in order to image an area somewhat wider than the camera's FOV. Fan-beam collimators have holes that converge along one axis but are parallel in the other axis (**Figure 7-14**). Cone-beam collimators are essentially converging collimators in that the holes converge in both axes, but they do not magnify as much as a standard converging collimator. Both are used for SPECT imaging of small organs, such as the heart or brain, and they improve sensitivity while also providing some degree of magnification (and therefore improved resolution), but at the expense of the FOV.

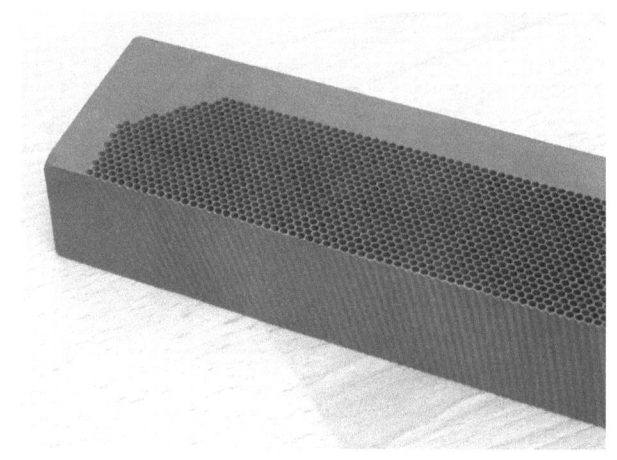

Figure 7-14 Cut-away view of a fan-beam collimator. Note that the holes slant toward the outside of the collimator, increasing the size of the FOV slightly in this axis. Photo courtesy of Nuclear Fields, Inc.

Summary

Collimators are essential to the image formation process in a gamma camera. Yet the collimator is the weakest link in the gamma camera, because it limits both resolution and sensitivity. Consideration of the design parameters of a collimator allows us to understand the trade-off between resolution and sensitivity. There are a variety of different types of collimators, each with advantages that apply to specific situations. It is important that the nuclear medicine technologist understand the uses and limitations of each type of collimator, so that the best images can be obtained. And the cardinal rule of keeping the collimator as close to the patient as possible should be kept in mind in almost all situations.

References

1. Bushberg JT, Seibert JA, Leidholdt EM, Boone JM. *The Essential Physics of Medical Imaging*. 2nd ed. Philadelphia, PA: Lippincott Williams & Wilkins; 2002:676, 685.
2. Yester M. Collimators. *Basic Science of Nuclear Medicine* [CD-ROM]. Reston, VA: Society of Nuclear Medicine; 2001.
3. Blend MJ, Patel BA, Byrom E. Collimator-induced defects in planar and SPECT gamma camera images: a multicenter study. *J Nucl Med Technol*. 1995;23: 167–172.
4. Anger HO. Scintillation camera with multichannel collimators. *J Nucl Med*. 1964;5:515–531.
5. Henkin RE, Boles MA, Dillehay GL, et al. *Nuclear Medicine*. St. Louis, MO: Mosby-Year Book; 1996:105, 127.

6. Cherry SR, Sorenson JA, Phelps ME. *Physics in Nuclear Medicine*. 3rd ed. Philadelphia, PA: Saunders; 2003:267–268.
7. Budinger T. Radionuclide enhancements above and beyond signal to noise: losing the background. Hal Anger Lecture, Society of Nuclear Medicine Annual Meeting, June 8, 2010.
8. McKitrick WL, Park HM, Kosegi JL. Parallax error in pinhole thyroid scintigraphy: a critical consideration in the evaluation of substernal goiters. *J Nucl Med*. 1985;26:418–420.
9. Tomas MB, Pugliese PV, Tronco GG, et al. Pinhole vs parallel-hole collimators for parathyroid imaging: an intraindividual comparison. *J Nucl Med Technol*. 2008;36:189–194.
10. Becker DV, Charkes ND, Hurley JR, et al. SNM Procedure Guideline on Thyroid Scintigraphy 2.0. Available at: http://interactive.snm.org/docs/pg_ch05_0403.pdf. Accessed August 18, 2011.
11. Rollo FD. *Nuclear Medicine Physics, Instrumentation, and Agents*. St. Louis, MO: Mosby-Year Book; 1977:413.

Additional Resources

Cherry SR, Sorenson JA, Phelps ME. *Physics in Nuclear Medicine*. 3rd ed. Philadelphia, PA: Saunders; 2003:Chapter 14.

CHAPTER 8

Image Characteristics and Performance Measures in Planar Imaging

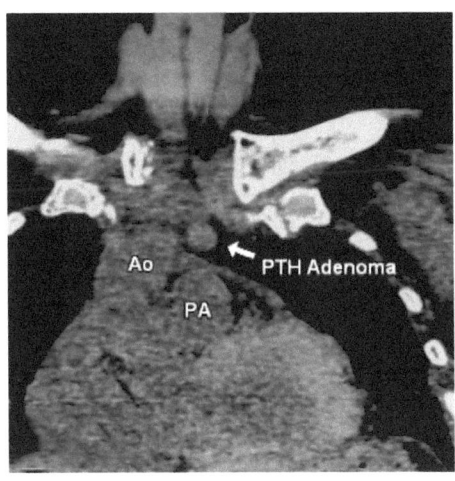

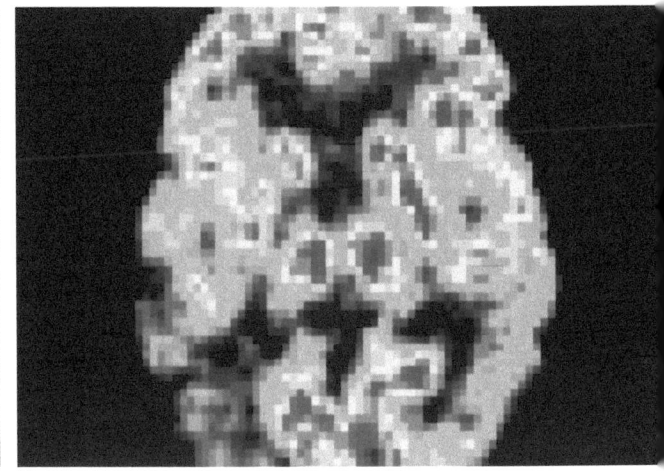

Learning Outcomes

1. Describe the origin and effect of each of the following planar image characteristics:
   a. Background
   b. Noise
   c. Third-dimension superposition
   d. Resolution loss with distance
   e. Photon attenuation and scatter
2. Discuss factors affecting contrast in planar imaging and how contrast can be improved.
3. List factors affecting gamma camera uniformity, sensitivity, and resolution.
4. Describe two methods used for measuring spatial resolution in a gamma camera; outline the measurement of the spatial full width at half-maximum (FWHM) using a line source of radioactivity, and calculate its value.
5. Define the modulation transfer function and discuss its application to evaluation of a gamma camera's performance.
6. Analyze the effect of changing each of the following acquisition parameters in a planar imaging situation:
   a. Total counts or time of acquisition
   b. Collimator
   c. Image matrix
   d. Energy window
   e. Object–collimator distance

Introduction

In theory, a gamma camera with an appropriate collimator ought to produce exactly correct images of a radioactive object. In practice, however, this is not true. Gamma cameras are subject to a number of limitations that negatively affect image quality. This chapter first considers the constraints on planar (two-dimensional, as opposed to tomographic) images and then discusses measures of gamma camera performance. The topic of resolution includes two techniques that allow us to quantify system resolution. Finally, we consider how choices of acquisition parameters affect planar images.

Characteristics of Planar Images

Planar gamma camera images have a number of characteristics that the operator must become familiar with. These characteristics must also be understood by the reader of the images in order to make an appropriate interpretation. Some are due to the properties of radioactive decay, others to issues of radiopharmaceutical biodistribution, and still others to the physics of imaging. Some of these characteristics can be mitigated with good technique, but most are not problems to be solved but rather limitations that we must live with.

Background

Previously, we introduced background as being those counts not coming from the source being measured. Moving to an imaging situation, we need to give this definition another facet. Most radiopharmaceuticals distribute not only to the organ(s) of interest, but also to other parts of the body. This nonspecific biodistribution thus obscures our vision of the organ of interest. It is the major constituent of background in a planar image. Background in a gamma camera image also includes gamma rays that penetrate the collimator septa, scattered gamma rays, and other types of mispositioned events. It is therefore affected to some extent by the choice of collimator and the width of the energy window. In fact, one of the major purposes of the collimator is to decrease that component of background that is due to scattered photons.

The only ways to decrease background due to the biodistribution of the radiopharmaceutical are to allow more time for clearance or to choose a different radiopharmaceutical. However, the visibility of background in an image can, to some extent, be decreased by changing the display parameters used.

Noise

Noise is an unwanted perturbation or variation in a wanted signal. Think, for example, of a radio signal that is being received from a distance. The audio feed from the station is the signal, and the static constitutes the noise. As we move farther from the radio tower, the noise becomes dominant, overwhelming the audio feed such that we can no longer distinguish it. Scientists use the concept of the *signal-to-noise ratio* (SNR) in many situations. An SNR of 1 means that the noise is equal in magnitude to the signal, in which case we cannot identify the signal. An SNR of 3 to 5 is needed to reliably identify and work with the signal in most circumstances.

What are the origins of noise in a nuclear medicine image? One is the random variability associated with radioactive decay and radiation detection. This kind of noise occurs with all types of radiation measurement, and it is best addressed through the application of counting statistics. A second source of noise is the graininess that results when we impose a digital format on an analog signal. In the imaging situation, the digital format is the image matrix. A photon that would project to the border between two pixels in an analog image must now be assigned to one or the other. This type of noise is called *quantum mottle*. Nuclear medicine images are noisier than other radiologic images because we have both types of noise.

The smaller the number of counts (N), the larger the variability ($\sigma = \sqrt{N}$) when expressed as a coefficient of variation. In an image we need to consider N not as the total number of counts in the image, but as the individual count-per-pixel values. This fact explains a common generalization about gamma camera imaging that "you can never have too many counts." An image with more counts will always have less noise and will look better than a similar image with fewer counts. More counts per pixel (N) means that the relative variability between pixels ($1/\sqrt{N}$) decreases. The best approach for decreasing noise, where practical, is to acquire the image for a longer time in order to accumulate more counts.

Third-Dimension Superposition

Planar images are two-dimensional, but the objects they depict are almost always three-dimensional. Activity in the third dimension is therefore superimposed within every planar image. While only the first few inches nearest the collimator face are seen well, there can be a contribution to the image from the opposite side of the body, especially from an area of increased activity. Planar imaging uses orthogonal views and oblique angles to adequately define the location of a focus of radioactivity in a patient's body (**Figure 8-1**).

Resolution Loss with Distance

One consequence of the use of a collimator is that parts of an object that are closer to the collimator will be seen

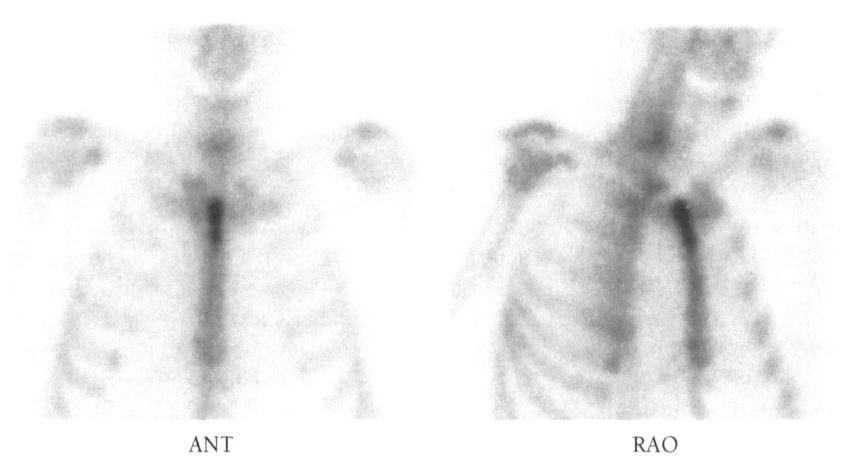

ANT RAO

Figure 8-1 Third-dimension superposition. Shown are anterior and right anterior oblique (RAO) views of the chest on a bone scan, in which a linear area of increased activity is shown to be in the sternum and not the spine. The images also demonstrate the loss of resolution with increasing distance (compare the clarity of the right shoulder with that of the left in the RAO view). Image courtesy of Virginia Mason Medical Center.

more clearly than parts of the object that are farther away. This can be clearly seen in Figure 8-1: the right shoulder, which is closest to the camera in the RAO view, is seen much more clearly than the left shoulder, which is at some distance from the face of the collimator. The reasons for this relate to the geometry of gamma rays passing through collimator holes. For planar imaging, keeping the camera as close to the patient as possible minimizes this loss of resolution; even so, because internal organs are internal, some resolution loss by necessity must occur.

Photon Attenuation and Scatter

A brief review of photon interactions with matter is helpful at this juncture (see also Appendix A). At energies used in nuclear medicine, gamma rays experience two types of interactions with atoms, namely, photoelectric and Compton interactions. In a photoelectric interaction, the kinetic energy of the gamma ray is completely absorbed, and an orbital electron of the absorbing atom is ejected. In a Compton interaction, the gamma ray is scattered by its interaction with an orbital electron, such that its direction is changed, but it retains kinetic energy and will undergo additional interactions. The likelihood of a photoelectric vs a Compton interaction depends on both the energy of the gamma ray and the atomic number(s) of the atoms with which it is interacting. **Table 8-1** shows the most likely interactions of gamma rays of energies encountered in nuclear medicine with different materials of significance in imaging.

Photon attenuation includes both absorption (photoelectric) and scattering (Compton) interactions. (Scatter is usually taken to indicate interactions within the object being imaged, rather than in the collimator.) Either results in the removal of a photon from the fraction of potentially detectable photons. Attenuation is the essence of x-ray and computed tomography (CT) imaging, but it is a significant hindrance in nuclear medicine, because it prevents gamma rays from being registered in the camera. Both normal anatomy and body habitus contribute to attenuation. In some cases, such as breast attenuation, the attenuating body part can be moved or repositioned, but in most cases we must live with the attenuation that the patient's body creates. Obviously, if an object external to the patient is causing attenuation or scatter, it must be removed. **Figure 8-2** shows several examples of internal and external attenuation.

The issue of scatter is complex. Table 8-1 shows that throughout the gamma ray energy range pertinent to nuclear medicine, Compton interactions are the most common interactions in soft tissue. In clinical imaging, a large percentage (sometimes more than one-half) of the total counts may be scattered gamma rays. Scatter has some relationship to the radiopharmaceutical biodistribution, in that a radiation source located deep in the object will generate more scattered gamma rays than one that is near the surface. The collimator rejects gamma rays coming at undesirable angles, but it is unable to eliminate gamma rays that have been scattered within the object but still pass through the collimator's holes (shown as path c in Fig. 5-2). The gamma camera's ability to exclude scattered photons depends on the energy window used, including both the width and the position of the window, as well as the energy resolution of the scintillator. Worst of all, scatter will tend to "fill in" an area of decreased activity, making detection more problematic for cold (non-radioactive) lesions than for hot spots.

Scatter subtraction has been used to try to account for and remove scatter from nuclear medicine images (1). In one version of this technique, a second energy window is set in the scatter region of the energy spectrum. Data from this window are appropriately scaled and then subtracted from the photopeak image on a pixel-by-pixel basis. While this method does improve contrast, it does so by decreasing the total number of counts, which increases image noise. In addition, the ratio of scattered to unscattered photons changes with depth in the patient, so the scatter image does not represent exactly the same view as the photopeak image.

Patient Motion

Some patient motion, particularly that due to respiratory and cardiac function, is unavoidable, due to the long acquisition times of nuclear medicine images. The blurring that patient motion adds to our images makes them look even more "fuzzy" than they would if such motion were not present. Because nuclear medicine is a functional rather than an anatomic imaging modality, this lack of anatomic detail is acceptable. It is, however, very important to avoid unnecessary motion. The nuclear medicine technologist must communicate to the patient the importance of not moving, both before starting the acquisition and during the imaging period.

Table 8-1

Most Likely Interactions of Gamma Rays with Different Materials

Gamma Ray Energy (Radionuclide)	Air	Soft Tissue	Sodium Iodide	Lead
80 keV (Tl-201)	Compton	Compton	Photoelectric	Photoelectric
140 keV (Tc-99m)	Compton	Compton	Photoelectric	Photoelectric
250 keV (In-111)	Compton	Compton	Photoelectric	Photoelectric
360 keV (I-131)	Compton	Compton	Photoelectric	Photoelectric
511 keV (annihilation photons)	Compton	Compton	Compton/photoelectric	Photoelectric

(a) Belt buckle

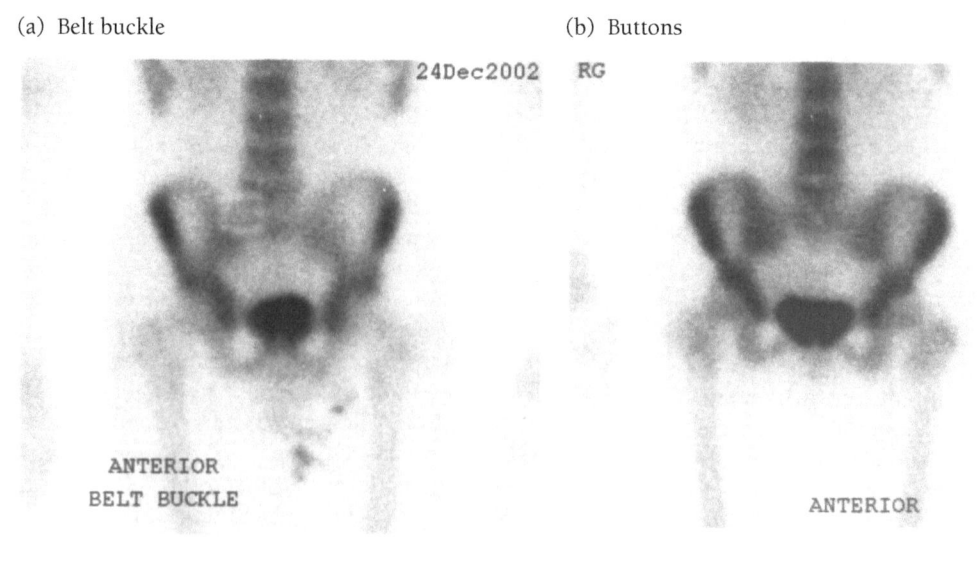

(b) Buttons

(c) Breast

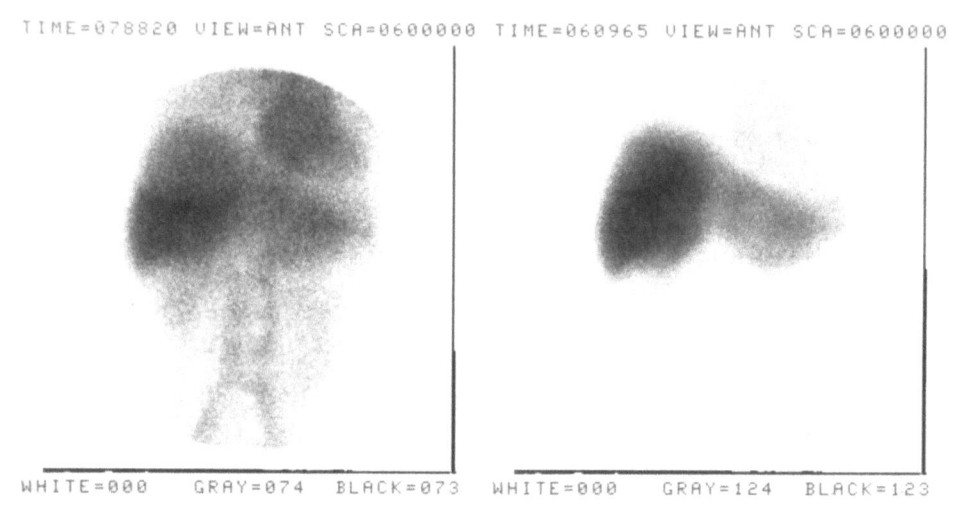

Figure 8-2 Examples of attenuation. Figure 8-2a shows a belt buckle and Figure 8-2b the buttons on blue jeans. Figure 8-2c shows an early image of a hepatobiliary study in which the right breast overlies the liver, creating a photopenic artifact. In the right-hand image, the patient elevated her breast to demonstrate normal appearance of the liver. Images courtesy of Virginia Mason Medical Center.

Contrast

Planar nuclear medicine images exhibit areas of greater or lesser radioactivity in the body, which reveals the underlying physiology and/or pathology. This relative quantitation is usually sufficient for image interpretation. (Absolute quantitation would require an external standard and an accounting of the effects of third-dimension superposition, scatter, and attenuation. It is rarely done in planar imaging.) *Contrast* refers to these relative differences in count density.

Contrast depends both on the properties of the object itself and on the image that the gamma camera registers. Let's consider planar images of a cylinder filled with radioactive solution, into which is placed a smaller, nonradioactive cylindrical insert. The object itself has inherent contrast that can be described mathematically as

$$C_{\text{object}} = \frac{O_{\max} - O_{\min}}{O_{\max} + O_{\min}} \tag{8-1}$$

where $O_{\max}$ and $O_{\min}$ are the actual count densities in µCi or kBq per cm³ in the cylinder and the insert, respectively. **Figure 8-3a** shows an activity concentration profile through such an object.

We are imaging the cylinder with a gamma camera, which is an imperfect imaging device. So the contrast seen in the image will not equal the contrast present in the object. But it can be defined similarly:

$$C_{\text{image}} = \frac{I_{\max} - I_{\min}}{I_{\max} + I_{\min}} \tag{8-2}$$

where $I_{\max}$ and $I_{\min}$ are the counts per pixel measured by the camera (Fig. 8-3b). Equations 8-1 and 8-2 yield values that can range from 0 (when maximum and minimum are the same) to 1 (when the minimum value is 0). The image contrast will always be less than or equal to the object contrast.

The image contrast must have some minimum value, if we are to visualize the object as distinct from the background. In

(a) Object contrast

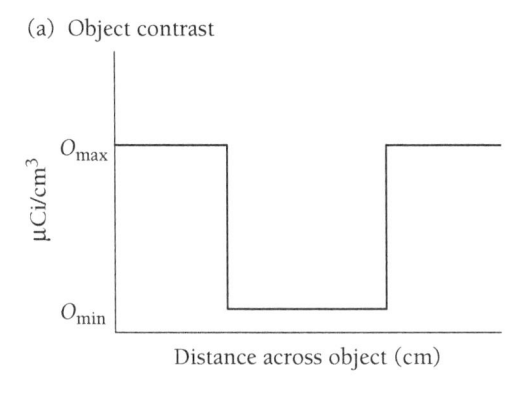

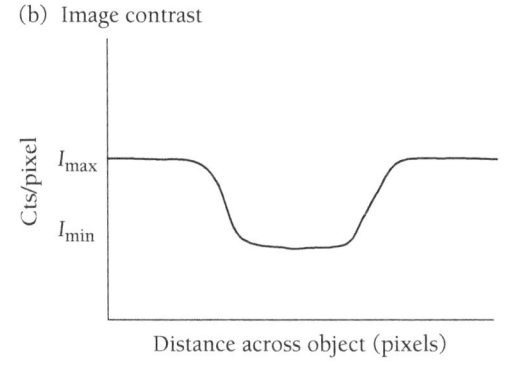

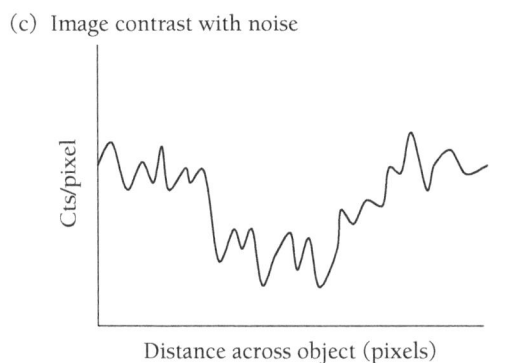

(b) Image contrast

(c) Image contrast with noise

Figure 8-3 Illustration of the concepts of contrast. In each figure, a count profile of a radioactive cylinder with a nonradioactive insert is shown. Figure 8-3a demonstrates object contrast. The insert has no radioactivity (that is, O_{min} is zero). Figure 8-3b shows the image contrast in a noise-free situation. Because of the imperfect imaging ability of the gamma camera, the difference between the insert and the cylinder is less in the image than in the object. Figure 8-3c shows that in the presence of noise, the image contrast between the insert and the cylinder is obscured.

the situation with no image noise, as illustrated in Figure 8-3b, that minimum value is as small as 0.10 (i.e., a difference between I_{max} and I_{min} that is 10% of the sum of I_{max} and I_{min} is visible). But in nuclear medicine, we do have noise, so we must also consider its effect on contrast. Intuitively, we recognize that the count difference between the insert and the cylinder must be significantly larger than the pixel-to-pixel variability if the lesion is to be seen (Fig. 8-3c). In most cases, the count difference between different parts of the image needs to be at least 3 times the statistical variability present in the image. This factor of 3 is known as the *Rose criterion* and is considered a minimum requirement for the *contrast-to-noise ratio* (CNR) in imaging (2).

Sample Calculation 8-1   Per-Pixel Statistics and the Rose Criterion

An image is acquired with a count density of 1,000 cts/cm² in a matrix that produces 0.3-cm pixels. What is the statistical variability of pixels with this count density? How many counts would a cold lesion need to have to be visible in this count density, according to the Rose criterion?

The count density is

$$\frac{1,000 \text{ cts}}{\text{cm}^2} \times \frac{(0.3 \text{ cm})^2}{\text{pixel}} \cong \frac{90 \text{ cts}}{\text{pixel}}.$$

The statistical variability of a pixel with 90 counts is $\sqrt{90} = 9$ cts. Given a Rose criterion of 3, a cold lesion would need to be $3 \times 9 = 27$ cts/pixel below the 90 cts/pixel density, or 63 cts/pixel, if we are to be sure to visualize it.

As noise increases, the count density difference between the insert and the cylinder needs to increase also, if the insert is to be visualized. Similarly, if we try this experiment with smaller and smaller inserts, visualization requires that the difference between I_{max} and I_{min} increase, given the same statistical variability. If we acquire the image for a longer time, we can decrease the statistical variability and therefore make the difference between I_{max} and I_{min} more obvious. An extensive discussion of the effect of various parameters on contrast and noise can be found in Reference 2 (pp. 259–267).

Image contrast ultimately depends on all the image characteristics discussed thus far. The main factor degrading contrast in planar imaging is the presence of underlying activity (3), referred to previously as third-dimension superposition. The loss of image contrast due to superimposed activity is a fact of life that we cannot avoid in planar imaging; the purpose of tomography is to remove this third-dimension superposition, thereby greatly improving contrast. The other image characteristics also degrade image contrast. Background, scatter, and patient motion all cause the difference between lesion and normal tissue to be less in the image than in the object. Resolution loss with distance impacts the sharpness of the boundary change between a hot area and a cold area. And it is clear from the discussion above that noise affects our ability to appreciate the image contrast that is present. Thus the concepts of contrast and CNR encompass all aspects of image quality.

Uniformity and Sensitivity

We now move to a discussion of *performance measures*, which provide quantitative ways to express the performance of a gamma camera. They give us ways to analyze gamma cameras and imaging situations, providing objective comparisons that complement our subjective assessments. Performance measures are generally evaluated with quality control tests.

Table 8-2

Typical Values of Various Performance Measures of Modern Gamma Cameras

Characteristic	Typical Value
Intrinsic uniformity	2.5–4.5% (at < 20,000 cts/sec)
	3.5–5.0% (at 75,000 cts/sec)
Extrinsic system sensitivity	150–350 cpm/μCi
Maximum intrinsic count rate	150,000–350,000 cts/sec
Dead time	1–2 μsec
Intrinsic spatial resolution	3.5–4.5 mm FWHM[1]
	6.5–9.0 mm FWTM[1]
Intrinsic spatial linearity	0.2- to 0.5-mm deviation
System spatial resolution at 10 cm	7- to 12-mm FWHM (collimator dependent)
Energy resolution	9–10% (Tc-99m)

[1] FWHM = full width at half-maximum, FWTM = full width at tenth-maximum; see Fig. 8-9 for a description of each. All tests performed according to NEMA specifications. Adapted from: Botti J. Gamma camera performance evaluation and quality control. In: Fahey R, Harkness B, eds. *Basic Science of Nuclear Medicine* [CD-ROM]. Reston, VA: Society of Nuclear Medicine; 2001.

We consider three performance measures that are easily performed in most nuclear medicine departments: uniformity, resolution, and sensitivity. These essential qualities of a gamma camera determine the camera's ability to produce high-quality nuclear medicine images. Uniformity in particular is essential for gamma camera imaging: if the gamma camera does not have acceptable uniformity, image interpretation will likely be incorrect. Resolution and sensitivity are both highly affected by the choice of collimator. All three quantities can be measured either intrinsically (without a collimator) or extrinsically (with a collimator installed). But because a collimator is required for imaging, the extrinsic values for resolution and sensitivity are more relevant than the intrinsic values. **Table 8-2** gives examples of typical values in modern gamma cameras.

Uniformity

Uniformity is defined as the ability to create an image showing uniform response to a uniform radioactive distribution. It is evaluated daily in most nuclear medicine departments, by acquiring and analyzing a flood image. Evaluation should include not only visual inspection but also a computer analysis, because the eye's ability to see nonuniformities decreases greatly below count differences of about 5%.

Modern gamma cameras are considerably more uniform than early gamma cameras. This is primarily due to energy, linearity, and uniformity correction tables applied to each image electronically. Degradation of the measured uniformity value may be caused by an electrical or mechanical problem with the camera itself, such as a photomultiplier tube (PMT) failure. Or it can be due to a variance between the stored correction tables and the camera's current performance. In most commercial systems, the first response to deteriorating uniformity is to reacquire the uniformity correction map.

Sensitivity and Count Rate

Sensitivity is the ability of a gamma camera to use efficiently all of the photons that are available to it in a given time period. It is measured as counts per minute per μCi or counts/min per kBq. The main determinant of intrinsic sensitivity is crystal thickness. Thicker crystals have greater detection efficiency for higher-energy gamma rays, according to the formula

$$\text{Sensitivity} \approx 1 - e^{\mu_\ell x} \tag{8-3}$$

where x is the crystal thickness and μ_ℓ is the energy-dependent linear attenuation coefficient for sodium iodide. This determinant of sensitivity is therefore a function of gamma ray energy as well as crystal thickness (**Figure 8-4**).

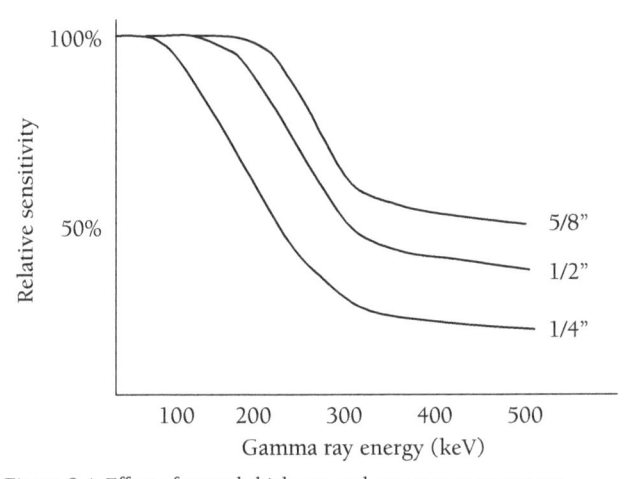

Figure 8-4 Effect of crystal thickness and gamma ray energy on sensitivity in sodium iodide. A crystal of ⅝-inch thickness is quite adequate to stop gamma rays up to about 200 keV, but at higher energies the efficiency for photoelectric and Compton interactions decreases dramatically. A ¼-in-thick crystal would give the best resolution but has inadequate sensitivity even for Tc-99m photons.

Obviously, the width of the energy window and the amount of scatter in the object affect sensitivity.

In the extrinsic gamma camera, the collimator has by far the greatest influence on sensitivity. In fact, it is best to think of sensitivity as a characteristic of the gamma camera/collimator combination. We can decrease the noise level of an image by acquiring more counts; this can be accomplished either by increasing the imaging time or by changing to a more sensitive collimator. The latter option requires that we give up some resolution.

As we consider sensitivity, we must also look at situations in which the gamma ray flux is higher than the system can manage. The specific problems we will run into are dead time, pulse pileup, and baseline shift. In a gamma camera, as in a single-PMT scintillation detector, the result of dead time is that the count rate we measure is less than the actual count rate.

The main cause of dead time in any sodium iodide detector is the time required for all of the scintillation photons from a single gamma ray interaction to be released. One method that gamma camera manufacturers have used to minimize this is called *pulse clipping* (**Figure 8-5**). In this technique, the signal at the PMT anode is terminated after the bulk of the scintillation photons have been registered, therefore allowing more counts to be registered. A pulse integration time of 0.4 (μsec) allows for collection of 81% of the total scintillation light from an event, compared to 98% for a 1-μsec pulse integration time. The downside of this technique is that it degrades energy resolution. Some systems have a toggle switch to turn on pulse clipping, while others use an algorithm that incorporates pulse clipping automatically at high count rates.

Pulse pileup and baseline shift are the consequence of pulse shaping at the amplifier (Fig. 4-10), in conjunction with a high count rate. These phenomena primarily affect the Z pulse, degrading energy resolution. But in a gamma camera, they can also generate mispositioned counts. Two Compton-scattered gamma rays, interacting simultaneously in the camera, may be registered as a single "event" whose "location" is *between* the interaction locations of the two gamma rays. An image of two point sources of high radioactivity shows not only the two sources but also a "bridge" of counts between the two. This, too, can be addressed electronically, using techniques such as pulse-tail extrapolation (**Figure 8-6**).

High count rates can therefore potentially result in not only decreased sensitivity, but also degraded uniformity, spatial resolution, and energy resolution. Fortunately, routine nuclear medicine practice only rarely generates high enough count rates for these problems to arise. One situation that does is a first-pass cardiac study. In this procedure, a bolus of radioactivity is imaged at a very fast framing rate (25–50 msec/frame) as it travels through the right and left sides of the heart for the first time. The goal of the study is to measure right- and left-ventricular ejection fractions, using just a few heartbeats for each measurement. A high-sensitivity collimator is required, as is a high radiopharmaceutical dosage, and count rates of 150,000 cps or more may be generated. It is important in a situation such as this to recognize the high count rate and to engage any mechanisms the camera has to compensate for it.

Spatial Resolution

Spatial resolution is defined as the ability of a gamma camera to reproduce the details of a nonuniform radioactive distribution. It is easy to conceptualize spatial resolution using a bar phantom. The smaller the bars visualized, the better the camera's resolution. Spatial resolution is measured in mm, and a smaller number indicates better resolution. Another way to conceptualize spatial resolution is to think of it as the amount of blurring that occurs when a point source or a thin line source is imaged with the camera.

Resolution boils down to the ability to put counts into their correct locations. In gamma cameras, resolution is limited by a number of factors. Statistical fluctuations in the amount of scintillation light detected, variations in detection efficiency, and mispositioning of events due to PMT nonlinearities are the main determinants of intrinsic resolution. Photons of higher energy produce more scintillation photons and therefore more precisely reflect the location of the gamma ray interaction (**Figure 8-7**). A thicker crystal requires the scintillation photons to travel farther before arriving at the PMTs, thus decreasing the accuracy of position determination for each event.

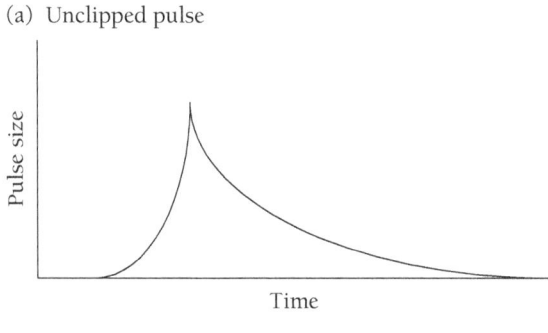

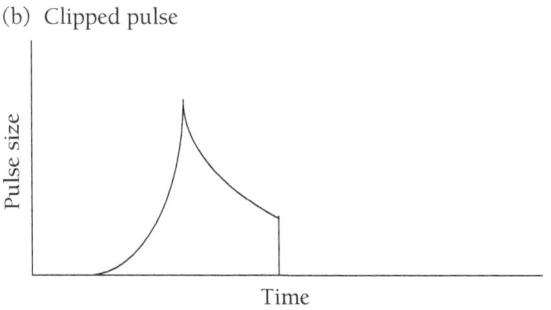

Figure 8-5 Pulse clipping. This technique reduces the time required to register each event by cutting off the voltage signal received from each PMT before it has returned all the way to baseline. It works because most PMT output pulses are shaped the same way, such that the total signal can be estimated from the part that is accepted before the clipping takes place. The chief disadvantage of this method is that the energy discrimination is less accurate, leading to increased (degraded) energy resolution.

(a) Pulse pileup

(b) Tail clipping and extrapolation

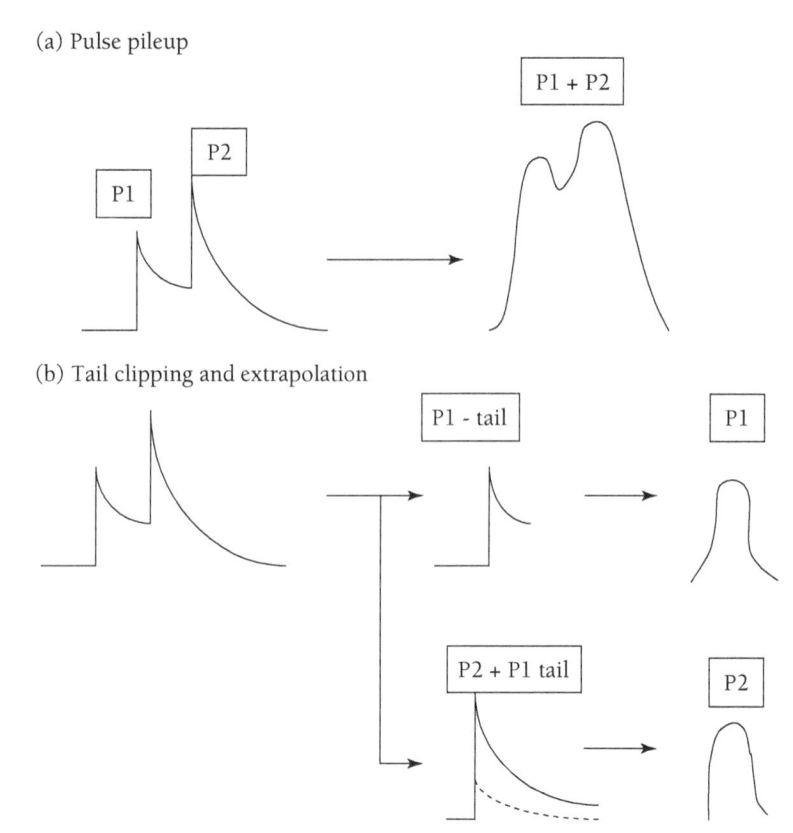

Figure 8-6 Electronic correction for pulse pileup. Figure 8-6a shows pulse pileup, in which two events are close together in time, such that the tail of the first pulse adds to the measured value of the second pulse. With pulse-tail extrapolation, the tail of the first pulse is extrapolated and then subtracted from the second pulse, so that each can be measured correctly (Fig. 8-6b). Modified from: Lewellen TK, Bice AN, Pollard KR, et al. Evaluation of a clinical scintillation camera with pulse tail extrapolation electronics. *J Nucl Med.* 1989;30:1554–1558. Used with permission of the Society of Nuclear Medicine.

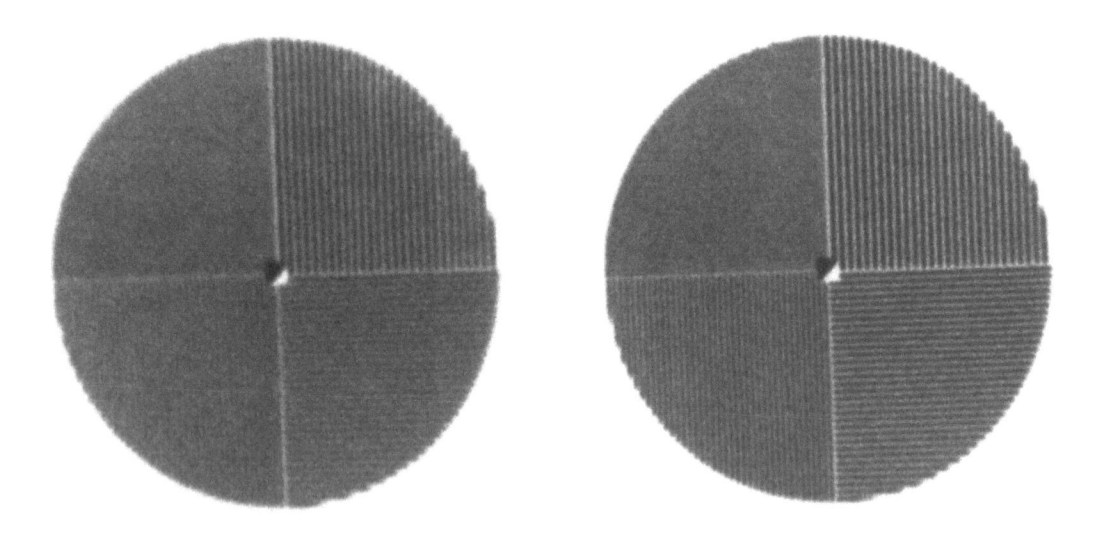

Figure 8-7 Effect of radionuclide energy on resolution. The figure shows intrinsic bar phantom images using Tl-201 (left) and Tc-99m (right). Resolution is degraded for the 80-keV photons of thallium compared to the 140-keV photons of technetium. Image courtesy of Virginia Mason Medical Center.

The collimator is the major determinant of a gamma camera's extrinsic resolution. Moreover, we can't take a picture with a gamma camera unless we have a collimator. So while we can measure the resolution of the intrinsic (uncollimated) camera, the more meaningful value is the extrinsic or system resolution. To be even more realistic, we should measure resolution at some distance from the collimator face and include some kind of scattering medium between the source and collimator. Thus the value quoted in Table 8-2 is the FWHM (see the following for a complete description of this measure of resolution) with the source 10 cm from the collimator and with scattering material in front of and behind the source. The degradation of image clarity with distance and scatter can be seen in **Figure 8-8**.

Image acquisition parameters can affect perceived resolution, but only up to the limits of the system's intrinsic resolution (4). Accumulation of more counts improves the eye's ability to visually appreciate the available resolution, but does not change the system's inherent capabilities. Digitization can degrade resolution (if the pixel size exceeds the system resolution) but cannot improve it. Magnification (via either a pinhole collimator or digital zooming) can improve resolution, but only up to the limit of the intrinsic resolution. In planar imaging, the only way resolution can truly be altered is by changing either the collimator or the object–collimator distance.

Bar Phantoms

The most commonly employed method for evaluation of resolution is acquisition and visual analysis of a bar phantom image. A variety of bar phantoms are available, the most common being the four-quadrant (see Fig. 9-5) and parallel-line equal-spacing (PLES) types. A bar phantom provides a semiquantitative measure of resolution, in that it defines a camera's resolution to a ballpark range (e.g., intrinsic resolution is better than 4 mm but not as good as 2 mm). It also allows us to look for nonlinearities (wavy lines), which may indicate that a PMT is beginning to fail. Most bar phantoms are engineered so that the lead strips are only thick enough to stop Tc-99m gamma rays, so they should be used with caution when imaging higher-energy gamma rays.

Bar phantoms are quite adequate for the routine evaluation of spatial resolution and linearity, but we would prefer a more quantitative measure for purposes such as comparing one gamma camera to another. The next two sections describe two methods used to more exactly describe this measure of gamma camera performance. Ultimately, as we shall see, all three measures of resolution are related to one another.

Line-Spread Function

A quantitative expression of resolution is obtained by acquiring a *line-spread function* (LSF). An LSF measurement on an intrinsic gamma camera requires a phantom with 1-mm-wide slits, illuminated by a point source. For the more realistic extrinsic measurement, the LSF is easily obtained by imaging a very thin activity source (e.g., a capillary tube filled with Tc-99m). (Similar results are obtained with a *point-spread function* [PSF], but a true point source is harder to create than a line source.) A computer is used to obtain a count profile (a graph of counts per pixel vs location across the FOV) perpendicular to the capillary tube.

From the count profile, we can measure the FWHM as the width of the peak of the count profile, measured at one-half the maximum height of the peak (**Figure 8-9**). It is measured in pixels and converted to mm or cm using the camera's pixel calibration value in cm/pixel. It is a representation of the width of the line source, as it is reproduced by the gamma camera. **Figure 8-10** shows the result of trying to separate sources that are closer together than the system FWHM.

When scatter is present, the tails of the LSF become more significant. In this case, one should also measure the *full width at tenth-maximum* (FWTM) (shown in Fig. 8-9b). The FWTM is an effective measure of septal penetration: if the FWTM is greater than 3 times the FWHM, then septal penetration is significantly degrading the system resolution (5). This is particularly important for high-energy collimators (6).

Sample Calculation 8-2   Calculation of FWHM and FWTM from a Line-Spread Function

The following counts-per-pixel values are obtained from a count profile across a line-spread function:

Pixel No.	Counts
209	8
210	44
211	97
212	172
213	298
214	425
215	305
216	217
217	190
218	108
219	48
220	12

The pixel dimension is 1.6 mm. Determine the FWHM and FWTM in mm.

Given the maximum of 425 cts/pixel, the half-height value is about 212 and the tenth-height value about 40 cts. The two values closest to the half-height are 172 cts (pixel 212) and 217 cts (pixel 216). The width of the peak is therefore approximately four pixels, which is

$$4 \text{ pixels} \times \frac{1.6 \text{ mm}}{\text{pixel}} = 6.4 \text{ mm}.$$

For the FWTM, pixels 210 and 219 are closest to the tenth-height value, corresponding to 9 pixels and a FWTM of about 14.4 mm.

Modulation Transfer Function

To accurately portray a radiopharmaceutical distribution in a patient, a gamma camera needs good resolution (relates to placement of counts) and good contrast (relates to variation in count density). We must have both of these

(a) Bar phantom imaged at increasing distance

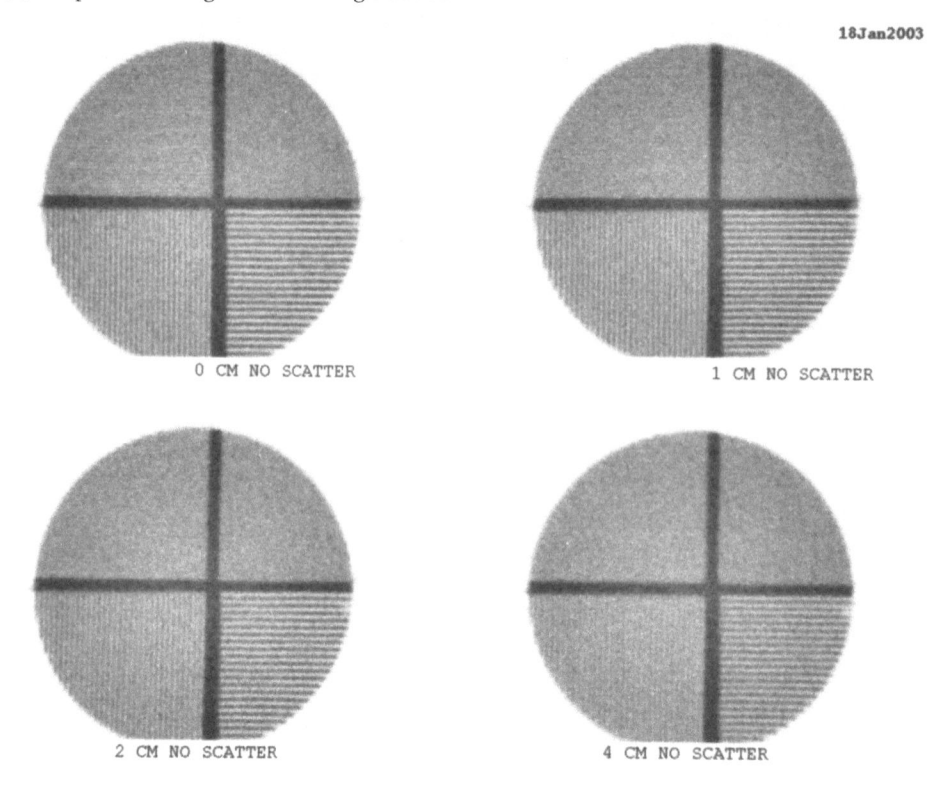

(b) Bar phantom imaged at increasing distance by interposing a scattering medium

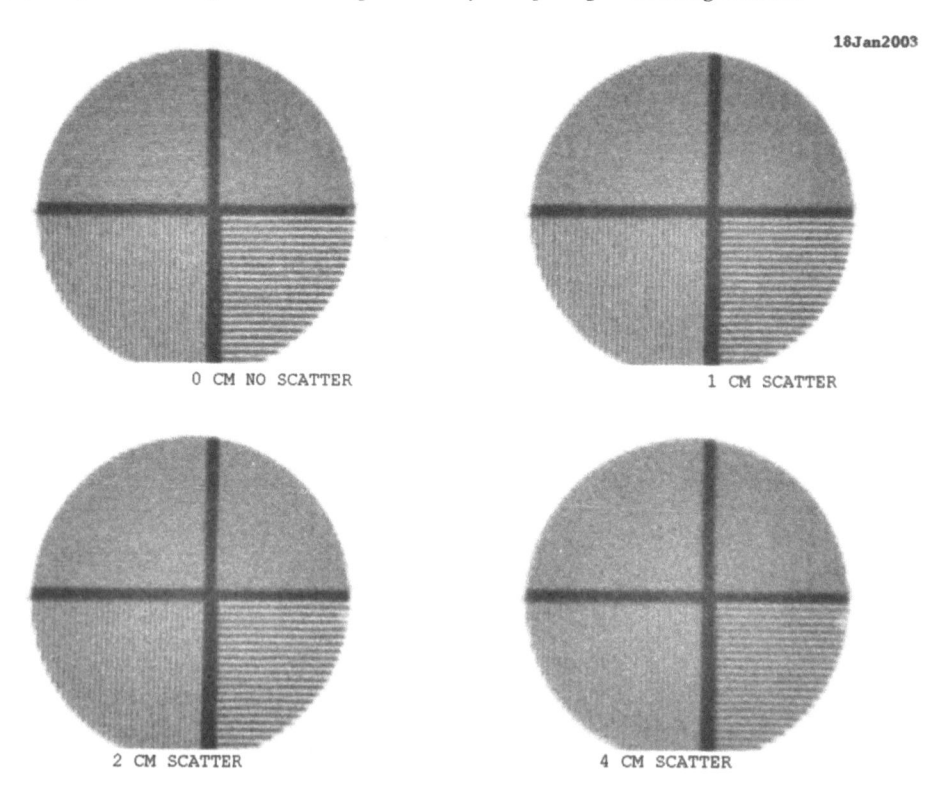

Figure 8-8 Effect of distance and scatter on resolution. Figure 8-8a shows extrinsic bar phantom images at the collimator surface (0 cm) and at a distance of 1, 2, and 4 cm from the collimator surface, with only air between the collimator and phantom. The third set of bars, in the upper left part of the phantom, is not resolved at 2-cm distance. Figure 8-8b shows the same distances, but with scattering material between the gamma camera and the bar phantom. Here, the third set of bars is not visualized with 1-cm scatter, and the second-largest bars (at the lower left) are barely distinguishable with 2-cm scatter. Images courtesy of Virginia Mason Medical Center.

(a) Physical setup for extrinsic line-spread function measurement

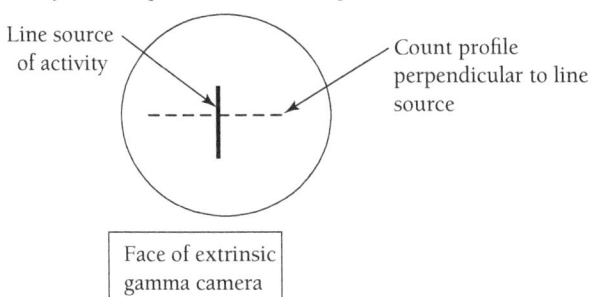

(b) Line-spread function showing FWHM and FWTM

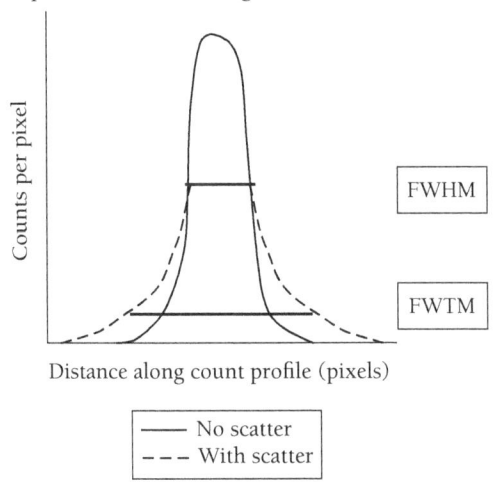

Figure 8-9 Measurement of the line-spread function. Figure 8-9a shows the physical setup. A capillary tube filled with Tc-99m is commonly used as a line source. The line-spread function with FWHM and FWTM is shown in Figure 8-9b. After a digital image is acquired, a count profile is drawn perpendicular to the line source. The width of the count profile is measured at one-half its maximum height to determine the FWHM and at one-tenth of the maximum height to determine the FWTM. Both measurements are in pixels and can be converted to mm using the gamma camera's pixel calibration factor. The presence of scatter may or may not affect the FWHM, but it always affects the FWTM.

qualities to see abnormalities in a clinical image. The *modulation-transfer function* (MTF) (7) combines these two qualities into a single assessment. The MTF measures the ability of a system to reproduce a source containing objects of varying contrasts at varying frequencies.

Many readers will be familiar with the concepts of frequency and modulation as they relate to a stereo or sound system: the medium (radio, audiotape, or compact disc) produces sounds of varying frequencies, and the graphic equalizer in the stereo system modulates the amplitudes of the various frequencies to produce an overall effect pleasing to the ear. In imaging, *frequency* refers to how rapidly counts are changing from point to point within the object being imaged. *Modulation* describes the loss of fidelity in reproducing that count change in the image created by the gamma camera. The gamma camera modulates image data in a frequency-dependent manner: as the frequency increases, the gamma camera's ability to reproduce the count changes decreases.

Figure 8-11 illustrates these concepts. Imagine a phantom containing radioactivity in amounts that vary sinusoidally. That is, there is a maximum photon flux/cm^2 and a minimum photon flux/cm^2 changing in a sine wave pattern, with "peaks" and "troughs" of radiation intensity. Imagine further that the peaks and troughs get closer and closer together; that is, the spatial frequency goes from a low value at one place in the phantom to a high value in another. Finally, imagine that we image such a phantom with a gamma camera.

At low frequencies, the peaks and troughs are far apart and are easily imaged by the camera. But as the frequency of radiation intensity change increases, the camera is less able to depict the difference between them. Using Equations 8-1 and 8-2, we would find that the image contrast decreases as frequency increases. The MTF compares C_{image} to C_{object} at a variety of frequencies:

$$\text{MTF}(f) = \frac{C_{\text{image}}(f)}{C_{\text{object}}(f)}. \qquad (8\text{-}4)$$

The (f) in Equation 8-4 reminds us that object contrast, image contrast, and MTF are all functions of frequency. At low frequencies, the image contrast is equal to the object contrast, and the MTF has a value of 1. As frequency increases (count density changes get closer together), the system is less capable of reproducing the object contrast, and the MTF decreases. A typical MTF graph is shown in **Figure 8-12**. Visibility of a pattern by the human eye becomes marginal at an MTF of approximately 0.1. When the frequency within the object exceeds the system's resolution, the MTF falls to 0, and the imaging system provides no usable information.

The value of the MTF lies in its ability to compare gamma cameras in different situations. **Figure 8-13** shows MTF graphs for three collimators at three distances. At the collimator surface, all three perform similarly. But as the object–collimator distance increases, the high-resolution collimator maintains image fidelity through higher frequencies than the other two collimators. The MTF graphs make clear the differences between the collimators.

Relationship Among Bar Phantoms, LSF, and MTF

The three ways used to measure resolution are all intertwined, which makes sense because each expresses an aspect of a gamma camera's ability to see details. First, let us consider the relationship between the bar phantom and the LSF. It should be obvious that if the FWHM of camera A is smaller than the FWHM of camera B, camera A will be able to resolve smaller bars than camera B. It has been shown empirically that the smallest bar size seen is about equal to the FWHM divided by 1.75. A camera with a 9-mm FWHM will allow visualization of 5-mm bars.

We can also relate the bar phantom to the MTF. A bar phantom is similar to the sinusoidal phantom used to create the MTF curve, in that the bars and spaces of the bar phantom provide a square wave variation in radiation

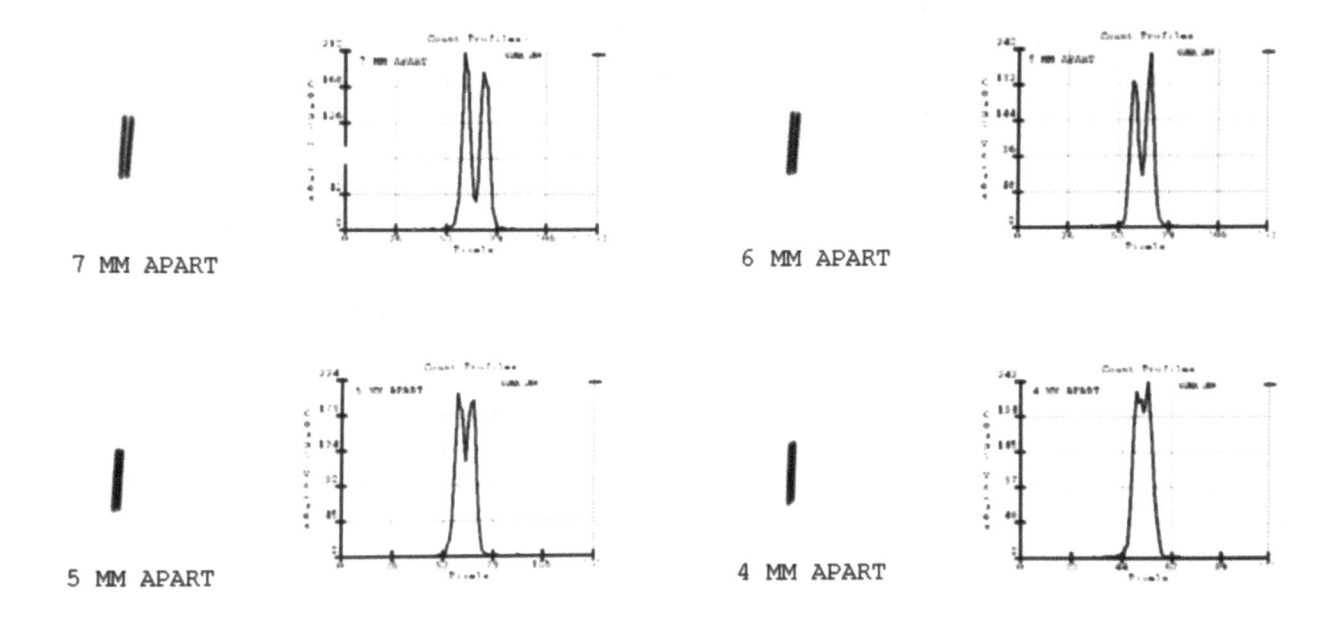

Figure 8-10 Images and count profiles of line sources with various separations. The measured FWHM on this camera is about 5 mm. As the line sources come closer together, they become indistinguishable and their count profiles merge. Images courtesy of Virginia Mason Medical Center.

intensity. A four-quadrant bar phantom essentially has four frequencies of the MTF curve. The four points superimposed on the MTF graph in Figure 8-12 represent the four primary frequencies of a bar phantom.

Finally, MTF curves can be generated mathematically from Fourier transformation of the LSF. The Fourier theorem states that any image can be described as the sum of sine and cosine waves of varying frequencies and amplitudes. The LSF thus contains information about the gamma camera's ability to image a wide range of frequencies, and Fourier transformation can be used to generate the MTF curve. Keep in mind that both the LSF and the MTF describe the system's contrast and resolution in a noiseless situation; that is, without considering the statistical variation inherent in nuclear medicine imaging (8).

Effects of Acquisition Parameters

Planar imaging uses only a few acquisition parameters, namely, the counts acquired in an image, the collimator, the image matrix, and the distance between the collimator and the object. We thus have only a few options for making changes to improve image quality or to decrease imaging time. Moreover, almost all of the changes that can be made involve trade-offs. This section considers how changes in each of the acquisition parameters affect the final image. **Table 8-3** considers the question from the standpoint of the desired result and how to bring it about.

Counts/Time

Planar gamma camera images are generally acquired for a given length of time or a specified number of counts. As the time of imaging is lengthened, the number of counts increases in a linear fashion. Image noise, or pixel-to-pixel variations in counts, decreases as the number of counts increases, so a longer imaging time always produces a less noisy image. As a general, static imaging protocols state the number of counts necessary for a particular image, and the image is acquired for the time needed to acquire that many counts.

But increasing time in order to decrease noise and improve image quality can increase the likelihood of patient motion. The most likely results of motion are degraded spatial resolution and blurring of the image. Thus, increasing the time of an image should be accompanied by stressing the importance of not moving. One could also consider adding immobilization devices (e.g., tape, sandbags, straps) to assist the patient in staying still.

A longer imaging time may also be inappropriate if radionuclide location changes during the imaging period. A gastrointestinal (GI) bleeding study with Tc-99m-labeled red blood cells is a good example. Labeled erythrocytes that bleed into the gastrointestinal lumen will subsequently move with the bowel contents due to peristalsis. If dynamic images are acquired at a relatively slow framing rate (such as 60 sec/frame), activity in the GI tract may move over the course of a single frame, spreading the counts out and lessening our ability to detect discrete evidence of bleeding. If the framing rate is shortened to 15 or 30 sec/frame, each image has fewer counts, but a collection of labeled erythrocytes in the intestinal lumen may be contained in a smaller volume and thus be more noticeable.

Choice of Collimator

The collimator used for a particular imaging situation depends on several factors. First, obviously, is the selection

(a) Illustration of frequency in the spatial domain, showing both the actual frequency and contrast within the objects (solid lines) and the amount of contrast seen by the imaging system (dashed lines)

Low frequency — dashed and solid lines overlap

Medium frequency — imaging system is unable to completely reproduce the object contrast

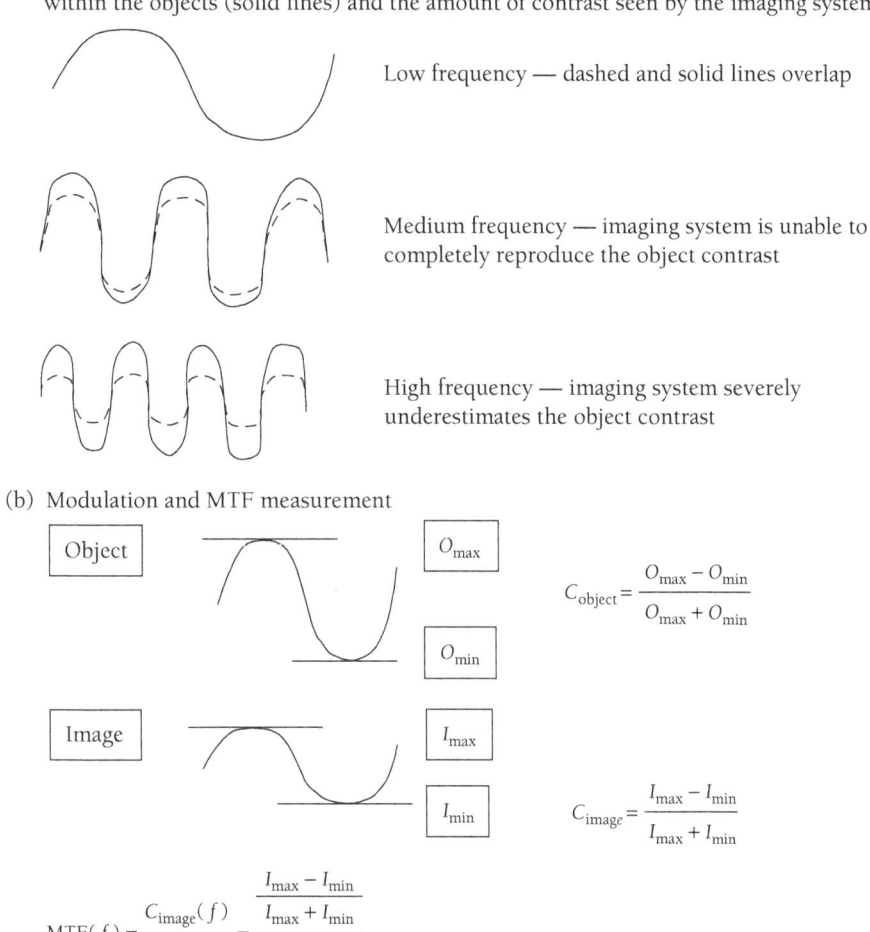

High frequency — imaging system severely underestimates the object contrast

(b) Modulation and MTF measurement

Object — O_{max}, O_{min}

$$C_{object} = \frac{O_{max} - O_{min}}{O_{max} + O_{min}}$$

Image — I_{max}, I_{min}

$$C_{image} = \frac{I_{max} - I_{min}}{I_{max} + I_{min}}$$

$$MTF(f) = \frac{C_{image}(f)}{C_{object}(f)} = \frac{\frac{I_{max} - I_{min}}{I_{max} + I_{min}}}{\frac{O_{max} - O_{min}}{O_{max} + O_{min}}}$$

Figure 8-11 Object contrast vs image contrast. In Figure 8-11a, areas of higher and lower counts within the object are shown as solid lines in count profiles. The contrast reproduced in the imaging system is shown as dashed lines. As frequency increases, the imaging system is less and less able to reproduce the contrast seen in the object. In nuclear medicine imaging, background (which changes slowly) is an example of a low-frequency image component, whereas sharply defined edges are examples of high-frequency components. The MTF compares the contrast visualized in the image (the bottom sinusoid in Fig. 8-11b) to that present in the object (the top sinusoid), both of which are functions of frequency.

of collimators available for a given camera. A second important factor is the energy of the radionuclide being imaged. One should generally choose a collimator with an energy rating at least as high as the radionuclide energy. The use of a low-energy collimator for a high-energy radionuclide results in star artifacts and loss of spatial resolution as gamma rays penetrate the too-thin septa of the collimator (see Fig. 7-7). Again, there is a trade-off: one can choose to use a collimator with a lower energy rating than the gamma ray energy, to obtain more counts in a given imaging time. One must then be aware that the image will have poorer resolution than if the "correct" collimator were used.

A camera may have more than one collimator applicable to low-energy gamma rays (< 150 keV). The collimator with smaller and/or longer holes will give improved spatial resolution, whereas that with larger and/or shorter holes will have increased sensitivity. Deciding which one to use depends on the goal of the imaging procedure.

When good spatial resolution is the primary goal, a higher-resolution collimator should be employed. When resolution is less important than quantitative information such as counts within a region of interest, a collimator with greater sensitivity may be a better choice.

Image Matrix

The choice of image matrix is once again a trade-off between sensitivity and resolution, but now on a pixel-by-pixel basis rather than a whole-image basis. Noise increases approximately geometrically as the matrix dimension increases (see Fig. 6-4). A given number of counts may be quite adequate to the imaging situation if a coarse image matrix is used, but produces a noisy image if a fine image matrix is required. An image matrix with pixels larger than the system resolution causes an unnecessary loss of image quality. The needs of the imaging protocol guide the choice of image matrix, based on considerations of noise and the desired resolution.

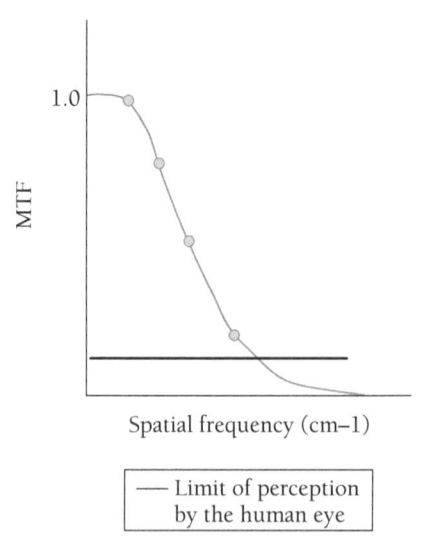

Figure 8-12 A typical MTF plot. An MTF value of 1.0 indicates that the image perfectly reproduces the object, a situation that happens only at low frequencies with gamma camera imaging. As the spatial frequency increases, the ability of the gamma camera to reproduce the object decreases. Ultimately, the gamma camera produces a flat image of a high-frequency pattern, such that C_{image} and therefore MTF equal 0. The four points shown on the graph represent the information obtained from a four-quadrant bar phantom; the MTF curve "fleshes out" the limited amount of information about camera performance that we get from the bar phantom image.

Energy Window

We can also try to improve image quality by using the PHA energy window to exclude scattered events. Again, a compromise is required: a narrower window excludes more scattered gamma rays, but requires longer imaging times and/or fewer counts, the latter resulting in increased image noise. In addition, the physics of the Compton interaction works against exclusion of scatter. A ±10% window at 140 keV accepts gamma rays scattered over angles as large as 50°. As the gamma ray energy decreases, even larger angles are included in the window, such that a ±10% window for the 80-keV photons of Tl-201 includes scattering angles up to 73°. Thus, narrowing the energy window has limited effectiveness at best.

Object–Collimator Distance

This is the one acquisition parameter that does not involve any trade-offs. Decreasing the object–collimator distance always improves resolution and affects sensitivity only slightly for most collimators (see Figs. 7-13a and 7-13b). For most imaging situations, this means bringing the camera in so close that it touches the patient. Good positioning may require extra time, but pays big dividends in terms of image quality.

Summary

Nuclear medicine images demonstrate poor resolution compared to other radiology modalities. A state-of-the-art gamma camera with a high-resolution collimator has about 5-mm resolution, whereas x-ray, CT, and magnetic resonance (MR) images all have spatial resolution of 0.1 mm or less. As a result, nuclear medicine is often given the derogatory label of "unclear medicine" and is sometimes treated as the poor stepsister of the radiology department.

What nuclear medicine does offer to the field of radiology is the ability to image function, and it does so in part by offering high contrast. One need only consider a stress fracture as seen on a bone scan, accompanied by a negative x-ray, to recognize this fact. The strength of nuclear medicine will always be its ability to image physiology.

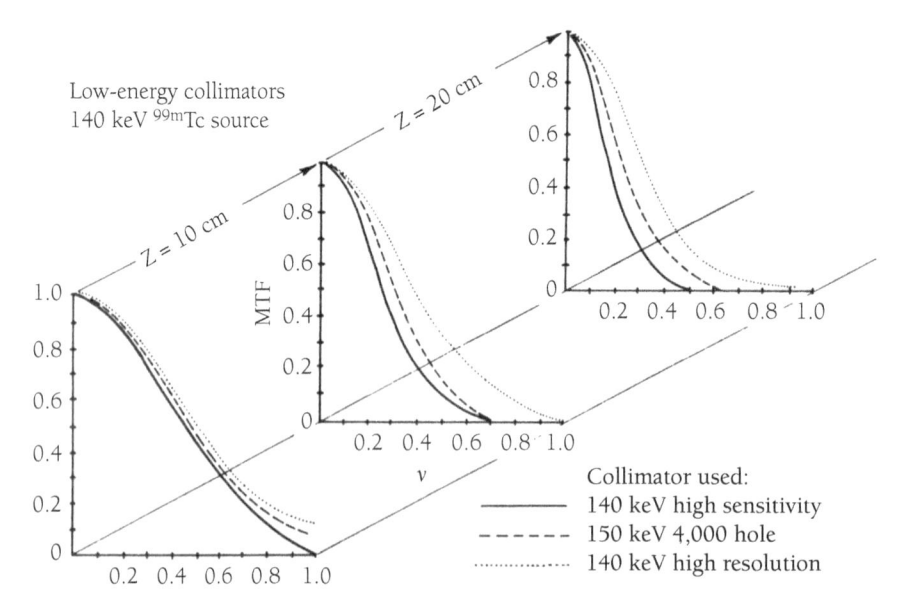

Figure 8-13 Use of the MTF in collimator evaluation. The set of curves on the left shows the MTFs for three collimators, with the source at the collimator surface. The middle set of curves shows the same three collimators imaging a source that is 10 cm away, and the right set with the source that is 20 cm away from the collimator surface. The MTF shows the improved resolution of the high-resolution collimator as the object–collimator distance increases. Reprinted from: Early PJ, Sodee DB. *Principles and Practice of Nuclear Medicine*. 1st ed. St. Louis, MO: Mosby-Year Book; 1985: 468. Used with permission from Elsevier.

Table 8-3

Improving Gamma Camera Images

Desired Result	Ways to Bring About	Caveats and Trade-offs
Less image noise	• More counts	• Longer imaging time
	• Collimator with greater sensitivity	• Degraded spatial resolution
	• Coarser image matrix	• Potential degradation of spatial resolution
Improved spatial resolution	• Collimator with better resolution	• Fewer counts and/or longer imaging time
	• Decrease in object–collimator distance	• None
	• Finer image matrix	• Fewer counts per pixel
Shorter imaging time	• Fewer total counts	• Increased image noise
	• Collimator with greater sensitivity	• Degraded spatial resolution

That being said, we can still maximize the information available in our images by paying attention to the image characteristics discussed in this chapter. Camera uniformity must be excellent, adequate time for radiopharmaceutical clearance must be allowed, and sufficient counts must be obtained. While resolution will never be as good as with other radiologic modalities, we can keep it as high as possible by keeping the distance between collimator and patient as small as possible. With attention to these aspects of planar images, we can ensure that the physiologic information they provide is as good as it can be.

References

1. Sandler MP, Coleman RE, Patton JA, et al. *Diagnostic Nuclear Medicine*. 4th ed. Philadelphia, PA: Lippincott Williams & Wilkins; 2003:54.
2. Cherry SR, Sorenson JA, Phelps ME. *Physics in Nuclear Medicine*. 3rd ed. Philadelphia, PA: Saunders; 2003:232, 264.
3. Heller SL, Goodwin PN. SPECT instrumentation: performance, lesion detection, and recent innovations. *Semin Nucl Med*. 1987;17:184–199.
4. Lee KH. *Computers in Nuclear Medicine: A Practical Approach*. 2nd ed. Reston, VA: Society of Nuclear Medicine; 2005:82.
5. Henkin RE, Boles MA, Dillehay GL, et al. *Nuclear Medicine*. St. Louis, MO: Mosby-Year Book; 1996:Chapters 7, 9.
6. Yester M. Collimators. In: Fahey R, Harkness B, eds. *Basic Science of Nuclear Medicine* [CD-ROM]. Reston, VA: Society of Nuclear Medicine; 2001.
7. Early PJ, Sodee BD. *Principles and Practice of Nuclear Medicine*. 1st ed. St. Louis, MO: Mosby-Year Book; 1985:Chapter 15.
8. Fahey F. Image quality. In: Fahey R, Harkness B, eds. *Basic Science of Nuclear Medicine* [CD-ROM]. Reston, VA: Society of Nuclear Medicine; 2001.

Additional Resources

Bushberg JT, Seibert JA, Leidholdt EM, Boone JM. *The Essential Physics of Medical Imaging*. 2nd ed. Philadelphia, PA: Lippincott Williams & Wilkins; 2002: Chapter 21.

Cherry SR, Sorenson JA, Phelps ME. *Physics in Nuclear Medicine*. 3rd ed. Philadelphia, PA: Saunders; 2003:Chapters 14, 15.

Graham LS, ed. *Nuclear Medicine: Self-Study Program II: Instrumentation*. Reston, VA: Society of Nuclear Medicine; 1996:12–21.

Henkin RE, Boles MA, Dillehay GL, et al. *Nuclear Medicine*. St. Louis, MO: Mosby-Year Book; 1996:Chapters 7, 9.

CHAPTER 9

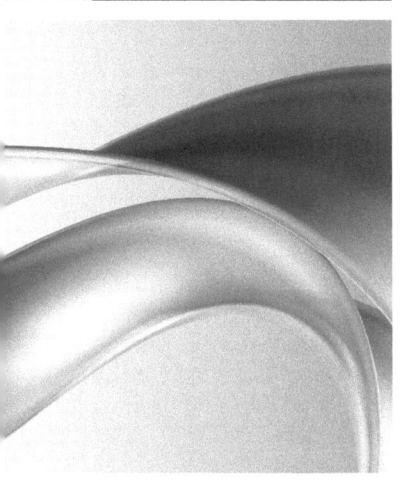

Departmental Quality Assurance and Quality Control of Gamma Cameras

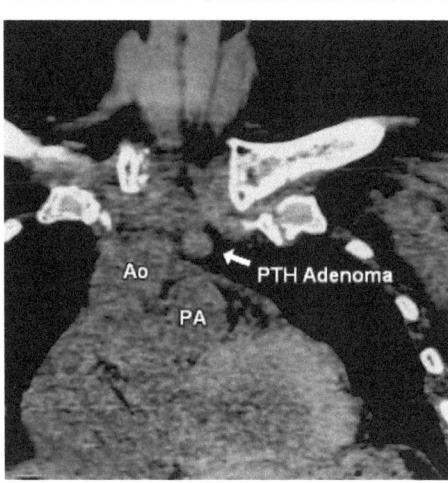

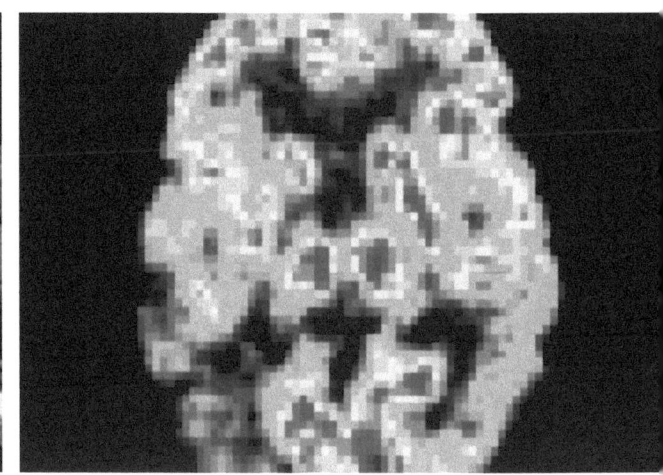

Learning Outcomes

1. Identify elements of departmental quality assurance, from the standpoints of individual study and departmental performance.
2. List the goals of a quality control program for a nuclear medicine department and discuss the use of action levels in conjunction with such a program.
3. Describe routine quality control testing of a planar gamma camera, including peaking, uniformity floods (both intrinsic and extrinsic methods), and bar phantoms; describe also the expected results in each case.
4. List and briefly describe the following nonroutine quality control tests for a gamma camera:
    a. Line-spread function
    b. Pixel size determination
    c. Sensitivity
    d. Collimator integrity
    e. Multiple-window spatial registration
    f. Count rate capabilities
5. Explain the purposes of National Electrical Manufacturers Association (NEMA) testing.
6. Define the terms *acceptance testing* and *benchmarking* and discuss how they fit into gamma camera purchase and installation.
7. Identify commonly encountered problems with gamma camera images and describe their appearance.

Introduction

Gamma cameras are quite complex in their construction and operation. It is necessary to test them daily to ensure that they are working properly. Other tests are done on a less frequent basis in order to uncover changes in performance over time. The amount of effort devoted to this aspect of nuclear medicine practice varies, but close attention to quality control saves time and money and can eliminate major causes of misdiagnosis of nuclear medicine studies. This chapter also discusses issues related to the purchase and initial testing of a gamma camera. The chapter concludes with a number of images illustrating camera artifacts. But let's begin by considering the larger question of overall department quality.

Quality Assurance

Quality control (QC) of equipment is only one aspect of a more comprehensive program of quality assurance. *Quality assurance* is the term used to describe how an organization knows that it is doing its job correctly. In medicine, it encompasses the quality of care given to patients, the appropriateness of diagnosis and treatment, and the level of patient satisfaction. In the United States, quality assurance is not just an ideal that all hospitals should strive for, but a requirement of The Joint Commission (TJC; formerly the Joint Commission on Accreditation of Healthcare

Organizations). Within the field of nuclear medicine, accrediting organizations, such as the American College of Radiology (ACR) and the Intersocietal Commission on Accreditation of Nuclear Laboratories (ICANL), offer mechanisms for nuclear medicine departments to prove their excellence, using a variety of quality assurance measures. Appendix F discusses laboratory accreditation in greater detail.

Procedural Quality Assurance

A comprehensive quality assurance program in nuclear medicine starts with the scheduling of an examination and ends with the final report of the results. We can see aspects of quality assurance throughout the entire timeline of a nuclear medicine procedure:

- Scheduling: Was the correct exam scheduled? Did the patient get appropriate information on the examination being done and the preparation needed? Are there contraindications that preclude the performance of the examination?
- Patient interview: Is this the correct patient? Is the patient pregnant or breastfeeding? Is the patient properly prepared (e.g., diet, medications)? What is the indication for performing the study, and can the requested study answer the clinical question?
- Radiopharmaceutical and dosing: Is this the correct radiopharmaceutical and dosage for this patient? Did the radiopharmaceutical preparation pass its quality control tests? Was the radiopharmaceutical administered at the correct time, via the correct route, and with good technique?
- Imaging: Is the study performed according to the department protocol? Is the image quality sufficient for the interpreting physician to provide a helpful interpretation? Are mathematical calculations and computer manipulations performed correctly and recorded in a logical fashion?
- Interpretation: Is the report clear and correct? How do the results of this examination compare with other studies done on this patient?
- Patient satisfaction: Is the patient satisfied with all aspects of interaction with the nuclear medicine department? Did the patient wait an overly long time? Is the patient happy with his or her treatment by the technical and medical staff in the department?

These questions are so important that if any *one* of them is not addressed correctly, the entire procedure may be rendered worthless. While technologists tend to focus on quality control issues, quality assurance questions are equally, if not more, important.

Departmental Quality Assurance

Beyond consideration of quality assurance on a study-by-study basis, a nuclear medicine department should consider its performance as a department. This aspect of quality assurance is evidenced not just by the absence of mistakes, but also by processes that examine outcomes and promote continuous improvement. Questions that can be asked in this regard include these:

- Compliance with regulations: What is the department's record with regard to radiation safety inspections? How can the department improve its day-to-day execution of radiation safety tasks? Are radiation exposures as low as reasonably achievable?
- Radiopharmaceutical administrations: What is the department's misadministration rate? What circumstances lead to misadministrations, and how can they be avoided?
- Procedures: Is the department's protocol manual up to date? How are protocol changes communicated to department members?
- Study interpretation: How do the results of nuclear medicine studies compare to other procedures that give similar information (e.g., lung scan vs pulmonary angiography, myocardial perfusion imaging vs cardiac catheterization)? What is the interobserver variability in a multiphysician department?
- Recordkeeping: Are the department's records up to date? Is information easily retrievable? Are records being saved for an adequate length of time?
- Continuing education: How are department members encouraged to attend educational offerings? How are suggestions gathered at such events incorporated into department protocols?

Departmental quality assurance, by necessity, must be done over a longer time frame than instrument quality control or procedural quality assurance. It can easily be forgotten as we concentrate on the day-to-day work. But it is only by asking questions such as these that a department can bring about lasting improvement.

Routine Quality Control Testing for Planar Gamma Cameras

Gamma cameras are particularly complex instruments compared to other types of imaging devices in the radiology department. They can fail in many different ways, and those failures directly impact the ability of the nuclear medicine physician to interpret the images produced. Routine quality control testing of gamma cameras is therefore a vital part of the operation of a nuclear medicine department. The "big picture" questions for quality control of equipment include the following (adapted from Reference 1):

- Is the camera operating within acceptable performance tolerances?
- How stable is the camera? Is it drifting from hour to hour or day to day? Are the changes erratic, or do they follow a discernible pattern?
- Are appropriate quality control images available to those interpreting the diagnostic images, in order to rule out artifacts?
- How does the performance of the camera compare with others in the department? With similar instruments around the country?
- Are the results of each day's evaluations used to provide a "go/no-go" answer for each instrument in

question? Can the feedback loops be made more effective?
- Is the current quality control program worthwhile? Does it provide useful information?

A good quality control program requires consistency in acquisition, analysis, and utilization of results. All personnel must do routine quality control tests in the same way, and consistent, accurate recordkeeping is essential. Written descriptions of QC procedures should include acceptable ranges for results. The department should set *action levels*, which are numeric values for test results that trigger corrective measures, and corrective actions to be taken when action levels are exceeded. Comparison to benchmark results and longitudinal records will be more valuable than simple day-to-day "eyeball" evaluations.

Table 9-1 provides a summary of suggested planar quality control procedures and the frequency for their performance, as given by a variety of references. These should be considered in light of specific guidance from the manufacturer of a given gamma camera, and one should abide by the manufacturer's recommendations where there is disagreement. The ultimate goal, of course, is to maximize image quality and therefore the information obtained from the nuclear medicine study; a department's quality control program should be scheduled with this in mind.

Peaking

The first QC test checks the alignment of the gamma camera's pulse height analyzer (PHA) window with the photopeak of the gamma ray being imaged, a process called *peaking*. Ideally, a gamma camera should be peaked in the morning for each isotope being used that day. Some manufacturers offer automated peaking (*autopeaking*), which works by adjusting the energy window position to equalize counts in two adjacent subwindows on either side of the photopeak, usually without operator intervention.

The peaking procedure should be done with a scatter-free source. In the intrinsic situation, the source can be made scatter-free by putting it on top of a lead brick on the floor and pointing the camera head down at it. An extrinsic source is usually scatter-free if it is resting on the collimator. Whether intrinsic or extrinsic, the source should expose the entire field of view (FOV). Peaking should never be done with a patient as the source, especially in an autopeaking situation, because this can potentially lead to an incorrect placement of the window (see Fig. 4-7). If possible, the energy resolution of the camera should be measured and compared to its benchmark value (although many systems do not have this capability).

It is normal for the position of the PHA window to vary from day to day, within a range of a few keV, due to fluctuations in high-voltage supply to the camera head and other factors. If a camera's photopeak location shifts significantly, the uniformity image for the day should be closely examined and a service call contemplated. For a multihead camera, the photopeak settings should not vary by more than a few keV from one head to another. The user should check the manufacturer's recommendations in this regard.

Some scientists have advocated routine use of an off-peak window (usually asymmetric to the high side of the photopeak) to decrease the amount of scatter accepted into the PHA window. Keep in mind, however, that an asymmetric window tends to make photomultiplier tubes (PMTs) visible on the uniformity flood image (**Figure 9-1**) and produce or accentuate nonuniformities. (In fact, off-peak images can be useful in evaluating detector tuning, loss of optical coupling, and crystal deterioration.) If an asymmetric window is to be used for patient studies, the service personnel must know that the department is using off-peak windows, so that the camera can be properly tuned to accommodate the practice. In addition, everyone in the department must agree on the amount of asymmetry to be used. Modern uniformity correction techniques may be able to maintain uniformity with asymmetric energy windows, but with the improved energy resolution of modern gamma cameras, there may be less reason to consider employing them.

Table 9-1

Recommended Quality Control Tests for Planar Gamma Cameras

Test	Recommended Frequency
Peaking	Daily[1-4]
Field uniformity	Daily[1-4]
With other radionuclides	Quarterly[5]
System uniformity (for all collimators)	Semiannually[2] Quarterly[3] Periodic[a,4]
Spatial resolution/linearity	Weekly[1-4]
Sensitivity	Quarterly[3] Semiannually[2] Periodic[a,4]
Dead time/maximum count rate	Quarterly[3] Semiannually[2] Annually[1] Periodic[a,4]
Multiple-window spatial registration	Quarterly[3] Annually[1] Periodic[a,4]

[a]Periodic = semiannually or when a problem is suspected.
[1]Botti J. Gamma camera performance evaluation and quality control. In: Fahey R, Harkness B, eds. *Basic Science of Nuclear Medicine* [CD-ROM]. Reston, VA: Society of Nuclear Medicine; 2001.
[2]Henkin RE, Boles MA, Dillehay GL, et al. *Nuclear Medicine*. St. Louis, MO: Mosby-Year Book; 1996:125, 140, 144.
[3]Graham LS. *Nuclear Medicine: Self-Study Program II: Instrumentation*. Reston, VA: Society of Nuclear Medicine; 1996:22.
[4]Zeissman HA, O'Malley JP, Thrall JH. *Nuclear Medicine: The Requisites*. 3rd ed. Philadelphia, PA: Mosby; 2006:47.
[5]Zanzonico P. Routine quality control of clinical nuclear medicine instrumentation: a brief review. *J Nucl Med*. 2008;49:1114–1131.

(a) Asymmetric low (upper left), asymmetric high (upper right), and on-peak (lower left) flood images

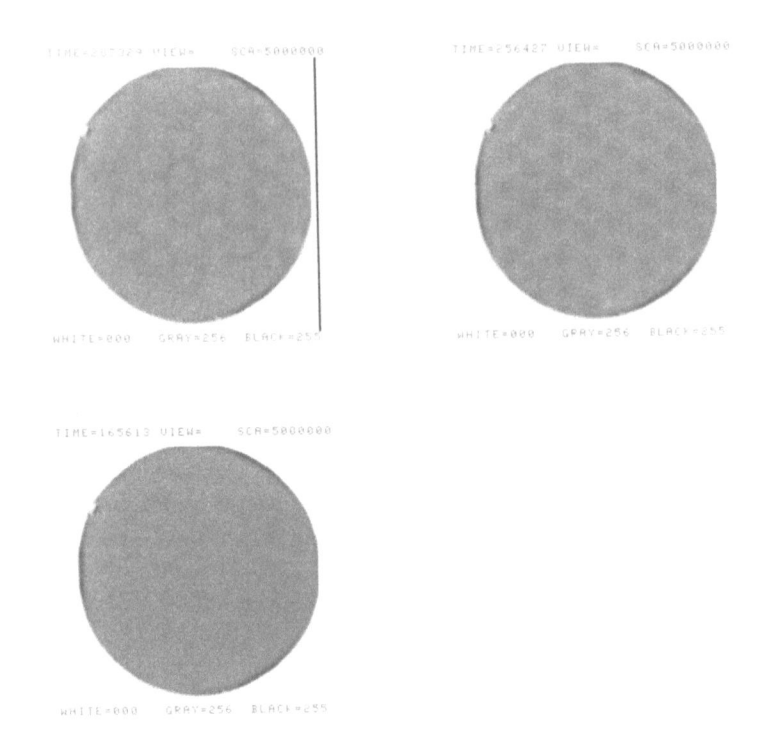

(b) On-peak (upper left), asymmetric low (upper right), and asymmetric high (lower left) flood images.

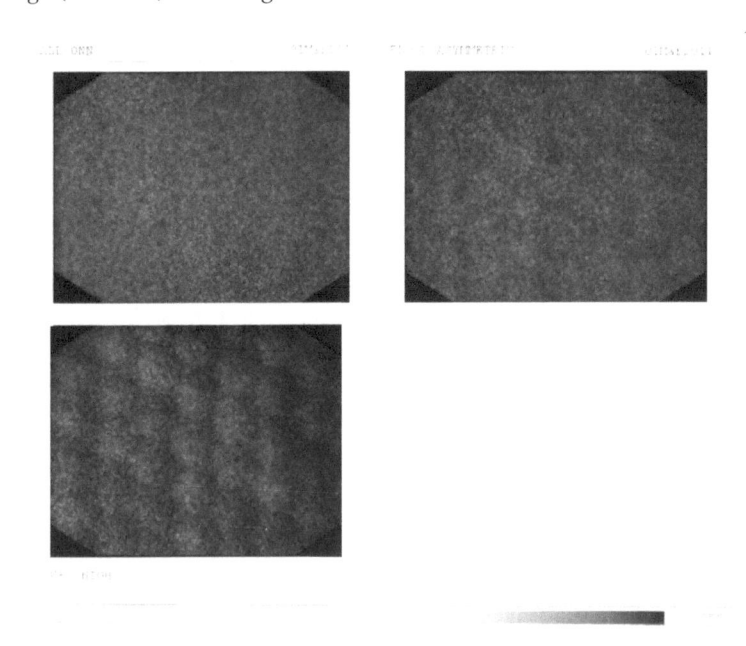

Figure 9-1 Asymmetric energy windows. In both cameras shown, PMTs are visible on both asymmetric high and asymmetric low images. In the second set of images, the integral uniformity increases from 6.1% for the on-peak flood to 7.1% (10 keV low) or 13.9% (10 keV high) for the asymmetric windows. Figure 9-1a courtesy of Virginia Mason Medical Center. Figure 9-1b courtesy of Swedish Medical Center.

Uniformity Flood

The evaluation of field uniformity is the most sensitive indicator of camera performance and stability. A flood image should be taken every day that the gamma camera is to be used for imaging patients. Floods are either *extrinsic* (with a collimator) or *intrinsic* (without a collimator); the two methods require quite different approaches.

For an intrinsic flood, the collimator is removed and a point source containing a small (<1 mCi or 37 MBq) amount of radioactivity (usually Tc-99m) is placed at a distance of at least five times the largest camera dimension from the camera face. This distance results in less than a 1% difference in photon flux between the center and the edges of the crystal, based on the inverse-square law. Intrinsic uniformity degrades with increasing count rate, so the source activity should be chosen so as not to exceed about 20,000 counts per second (cps). In some systems, a separate edge mask may be required if the edge mask is normally incorporated into the collimator for clinical imaging. For some multi-head cameras, a very low activity source is placed between the camera heads. This produces a nonuniform photon flux at the face of the crystal, which must be corrected before evaluating uniformity. In an intrinsic setting, any nearby radioactive source will cause a noticeable artifact (**Figure 9-2**).

To obtain an extrinsic flood, the collimator is left on (it should not affect the uniformity measurement unless it is damaged) and a flat-field flood source is placed on the collimator face. The flat-field flood source may be a Plexiglas phantom into which water and 5 to 15 mCi (185–555 MBq) of radioactivity (usually Tc-99m) are added, or a solid Co-57 sheet phantom made to very fine tolerance in terms of photon flux (counts/min/cm^2). Both of these have disadvantages. Some commercially available fillable phantoms have a tendency to bulge, providing a nonuniform photon flux that is unacceptable for modern uniformity correction programs. These phantoms can also be nonuniform due to air bubbles or inadequate mixing. The solid Co-57 phantom takes longer to acquire an adequate number of counts, is expensive, and must be replaced on a regular basis (about every 2 years). In addition, the energy spectrum of a Co-57 flood source may change over time, due to Co-58 and Co-59 impurities (2). The main advantage of the extrinsic flood method is that it is quicker and eliminates the need to expose the crystal.

Figure 9-2 Presence of an extraneous source in an intrinsic flood. The rim of the camera housing creates the shadow effect on the left side of the image, the direction from which the extraneous source is exposing the crystal surface. Image courtesy of Virginia Mason Medical Center.

The choice between intrinsic and extrinsic floods is dependent on department policy and manufacturer's recommendations. Whichever is done routinely, the other should be done on a less frequent (i.e., weekly, monthly, or quarterly) basis. It is also a good idea to look at flood images with and without corrections, if possible, in order to track the camera's uncorrected performance. Floods using other radionuclides that are imaged with the camera should be performed at least quarterly. This verifies the uniformity of the system with these radionuclides, checks the isotope-specific uniformity correction maps, and prompts the acquisition of new uniformity correction maps if the flood quality is not high.

Flood images should be evaluated both visually and quantitatively. An image containing 2 to 6 million counts (cts) is adequate for visual inspection, but visual inspection will not detect nonuniformities with count differences that are less than about 5% variation from the average. Quantitative analysis of uniformity requires 30 to 120 million cts to overcome the statistical variability inherent in a radionuclide image.

Two formulas are used to quantify the degree of variation in a flood acquisition. *Integral uniformity* searches the entire flood to find the maximum and minimum ct/pixel values:

$$\text{Integral uniformity} = \frac{\max \text{cts/pixel} - \min \text{cts/pixel}}{\max \text{cts/pixel} + \min \text{cts/pixel}} \times 100\%. \quad (9\text{-}1)$$

Increasing values of this number indicate worsening uniformity.

Sample Calculation 9-1 Integral Uniformity

A flood image is acquired for a mean count density of 10,000 cts/pixel. The flood is completely uniform, such that the only variability in the count density is that due to Poisson statistics. Calculate the count density of pixels that are 2 standard deviations higher and lower than the mean, and use them to estimate the integral uniformity.

The standard deviation of 10,000 cts is 100 cts, so the 2 standard deviation values are 9,800 and 10,200 cts. The integral uniformity is

$$\frac{10,200 - 9,800}{10,200 + 9,800} \times 100\% = \frac{400}{20,000} \times 100\% = 2\%.$$

Thus, even a "perfect" flood with only statistical variability has an integral uniformity of about 2%.

Differential uniformity looks at changes in cts/pixel values over short segments of the flood:

$$\text{Differential uniformity} = \frac{\text{high} - \text{low}}{\text{high} + \text{low}} \times 100\% \quad (9\text{-}2)$$

where *high* and *low* refer to the highest and lowest ct/pixel values, respectively, within a five-pixel segment. The value reported for differential uniformity is the largest value found for this formula when all five-pixel segments in the flood are considered. Some analysis programs report separate row and column differential uniformity values. Thus, integral uniformity provides a global measure of the flood quality, whereas differential uniformity indicates the greatest (worst-case) nonuniformity over a short distance. Integral uniformity will always be greater than or equal to differential uniformity.

Typically, commercially available computer programs evaluate integral and differential uniformity over both the *useful field of view* (UFOV), usually defined as 95% of the exposed camera face, and the *central field of view* (CFOV), defined as the center 75% of the UFOV. Gamma camera performance degrades near the edges of the FOV, so the UFOV uniformity value will always be greater than or equal to the CFOV value. Two examples of commercially available uniformity analysis programs are shown in **Figure 9-3**. The analysis program should report integral and differential uniformity values for useful and central

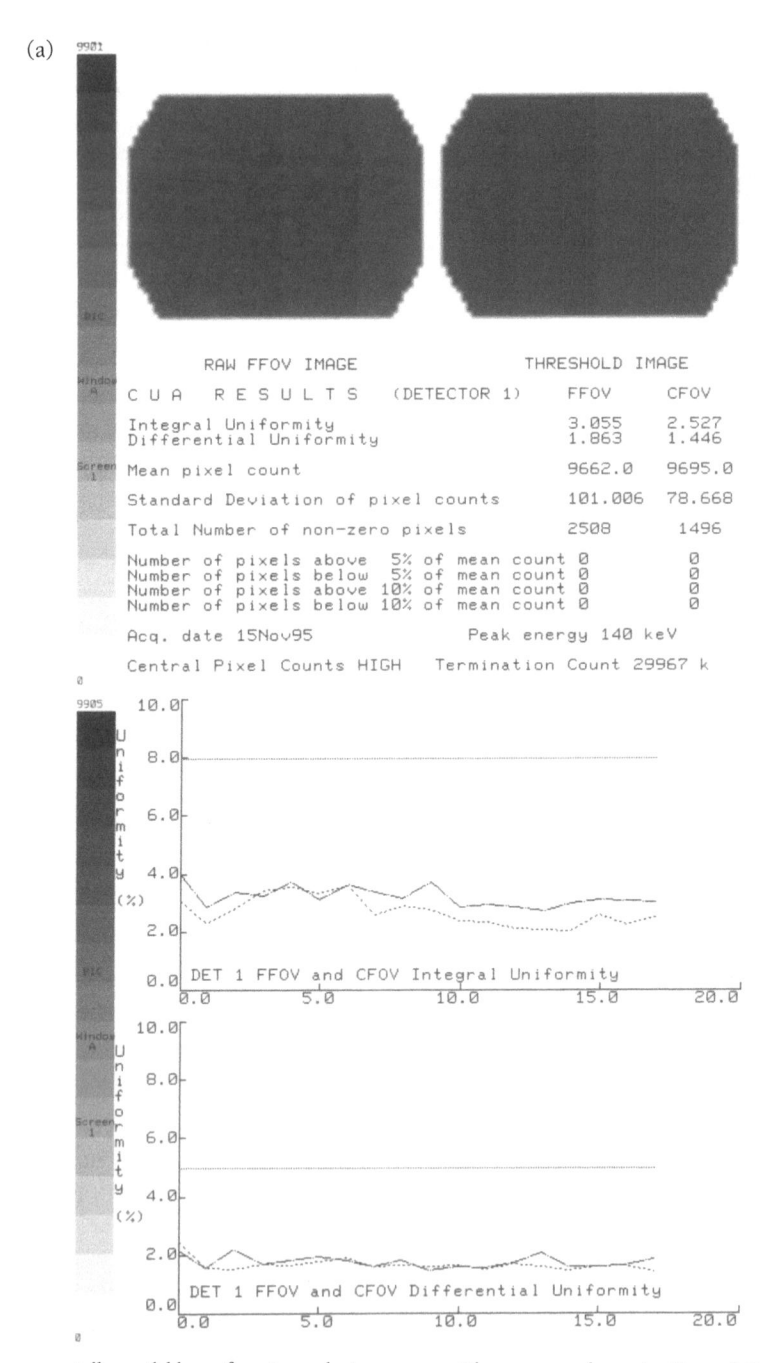

Figure 9-3 Two examples of commercially available uniformity analysis programs. The program shown in Figure 9-3a includes Levy–Jennings plots of integral and differential uniformity, making it easy to spot trends. The program shown in Figure 9-3b identifies the areas that are the most nonuniform (the boxes indicate areas of integral nonuniformity, and the lines indicate areas with the greatest differential nonuniformity). The operator can then check to see if the same area is being marked day after day. Images courtesy of Virginia Mason Medical Center.

Chapter 9: Departmental Quality Assurance and Quality Control of Gamma Cameras

(b)

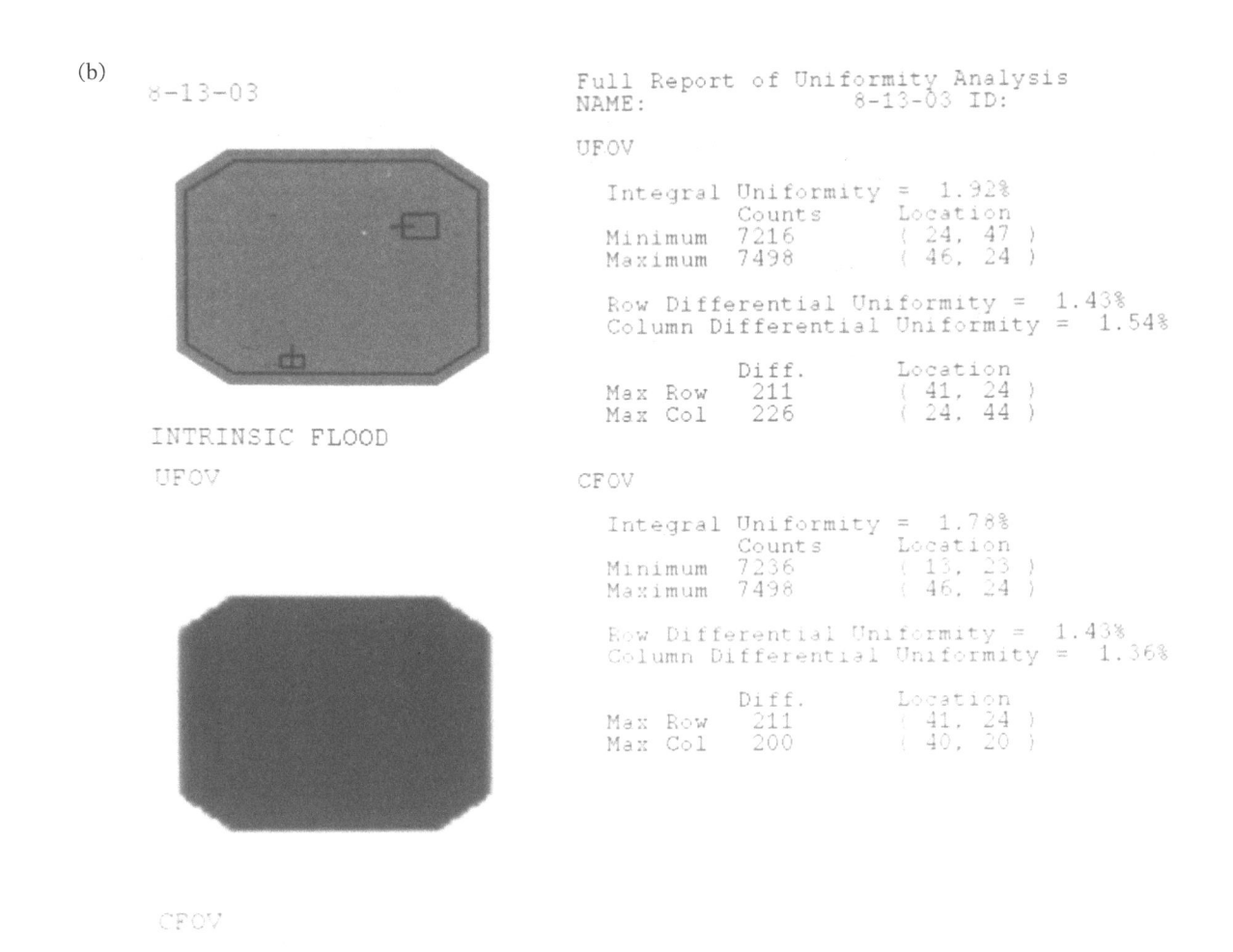

```
8-13-03                    Full Report of Uniformity Analysis
                           NAME:              8-13-03 ID:
                           UFOV
                              Integral Uniformity =  1.92%
                                       Counts        Location
                              Minimum   7216         ( 24, 47 )
                              Maximum   7498         ( 46, 24 )

                              Row Differential Uniformity =  1.43%
                              Column Differential Uniformity =  1.54%
                                         Diff.        Location
                              Max Row    211         ( 41, 24 )
                              Max Col    226         ( 24, 44 )
INTRINSIC FLOOD
UFOV                       CFOV
                              Integral Uniformity =  1.78%
                                       Counts        Location
                              Minimum   7236         ( 13, 23 )
                              Maximum   7498         ( 46, 24 )

                              Row Differential Uniformity =  1.43%
                              Column Differential Uniformity =  1.36%
                                         Diff.        Location
                              Max Row    211         ( 41, 24 )
                              Max Col    200         ( 40, 20 )

CFOV
```

Figure 9-3 (continued)

FOVs and should indicate the area(s) demonstrating the greatest nonuniformities. Ideally, the program includes a graph (such as a Levy–Jennings plot, seen in Fig. 9-3a) that shows the change in the reported value(s) over time; this is the best way to see slow drifts in camera performance. A specific level of uniformity should be set as an action level, such that when measured uniformity rises above the action level, some form of corrective action is taken.

Integral flood uniformity should run between 1% and 5% for a well-tuned camera with all corrections in force. Uniformity values of 3% or lower are desirable for single-photon emission computed tomography (SPECT) imaging. Extrinsic flood uniformity tends to be a little higher (4–6%), but this may be due in part to the inherent nonuniformity in the flood source rather than an effect of the collimator. An action level of 5% for integral and differential uniformity is recommended (3). An elevated or rising uniformity measurement is often improved following acquisition of a new uniformity correction map (3). It is generally recommended that new uniformity correction maps be acquired monthly or quarterly for all radionuclides in routine use. Floods with nonroutine radionuclides may routinely demonstrate higher uniformity values and may therefore have a higher uniformity action level. When these floods exceed their action level, the uniformity correction maps for the specific radionuclides should likewise be reacquired.

Count profiles are very useful in assessing gamma camera performance. A *count profile* displays graphically the counts per pixel along a straight line across the FOV that has been defined by the user. Most computer systems allow the line to be drawn at any angle and to be 1 or more pixels thick. An example of a count profile across a flood image is shown in **Figure 9-4**. The figure shows that even a uniform-appearing flood image has a fair amount of pixel-to-pixel variability (ct/pixel values range from 25 to 50, around an average of 38 cts/pixel). Count profiles are employed in several of the tests discussed in the following sections.

Bar Phantoms and Other Measures of Spatial Resolution

Most nuclear medicine departments utilize a bar phantom of some kind for routine, semiquantitative determination of gamma camera spatial linearity and resolution (**Figure 9-5**). The "semiquantitative" qualification is due to the fact that bar phantoms have only a few, finite bar widths. We can speak of resolution being better than the smallest bar visualized, but not as good as the largest bar not visualized. *Linearity* refers to the gamma camera's ability to reproduce a straight line. While a bar phantom is certainly helpful in this respect, the uniformity image

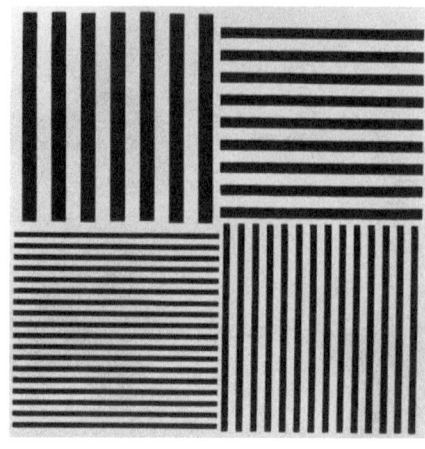

Figure 9-5 Bar phantom. The four-quadrant bar phantom must be rotated four times to evaluate resolution and spatial linearity in all four quadrants. Photo courtesy of Capintec, Inc.

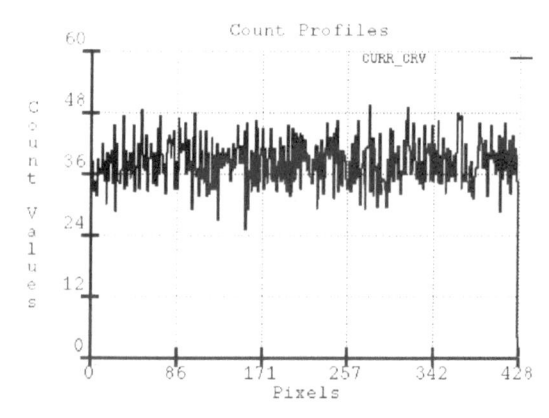

Figure 9-4 Count profile of a flood image. The X-axis of a count profile is the location in pixels, from the beginning to the end of the user-defined line. The Y-axis shows the counts per pixel (or multiple pixels if a thickness greater than 1 pixel is chosen). Images courtesy of St. Joseph Medical Center.

may actually be more valuable in the evaluation of linearity: a deviation of 0.4 mm from linearity produces a nonuniformity of 8% (4).

Because the collimator has a large effect on resolution, it is necessary to use different bar phantoms for intrinsic vs extrinsic situations. Beyond the issue of obtaining an accurate evaluation of resolution, an inappropriate choice of bar phantom can also produce *Moiré patterns* (**Figure 9-6**). When the width of the bars approaches the collimator's hole diameter, the bars and holes set up interference patterns, producing apparent "bars" that are oriented differently than the physical bars of the phantom, as well as other interesting patterns. Reference 5 has a good description of the origin of this phenomenon. The term *Moiré* is the French word for "watered," because the patterns are said to resemble watered silk fabric. Moiré patterns are commonly seen with high-sensitivity and medium- and high-energy collimators and can also be seen when the matrix dimension of a digital acquisition is similar to the bar size. They have not been reported in clinical images. One should always look closely at the orientation of the bars in a bar phantom image to be sure they match the physical orientation of the bars in the phantom.

System spatial resolution should be evaluated both at the surface of the collimator and at 10-cm distance. The surface measurement is most often done with a bar phantom, while the 10-cm measurement of the line-spread function (LSF) (see the following paragraph) provides a more realistic measurement. The 10-cm measurement can be performed with a scattering medium (such as water or lucite) between the source and the collimator, which more accurately reflects the system's resolution in actual imaging situations. The bar phantom images should include at least 5 million cts, and the image matrix should be 512×512, so that the bar phantom image evaluates the camera's resolution and not the resolution of the computer. The full width at tenth-maximum (FWTM) is much more affected by scatter and septal penetration than is the full width at half-maximum (FWHM).

Spatial resolution can be quantified in an absolute fashion using a *line-spread function* measurement. An LSF measurement is performed using a thin line source of radioactivity, such as a capillary tube filled with a few μCi of a Tc-99m solution. (Use some kind of soft putty to seal the ends of the tube; the putty used to seal microhematocrit tubes, commercially available as Critoseal® [Sherwood Medical Industries], works nicely.) The diameter of the line source should be less than one-half the width of the smallest bars that can be seen with the system, or less than one-quarter of its FWHM. The line source is imaged extrinsically (again with a 512×512 matrix), a count profile is drawn across it perpendicularly, and the FWHM and FWTM of the line source are calculated (see Fig. 8-9). There should ideally be at least five data points between the two intersection points of the half-maximum line. The

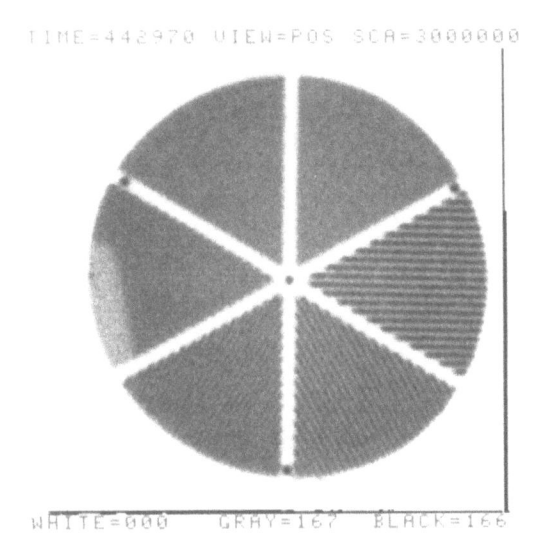

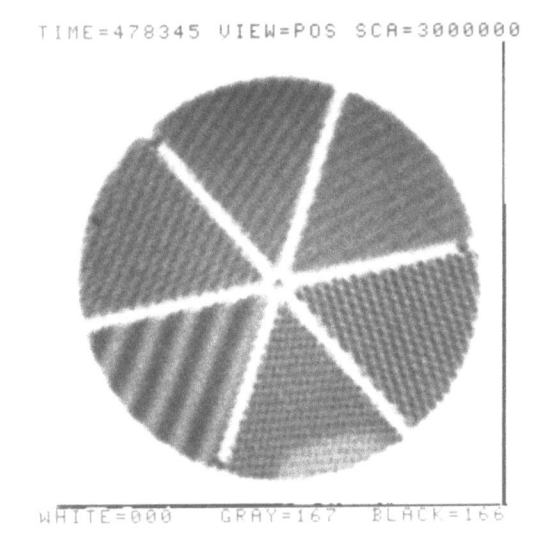

Figure 9-6 Moiré patterns. The image on the left is an extrinsic image of a six-sector bar phantom, using a low-energy high-resolution collimator. The image on the right is the same bar phantom, imaged with the high-energy collimator. Note that in some sectors, the bars still appear to be bars, but they are not pointing in the correct direction. Images courtesy of Virginia Mason Medical Center.

FWHM is measured in pixels and converted to cm based on the pixel size (see the following pixel size determination).

A "quick and dirty" estimate of the FWHM can be obtained by multiplying the width of the smallest bars seen on a bar phantom image by 1.75. This is not as accurate as the LSF measurement because the bar phantom has only limited choices for bar widths. If we can visualize 5-mm bars but not 3-mm bars, then we know only that the FWHM is between 5 and 9 mm. We cannot state the FWHM exactly using this method.

Nonroutine Quality Control Tests

The following tests are performed infrequently in most nuclear medicine departments. A marked change in system performance may require that one or more of these tests be done. Some experts recommend that these procedures, or some portion of them, be done quarterly or annually.

Pixel Size Determination

In a digital image, distances can be measured in pixels, making it necessary to know the size of each pixel. While the pixel size can be calculated from the dimensions of the FOV, it can also be verified quite easily. Two 10-cm lines are drawn at right angles to each other on a sheet of cardboard. A drop of radioactivity is placed at each end of each line. The cardboard is laid on the collimator surface with the two lines aligned with the camera's X- and Y-axes and imaged. On the computer, a count profile is drawn to include the two point sources at the ends of one of the lines. Two peaks are seen; the distance between them, measured in pixels, is equal to 10 cm. The analysis is repeated with the other line to verify pixel size in the other axis; the values for the two directions should be within a few pixels of each other. In a dual-head system, the pixel size between the two heads should not vary by more than 0.5% (6).

Sensitivity Check

Sensitivity is commonly measured extrinsically, by putting 1 to 2 mCi (37–74 MBq) of Tc-99m solution into a petri dish and then diluting the solution so that it has about a 3-mm depth. The syringe used to dispense the radioactive solution should be assayed in a dose calibrator both before and after dispensing to the petri dish, so that the activity in the petri dish is known exactly. One may also use a Co-57 sheet source in an extrinsic setting (4); the actual activity may deviate from the calculated value if the sheet source has (or had) radionuclidic contaminants. The petri dish or sheet source is placed on the collimator surface, and 10 count measurements of 1 min each are acquired. The count rate should be less than 10,000 cps. A 1-min background measurement is also made. The mean of the 10 measurements is calculated, background counts are subtracted, and sensitivity is expressed as cpm/µCi (see Sample Calculation 9-2 on p. 120):

$$\text{Sensitivity} = \frac{\text{mean cpm} - \text{bkg cpm}}{\text{source activity } (\mu\text{Ci})}. \quad (9\text{-}3)$$

To compare sensitivity measurements on a camera over time, they must be done under the exact same conditions: same energy window width, same collimator, same applied corrections. Sensitivity is more a test of the collimator than of the camera; it should be checked on a quarterly or semiannual schedule, but it is generally quite stable (4). Multiple-head systems should demonstrate no more than 5% difference in sensitivity between heads (2).

Collimator Integrity

In addition to regular inspection of extrinsic uniformity flood images, one can evaluate collimator integrity by positioning a point source (e.g., 20 mCi of Tc-99m) at least 20 ft away from the camera and acquiring a 1 million to

Sample Calculation 9-2 Sensitivity Determination

A sensitivity test is performed as follows:

- Activity in syringe before dispensing = 1.81 mCi
- Activity in syringe after dispensing = 0.03 mCi
- Background = 98 cpm
- Count measurements of activity in petri dish (1 min each):
    1. 348,919
    2. 352,004
    3. 349,187
    4. 351,992
    5. 350,457
    6. 347,804
    7. 349,119
    8. 348,775
    9. 351,676
    10. 349,623

What is the camera's sensitivity?
The average count rate is 349,955, or 349,857 cpm after background subtraction. The activity in the petri dish is 1.81 − 0.03 mCi = 1.78 mCi or 1,780 µCi. The sensitivity is thus

$$\text{Sensitivity} = \frac{349{,}857 \text{ cpm}}{1{,}780 \text{ µCi}} = \frac{196 \text{ cpm}}{\text{µCi}}.$$

2.5 million count image. This is most easily accomplished by taping the source to a wall and directing the camera face toward it. With the source at such a great distance, the gamma rays that reach the camera are essentially parallel. They cannot enter the scintillation crystal unless the collimator holes are also parallel and oriented in the same direction as the gamma rays. The appearance of the point source should be a large, radially symmetric area of activity, as in the lower image in **Figure 9-7**. The source may need to be repositioned several times to check the entire face of the collimator. This procedure reportedly shows defects more readily than the extrinsic high-count flood image (7).

Collimator evaluation should be included on a regular QC schedule, so that it is performed monthly, quarterly, or biannually. But one should also perform this test if there is any possibility that a collimator may have been damaged. Collimators should be visually inspected on a regular basis for signs of damage. If a gamma camera is to produce optimal images, the collimator uniformity must approach the intrinsic uniformity (7).

Multiple-Window Spatial Registration

When a radionuclide with more than one photopeak, such as In-111 or Ga-67, is used for imaging, it is important to know that the events in the different photopeaks are being assigned to the same location. Multiple-window spatial registration (MWSR) evaluates whether this is true. The

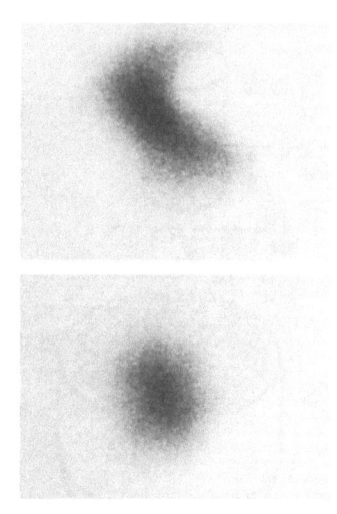

Figure 9-7 Collimator evaluation. The image is obtained using a point source of radioactivity positioned a large distance from the collimator. When the collimator holes are no longer perpendicular to the crystal face and parallel to one another, gamma rays hitting the collimator perpendicularly cannot enter them. This is seen in the upper image, while the lower image shows an undamaged collimator. Reprinted from: Early PJ, Sodee DB. *Principles and Practice of Nuclear Medicine*. 2nd ed. St. Louis, MO: Mosby-Year Book; 1995: 267. Used with permission from Elsevier.

test uses drops of a multiple-energy isotope at four locations on a cardboard phantom. The phantom is imaged using each energy window separately, and the resulting images are subtracted from one another. If the system is not correctly locating the events, the dots will not superimpose exactly. One can alternatively analyze the images by drawing count profiles through each pair of dots and determining the pixels containing the maximum counts for each energy window. If the events are not being correctly located, the pixels containing the maximum counts will not be the same (**Figure 9-8**). This test should be done every 3 to 6 months, because this is a relatively common problem for gamma cameras (2, 4).

Another way to evaluate MWSR is to intrinsically image a bar phantom using each photopeak separately. The images obtained from the different photopeaks, when summed into a composite image, should appear as clear as the image using only the lowest photopeak. Any misregistration will also be apparent as a double exposure in the composite image. A knowledgeable physician or technologist may be able to recognize a similar effect on clinical images. An MWSR deviation greater than 2 mm will cause a loss of spatial resolution and contrast (2).

Count Rate Capabilities

All systems should have a dead time measurement at least at the time of acceptance testing. If high-count-rate studies such as first-pass radionuclide angiograms are performed, the determination of count rate performance is an important quality control parameter. This is most easily evaluated with the two-source method (8):

- Prepare two Tc-99m sources, each of which produces a count rate of about 20,000 cps, or so that the combined sources produce a count rate approximately

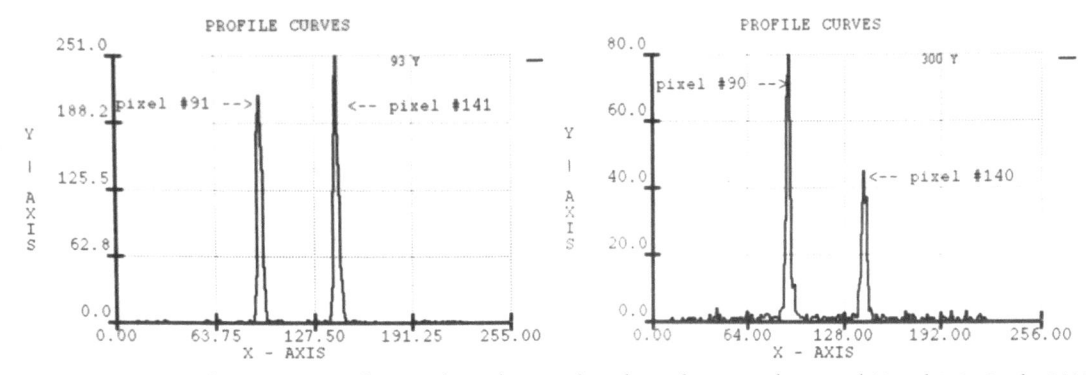

Figure 9-8 Multiple-window spatial registration. In this test, the 93-keV window shows the two peaks at pixel 91 and 141. On the 300-keV peak, they are at pixels 90 and 140. While the error in this system is small, larger misregistrations can occur and are detrimental to image interpretation. Image courtesy of Virginia Mason Medical Center.

equal to the vendor-specified 20% loss count rate. The two sources should be approximately equal in activity and should be placed in a phantom that simulates tissue scattering.
- If a high-count-rate mode can be enabled, it should be turned on. The energy window should be set at 20%. This measurement can be performed intrinsically or extrinsically.
- Using a counting time of 100 sec, determine the count rate of source 1 alone, sources 1 and 2 together, and source 2 alone. Repeat in the reverse order as a control. Subtract background from all measurements.
- Calculate the dead time using the following formula:

$$\tau (\mu sec) = \left[\frac{2R_{12}}{(R_1 + R_2)} \ln \left(\frac{R_1 + R_2}{R_{12}} \right) \right] \times 10^6 \quad (9\text{-}4)$$

where R_1, R_{12}, and R_2 are the count rates from source 1 alone, sources 1 and 2 together, and source 2 alone, respectively.
- Calculate the actual count rate for a 20% loss of counts, using the formula

$$R_{20\% \text{ loss}} = \frac{0.2231}{\tau}. \quad (9\text{-}5)$$

This value should be compared to that specified by the vendor.

Measured dead time depends on the ratio of counts accepted by the PHA to total counts seen by the camera, because the system components that determine dead time are located prior to the PHA. Therefore, the window width and the presence or absence of scatter will significantly alter the result obtained by this measure. Similarly, the use of an electronic edge mask means that the measured count rate is much lower than the count rate the camera is actually dealing with. All of these variables need to be considered in evaluating the results of this measurement.

Alternatively, the camera's count rate performance may be evaluated by generating the relationship between true and observed count rate (5). A 20-mCi Tc-99m source is placed 150 cm from the intrinsic camera face (which has the edge packing masked, either electronically or with lead shielding). Twenty-five 1-mm copper plates are placed in front of the Tc-99m source. The count rate is measured as the copper plates are removed, one by one. At low count rates, the observed rate is equal to the actual count rate. As more copper plates are removed, the observed count rate does not increase as much, because counts are lost due to dead time. The copper plates should be removed until the observed count rate decreases, so that the entire count rate curve is documented.

The data from this procedure are used to create a graph like that shown in **Figure 9-9**. From the low-count-rate

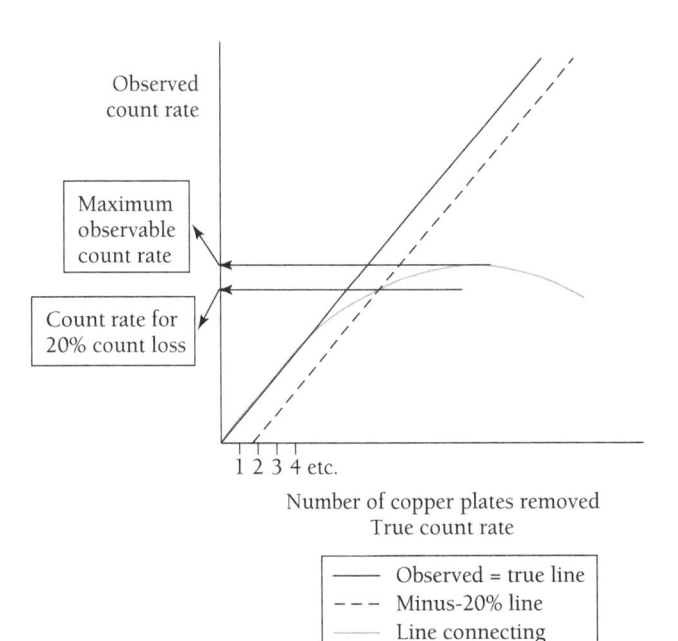

Figure 9-9 Maximum count rate and 20% loss value. The count rate curve (the light-gray line) represents the data points generated in the experiment described in the text. The X values for each point are initially graphed relative to the number of copper plates removed. But because there is no dead time at low count rates, we can use the observed count rate in this region as the true count rate and thus correlate with the copper-plate scale. The rest of the "observed = true" line is extrapolated from the low-count-rate data points. The maximum observable count rate is the peak of the count rate curve, read from the Y-axis. The 20% count rate loss is the point at which the minus-20% line crosses the count rate curve.

data, the "observed = true" line is created by extending the straight-line portion of the observed count rate. A second line, 20% lower than the "observed-true" line, is then drawn on the graph. The maximum observable count rate is determined from the peak of the count rate curve. The 20% loss value is where the count rate curve crosses the minus-20% line. No additional useful image information is being gained when the 20%-loss count rate is exceeded.

Camera Purchase and Acceptance Testing

When preparing to acquire a new gamma camera, the purchaser needs first to stipulate the specific characteristics required and then solicit proposals from manufacturers. These characteristics may include camera performance parameters such as spatial resolution as well as the types of collimators needed, the ability to perform specific clinical studies, compatibility with existing computer systems, and even physical dimensions. The expectations for service and preventive maintenance should be clearly spelled out, as should arrangements for hardware and software upgrades. Delineation of the user's needs and desires provides a starting framework from which the user and manufacturer can negotiate.

NEMA Standards

Newly purchased gamma cameras must meet standards for performance that are established by NEMA and updated periodically (9). This association of vendors has reached consensus on both the measures of performance and the methods by which gamma cameras are to be evaluated and compared to one another. Gamma camera testing according to NEMA standards requires equipment and software that are not generally available to nuclear medicine technologists (although the vendor may supply both) as well as experience that nuclear medicine technologists generally do not have. For these reasons, the NEMA tests themselves are not discussed in detail.

Gamma cameras must undergo testing to verify their performance before they leave the factory. NEMA publication NU 1-2007 describes the measurements and methods to be used for testing (2, 9). Some NEMA parameters are expected to be typical of system performance of a particular class of gamma cameras. The manufacturer performs these tests on a limited number of each model of gamma camera to demonstrate that the model meets these standards. Other NEMA parameters must be met or exceeded on every gamma camera, and hence the manufacturer must substantiate them for each camera shipped to a buyer. (Older NEMA terminology used "class standard" for the first situation and "performance standard" for the second.) Note that NEMA standards are regarded as minimum acceptable standards; a system meeting a NEMA specification should perform at least as well as the standard indicates.

Acceptance Testing and Benchmarking

Once the system is reassembled on site and deemed by the vendor to be ready for clinical studies, it should undergo *acceptance testing*, as required by TJC (4). Acceptance testing provides a quantitative measure of gamma camera performance and verifies that the system as installed meets the vendor specifications. It answers the question, "Did we get what we paid for?" Acceptance testing should be performed by an experienced medical physicist and should follow NEMA specifications. **Table 9-2** lists tests that should be performed in this process.

In addition to testing the gamma camera, acceptance testing verifies that it has the proper environment. The initial conditions for temperature, airflow, and electric power must meet manufacturer specifications. After installation, it becomes the job of the technologist to recognize when these conditions have changed and whether the changes might be affecting the gamma camera's performance.

Benchmark testing is done immediately after the institution accepts the gamma camera. It should include all of the routine quality control tests that will be performed on the gamma camera. The results provide the benchmark against which future quality control results will be compared. Therefore, benchmark test results should be stored permanently, but should also be readily accessible. It is advisable to repeat and rearchive benchmark testing after major service. In an ideal world, the NEMA protocols performed at the time of acceptance testing would be repeated every 1 to 3 years, and new benchmarks acquired after the gamma camera's performance has been optimized.

Note that "imaging recording and display modules" are listed in Table 9-2. While nuclear medicine images do not require a particularly high-quality monitor, video display terminal (VDT) performance should not be ignored. Quality control procedures can be patterned after protocols used in the radiology department (10). A common test pattern for medical image display devices, produced by the Society of Motion Picture and Television Engineers (SMPTE), is shown in **Figure 9-10** (11).

Troubleshooting Gamma Cameras

The last section of this chapter is devoted to images of gamma cameras with problems. It is not intended to be all-inclusive, because as electronics in gamma cameras advance, they may produce new types of artifacts. Rather, it will provide examples of specific known artifacts to demonstrate the range of possible ways in which gamma cameras can malfunction.

1. Wrong energy window (**Figure 9-11**): When an image "doesn't look right," a common reason is that the photopeak does not correspond to the radionuclide being imaged. Even student technologists with less than 1 year of experience in nuclear medicine may be able to spot this problem. When in doubt, go back to the spectrum display to be sure that the window is correctly aligned with the photopeak.

Table 9-2

Measures of Planar Gamma Camera Performance to Be Determined in Acceptance Testing

Planar performance measures	• Intrinsic uniformity
	• On-peak and off-peak
	• With and without corrections
	• Clinical isotopes
	• Intrinsic spatial resolution
	• Intrinsic and system count rate performance (maximum count rate and dead time)
	• Intrinsic spatial linearity
	• Intrinsic energy resolution
	• System spatial resolution (with and without scatter)
	• System sensitivity (for each collimator)
	• Multiple-window spatial registration
	• Collimator uniformity
Environmental conditions	• Room temperature
	• Voltage and current of camera supply line
	• Ventilation rate and room humidity
Mechanical and safety checks	• Emergency stop and motion/pressure sensor mechanisms
	• Collimator-changing mechanisms and devices
	• Electrical grounding, cabling, and connections
	• Functionality of hand switches and controls
Functionality checks	• Image recording and display modules
	• Angle indicators
	• Camera head shielding
	• Operational status and alignment of scanning table and other peripherals

Early PJ, Sodee BD. *Principles and Practice of Nuclear Medicine*. 2nd ed. St. Louis, MO: Mosby-Year Book; 1995:279–284.
Siegel JA, Benedetto AR, Jaszczak RJ, et al. AAPM Report No. 22. Rotating scintillation camera SPECT acceptance testing and quality control. New York, NY: American Institute of Physics; 1987.
AAPM Report No. 9. Computer-aided scintillation camera SPECT acceptance testing. New York, NY: American Institute of Physics; 1982.

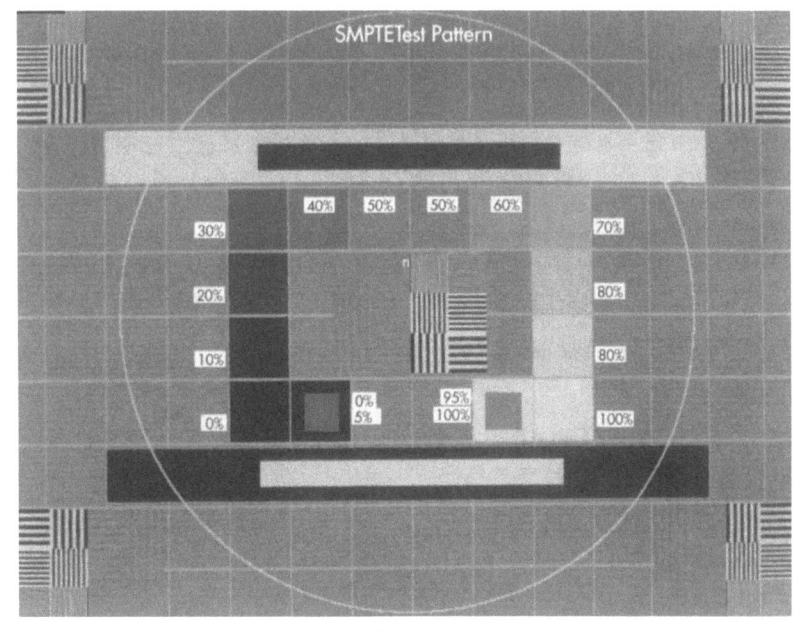

Figure 9-10 Medical diagnostic imaging test pattern. This pattern, produced by the Society of Motion Picture and Television Engineers (SMPTE), is used by companies and service personnel to determine the proper functionality of video display monitors. Reprinted from: Papp J. *Quality Management in the Imaging Sciences*. 3rd ed. St. Louis, MO: Mosby-Elsevier; 2006: Fig. 9-17. Used with permission of Elsevier.

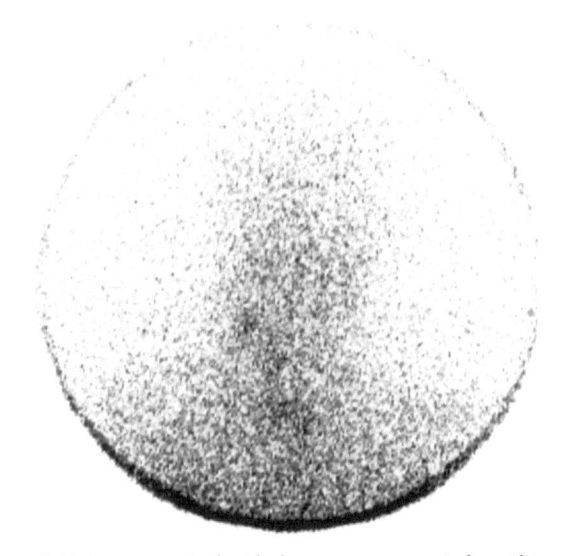

Figure 9-11 Image acquired with the wrong energy window. This radionuclide is I-131, but the energy window was accidentally left on 140 keV. The image is an anterior head–neck view looking for thyroid cancer metastases. Image courtesy of Virginia Mason Medical Center.

2. PMT problems (**Figure 9-12**): This is the most common problem affecting gamma cameras. PMTs can fail for a number of reasons, including loss of vacuum, high voltage changes, and failure of the preamplifier. A poorly functioning PMT affects not only its location but also the surrounding area, as events are incorrectly positioned due to the absence of the failed PMT's input into the position circuit. Even greater regional effects are seen in systems that tune the PMTs relative to one another (Fig. 9-12b). The ability to visualize a failed PMT depends greatly on the system; in some, it may be immediately obvious that a tube has failed, while in others the changes may be subtler, and in still others multiple PMTs may be affected via autotuning circuits. Uniformity corrections will not be able to completely cover up a PMT failure.

3. Cracked crystal (**Figure 9-13**): Even a small crack produces a wide defect because photons are reflected away from the crack. A cracked crystal will show edge packing around the crack. A cracked crystal must be replaced, and scintillation crystals are very expensive.

4. Measles (**Figure 9-14**): When a scintillation crystal starts to absorb water, these characteristic spots are seen. The ability to visualize the spots is improved if an off-peak window is used. This phenomenon is also called *yellowing* of the crystal. A yellowed crystal may cause subtle problems with clinical images.

5. Loss of automated corrections: The loss of a camera's energy, linearity, or uniformity correction map is usually apparent as a significant deterioration in both uniformity and spatial linearity. **Figure 9-15** shows a thallium uniformity flood before and after acquisition of a new uniformity correction map.

6. Off-peak windows (Figure 9-1): Typically, if the window is off-peak on the high side, the tubes will appear hot, whereas if it is on the low side, they will appear cold. However, with modern correction systems, a variety of artifacts may be seen. With some cameras, the use of a source with activity higher than the recommended amount will cause similarly aberrant flood images.

7. Poor coupling of PMTs to scintillation crystal (**Figure 9-16**): As the coupling deteriorates, a variety of artifacts may result. Poor coupling can sometimes

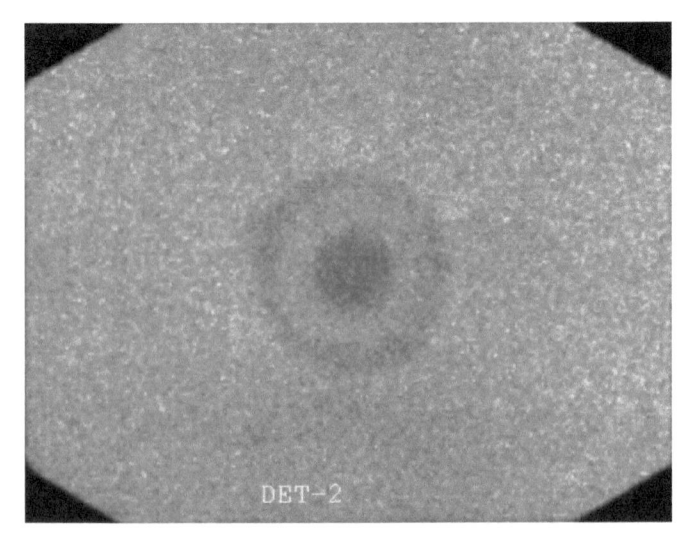

(a) Malfunctioning preamplifier in center PMT of a gamma camera

(b) Malfunctioning PMT in a gamma camera that tunes PMTs relative to each other

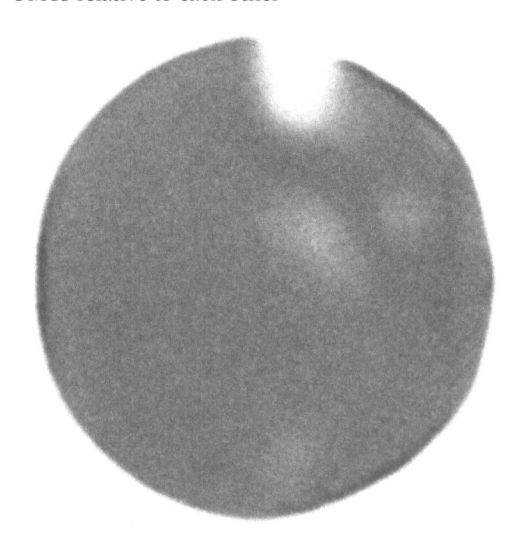

Figure 9-12 Two examples of malfunctioning PMTs. When a PMT fails, it has effects on not just its own area, but on a fairly large region of the camera. The camera on the right is a type that tunes PMTs relative to one another, so that when one fails, the camera adjusts other PMTs out of tune as it tries to compensate. Figure 9-12a courtesy of Swedish Medical Center. Figure 9-12b courtesy of Virginia Mason Medical Center.

Small imperfection   Cracked crystal

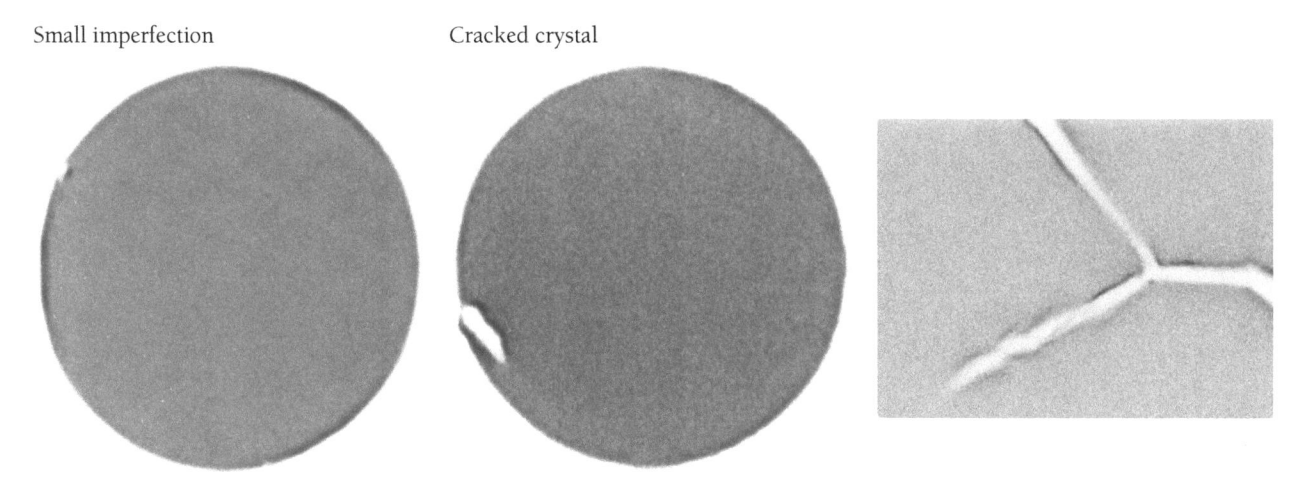

Figure 9-13 Crystal defects. The crystal on the left had a ball bearing caught between the collimator and the crystal. The crystal in the middle had a collimator dropped on it. The crystal on the right was damaged by an impact from a bar phantom. Note the edge packing around the fracture in all cases. Courtesy of Virginia Mason Medical Center.

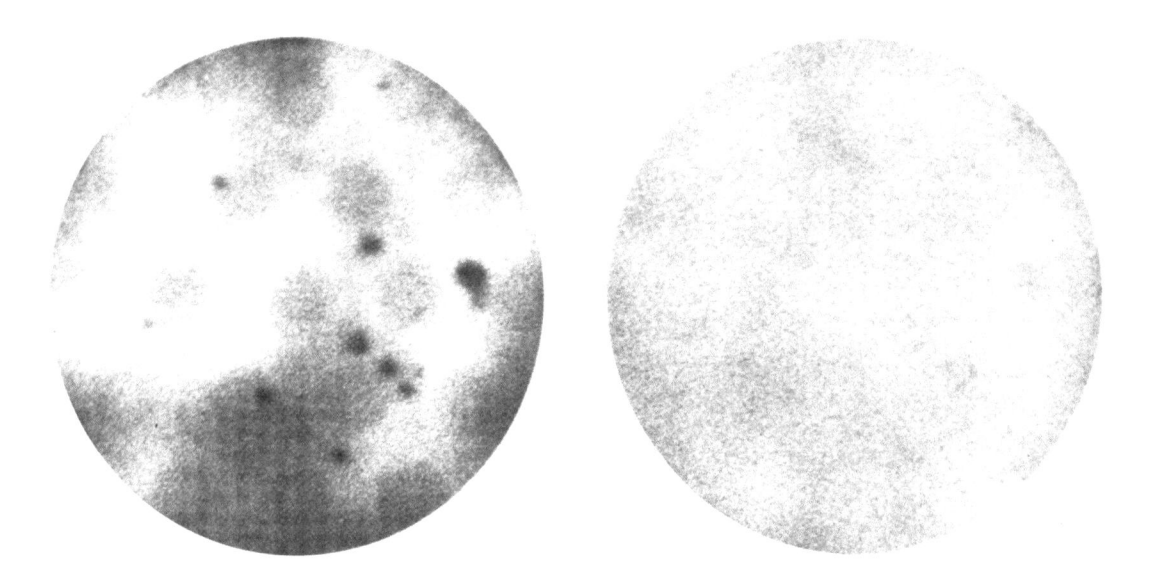

Figure 9-14 Measles. The image on the left is taken using an asymmetric window, showing the yellowing spots much more clearly than the on-peak image on the right. Reprinted from: Early PJ, Sodee DB. *Principles and Practice of Nuclear Medicine.* 2nd ed. St. Louis, MO: Mosby-Year Book; 1995: 270. Used with permission from Elsevier.

be seen on an off-peak image, but may be detectable only by comparison to benchmark images.

8. Collimator artifacts (**Figure 9-17**): Small artifacts in collimators may be difficult to appreciate, even on high-count extrinsic flood images.
9. Fillable flood phantom problems (**Figure 9-18**): Fillable flood phantoms can suffer from poor mixing, bulging, and the presence of air bubbles.
10. Photographic system problems (**Figure 9-19**): Photographic systems, whether incorporated into the gamma camera or as stand-alone devices, can suffer problems of their own. Periodically they should be vacuumed to remove dust. The lenses of photographic devices should be cleaned and realigned, and a test pattern evaluated regularly as a part of a preventive maintenance contract. One way to determine that an artifact originates in the photographic system is to repeat the image after rotating the camera orientation by 90°. If the artifact does not move, it must be in the photographic system.

Summary

The following quote from Reference 1 summarizes this chapter: "Quality control testing does not, in and of itself, assure quality. The quality control measurements provide a framework for the personnel to effectively make decisions concerning the usability and adequate performance of a given piece of equipment." In other words, quality control requires not only doing the tests, but also evaluating

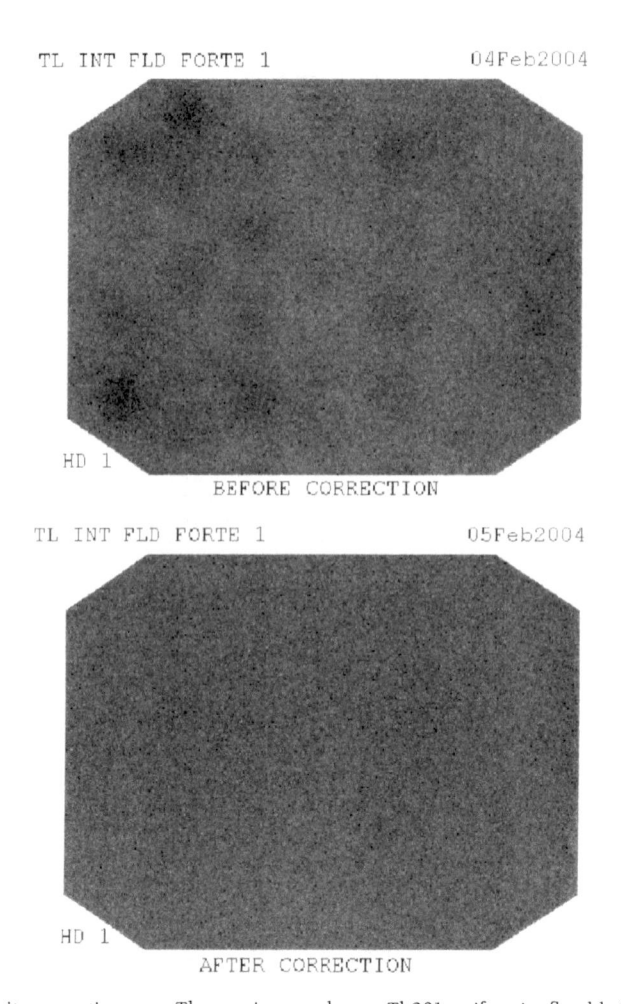

Figure 9-15 Need for updated uniformity correction map. The two images show a Tl-201 uniformity flood before (above) and after (below) acquisition of a new uniformity correction map. A gamma camera's uniformity should be checked with every isotope imaged by that camera; a camera may have excellent uniformity with one radionuclide and noticeable nonuniformities with another. Courtesy of St. Joseph Medical Center.

(a) Prior to recoupling of PMTs to crystal

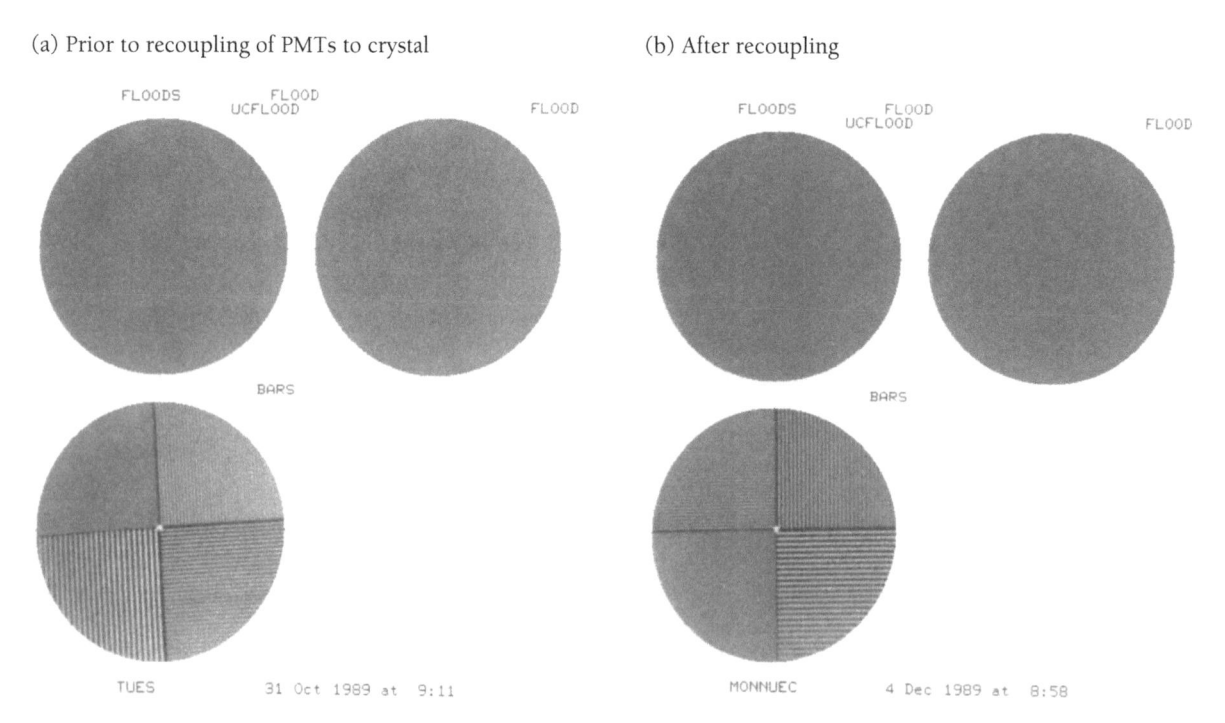

(b) After recoupling

Figure 9-16 Poor coupling of PMTs to the crystal. Figure 9-16a shows the camera before recoupling. The images show a gradation from darker to lighter. Figure 9-16b shows improvement after recoupling. Courtesy of Virginia Mason Medical Center.

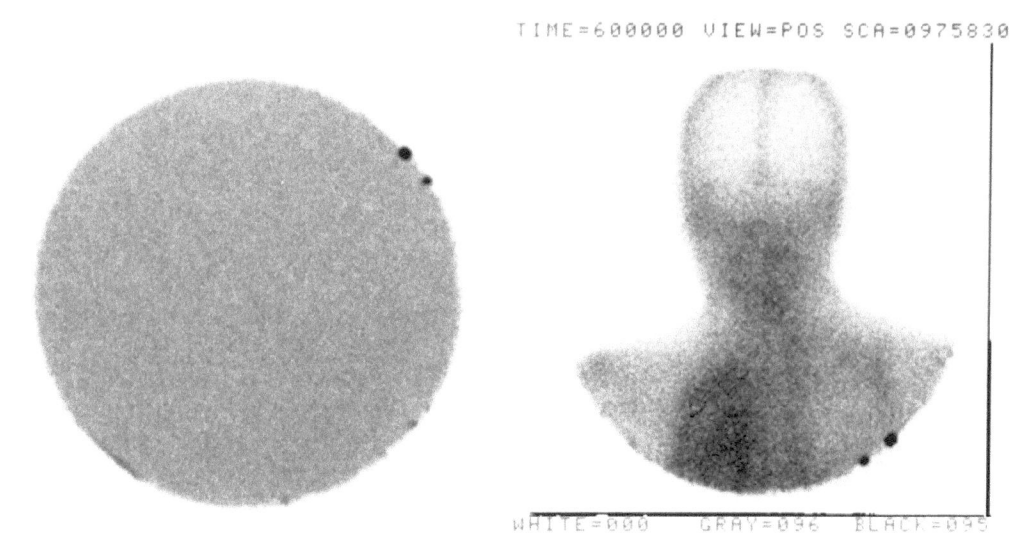

Figure 9-17 Collimator defects. In this case, damage to the collimator has pushed septa together, leaving two larger holes that allow many gamma rays to reach the crystal. Courtesy of Virginia Mason Medical Center.

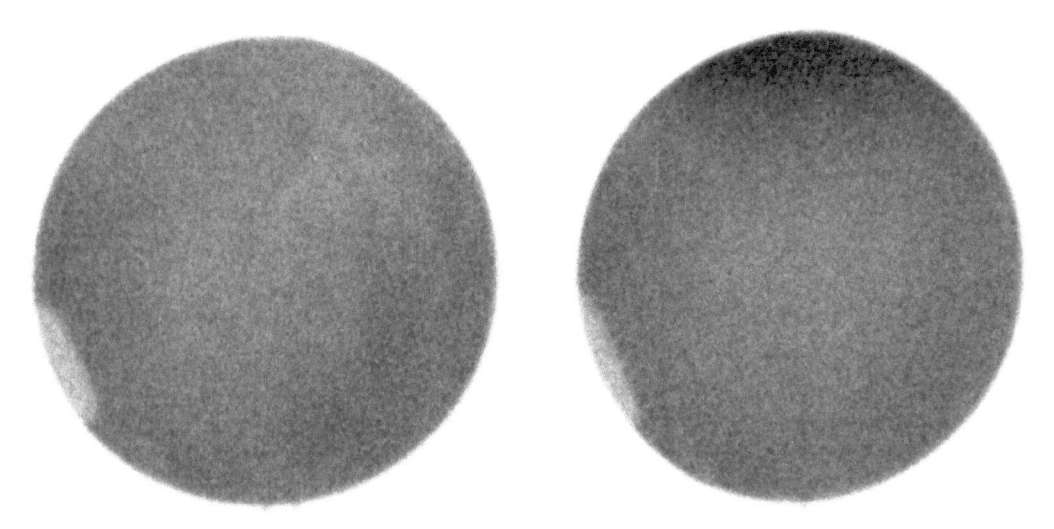

Figure 9-18 Fillable flood phantom artifacts. Note the lack of uniformity and the large air bubble in both images. Courtesy of Virginia Mason Medical Center.

Figure 9-19 Dust in photographic system. Several "photopenic" areas on this flood are actually "dust bunnies" within the photographic system. Courtesy of Virginia Mason Medical Center.

Summary 127

the results and understanding their meaning, and, most importantly, taking action based on the results.

It should be clear to the reader at this point that a planar gamma camera is an intricate device in which any number of problems can occur. Clinical nuclear medicine images depend on the absence of abnormalities in the gamma camera itself. The need for optimal performance will become even more important in SPECT imaging. But even planar images require careful attention to underlying system performance.

References

1. Rhodes BA, ed. *Quality Control in Nuclear Medicine*. St. Louis, MO: C.V. Mosby; 1977:286–287.
2. Botti J. Gamma camera performance evaluation and quality control. In: Fahey R, Harkness B, eds. *Basic Science of Nuclear Medicine* [CD-ROM]. Reston, VA: Society of Nuclear Medicine; 2001.
3. Zanzonico P. Routine quality control of clinical nuclear medicine instrumentation: a brief review. *J Nucl Med.* 2008;49:1114–1131.
4. Henkin RE, Boles MA, Dillehay GL, et al. *Nuclear Medicine*. St. Louis, MO: Mosby-Year Book; 1996:125, 140, 144.
5. Early PJ, Sodee BD. *Principles and Practice of Nuclear Medicine*. 2nd ed. St. Louis, MO: Mosby-Year Book; 1995:279–284.
6. Siegel JA, Benedetto AR, Jaszczak RJ, et al. AAPM Report No. 22. Rotating scintillation camera SPECT acceptance testing and quality control. New York, NY: American Institute of Physics; 1987.
7. Blend MJ, Patel BA, Byrom E. Collimator-induced defects in planar and SPECT gamma camera images: a multicenter study. *J Nucl Med Technol.* 1995;23:167–172.
8. AAPM Report No. 6. Scintillation camera acceptance testing and rotating scintillation camera SPECT acceptance testing and quality control. New York, NY: American Institute of Physics; 1987.
9. National Electrical Manufacturers Association. *Performance Measurements of Gamma Cameras*. Publication NU 1-2007. Rosslyn, VA; 2007.
10. Parker JA, Wallis JW. Systems for remote interpretation of emergency studies. *Semin Nucl Med.* 2003;33:324–330.
11. Papp J. *Quality Management in the Imaging Sciences*. 3rd ed. St. Louis, MO: Mosby-Elsevier; 2006:142.

Additional Resources

Early PJ, Sodee DB. *Principles and Practice of Nuclear Medicine*. 2nd ed. St. Louis, MO: Mosby; 1995:Chapter 13.

Henkin RE, Boles MA, Dillehay GL, et al. *Nuclear Medicine*. St. Louis, MO: Mosby-Year Book; 1996:Chapter 9.

IAEA. *Quality Control Atlas for Scintillation Camera Systems*. Vienna: Internal Atomic Energy Agency; 2003.

NEMA Publication NU 1-2007. Performance measurements of gamma cameras. Rosslyn, VA: National Electrical Manufacturers Association; 2007.

Zanzonico P. Routine quality control of clinical nuclear medicine instrumentation: a brief review. *J Nucl Med.* 2008;49:1114–1131.

PART III

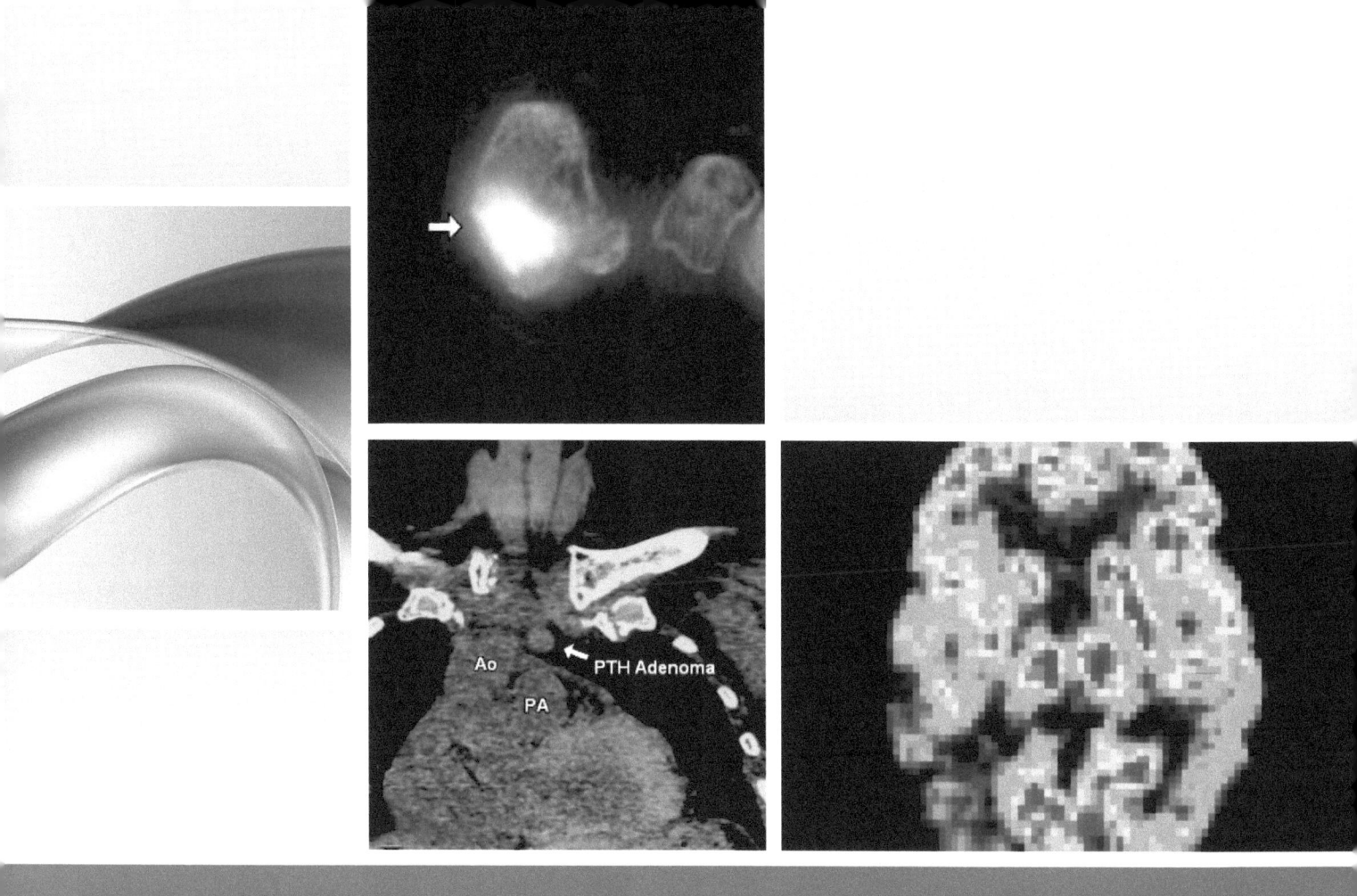

Single-Photon Emission Computed Tomography (SPECT)

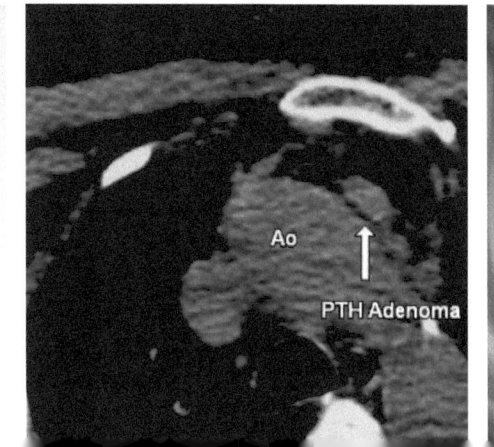

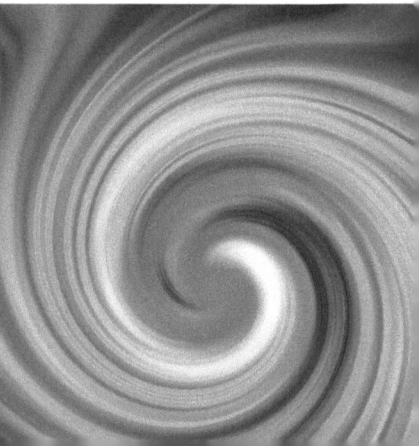

CHAPTER 10

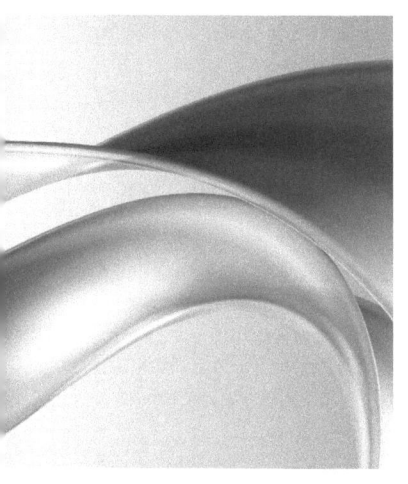

Single-Photon Emission Computed Tomography (SPECT)

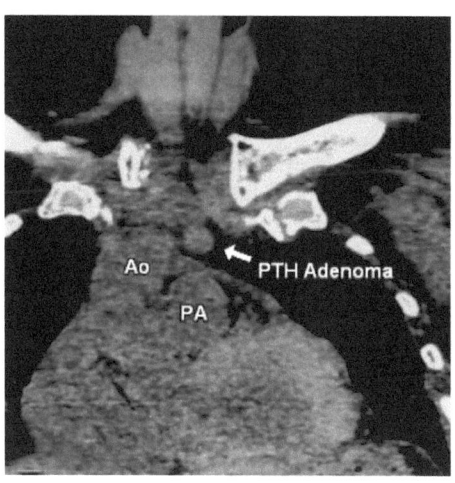

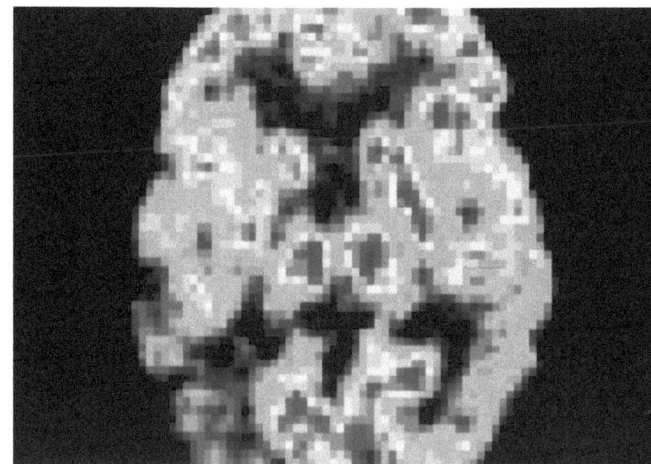

Learning Outcomes

1. Outline the basic concepts behind computed tomography, including Radon's theory and its application to nuclear medicine imaging.
2. List the acquisition parameters that must be specified for a SPECT study and assumptions inherent to SPECT reconstruction.
3. Describe a nuclear medicine image from the standpoint of the spatial frequencies found within it.
4. Define the Nyquist frequency, and calculate its value, given the pixel size.
5. Discuss the concept of backprojection and why filters are needed for reconstruction based on backprojection.
6. Illustrate ramp and low-pass filters on a frequency-domain graph, and relate these to the frequencies found in nuclear medicine images; discuss the need for both the ramp and the low-pass filter.
7. Diagram the iterative cycle, including the modeling of the laws of physics and the properties of a gamma camera.
8. Contrast the concepts of iterative reconstruction with filtered backprojection, and discuss the advantages for SPECT imaging.
9. Describe two- and three-dimensional ways of displaying SPECT images.

Introduction

The main limitation of planar images is third-dimension superposition, such that over- and underlying structures often obscure the area of interest. Contrast would be greatly improved if we could eliminate this superposition of tissues and consider only the part of the object that contains the area of interest. *Tomography* is the imaging of the body in multiple slices. The word comes from the Greek roots *tomo* (to cut) and *graphein* (to write or display). In nuclear medicine, two types of tomography are routinely employed. Single-photon emission computed tomography (SPECT), which is generally performed with a gamma camera, is the topic of this chapter. The other tomographic nuclear medicine technique, positron emission tomography (PET), is a topic unto itself.

This chapter covers the basics of SPECT imaging. The major issue is how to combine a series of two-dimensional (2D) projections of the object of interest in order to generate a three-dimensional (3D) spatial representation. There are two quite different approaches to this process, both of which are discussed at length in this chapter.

Development of Computed Tomography Techniques

The mathematical principles underlying tomographic imaging were developed in 1917 by Johann Radon (1). He proved mathematically that the internal structure of an unknown object could be reproduced from an infinite number of projections (i.e., external views from different angles) of the object. The set of projections of the object is called the *Radon transform*. The objective, then, is to recreate a 3D representation of the object itself from the projections.

The first practical application of Radon's theorem was in the 1950s in the field of astronomy (2). An early version of 3D reconstruction of nuclear medicine images was developed by Kuhl and Edwards in the early 1960s (3). But it was the invention of the x-ray computed tomography (CT) scanner in the early 1970s that showed the clinical utility of this technique for diagnostic imaging. The credit and the Nobel Prize for this work were given to Godfrey Hounsfield of England, who developed the first scanner (4), and Allan Cormack of South Africa, who conceived the analytic approach to reconstruction (5, 6). However, it was actually David Kuhl who produced not only the first nuclear medicine tomography images, but also the first transmission CT images, using an Am-241 source (7). His aim was to correlate the nuclear medicine images with radiographic anatomy, an idea that is at the forefront of nuclear medicine today, more than 40 years later.

Two earlier tomographic techniques set the stage for the advent of computed tomography. The first is focal-plane tomography, a procedure commonly used with x-ray imaging (and briefly employed in nuclear medicine). X-ray focal-plane tomography moves the film cassette in one direction as the x-ray tube pivots in the opposite direction. The fulcrum or pivot point is in a single body plane throughout the exposure, and that plane is the only one to stay in focus, while other body planes are blurred. The second antecedent is coded-aperture tomography, in which a limited number of views of an object from different angles are summed to create a set of tomographic slices. An application of this concept to nuclear medicine, called *seven-pinhole tomography*, was employed for myocardial perfusion imaging in the late 1970s. It demonstrated that the power of tomography could be used to improve the diagnostic capabilities of scintigraphic imaging.

Computed tomography techniques, as understood today, involve reconstruction of a 3D image following the acquisition of information from many different angles around the object. X-ray CT (which is typically referred to as "CT" without any additional descriptor) is an example of *transmission tomography*, because it measures the transmission of x-rays through the body. Nuclear medicine forms of computed tomography are referred to as *emission tomography*, because they image gamma rays that are emitted from the patient. Emission tomography must deal with several issues that are not found in x-ray CT:

- The use of an administered radiopharmaceutical limits the number of emissions and increases the time needed to acquire sufficient information.
- The statistical nature of radioactive decay and the low photon flux of nuclear medicine images result in a significant amount of image noise.
- Camera parameters and patient tolerance further limit the ability to obtain adequate information.
- Attenuation, rather than being the desired information as in CT scanning, is a significant interfering factor.

Emission tomography employing single-photon-emitting radionuclides such as Tc-99m is called *single-photon emission computed tomography* (abbreviated SPECT in the United States and SPET in Europe). Emission tomography that utilizes the coincidence properties of annihilation photons resulting from positron decay is called *positron emission tomography* (PET).

The great majority of SPECT studies are acquired using a rotating gamma camera with a collimator. There are several SPECT-only systems that are not based on use of a planar gamma camera. In this text, the term *tomograph* is used to designate the imaging device used to acquire the tomographic images. While this terminology is not in common use, it is consistent with the definitions given in both Mosby's and Taber's medical dictionaries, and with that found in the online encyclopedia Wikipedia. It is also the term used by the National Electrical Manufacturers Association (NEMA). *Tomograph* avoids the confusion of the words *scanner* (which can be used to indicate the operator of the tomograph) and *system* (which implies the imaging device plus a processing computer and other add-ons).

Overview of the SPECT Process

The essence of SPECT is to obtain many 2D images, called *projections*, from different angles around the object being imaged; to reconstruct from those images the object's activity distribution into a 3D image matrix; and then to display sets of 2D slices of the 3D image matrix. The 3D image matrix represents the radioactivity distribution within the object, although that representation is modified by the characteristics of the raw planar images and by the nature of the reconstruction process employed. Throughout the discussion of SPECT, the terminology of 2D projections (the raw projection images), 3D image matrix (the reconstructed study), and 2D slices (the plane-by-plane views of the 3D image matrix) will be used.

Acquisition

The first requirement for SPECT is a gamma camera that can rotate in a circle. Virtually all gamma cameras manufactured since the early 1990s have this capability (see examples in Fig. 5-6). **Figure 10-1** illustrates the typical geometry of a rotating gamma camera. Using such a camera, multiple projections are acquired. A typical acquisition might consist of 128 two-dimensional projections, evenly spaced over 360°, each projection putting counts into an image frame that has a 128 × 128 matrix. The

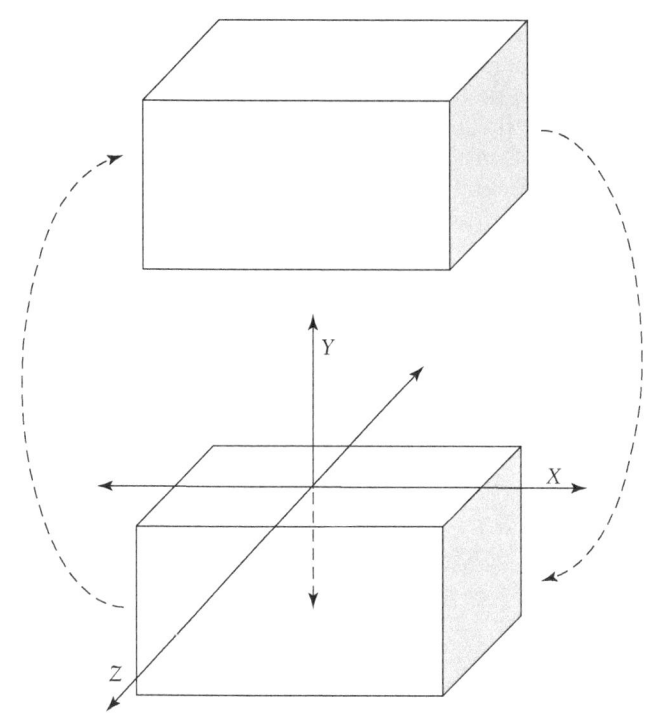

Figure 10-1 Axes as they are usually designated for SPECT imaging (Ref. 8). The *X-Y* plane is the transaxial or cross-body plane. The Z-axis is defined by the axis of rotation of the gamma camera and the head-to-toe direction of the patient. It is sometimes referred to as the longitudinal direction.

projections are most commonly acquired in a step-and-shoot format, in which the camera is stationary while acquiring a projection and then not imaging as it rotates to the next acquisition angle.

All of the images must be acquired for the same length of time in order for reconstruction to work properly. Further, the reconstruction process assumes that the radiopharmaceutical does not move and the patient stays still during the study, so that radioactivity will be seen at the same location in different projections. Many SPECT studies require the patient's arms to be above the head, out of the imaging field. The time per image is therefore a compromise between the need for a reasonable number of counts in each image, on the one hand, and patient tolerance for a long scanning time, on the other, such that most studies are acquired over 15 to 45 minutes (min).

SPECT imaging can be combined with the gating technique. This is commonly done for myocardial perfusion imaging. Each 2D projection is treated as an eight-frame gated study, and counts are acquired into the eight frames over a number of heartbeats, based on the patient's electrocardiographic R wave. The gated information is then included in the resulting reconstruction, producing what amounts to a four-dimensional (4D) display (i.e., the three dimensions of space, plus time).

Reconstruction

Acquisition of 2D projections is the easy part of SPECT; the hard part, from the standpoint of comprehension, is the process of reconstructing a 3D representation of the radiopharmaceutical distribution in the object, using the 2D projections. Reconstruction is the crucial step in all forms of computed tomography, but is of particular importance to SPECT because of the limitations discussed. Two different approaches have been used; both are described briefly here and are discussed at length in the next two sections.

The first approach, called *filtered backprojection* (FBP), has been in use since the early days of SPECT. It is an example of an *analytic* method of reconstruction, meaning that it applies mathematical formulas to the count/pixel values from the 2D projections, in order to generate the 3D image matrix. This technique does not require a high-powered computer, and for this reason it has been the more commonly used reconstruction method throughout the 1980s and 1990s.

As we shall see below, FBP requires manipulation, or *filtering*, of the data to account for the inability of the mathematical functions to reconstruct the object correctly. To appreciate how to manipulate the filters used in FBP, it is necessary to understand the conversion from the spatial domain into the spatial frequency domain as well as the process of backprojection. In actual practice, the computer does all of the mathematical heavy lifting. But we will spend some time explaining how FBP works, while keeping the math at the descriptive level as much as possible.

An assumption inherent in analytic reconstruction is that the count/pixel values in the 2D projections are exactly correct, that is, without variation due to statistical considerations, such that the mathematical formulas will invariably produce the correct 3D image matrix. In other words, FBP assumes that all we need to do is to apply the pixel values in the 2D projections into the mathematical formulas used for reconstruction, and the "right" 3D image matrix will be generated. This assumption is not met in gamma camera images because individual pixel values may be affected by noise. *Iterative* methods do not make this assumption; instead they assume that gamma camera images are subject to the laws of physics and statistics. This different approach, along with improvements in computing power, has moved iterative reconstruction techniques to the forefront of SPECT.

Iterative reconstruction begins with a guess as to the radiopharmaceutical distribution in the object, called an *estimated 3D image matrix*. The computer generates *2D estimated projections* (what it thinks the gamma camera looking at the estimated 3D image matrix would see). The laws of physics, as well as consideration of attenuation and scatter, can be taken into account in this step. The estimated 2D projections are then compared to the *measured 2D projections* (i.e., the images actually obtained by the gamma camera), and the comparison is used to correct the estimated 3D image matrix. Many cycles, or *iterations*, of this process are required to reach a good approximation of the radiopharmaceutical distribution in the object.

The 3D Image Matrix

The end result of the reconstruction process is the 3D image matrix, which represents the distribution of the radiopharmaceutical in the object. The smallest unit of the 3D image matrix is a *voxel* (volume element), the 3D analog of the pixel. Most acquisition protocols are designed to produce cubical voxels. The 3D image matrix can then be displayed in a variety of ways, which are discussed at the end of this chapter.

Analytic Reconstruction

We begin by considering the geometry of a single projection (**Figure 10-2**). With the gamma camera at an angle θ, each location on the camera face "sees" a column of tissue. The black line shows one such column (it is perpendicular to the camera face because a parallel-hole, nonslanted collimator is being used). This column of tissue has some amount of radioactivity in each small subsection; the total amount of radioactivity in the column is called its *ray-sum*.

The value s registered by the gamma camera is therefore related to the ray-sum. This is not an exact relationship, because the gamma rays coming from the object are subject to attenuation and scatter, both of which are more likely for subsections of the column more distant from the camera face. In addition, gamma rays from other parts of the object (not in the column shown) may contribute to the value of s, as a result of scatter and the depth-dependent loss of resolution. These complications will become issues to be dealt with as we try to improve SPECT image quality, but for the moment we can ignore them.

A single 2D projection, then, consists of a number of pixels, each of which estimates a ray-sum value. Note that the count profile in Figure 10-2 shows a 1D representation (a single row of pixels) from one transaxial slice of the object, whereas in fact the projection is 2D and the object is 3D. This simplification will suffice for the discussion of backprojection, because it works on a slice-by-slice basis, after which the individual slices are appended together to create the 3D image matrix. But that part comes after; right now the question is, How do we get from a set of projections around the object to the reconstruction of a 2D slice of the object?

Unfiltered Backprojection

A simplistic way to go about reconstruction is to take the value s in each pixel and apply it to all of the points along the equivalent column in the reconstructed 3D image matrix. Consider **Figure 10-3**. A single hot spot within a circular object is imaged in four projections (Fig. 10-3a). In each projection, the hot spot is seen as an area of increased activity, which is presented as a peak in each of four count profiles, one from each projection. In Figure 10-3b, the count profiles are backprojected into the image matrix. But absent knowledge of the location of the hot spot, the pixel value from the count profile is instead put into every voxel in the column perpendicular to the projection plane. We will call this *unfiltered backprojection* (UBP), to distinguish it from FBP. It can be compared to using a paint roller, in that the intensity of a given point in the count profile is paint-rolled or backprojected across the entire image.

Unfiltered backprojection therefore produces an image in which the count value at a particular location is the total of all the ray-sum estimates passing through that point. Where the hot spot is, the ray-sums are all high, so the corresponding location in the reconstructed image is also high. Backprojection is essentially a summation algorithm. It is easily accomplished and does not require a computer; Kuhl and Edwards used it in their early attempt at SPECT imaging.

But UBP by itself has two significant drawbacks. First, UBP puts counts in the 3D image matrix where there was no activity in the corresponding area of the object, and even outside of the object. Second, the area of elevated count density is larger than the area of increased activity in the object, and its size increases as we add more projections. Each backprojection in UBP contributes a ray of activity that extends across the entire image space. With a few projections, the rays appear as a star. With many projections, the star blurs into a general fogging of the image (Fig. 10-3c).

The more projections we add, the larger the star gets and the more blurring there is (**Figure 10-4**). Figure 10-4a shows a point source of activity (essentially the same as in Fig. 10-3a), imaged over 128 projections and reconstructed with UBP. The solid line of Figure 10-4c is a count profile through this image. The shape of the count profile can be described by the equation $y = 1/r$, where r is the radius of a circle centered on the point of highest count density. The number of counts at any point in the count profile is inversely proportional to its distance from the peak activity. This additional elevated count density, extending far beyond the point source itself, is the result

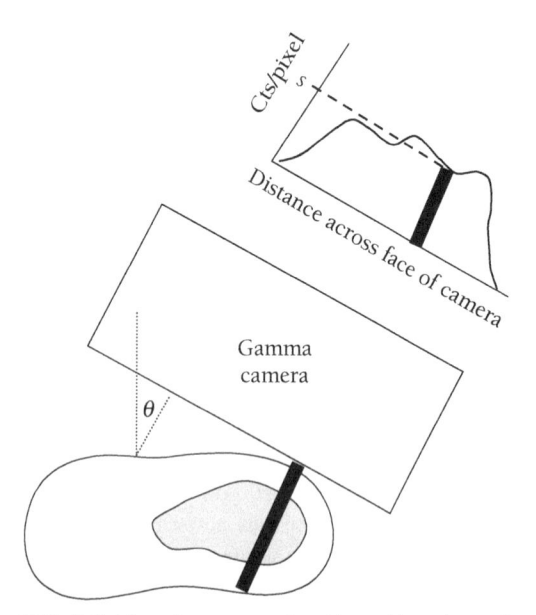

Figure 10-2 Definition of a ray-sum. An object with an internal organ is shown in transaxial cross section (the *X-Y* plane of Fig. 10-1), with a gamma camera positioned at an angle θ above it. One column of tissue perpendicular to the camera face is indicated by the black stripe. The total activity within this column is its ray-sum. The value s in the corresponding pixel of the 2D projection at θ (shown in the count profile above the camera) is an estimate of the ray-sum's value.

(a) Count profiles in four projections around a point source contained in a cylindrical object

(b) Unfiltered backprojection of the four projections

Boundary of 3D image matrix

Boundary of object being imaged

(c)

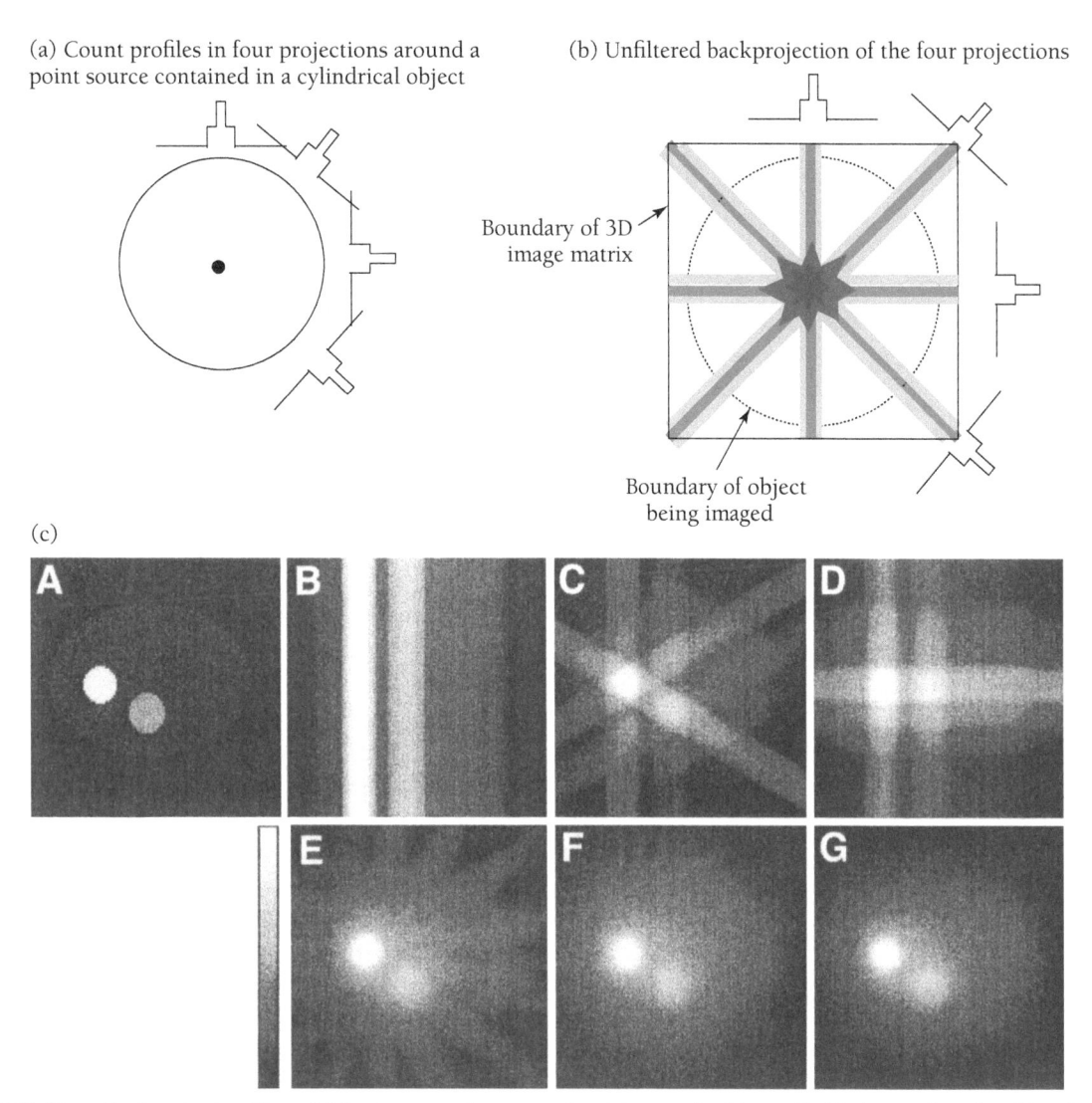

Figure 10-3 Unfiltered backprojection. Figure 10-3a shows a point source of activity contained in a cylindrical nonradioactive object (again shown in transaxial cross section) and the count profiles from four different angles around the object. Figure 10-3b shows that the four ray-sums, when backprojected, cross at the location of the point source in the 3D image matrix. But the backprojection process puts counts in many other parts of the 3D image matrix that do not correspond to any activity in the object. (As in Fig. 10-2, a 2D image matrix is shown, but in reality we have more 2D image matrices in front and behind this one, so we can refer to this 2D diagram as a 3D image matrix.) Figure 10-3c shows a computer simulation of an object with two areas of increased activity and backprojection of 1, 2, 3, 4, 8, 32, and 128 projections. Note that the two areas of increased activity are clearly seen, but that their edges are indistinct, and that the object itself is larger than it is in the original. Figure 10-3c reprinted from: Bruyant, PP. Analytic and iterative reconstruction algorithms in SPECT. *J Nucl Med.* 2002;43(10):1343–1358, Figure 6.

of the UBP process superimposing many backprojections, and it is called *1/r blurring*. It is essentially the spillover of counts from the area of increased count density into neighboring voxels. This blurring makes the reconstructed image difficult to interpret, and for this reason UBP is unacceptable as a method of reconstruction for SPECT.

Mathematicians would describe the UBP image as the convolution of the true image with the function 1/r. The "true image" is the reconstructed image matrix that would be obtained without the blurring added by the UBP process. This is what we're aiming to produce. *Convolution* is a mathematical operation that multiplies two functions that are both in the spatial domain (i.e., 1D, 2D, or 3D space). **Figure 10-5** shows a simple 2D example of the convolution of two functions, an input function and a system function. The system function acts on each data point of the input function to generate the output function. In UBP, the input function is the count densities from the 2D projections, and the system function is the 1/r blurring (the latter extending across the entire image, not just within a confined area, as is shown for the system function in Fig. 10-5).

We would like to separate out and remove the 1/r blurring to retain only the true image. Deconvolution accomplishes this. Deconvolution of two functions in the spatial domain is computationally complex, but it becomes quite easy if the data are converted to the spatial frequency domain. The next section delves into the subject of frequency, after which we discuss the FBP method of SPECT image reconstruction.

(a) 128 projections, unfiltered backprojection

(b) 128 projections with ramp filter

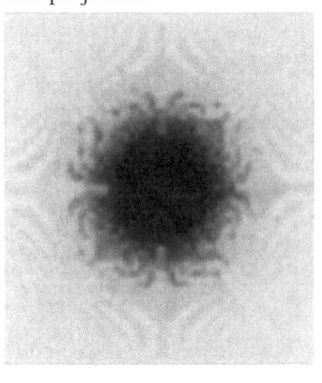

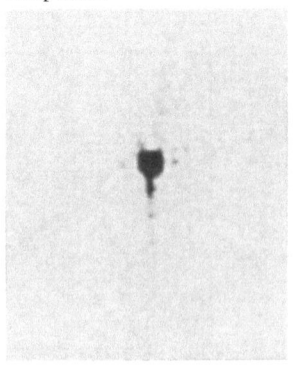

(c) Count profile through Figure 10-4a (solid line) and Figure 10-4b (dashed line)

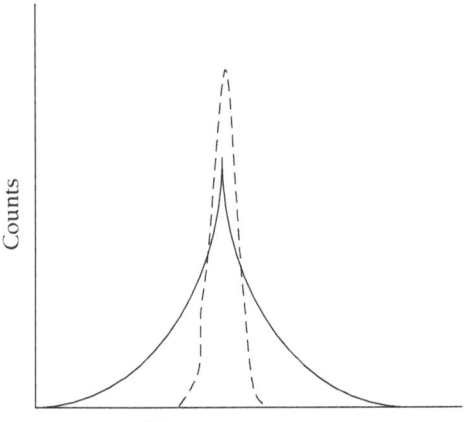

Figure 10-4 Result of the backprojection process. The image in Figure 10-4a shows a slice from the unfiltered backprojection of a point source imaged with 128 projections. Note that the size of the reconstructed point source increases as the number of projections increases, just as in Figure 10-3c. Figure 10-4b shows backprojection with a ramp filter. The effect of the ramp filter is to subtract out the extra activity contributed by the backprojection process, generating a point of activity rather than the blur of Figure 10-4a. Figure 10-4c shows count profiles through Figures 10-4a and 10-4b. The shape of the solid-line count profile is quite similar to the shape of the function $y = 1/r$, leading to the name *1/r blurring*. Reprinted from: Henkin RE, Boles MA, Dillehay GL, et al. *Nuclear Medicine*. St. Louis, MO: Mosby-Year Book; 1996: Fig. 18-6. Used with permission from Elsevier.

The Frequency Domain

We typically think of frequency as a quantity of time. For example, a musical pitch has a specific frequency, measured as the number of sound waves passing a location (such as an eardrum) per unit time. In the imaging context, we can think of our images in the *spatial frequency domain*, in which frequency is measured as how fast count densities are changing as we move across the image. The units of spatial frequency are cm^{-1} or mm^{-1}. If we envision a 2D image as a series of count profiles (one for each row of pixels), the changing slopes of the count profiles represent frequency. A steep slope (either positive or negative) represents a high frequency, while a flat portion of the count profile represents a low frequency. The term *frequency domain* will be used here equivalently with spatial frequency domain (some authors also refer to the spatial frequency domain as *frequency space*).

All nuclear medicine images can be displayed in the spatial frequency domain as well as in the *spatial domain* (also known as *object space*). However, our eyes are, for the most part, unable to interpret a spatial frequency domain image in a meaningful way. An analogy to music is again instructive, in an inverse sort of way (8). A musical piece is a collection of sound waves of different temporal frequencies. Our ears are attuned to these frequencies, so we hear the sound waves as music. The music can be represented on paper, but only those with some training in music can make sense of that representation. Our eyes, on the other hand, are well trained to appreciate objects in the spatial domain, and images of those objects, but not to "see" frequencies. Our sensory context for understanding images extends only to the spatial domain, and not to the spatial frequency domain.

Because we cannot visualize frequencies, we need a way to categorize the frequencies found in a nuclear medicine image. For the purpose of this discussion, we can think of three broad categories of spatial frequency (9):

- *Low frequencies* include components of an object that are large and homogeneous and thus depict the general shape of an object. Background activity usually

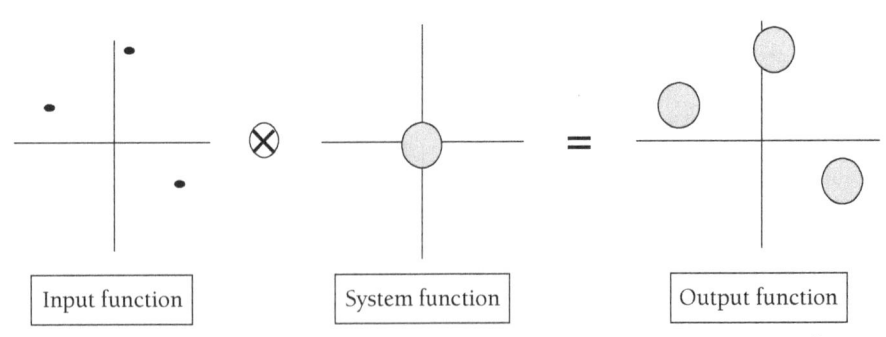

Figure 10-5 Convolution. This figure shows how a system function acts on an input function to generate an output function, a process called *convolution*. In the example, the system function (a large circle) acts on each of the small points of the input function. Essentially the system function interferes with our ability to determine the input function, because we can't determine precisely where the three points are. Both the input function and the system function are in the spatial domain. If we have the output function and wish to retrieve the input function, we must reverse the operation, which is called *deconvolution*. Deconvolution is most easily done in the spatial frequency domain.

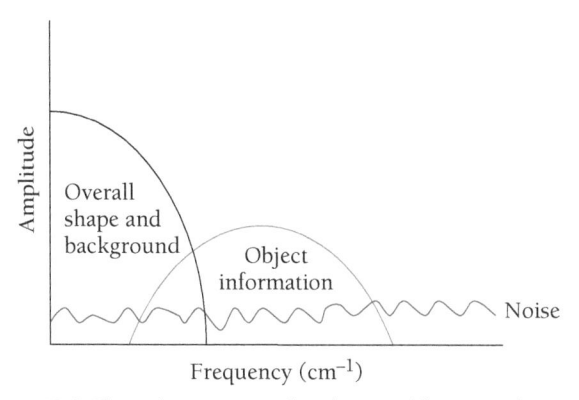

Figure 10-6 Object data represented in the spatial frequency domain. We can think of the information contained in the object as belonging to one of three categories: background, object data, and noise. These are represented on a graph with axes of frequency and amplitude (i.e., how much each frequency contributes to the object). Note that the three regions overlap significantly and that noise becomes dominant at high frequencies. This graph can be compared to the modulation transfer function (MTF) graph (Fig. 8-12), which uses similar axes.

has very low frequency, because it is relatively constant across the image.
- *Middle frequency* refers to areas in which counts are changing moderately quickly; this is often where the desired object information is.
- *High frequency* refers to areas where counts are changing quickly. Small objects and sharp edges are found here, as is image noise.

Figure 10-6 shows these three ranges in a frequency graph. The exact points of division or overlap between the three ranges depend on the radiopharmaceutical biodistribution, the study acquisition parameters, and the individual patient.

The *Fourier transform* is a mathematical operation that converts a function from a spatial domain representation to its frequency domain representation. It changes Cartesian (x, y) coordinates to the coordinates of the frequency domain, which are frequency (cycles/cm) and amplitude (usually expressed on a fractional scale). The Fourier transform works by expressing the image data as a series of sine waves of many frequencies and amplitudes. This is illustrated graphically in **Figure 10-7**. Figure 10-7a shows a square wave and Figure 10-7c an approximation of the square wave created by summing the four sine wave functions shown in Figure 10-7b. It is easy to see that the low-frequency wave generates the basic form of the square wave, and that the higher-frequency additions give it detail.

A *power spectrum* is a graph that shows the frequencies that compose an image on the X-axis and the amplitude or contribution of each on the Y-axis. Figure 10-7d shows the power spectrum for the waveform in Figure 10-7c. The height of each column in Figure 10-7d corresponds to the multiplier in front of the sine terms in each equation of Figure 10-7b. This simple waveform shows only a few discrete frequencies in its power spectrum. To reproduce the exact shape of the square wave, we would need many additional sine waves, and a continuous power spectrum would be seen. To reiterate the main point, low frequencies determine the overall appearance of the image, and high frequencies add detail. Fourier transformation is used to determine the frequency components of the image.

The power spectrum of a given imaging situation is modified by the camera characteristics and by the presence of noise (**Figure 10-8**). The object power spectrum (i.e., the spatial frequencies found in the object itself) is multiplied by the blurring effects of the gamma camera, as expressed by the MTF graph. Noise, which occurs across the power spectrum with approximately equal amplitudes, is added to the camera-blurred power spectrum to produce the final image power spectrum. Note that the contribution of noise becomes significant only at high frequencies, where the object has little information. An actual power spectrum of a bar phantom image is shown in Figure 10-8e.

The Nyquist Frequency

Most objects have frequencies across a wide range. However, we are not able to utilize all of the high frequencies of the image power spectrum in the SPECT reconstruction process, because of the finite size of the pixels. The *Nyquist frequency* is the highest frequency that can be represented by the imaging system. It is determined by the pixel size used in acquiring the projections:

$$\text{Nyquist frequency} = \frac{1}{2 \times \text{pixel dimension (mm)}}. \quad (10\text{-}1)$$

This definition is based on the sampling theorem, which states that visualization of a repeating cycle requires a minimum of 2 pixels per cycle (**Figure 10-9**). The usual

---

Sample Calculation 10-1   Nyquist Frequency

The camera described in Sample Calculation 6-1 has pixel dimensions of 7.8, 3.9, and 2.0 mm for 64×64, 128×128, and 256×256 image matrices, respectively. What is the Nyquist frequency for each matrix?

For the 64×64 matrix, the Nyquist frequency is

$$\frac{1}{(2)(\text{pixel dimension})} = \frac{1}{(2)(7.8 \text{ mm})} = 0.064/\text{mm}.$$

For the 128×128 matrix, it is

$$\frac{1}{(2)(3.9 \text{ mm})} = 0.13/\text{mm}.$$

And for the 256×256 matrix,

$$\frac{1}{(2)(2.0 \text{ mm})} = 0.25/\text{mm}.$$

As the pixel dimension decreases, the highest measurable frequency increases.

statement of the sampling theorem is that the sample size (i.e., the pixel size) should be no larger than one-half of the highest frequency we wish to visualize. Another way of thinking of it is that there must be at least 1 pixel between two peaks of a high-frequency object if we are to observe them as separate peaks.

In nuclear medicine, we have only a few choices for the sampling frequency, so we can turn the sampling theorem around to say that the pixel size creates a limit in terms of the maximum frequency that can be included in the reconstruction. If we fail to take the Nyquist frequency limitation into account, we may generate an aliasing artifact.

To summarize the process so far: backprojection is a method by which we can take the information from the 2D projections and reconstruct a 3D image matrix. But the 3D image matrix that results from UBP is very fuzzy, the result of the convolution of the object information

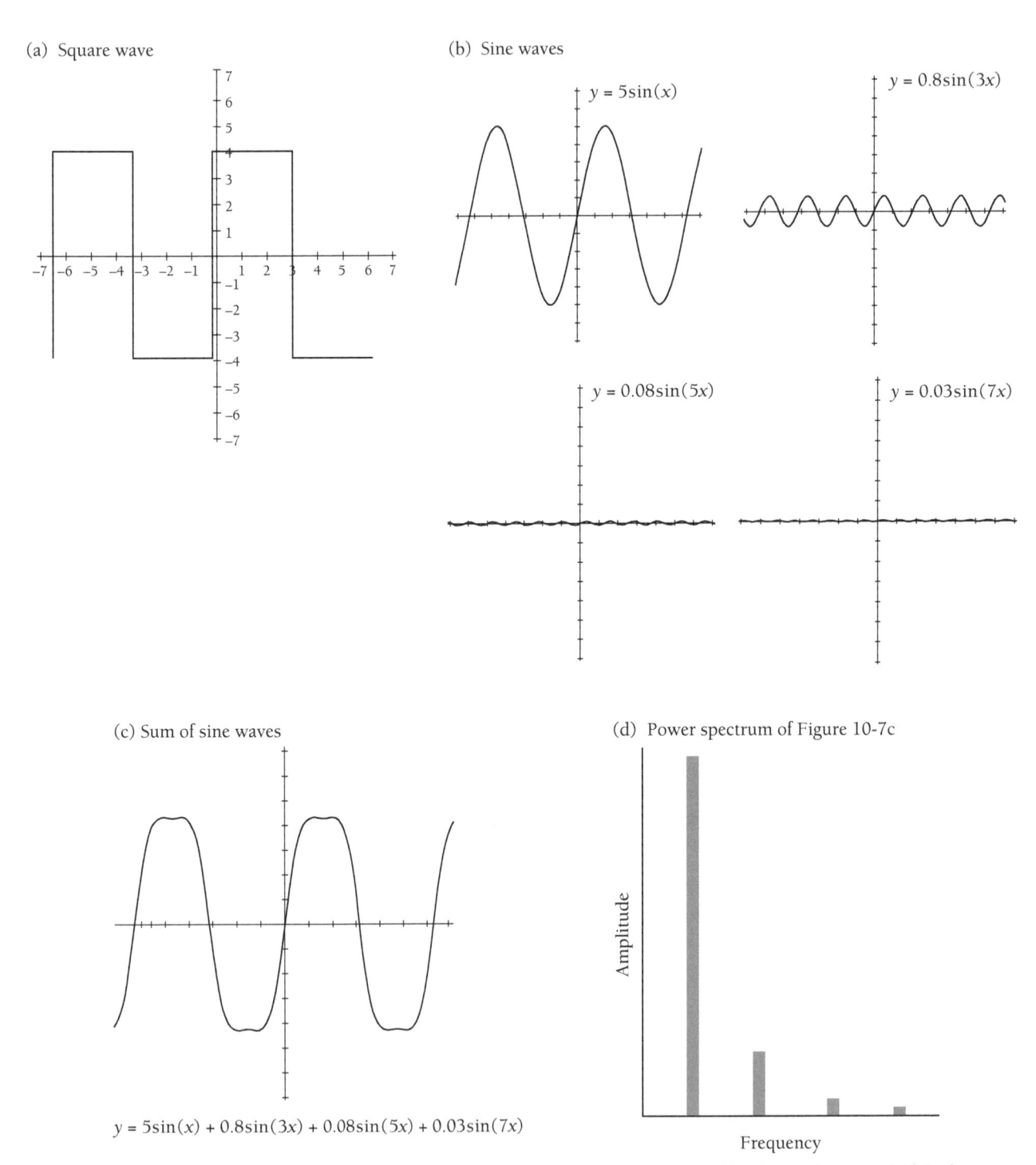

(a) Square wave

(b) Sine waves

$y = 5\sin(x)$

$y = 0.8\sin(3x)$

$y = 0.08\sin(5x)$

$y = 0.03\sin(7x)$

(c) Sum of sine waves

$y = 5\sin(x) + 0.8\sin(3x) + 0.08\sin(5x) + 0.03\sin(7x)$

(d) Power spectrum of Figure 10-7c

Figure 10-7 Square wave as a sum of sine waves. The square wave of Figure 10-7a can be approximated by the sum (Fig. 10-7c) of the four sine waves shown (Fig. 10-7b). The power spectrum (Fig. 10-7d) shows the relative contributions of each of the four sine waves to the not-quite-square wave in Figure 10-7c.

(a) Object frequency spectrum × (b) Gamma camera MTF + (c) Noise spectrum = (d) Image power spectrum

(e) Power spectrum of planar bar phantom

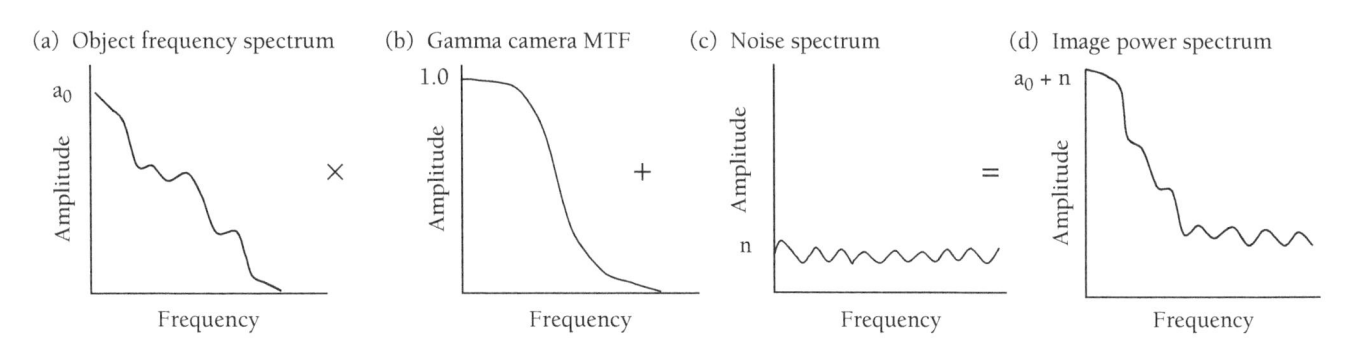

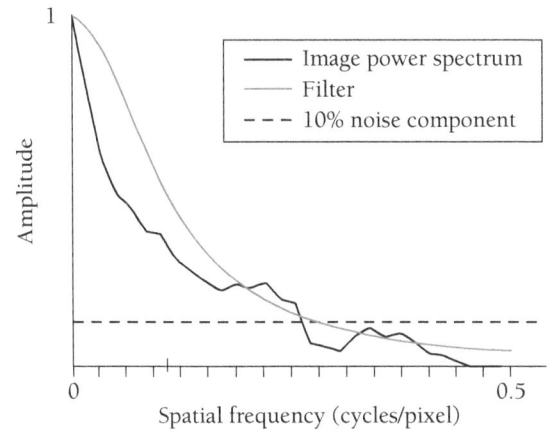

Figure 10-8 Contributions to a nuclear medicine image. The final power spectrum (Fig. 10-8d) is the result of the spectrum of frequencies present in the object (the object power spectrum, Fig. 10-8a) multiplied by the gamma camera's modulation transfer function (Fig. 10-8b), with noise added (Fig. 10-8c). Figure 10-8e shows an actual power spectrum that is generated by one commercial gamma camera computer system. The heavy line represents the image power spectrum, the less heavy line a suggested filter. The dashed line represents a 10% noise value, which is arbitrarily shown on all power spectra by this computer system. Adapted from: Groch MW, Erwin WD. SPECT in the year 2000: basic principles. *J Nucl Med Technol*. 2000; 28:233–244. With permission from the Society of Nuclear Medicine. Figure 10-8e courtesy of Harborview Medical Center.

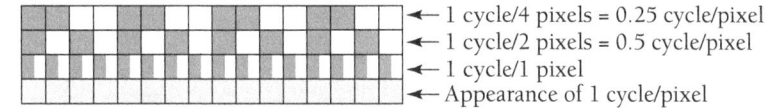

← 1 cycle/4 pixels = 0.25 cycle/pixel
← 1 cycle/2 pixels = 0.5 cycle/pixel
← 1 cycle/1 pixel
← Appearance of 1 cycle/pixel

Figure 10-9 Illustration of the Nyquist frequency. A series of repeating patterns is shown, with one cycle including both dark and white. In the last repeating pattern (1 cycle/pixel), both the dark and white parts of the pattern are within 1 pixel, and therefore all of the pixels appear gray (bottom row). Thus, at least 2 pixels are required to determine a cycle, and then only in the best-case scenario, in which the color change from dark to white lines up exactly with the pixels. The Nyquist frequency—the maximum frequency that can be distinguished for a given pixel matrix—is thus 1 cycle in 2 pixels, or 0.5 cycle/pixel.

with 1/r blurring. We need to use a deconvolution process to remove the 1/r blurring. Deconvolution is mathematically easy to accomplish in the spatial frequency domain, and the Fourier transform is the algorithm that converts each 2D projection into that domain. When we convert to the spatial frequency domain, we can calculate the Nyquist frequency, which is the highest frequency that the system can reproduce. The Nyquist frequency will become important as we consider the application of filters to the UBP process.

Filters

With this additional background information on frequency, we can proceed to the part of FBP that distinguishes it from UBP, namely, the filter. The filters used in FBP are simply mathematical equations that vary with frequency. The essence of filtering in FBP is that the filter allows us to control how much weight is given to data of low, medium, and high frequencies, in order to extract the relevant information and use it in the backprojection process. The filter accomplishes this by modifying the amplitudes of the spatial frequency components included in the reconstruction. With a filter, we can choose to include or exclude image data, based on their frequency, to improve image appearance.

As we have seen, the UBP process produces a blurred image, with counts in incorrect locations; this occurs because UBP uses the low-frequency data repeatedly as it backprojects the 2D projections. To correct for this, we need to apply a filter called the *ramp filter*. The ramp filter multiplies the image data at each frequency by a weighting factor that increases linearly with frequency (**Figure 10-10**). Low-frequency image data are suppressed and high-frequency image data are amplified, thus

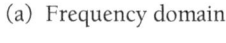

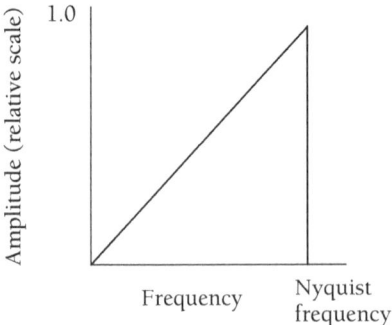

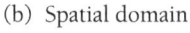

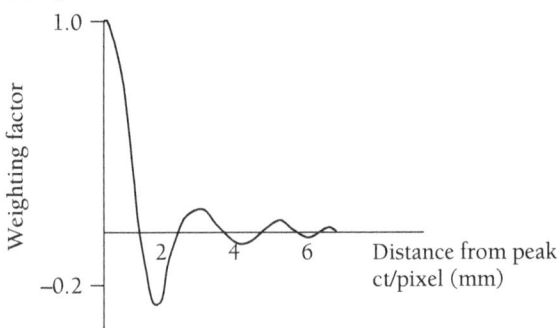

Figure 10-10 The ramp filter. Figure 10-10a shows the ramp filter in frequency domain (frequency as the X-axis and amplitude as the Y-axis of the graph). The ramp filter takes on the value of the frequency, that is, a $y = x$ line. The data at each frequency are multiplied by a weighting factor proportional to that frequency. Figure 10-10b shows the ramp filter in the spatial domain. This representation is often called a *kernel*. It shows the multiplication factor to be applied to the pixels near to the area of peak counts. The negative lobes serve to counteract the rays created by backprojection from other angles.

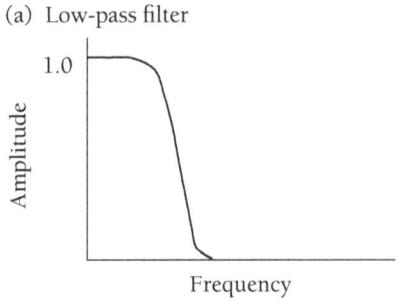

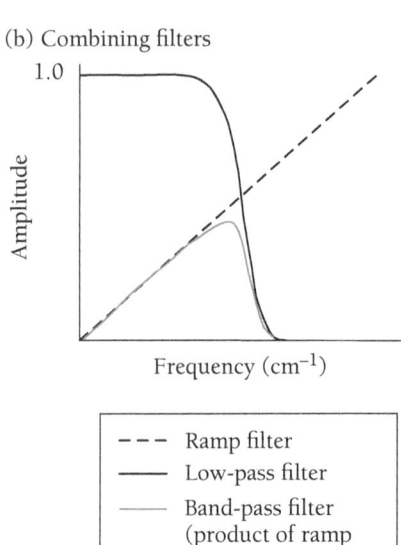

Figure 10-11 Roll-off filters, shown on amplitude–frequency graphs. A low-pass filter is pictured in Figure 10-11a (although filters can take on a variety of shapes, not just that shown). A low-pass filter allows only low frequencies to pass; a high-pass filter allows only high frequencies to pass. The ramp filter can be considered a high-pass filter, because it passes more high-frequency data than low-frequency data. The combination of filters simply involves their multiplication in the spatial frequency domain. Figure 10-11b shows how the combination of a ramp filter with a low-pass filter creates a band-pass filter that preferentially accepts frequencies in a narrow range.

compensating for the overuse of low-frequency data in the UBP process. The spatial domain representation of the ramp filter (Fig. 10-10b) shows that the filter adds negative lobes around areas of rapid counts/pixel change. These negative lobes decrease the count densities on either side of an area of increased activity, counteracting the overlapping backprojection rays seen in Figure 10-3b. The ramp filter is sufficient to remove the $1/r$ blurring that UBP produces, and restores sharp edges to the 3D image matrix (see Fig. 10-4b and the dashed line in Fig. 10-4c). The ramp filter is applied only in the transaxial or X–Y plane, because that is the only plane that experiences $1/r$ blurring in UBP (10).

If our images had no noise, we could stop with the ramp filter. But recall that nuclear medicine images always have noise, and this noise is most prominent in the high-frequency part of the image (Figs. 10-6 and 10-8). Application of the ramp filter therefore not only amplifies sharp edges and makes small objects visible, but also amplifies image noise to an unacceptable level. We must find a trade-off point between keeping detail that is important to the image and including noise in the reconstruction. "It is necessary to cut off the linear ramp around the point where the frequencies corresponding to patient data disappear into the noise" (11). For this reason, the ramp filter is combined with a second filter that "rolls off" the ramp filter.

There are several kinds of roll-off filters. *Low-pass filters* have their highest amplitude at low frequencies (**Figure 10-11a**). *Band-pass filters* have their highest amplitude in a mid frequency range, and *high-pass filters* in the high-frequency range. Figure 10-11b shows the ramp filter (which is a high-pass filter), a low-pass filter, and the band-pass filter that results when the two are multiplied together. (The filters used in SPECT imaging are sometimes called *windows*, because they allow only portions of the image data to "show through.") The ramp filter removes some of the low-frequency weighting that is exaggerated by the backprojection process. By removing noise, the low-pass filter performs a smoothing function. Changing the shape of the low-pass filter can thus increase or decrease the amount of smoothing in the reconstructed images.

A number of low-pass filters have been applied to SPECT images. Each is described by a mathematical formula that can be manipulated by modifying the value of one or more variables. They are usually known by the name of the developer; two common filters used for nuclear medicine studies are the Hann and the Hamming filters.

For many low-pass filters, the only variable in the mathematical formula that can be modified is the *cutoff frequency*, which is the frequency at which the filter function reaches zero. The cutoff frequency determines the maximum frequency that is retained in the filtered image, and thus the point of compromise between preserving image sharpness and removing the effects of image noise. A lower cutoff frequency increases the influence of the surrounding data points and therefore the amount of smoothing in the final reconstruction. A higher cutoff frequency increases the contribution of sharp count density changes, be they actual image information or noise.

The Butterworth filter function, which has two variables rather than one, has the greatest flexibility and is most commonly employed in SPECT, so we use it to illustrate the workings of these low-pass filters (**Figure 10-12**). The Butterworth filter has several mathematical formulations; the computer operating manual should specify its exact form for that system. The classic formula (12) is

$$\omega(f) = \sqrt{\frac{1}{1 + (f/f_c)^{2n}}} \quad (10\text{-}2)$$

where f is the frequency variable, $\omega(f)$ is the value of the filter function at f, f_c is the *critical frequency*, and n is the *order* (some references refer to the exponential term $2n$ as the *power*). The Butterworth filter has a transition zone in which the amplitude $\omega(f)$ drops from 1 down to 0 (Fig. 10-12a). The critical frequency is defined as the frequency at which $\omega(f) = 0.707$. It therefore determines the location of the transition zone along the X-axis. The order determines its steepness, such that a higher order produces a narrower transition zone. Figures 10-12b and 10-12c show how the Butterworth filter function changes as these two parameters change. By varying the two parameters, the Butterworth filter can be made to mimic most of the other types of low-pass filters that have been applied in SPECT. We later discuss how modification of these two parameters can be used to affect image quality. For now, it is enough to know that a roll-off filter is necessary in FBP in order to keep the noise out of the reconstructed 3D image matrix.

Filtering is thus required when using backprojection as the reconstruction method, because it corrects for the inherent inadequacies of UBP. We need both the ramp filter, which removes the 1/r blurring, and a roll-off filter, to keep the high-frequency components of the 2D projection from overpowering the reconstructed image. We can think of the filter function in Figure 10-11b as a weighting function in which each frequency has a different weighting factor. Because the roll-off filters are all based on mathematical functions, we can manipulate them to control the weighting factors assigned to each frequency, which ultimately controls the appearance of the final 3D image matrix.

It is crucial that the band-pass filter (the product of the ramp and low-pass filters) reach zero amplitude at a frequency no higher than the system's Nyquist frequency. When frequencies greater than the Nyquist are included in the reconstruction, an aliasing artifact results. To ensure that this does not occur, the filter must reach the X-axis before the value of the Nyquist frequency is reached. Thus, the critical frequency (of a Butterworth filter) or cutoff frequency (of other filters) is an important parameter in obtaining a quality image.

(a) General shape of Butterworth filters

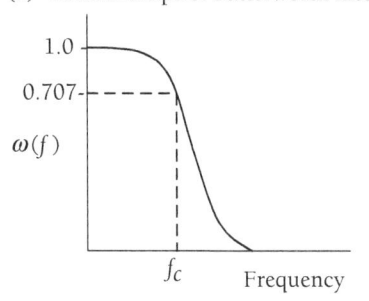

(b) Order = 10, change critical frequency

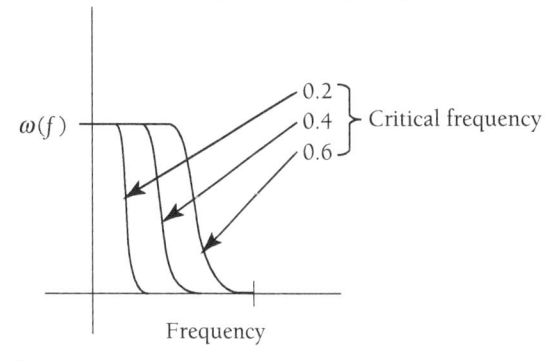

(c) Critical frequency = 0.4/cm, change order

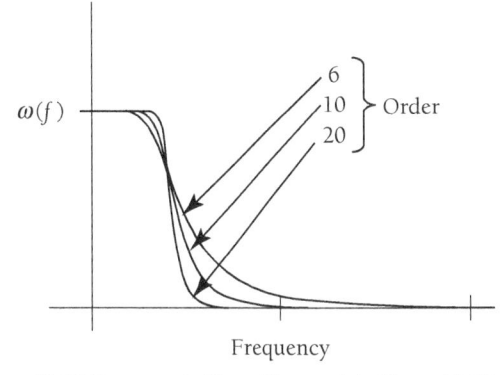

Figure 10-12 Butterworth filters. The graph in Figure 10-12a illustrates the general shape of the Butterworth filter, including the value of the critical frequency f_c. Figure 10-12b shows the effect of changing the critical frequency while keeping the order constant. Figure 10-12c shows the effect of changing the order while keeping the critical frequency constant. As can be seen from these examples, the order determines the shape of the transition zone, and the critical frequency determines its location.

A concise summary of FBP is quoted with permission from Reference 13:

> Analytical reconstruction uses the technique of FBP in which counts detected at a particular angle are then known to lie somewhere along a perpendicular ray through the object (back projection lines). From views obtained at various angles, the locations of overlap of the rays are determined, corresponding to the locations of the highest and lowest count point sources. However, for a variety of reasons this method by itself (simple [or unfiltered] back projection) results in loss of resolution and contrast, and yields a strongly blurred version of the original count distribution, with a characteristic "star artifact." By converting an image into its mathematical frequency components (i.e., a Fourier representation), removing the lower frequency components (i.e., ramp filtering), and performing an inverse Fourier transform, a 3D-count distribution with less blurring is obtained. At the same time, as approximately 10% of a nuclear image is from random noise, an additional mathematical smoothing filter is applied, resulting in the images customarily used for interpretation.

Incorporation of Filters in the Reconstruction Process

Filtering can be worked into the reconstruction process at a variety of different points. Filters may be used to modify the data before backprojection is performed (prefiltering), or alternatively may be applied to the reconstructed slices or the entire 3D image matrix after backprojection (postfiltering). The various methods are mathematically equivalent, but in practice a common choice is to convert the 2D projections to the spatial frequency domain, filter with the ramp filter modified by the low-pass filter, convert back to the spatial domain, and then backproject (12, 14). Often a Z-axis smoothing filter is applied after reconstruction to soften sharp count/voxel changes between transaxial planes, so that sagittal and coronal images appear less disjointed.

Iterative Reconstruction

Radon's original mathematics assumes that the 2D projections are correct representations of the 3D object. This is not true for 2D projections obtained with a gamma camera, because they are affected by attenuation, scatter, resolution loss with distance, and noise. In particular, the mathematics described by Radon assumes that the count values of each pixel in each 2D projection are exactly correct, and that a single correct solution exists to the problem of reconstruction into a 3D image matrix. While this produces reasonably good SPECT images, the underlying assumption is faulty. The count values in each pixel have statistical variability, or *noise*. The presence of noise implies that more than one set of 2D projections could be obtained from a given radiopharmaceutical biodistribution in the object being imaged. In addition, patient-specific attenuation maps, which indicate the densities of tissues through which gamma rays must pass, are not easy to incorporate into the FBP process. The desire to more accurately correct SPECT images for attenuation has pushed the development of a different family of reconstruction techniques called *iterative* methods.

The essence of iterative methods is to make a series of estimates of the radiopharmaceutical distribution in the object. Each estimate in turn is modified, based on comparison to the acquired projections, to produce the next estimate, such that the process over many iterations approaches the "best" match to the acquisition data. The algorithms used in the comparison process assume that the pixel values in the 2D projections are each a Poisson function of the true value for that pixel. The algorithm thus takes into account the statistical variability that is inherent in nuclear medicine images. While iterative algorithms have been applied to nuclear medicine images for over 25 years, their routine incorporation into SPECT reconstruction has only become possible with recent improvements in computer power and speed. Iterative methods present both new benefits and new challenges compared to FBP.

The Iterative Cycle

A schematic of the basic process of iterative reconstruction is shown in **Figure 10-13**. It starts with an initial guess as to the radiopharmaceutical distribution; this guess may be as simple as assuming a uniform biodistribution, or it may use a backprojection of the measured projections. This is the first *estimated 3D matrix*. The computer then creates *estimated 2D projections* using the initial guess, additional information related to the physics of imaging, and a patient-specific attenuation map. These estimated projections are then compared to the *measured 2D projections* obtained in the study, and the discrepancies between the two are used to modify the estimated 3D image matrix. The modified image matrix is then used as the starting point for the next iteration. The process is repeated until it *converges*, meaning that the estimated projections are very similar to the measured projections. Each trip through this cycle counts as one iteration.

The iterative cycle has two key steps. The *forward-projection* step models the image acquisition process. It creates the estimated 2D projections based on the count distribution in the estimated 3D image matrix. It attempts to determine the projections that would be expected, given the estimated 3D image matrix and the laws of physics that govern gamma ray travel and detection. The value of an individual pixel d of a given estimated 2D projection is determined according to an equation of the form:

$$P_d = \sum_b M_{b,d} A_b \tag{10-3}$$

in which P_d is the counts in pixel d of a specific estimated 2D projection, arising from activity A_b in voxel b of the estimated 3D image matrix. The term $M_{b,d}$ represents a model of photon detection based on the relative locations of voxel b and pixel d. Into this model can be incorporated

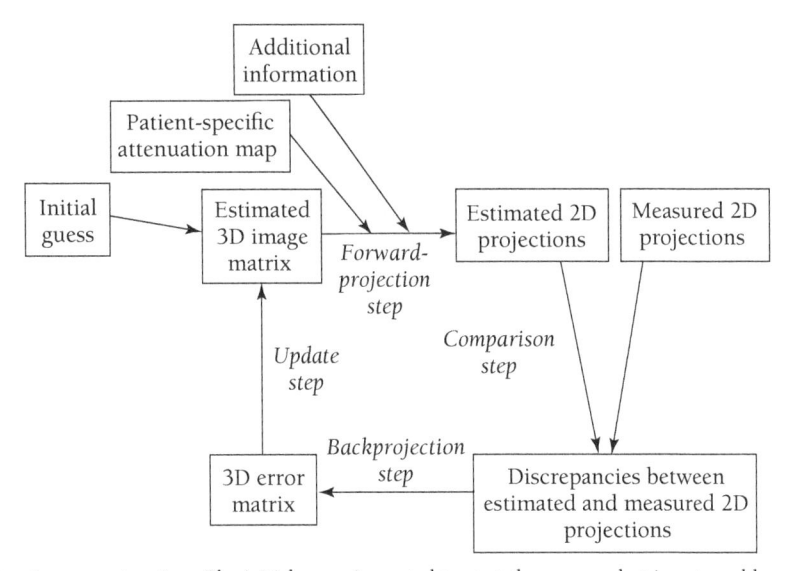

Figure 10-13 Schematic of iterative reconstruction. The initial guess is created to start the process, but is not used beyond that point. Each trip through the cycle is one iteration. The cycle is terminated when either (1) convergence is reached, meaning that the estimated and measured projections are acceptably close, or (2) a stopping rule, usually a maximum number of iterations, is reached. The major advantage of iterative reconstruction is the ability to incorporate a patient-specific attenuation map and our understanding of physics and statistics into the reconstruction algorithm.

the known attenuation (i.e., a patient-specific attenuation map), as well as the possibility of scatter and the depth-dependent resolution loss that is characteristic of gamma cameras. Therefore $M_{b,d}$ indicates the probability that activity in voxel b will be seen in pixel d of the 2D projection in question. The summation term shows that the final value for pixel d in an individual projection is based on consideration of all voxels in the estimated 3D image matrix. When all voxels have been considered for their contribution to each pixel of the 2D projection, the result is an estimate of what the projection should look like.

Once the estimated 2D projections have been created, they are compared to the measured 2D projections. The *comparison* step is the second key step of the iterative process, and how it is done depends on the algorithm used. The most popular iterative algorithm, *expectation maximization* (EM), is a statistical procedure that assumes that the number of counts in each pixel in the measured 2D projections is not a single value but rather is affected by Poisson statistics. It thus allows for the noise that we know is present in the measured 2D projections, and it attempts to find not a single "correct" solution but rather a 3D image matrix that is *likely* to produce the measured 2D projections.

The result of the comparison step is a set of errors (either ratios or differences) between the estimated and measured 2D projections. These error projections are backprojected to create an *error 3D image matrix*. The reconstruction algorithm weights the pixels in the error projections according to the likelihood that they actually contribute to each voxel in the 3D image matrix (15). That is, the system model $M_{b,d}$ is used to backproject the errors into the 3D error matrix. Thus the physics of imaging is modeled in the backprojection step as well as the forward-projection step. Finally, the 3D error matrix is either multiplied by or added to the estimated 3D image matrix in the *update* step, to produce a new estimate.

MLEM and OSEM

While there are several statistical outcome parameters that can be applied to the EM procedure, the one that has become the most popular is the *maximum-likelihood* (ML) parameter, which attempts to maximize a statistical quantity called the *likelihood*. This quantity is highest when the ratio between the estimated and measured 2D projections approaches 1. Another way to say it is that the goal of the maximum-likelihood expectation maximization (MLEM) algorithm is to find the activity distribution that has the highest probability of generating the measured projections.

In its pure form, the MLEM process uses all of the projections in each iteration. This causes it to converge slowly, requiring as many as 50 to 100 iterations. Each iteration takes considerably longer than a complete FBP reconstruction (16). An alternative method called *ordered-subsets expectation maximization* (OSEM) breaks the whole set of projections into a large number of subsets. For example, a 64-projection study might be broken into 16 four-projection subsets, with the four projections in each subset being evenly spaced within the 64 total projection images. The OSEM algorithm compares the first subset of estimated projections to the measured projection subset and updates the 3D image matrix, after which the next subset is considered. A full iteration has been completed when all subsets have been considered, but the updating of the estimated 3D image matrix is performed after each subset. This algorithm converges much more quickly than the MLEM method, requiring only about 2 to 10 iterations. **Figure 10-14** shows a slice from a myocardial perfusion study reconstructed with different numbers of iterations.

In MLEM and OSEM reconstruction, as the number of iterations increases, so does the amount of noise in the estimated 3D image matrix. The added noise has a characteristic

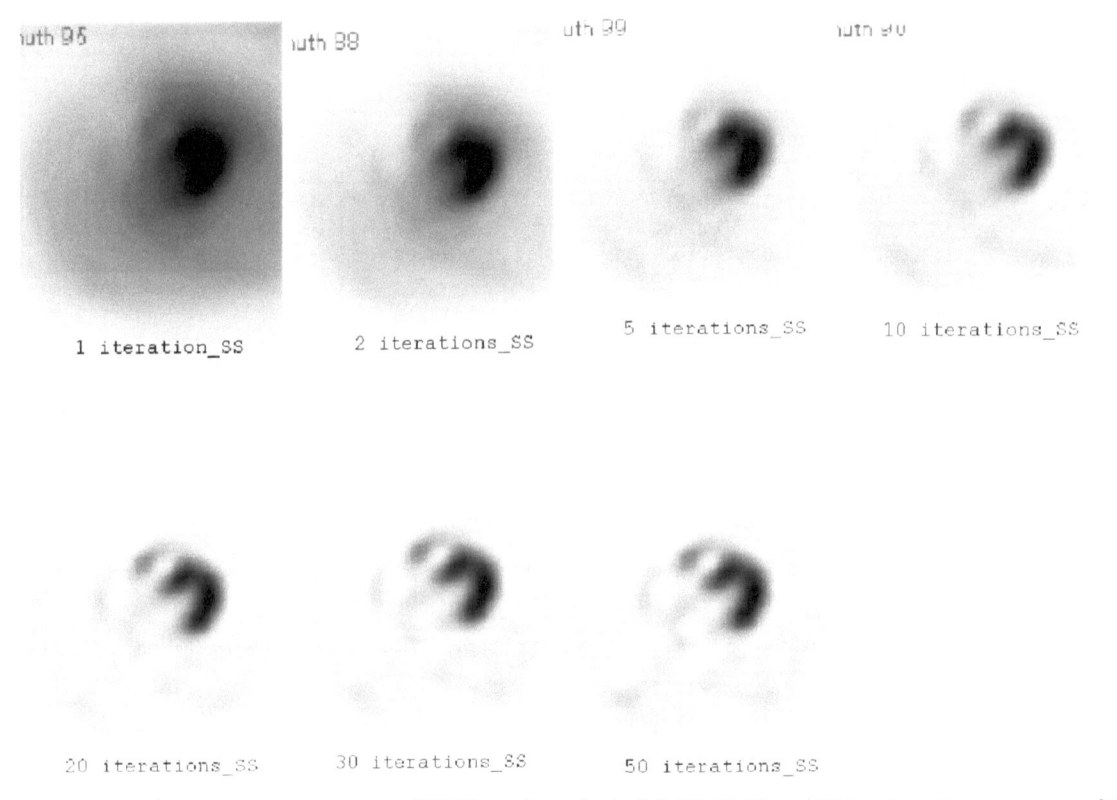

Figure 10-14 Iteration number. Iterative reconstructions (OSEM) are shown for 1, 2, 5, 10, 20, 30, and 50 iterations. Images courtesy of St. Joseph Medical Center.

"checkerboard" appearance (17). This "noise breakup phenomenon" is typical with statistical estimation algorithms. There is a point of compromise between the "best" 3D image matrix according to the statistical algorithm and the best choice from an appearance/readability standpoint. As a consequence, the usual procedure is to stop after a specified number of iterations. Another option is to apply a smoothing filter after reconstruction. This *postfiltering* allows for optimization of the number of iterations for a given type of study in order to maintain image detail, while still suppressing noise in the final product. Most vendors include the option of postreconstruction filtering in their iterative reconstruction packages.

Image Display

The final step in a SPECT study is display of the 3D image matrix. Display devices are almost entirely 2D. But because our information is in three dimensions, we will want to display it in ways that convey the 3D spatial relationships of the structures. Consequently, SPECT image display will utilize all the "tricks" in the nuclear medicine computer's "bag."

Two-Dimensional Display Techniques

Once the 3D image matrix has been reconstructed, the tomographic slices are immediately available (**Figure 10-15a**). We can view *transverse* slices (the X–Y plane of Fig. 10-1), which cut perpendicularly across the long axis of the body.

We can also consider the X–Z (or *coronal*) and the Y–Z (or *sagittal*) planes. We can display each plane as a series of 2D slices of the 3D image matrix (**Figure 10-16a**). Most systems also have the ability to display 2D slices that are 2 or more pixels thick. When compared to the 3D display techniques discussed below, the 2D slices represent the highest-resolution version of the data (8).

We may not, however, want to use the planes defined by the camera's rotation. We may instead want to tweak the planes because the patient's body is not exactly oriented to the camera's axes. Or we may want to use an entirely different set of orthogonal planes that are relative to the position of a particular organ, as is done with the heart (Fig. 10-15b). Computer display algorithms generally allow the user to reorient the study according to user-defined reference lines. Internally, the 3D image matrix is rotated to accomplish this *oblique reorientation*. Once reoriented, however, the voxels no longer line up in neat planes. A trilinear interpolation, essentially a smoothing operation in three dimensions, is used to determine the count densities of the reoriented voxels. The result is a reoriented 3D image matrix that can be sliced along the redefined orthogonal planes (Fig. 10-16b), with a slight loss of resolution due to the additional smoothing. If multiple oblique reorientations are performed, errors due to this loss of resolution can accumulate.

In nuclear medicine practice, identification of an abnormality is considered definitive only when the abnormality is seen in at least two orthogonal planes. *Dynamic triangulation* allows the reader to select a point in one slice of

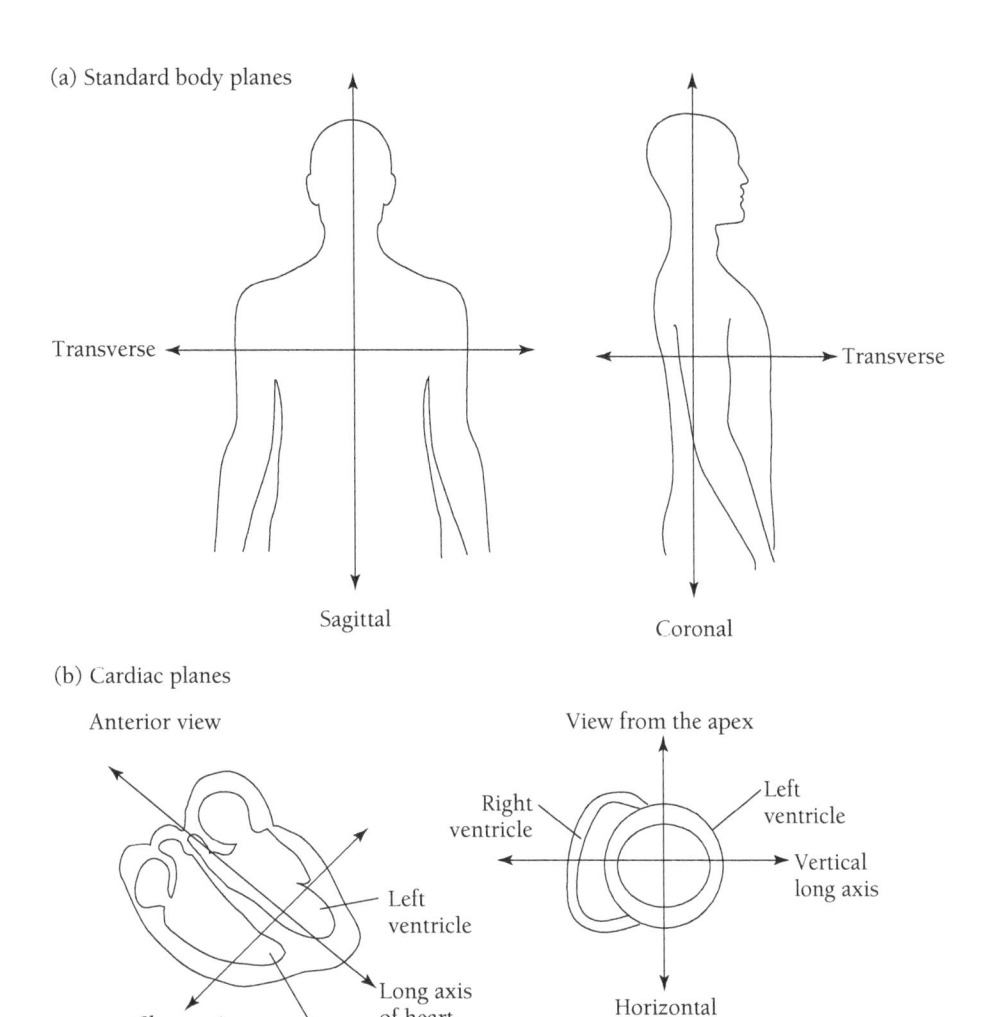

Figure 10-15 Tomographic planes in the body and in the heart. The lines show the orientation of each set of orthogonal planes; the reader may visualize a series of parallel lines corresponding to the 2D slices shown in Figure 10-16. Figure 10-15a shows standard body planes, and Figure 10-15b shows cardiac planes as defined by the American College of Cardiology. The use of axes oriented with the cardiac apex allows for myocardial perfusion images to be compared from one patient to another, even though the exact location and orientation of the heart in the thorax varies from patient to patient.

the 3D image matrix and click on it with the cursor; the computer then displays the two orthogonal slices containing the same voxel (**Figure 10-17**). A display of several slices around the point in each plane may be provided. Dynamic triangulation is exceptionally helpful in SPECT, because the limited amount of anatomic information in the images makes all three planes necessary for image interpretation.

Three-Dimensional Display Techniques

Display of 2D slices requires that the viewer mentally put them together in order to understand the spatial information in three dimensions. Several techniques are commonly employed to show visually realistic representations of the 3D image matrix in a 2D format. (Unfortunately, these techniques do not lend themselves to 2D display and so are not illustrated here.) *Surface rendering* generates a solid "model" of the exterior pixels, hiding the interior pixels from view and using light shading to convey the object's shape (8). The first step in surface rendering is to identify the surface of the organ(s) by segmenting the image into either "object" or "background," using count threshold and edge detection techniques. A boundary-tracking algorithm is then used to identify the boundary between object and background, and it "connects the dots" between slices, to create a wire-frame model of the surface. The surface generated is highlighted according to its light reflection capabilities, as if it were a solid object illuminated by external light. Surface rendering is helpful when the organ being imaged is most easily seen as a continuous surface; photopenic areas are then seen as "holes" in that surface.

Volume rendering essentially reprojects the 3D image matrix to create 2D projections, which can then be viewed in a rotating *cine display* (continuous-loop movie) or from a specific angle. The reprojection is accomplished with a ray-tracing technique, using a weighted sum of voxel counts along a particular viewing line. The weighting

(a)

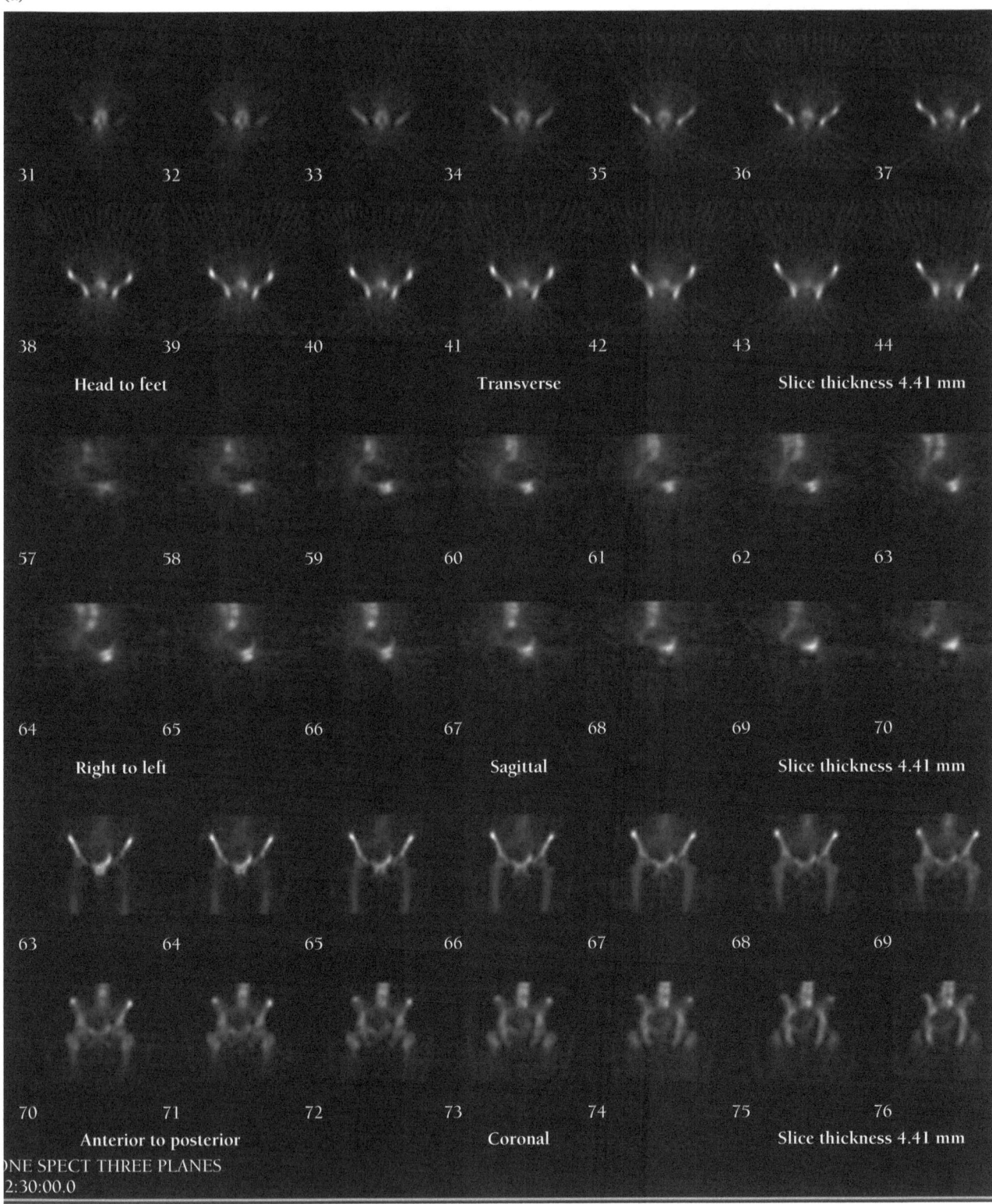

Figure 10-16 Two-dimensional slices. Figure 10-16a shows 2D slices from a bone SPECT study. The standard 2D slices for body and brain nuclear medicine studies correspond to the body axes shown in Figure 10-15a. In these types of studies, reorientation is performed to achieve left–right symmetry. In the heart, the long axis of the heart is used to define the correct orientation (Fig. 10-15b). As is standard with myocardial perfusion imaging, Figure 10-16b shows two sets of slices, the upper row of each pair showing the heart at stress and the lower row showing the heart at rest. Images courtesy of Virginia Mason Medical Center.

(b)

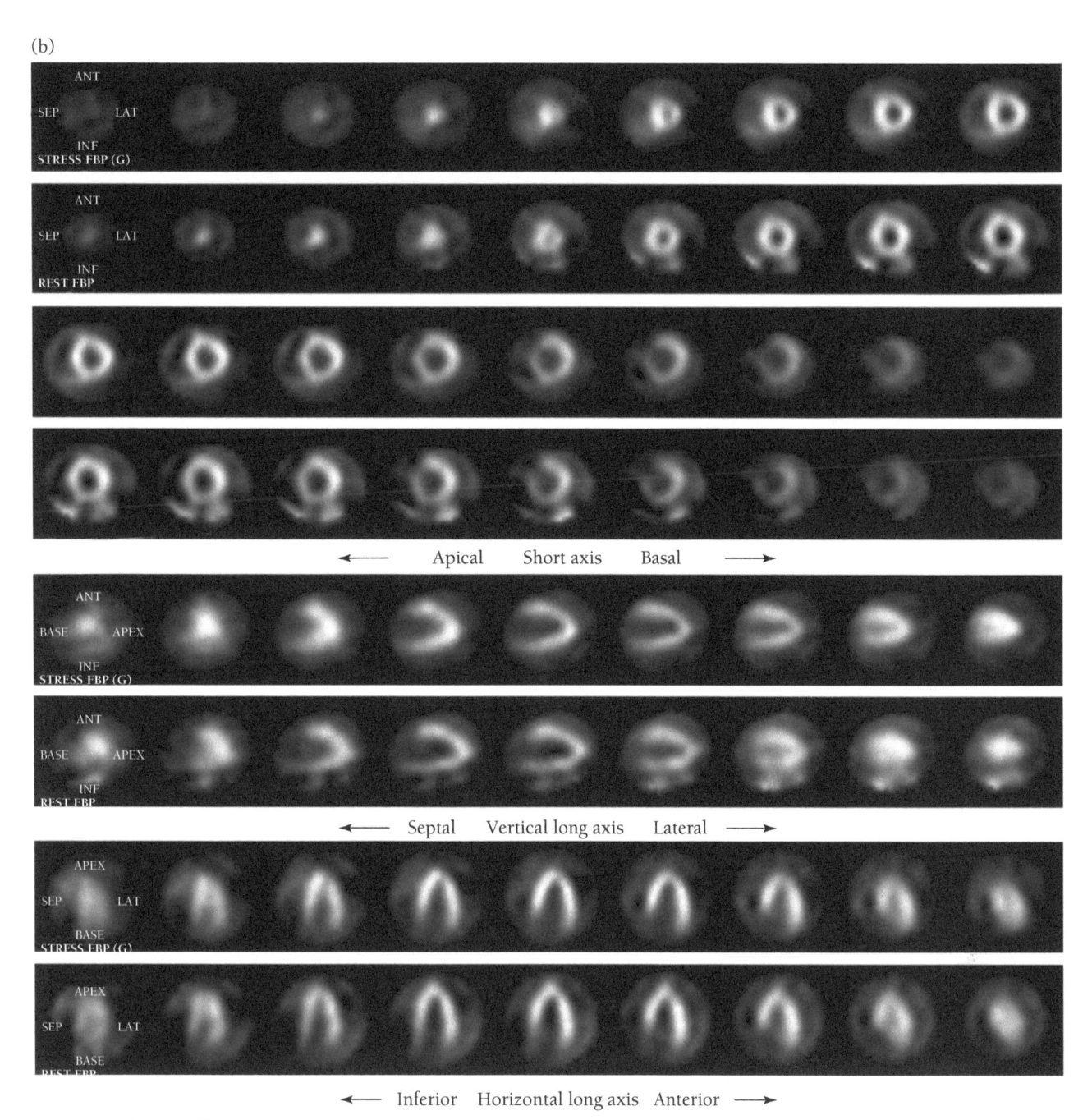

[Figure: SPECT cardiac images in short axis, vertical long axis, and horizontal long axis views, showing STRESS FBP (G) and REST FBP rows with orientation labels ANT/SEP/LAT/INF, BASE/ANT/APEX/INF, and APEX/SEP/LAT/BASE]

←— Apical   Short axis   Basal —→

←— Septal   Vertical long axis   Lateral —→

←— Inferior   Horizontal long axis   Anterior —→

Figure 10-16 (continued)

takes distance from the viewer into account, such that more distant voxels along the viewing line are given less weight than closer voxels. Rays are traced at different angles and different locations; all of the ray tracings at a particular angle can be combined to form a reprojection of the 3D image matrix. The process results in images that are quite similar to the raw SPECT projections, but with lower noise and greater contrast (8). Count thresholding may be used to eliminate background counts, and light reflection, gradient shading, and other ways of illustrating changing voxel counts are applied. In contrast to surface-rendered images, volume-rendered images are semitransparent, allowing the viewer to see one structure "through" another. The resulting image, when displayed in rotating cine format, gives the impression of organ volume and depth. Volume rendering retains somewhat more of the information of the 3D image matrix than does the surface-rendering technique and does not require identification of the object's surface, but it is more time-consuming to generate.

A related technique is the *maximum-intensity projection* (MIP) image (18). It is very similar to the volume-rendered image, except that instead of considering the sum of counts along a viewing line, the MIP image uses only the hottest voxel along each ray to generate the projections. Again, a weighting algorithm accounts for the depth

Image Display   147

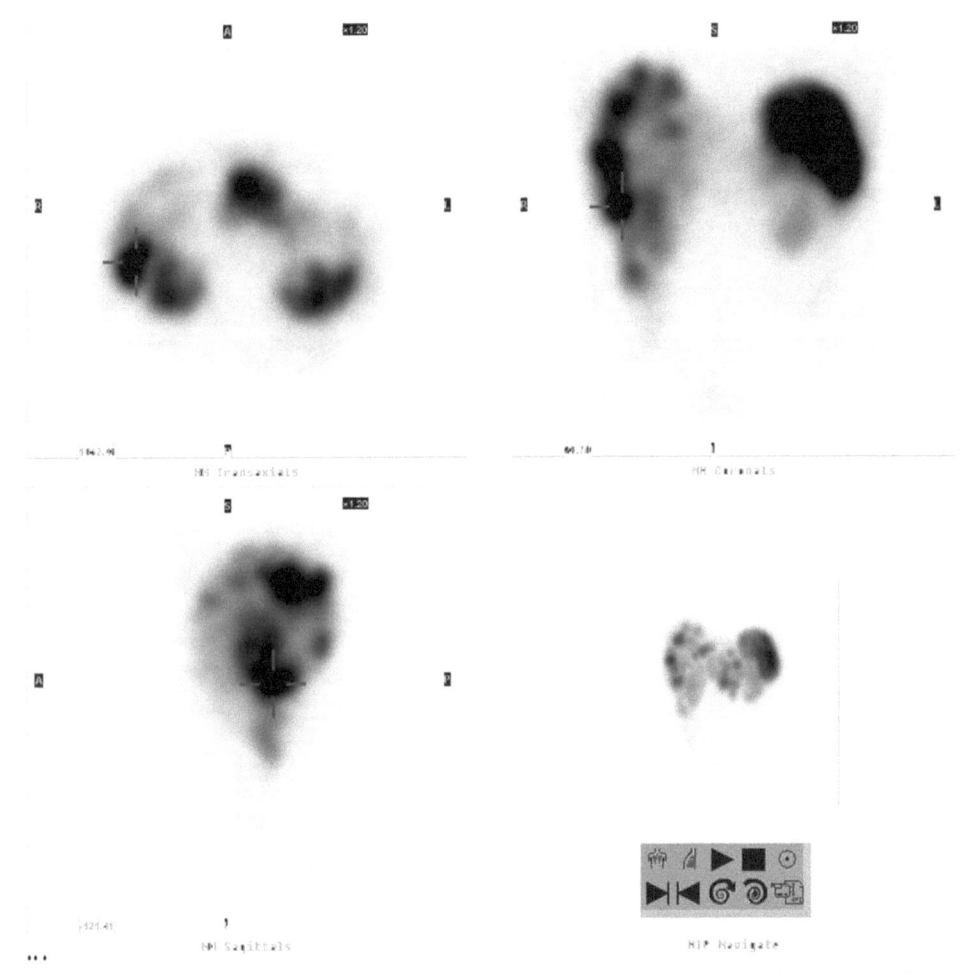

Figure 10-17 Dynamic triangulation. Dynamic triangulation allows the user to locate a particular area simultaneously in all three orthogonal planes. The small image at the lower right is a maximum-intensity projection (MIP) image of an In-111 octreotide study. The crosshairs have been placed on an area of increased activity in the liver. The larger images are the transverse, coronal, and sagittal slices that correspond to the location of the crosshairs. Images courtesy of Virginia Mason Medical Center.

of the hottest voxel, and projections are created and displayed in rotating cine fashion. The anterior MIP projection is often shown as a planar image and used for dynamic triangulation (see, for example, the small image in the lower right of Fig. 10-17). MIP images are very helpful for hot-spot imaging, because the areas of increased activity can be correlated to their correct 3D location. But MIP images also work for studies in which the abnormal area is cold. This area disappears, and the viewer has the impression of "seeing into" the organ through the cold spot.

Cine Modes

The three-dimensional nature of a SPECT study is often best appreciated by viewing a cine display of the data. Viewing the rotating raw 2D projections or a volume- or surface-rendered display allows the viewer to get a feel for the location and depth of abnormal areas. In a gated SPECT study, the 3D image matrix showing myocardial perfusion is generated after the eight gated frames of each 2D projection are added together, thus maximizing the information that the study is intended to provide.

Myocardial perfusion imaging generally includes at least one set of gated SPECT images, providing a 4D image set that combines the three spatial dimensions with the repeating myocardial contraction. The reconstructed 4D information is played in a cine format to evaluate myocardial wall motion. Visualization of functional data in gated SPECT studies is enhanced through the use of polygon "mesh" or "cage" structures to show the inner and/or outer surfaces of the myocardium at end diastole. The myocardial motion is then displayed in cine fashion, and the cages provide a reference for gauging the amount of motion in each wall of the left ventricle.

Viewing Recommendations

When viewing these further manipulations of the SPECT-derived 3D image matrix, one must remember that they are several steps removed from raw data. Pixel counts may reflect activity only in a relative way. In particular, the count density information that is at the heart of quantitative analysis in nuclear medicine may no longer be valid. For example, the segmentation into "object" or "background" that is done in surface rendering removes the actual count density information.

Validation of a particular 3D image display technique is difficult to accomplish and is not commonly done. Moreover, the realistic appearance of the 3D display techniques makes it easy to sidestep the issue of validation. It is therefore important that the impressions gained by viewing such derived images be confirmed by inspection of the 2D tomographic slices generated directly from the 3D image matrix. Similarly, the use of color scales to enhance SPECT images can be visually appealing but can leave an incorrect impression of their diagnostic meaning. As much as possible, display techniques and image normalization should be standardized so that the interpreting physician can read them in a consistent fashion.

Finally, it is important to mention that film or other forms of hard-copy images should not be the only means of image display for SPECT. The complexities of these studies exceed the ability of printed images to present them, in terms of color scale capabilities, flexibility, and ease of use. A computer display terminal is considered essential to the task of analyzing SPECT images. Manipulation of gray and color scales, dynamic triangulation, and cine displays are indispensable to the process of image interpretation in a 3D setting. In short, reading from a computer monitor is considered the standard of practice, and film is only a backup/storage methodology for SPECT (19).

Summary

Tomography has become widely accepted in radiologic imaging, particularly for CT, MRI, and nuclear medicine. Its application to nuclear medicine begins with a series of planar images acquired at various angles around the object being imaged. The resulting set of 2D projections is reconstructed, using either FBP or iterative reconstruction, into a 3D representation of the radiopharmaceutical biodistribution in the object. That 3D representation is then viewed in a variety of ways. It would appear at this juncture that iterative reconstruction produces better image quality and will become the reconstruction method of choice over time.

In contrast to the other tomographic imaging modalities such as CT and MRI, SPECT requires greater operator interaction in the reconstruction process. This is largely due to patient-to-patient variability in terms of body habitus and radiopharmaceutical biodistribution, both of which affect the count densities obtained in the 2D projections. These variations are accommodated in FBP by modifying the choice and/or qualities of the low-pass filter applied in the reconstruction process. Iterative reconstruction was developed in part to provide a less subjective "fix" to this problem.

The concepts of 3D image reconstruction are complicated and difficult to comprehend, whichever method is used. It is possible to let the computer perform image reconstruction without understanding the principles behind it. But such an approach limits our ability to modify the reconstruction if the final image appearance is not satisfactory. It is far better to achieve an understanding of how both FBP and iterative methodologies work, so that appropriate interventions can be made to improve image quality.

References

1. Radon J. Über die bestimmung von funktionen durch ihre integralwerte langs gewisser mannigfaltigkeiten. *Ber Verh Sachs Akad Wiss Leipzig*. 1917;69:262–277.
2. Bracewell RN. Strip integration in radio astronomy. *Aust J Phys*. 1956;9:198–217.
3. Kuhl DE, Edwards RQ. Image separation radioisotope scanning. *Radiol*. 1963;80:653–661.
4. Hounsfield GN. Computerized transverse axial scanning (tomography): part I. Description of system. *Br J Radiol*. 1973;46:1016–1022.
5. Cormack AM. Representation of a function by its line integrals with some radiological applications. *J Appl Phys*. 1963;34:2722–2727.
6. Cormack AM. Representation of a function by its line integrals with some radiological applications: II. *J Appl Phys*. 1964;35:2908–2913.
7. Kuhl DE, Hale J, Eaton WL. Transmission scanning: a useful adjunct to conventional emission scanning for accurately keying isotope deposition to radiographic anatomy. *Radiol*. 1966;87:278–284.
8. Lee K. *Computers in Nuclear Medicine*. 2nd ed. Reston, VA: Society of Nuclear Medicine; 2005:92, 155, 156.
9. Van Laere K, Koole M, Lemahieu I, Dierckx R. Image filtering in single-photon emission computed tomography: principles and applications. *Comput Med Imaging Graph*. 2001;25:127–133.
10. Christian PE, Waterstram-Rich KM. *Nuclear Medicine and PET/CT: Technology and Techniques*. 6th ed. St. Louis, MO: Mosby-Year Book; 2007:283.
11. Groch MW, Erwin WD. SPECT in the year 2000: basic principles. *J Nucl Med Technol*. 2000;28:233–244.
12. Gelfand MJ, Thomas SR. *Effective Use of Computers in Nuclear Medicine*. New York, NY: McGraw-Hill; 1988:48, 56.
13. Travin MI. Cardiac cameras. *Semin Nucl Med*. 2011;41:182–201.
14. Cherry SR, Sorenson JA, Phelps ME. *Physics in Nuclear Medicine*. 3rd ed. Philadelphia, PA: Saunders; 2003:280.
15. King MA, Tsui BMW, Pan TS, et al. Attenuation compensation for cardiac single-photon emission computed tomographic imaging: part 2. Attenuation compensation algorithms. *J Nucl Cardiol*. 1996;3:55–63.
16. Vandenberghe S, D'Asseler Y, Van de Walle R, et al. Iterative reconstruction algorithms in nuclear medicine. *Comput Med Imaging Graph*. 2001;25:105–111.
17. Katoh C, Ruitsalainen U, Laine H, et al. Iterative reconstruction based on median root prior in quantification of myocardial blood flow and oxygen metabolism. *J Nucl Med*. 1999;40:862–867.
18. Henkin RE, Boles MA, Dillehay GL, et al., eds. *Nuclear Medicine*. St. Louis, MO: Mosby-Year Book; 1996:258.
19. Wagner HN, Szabo Z, Buchanan JW, eds. *Principles of Nuclear Medicine*. 2nd ed. Philadelphia, PA: WB Saunders; 1995:338–339.

Additional Resources

Bailey DL. Transmission scanning in emission tomography. *Eur J Nucl Med*. 1998;25:774–787.

Brooks RA, DiChiro G. Principles of computer assisted tomography (CAT) in radiographic and radioisotopic imaging. *Phys Med Biol*. 1976;21:689–732.

Bruyant PP. Analytic and iterative reconstruction algorithms in SPECT. *J Nucl Med*. 2002;43(10):1343–1358.

Christian PE, Bernier DR, Langan JK. *Nuclear Medicine and PET Technology and Techniques*. 5th ed. St. Louis, MO: Mosby-Year Book; 2004:Chapter 9.

English RJ. *Single-Photon Emission Computed Tomography: A Primer*. 3rd ed. Reston, VA: Society of Nuclear Medicine; 1995:Chapters 2, 5.

Henkin RE, Boles MA, Dillehay GL, et al., eds. *Nuclear Medicine*. St. Louis, MO: C.V. Mosby; 1996:Chapter 21.

Hutton BF, Hudson HM, Beckman FJ. A clinical perspective of accelerated statistical reconstruction. *Eur J Nucl Med*. 1997;24:797–808.

Lee K. *Computers in Nuclear Medicine*. 2nd ed. Reston, VA: Society of Nuclear Medicine; 2005:Chapter 11.

Madsen MT. Recent advances in SPECT imaging. *J Nucl Med*. 2007;48:661–673.

Travin MI. Cardiac cameras. *Semin Nucl Med*. 2011; 41:182–201.

Vandenberghe S, D'Asseler Y, Van de Walle R et al. Iterative reconstruction algorithms in nuclear medicine. *Comput Med Imaging Graph*. 2001;25:105–111.

Van Laere K, Koole M, Lemahieu I, Dierckx R. Image filtering in single-photon emission computed tomography: principles and applications. *Comput Med Imaging Graph*. 2001;25:127–133.

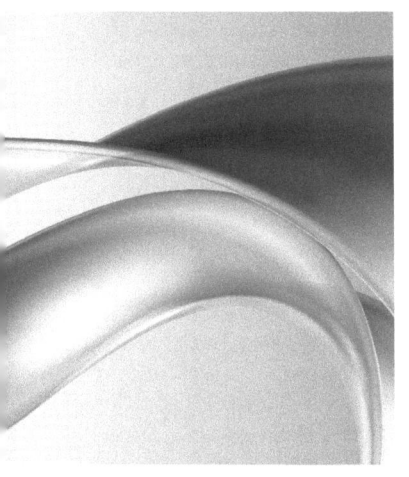

CHAPTER 11
Image Characteristics and Effect of Acquisition Parameters in SPECT Imaging

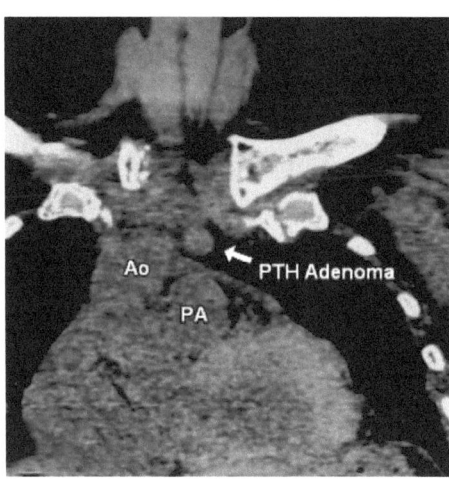

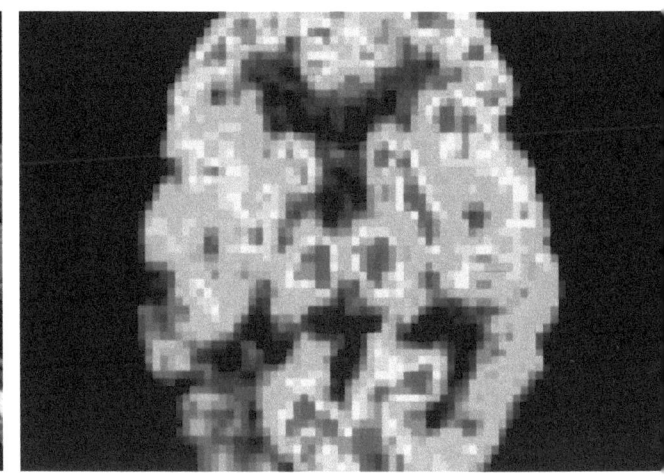

Learning Outcomes

1. State the main reason that SPECT images are improved compared to planar images.
2. Describe each of the following image characteristics as they relate to SPECT images:
   a. Resolution loss with depth
   b. Background
   c. Noise
   d. Attenuation and scatter
   e. Patient motion
3. Define the partial volume effect and describe its manifestation in SPECT images.
4. Discuss the measurement of spatial resolution in SPECT.
5. Analyze the effect of changing each of the following SPECT acquisition parameters:
   a. Collimator
   b. Energy window
   c. Image matrix
   d. Digital zoom
   e. Detector orbit
   f. Time/stop
6. Describe changes that can be made in the low-pass filter (used in filtered backprojection) to improve image quality.
7. Briefly describe the Gibbs phenomenon and aliasing artifacts, as they apply to SPECT imaging.

Introduction

The chief goal of SPECT imaging is to improve the ability to detect abnormal radionuclide distributions that are deep in the object being imaged. It removes the third-dimension superposition that is a major limitation of planar imaging. This results in a dramatic improvement in contrast compared to planar images. We must, however, examine the other characteristics of planar images (as discussed in Chapter 8), to see how they apply in SPECT. We must also consider how to apply the concepts of uniformity and spatial resolution to SPECT. The latter half of this chapter discusses how changes in acquisition parameters and filters affect the characteristics of the resulting SPECT images.

Image Characteristics in SPECT

With the exception of third-dimension superposition, the same factors that affect planar images (see Chapter 8) also impact SPECT. But the SPECT reconstruction process, which combines many images, amplifies them in the three-dimensional (3D) image matrix. In addition, the method used to reconstruct the projections plays a crucial role in determining what effect these image characteristics will have in the 3D image matrix. Throughout this chapter, there is an underlying assumption that the gamma camera has excellent uniformity and good rotational mechanics.

Chapter 13 addresses the issues of quality control and image appearance when this assumption is not true.

Background

Background can be defined as "nonspecific radionuclide distribution." The projections used to create a 3D image matrix have this kind of background. But a small count-density change in a background region may potentially appear significant in a SPECT study simply because it is seen from many different angles. A cleaner biodistribution yields an even greater degree of clarity in SPECT than it does in planar images.

Filtered backprojection (FBP) creates another kind of background as well, namely, counts from regions of increased activity that are spread across the 3D image matrix during the backprojection process. This is called *structured background*, and it is this background that the ramp filter is working to limit. Use of iterative reconstruction methods may reduce or eliminate structured background.

Noise

Noise—the statistical variations in the number of counts registered—is also present in the projections acquired in SPECT imaging. In fact, noise is a more significant factor in SPECT imaging than in planar imaging, for several reasons. First, the projections are acquired over a relatively short time (15–45 sec), in order to make the total imaging time tolerable. Each projection has fewer counts than would be obtained in a planar image, such that noise is a greater percentage of the total counts. Noise must be considered as a function of the individual projections, rather than the total counts acquired in the study.

Second, the FBP reconstruction process amplifies noise, in that the noise in the individual projections is propagated into the 3D image matrix. If a given pixel of a projection has a high count value due to noise, FBP reconstruction will cause other voxels in its immediate vicinity to also have higher count densities than they should. Noise thus contributes to the structured background mentioned above.

Noise is also an important consideration in setting filter parameters in FBP reconstruction. It is a significant component of the high-frequency end of the frequency spectrum, which is maximally amplified by the ramp filter. To decrease its contribution to the final 3D image matrix, FBP must employ a roll-off filter in addition to the ramp filter. The problem with this scheme is that we cannot define exactly what is noise and what is a significant count-density change in the object, either on the frequency spectrum or in the image. Therefore, we always run the risk of keeping too much or too little information, depending not only on the study being done but also on the characteristics of each individual patient.

The use of iterative techniques makes some of these issues disappear. In iterative reconstruction, specifically the maximum-likelihood expectation maximization (MLEM) technique, measured count density is treated as a Poisson function of the actual radioactivity distribution rather than a single defined value. Iterative techniques using the MLEM algorithm or its derivatives should therefore deal more effectively with the noise inherent in the 2D projections.

On the other hand, these algorithms are subject to increasing noise as the number of iterations increases. So no matter which reconstruction method is used, noise is an important characteristic of SPECT images and is a limiting factor in terms of quantitative accuracy. When considering any change in acquisition parameters, we must take the possibility of increased noise into account.

Resolution Loss with Distance

Resolution loss with distance is more of a problem for SPECT than for planar imaging because of the additional object–collimator distance needed to ensure that the camera can rotate around the object. Spatial resolution is worse overall in SPECT compared to planar imaging for this reason. Fortunately, there are ways to improve the resolution of the SPECT study. The use of body contour orbits and long-bore collimators is addressed in this chapter. Resolution loss can also be dealt with in reconstruction, specifically in the forward-projection step of the iterative reconstruction process. Such modeling is included in many newer reconstruction programs.

Attenuation and Scatter

These two image characteristics degrade SPECT images significantly. As much as 25% of Tc-99m gamma rays are lost to photoelectric absorption, and up to 50% of the gamma rays registered have undergone Compton scattering. Attenuation distorts the count-density information that is the essence of nuclear medicine imaging; it also increases the relative contribution of noise by decreasing the total number of counts registered. Scatter decreases contrast by putting counts in incorrect locations, especially in low-count-density areas bordering regions of increased count density. Because their effects are so profound, attenuation and scatter are addressed separately.

Patient Motion

Motion is a much bigger issue in SPECT than in planar imaging, because it causes the same source of radioactivity to be seen in two different places, and therefore to be reconstructed at two different locations in the 3D image matrix. The issue is compounded when transmission-based attenuation correction is used, because any motion affects two reconstructions instead of just one. The most significant source of motion in SPECT studies is whole-body (as opposed to cardiac or respiratory) motion. It is vitally important that the technologist make every possible effort to prevent whole-body motion, by making the patient as comfortable as possible before starting the acquisition and by reminding the patient not to move during the study.

It is also essential to evaluate the study for motion after it has been acquired and before the patient is allowed to leave. Various methods have been used to identify and correct for motion, including the use of fiducial markers and tracking of specific structures from projection to projection. One way to quickly check for motion is to view the raw projections in cine format (keeping in mind that a fast cine rate will decrease the eye's sensitivity to motion). An alternate way to evaluate motion is to create a *sinogram*, which is an image created by taking the same pixel row

(a) Creation of a sinogram

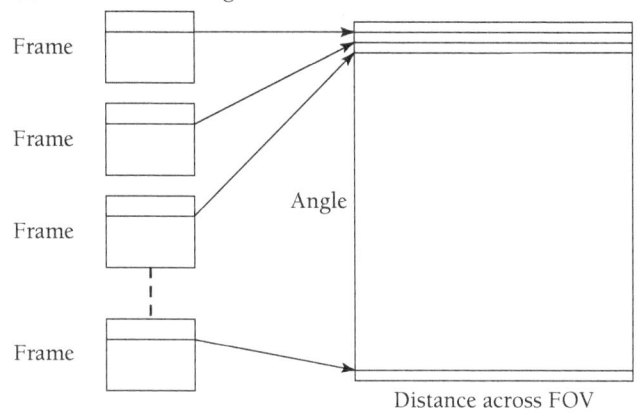

(b) Sinogram showing motion

Motion artifact on sinogram

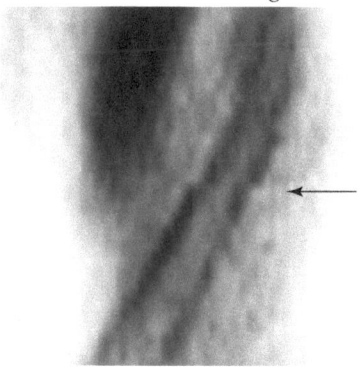

(c) Correction of motion using a sinogram

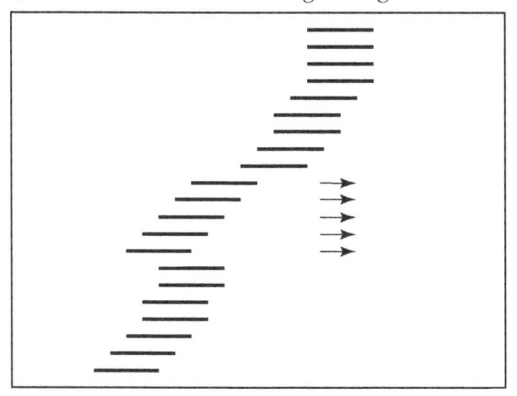

Figure 11-1 SPECT sinogram. A sinogram is created by taking the same row of pixels from each projection and stacking them in order from the first to the last frame to create a new "image" (Fig. 11-1a). An area of high activity should transition in a sine wave fashion from the top to the bottom of the sinogram; motion is seen as a sharp jag in that smooth transition (Fig. 11-1b). Motion correction programs shift the projections that are out of line (see arrows in Fig. 11-1c), to recreate the sine wave shape expected in the sinogram. Figure 11-1b courtesy of Virginia Mason Medical Center.

from each projection and stacking the rows one on another in a 2D image matrix (**Figure 11-1**). As the camera rotates around the object, the position of an internal structure should move in a smooth fashion from the top to the bottom of the sinogram. If the patient has moved, this smooth change in position is interrupted. Recent-generation nuclear medicine computer systems have excellent motion correction programs that should be employed as needed.

Partial Volume Effect

In any kind of 3D imaging, voxels have some finite size, and that size limits the degree of detail that may be seen. This mismatch between voxel size, on one hand, and count-density change, on the other, affects both the visibility of small objects and their perceived intensity. If a voxel's location corresponds to a region with only one type of tissue, then the reconstruction process should represent it correctly. But if a voxel contains two tissues with different radioactivity concentrations, the information about those two tissues will, by necessity, be averaged within the voxel. Thus, detail is lost at the boundary between two types of tissue. The *partial volume effect* (PVE) is the within-voxel averaging that occurs in any 3D imaging situation due to the finite size of the volume elements used.

The PVE is much more significant in SPECT than in CT, for two reasons. First, voxels are considerably larger in SPECT than in CT. Second, the limited resolution and the smoothing inherent in the reconstruction techniques lead to a spillover of counts from one slice to the next. "Individual slices always contain data from adjoining slices" (1). Spillover can go both ways: from an area of interest into the surrounding tissues and from surrounding tissues into the area of interest. Most of the time, these two are not balanced (2). Spillover increases the size of hot or cold areas, so that accurate volume measurements are hard to generate and contrast is decreased. Within a voxel, the intensity no longer accurately represents activity concentration. As a general rule of thumb, the count density of objects with a size dimension less than twice the imaging system's full width at half-maximum (FWHM) will be influenced by the surrounding structures. For an object that is twice the FWHM or larger, PVE is only a problem at the edges of the object. This is clearly shown in **Figure 11-2**.

Contrast

As with planar imaging, the goal of SPECT is to be able to visualize differences in count densities between normal and abnormal structures. We can define this visualization quantitatively as *contrast*. Let us consider the hardest type of lesion to visualize, and the type for which SPECT is most useful, namely, the cold (nonradioactive) lesion embedded in a hot background. For a cold lesion, the contrast formula (Eq. 8-2) can be written as

$$C_{\text{Lesion}} = \frac{I_{\text{Bkg}} - I_{\text{Lesion}}}{I_{\text{Bkg}} + I_{\text{Lesion}}} \quad (11\text{-}1)$$

where C_{Lesion} is the lesion contrast, I_{Bkg} is the background count density, and I_{Lesion} is the lesion count density. In a perfect system, I_{Lesion} is registered as 0 and C_{Lesion} equals 1. If I_{Lesion} equals I_{Bkg}, then C_{Lesion} equals 0. Thus, C_{Lesion} varies between these two extremes.

An early experimental result demonstrated the power of SPECT to improve contrast over planar imaging (3). A liver phantom with cold spheres 1.0 and 1.5 cm in diameter was imaged using both planar and SPECT methods, with the spheres positioned both centrally and peripherally. For planar images of 1 million counts, C_{Lesion} was less than 0.08

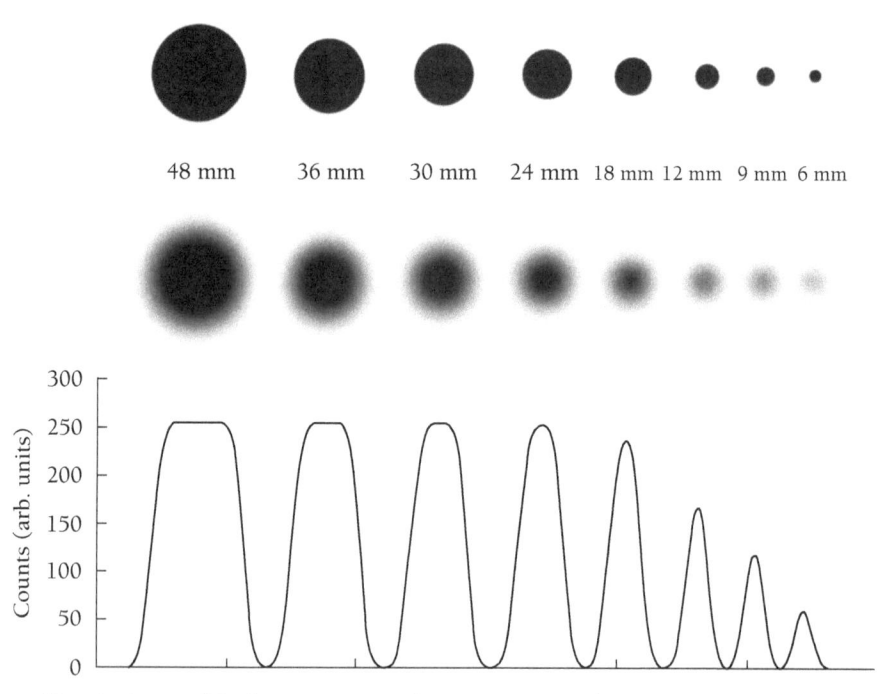

Figure 11-2 Partial volume effect. At the top of the figure are a series of source containers, shown in transverse cross section, with diameters as shown. All source containers have the same radioactivity concentration. The second row shows SPECT reconstructions of the source containers, and the graph at the bottom is a count profile through the middle of the images in that row. The system has a FWHM of 12 mm. When the container diameter is at least twice the FWHM, the maximum count-density values accurately represent the activity concentration (note the flat tops on the first several count profiles), except at the edges of the container. When the container diameter is smaller than twice the system FWHM, the partial volume effect becomes significant, and the count profiles show decreased counts per pixel and increased container size relative to the actual source containers. Reprinted from: Cherry SR, Sorenson JA, Phelps ME. *Physics in Nuclear Medicine*. 3rd ed. Philadelphia, PA: Saunders; 2003:318, Fig. 17-6. Used with permission from Elsevier Science.

(i.e., there was an 8% difference between the lesion and the liver background), in both central and peripheral locations. SPECT imaging yielded lesion contrast of 0.32 to 0.54, depending on the size and location of the spheres. Thus, in an idealized situation, SPECT enhances contrast by a factor of 4 to 7 compared to planar imaging. This study illustrates the most significant power of SPECT, namely, its ability to improve contrast.

Performance Measures in SPECT

We shall use the same performance measures as for planar imaging, particularly uniformity and spatial resolution, to describe SPECT systems. But they will be determined differently than for the planar situation. The formula for measurement of uniformity is the same as for planar imaging, but for SPECT it is measured on a transaxial slice of the reconstructed, attenuation-corrected 3D image matrix obtained from a cylindrical source of uniform activity concentration (4). Even in this idealized situation, in gamma cameras with excellent planar uniformity, SPECT uniformity is quite poor; values of 10 to 30% are routinely obtained (5).

Spatial resolution is measured using a tomographic acquisition of one or more line sources of radioactivity, either in air or in a scattering medium such as water, and is quantified using the FWHM of the resulting line-spread function (LSF). Resolution in a SPECT study depends on the camera's intrinsic and collimator resolution, the number of stops per 360° rotation, the matrix size, and the shape and cutoff frequency of the reconstruction filter. In contrast to planar images, in which resolution is strongly depth dependent, SPECT resolution in rotating gamma camera tomographs is about the same in all locations in the 3D image matrix (6).

Note, however, that spatial resolution is not improved with SPECT compared to planar imaging. In fact, it is usually worse, at approximately 8 to 15 mm for SPECT vs 7 to 12 mm for planar, both highly collimator dependent. (Significantly better values for SPECT FWHM have recently been published using iterative reconstruction and attenuation correction, scatter compensation, and resolution recovery.) Resolution degradation is primarily due to the increased object–collimator distance and the increased noise. Further, reconstruction methods that reduce noise, such as filters with lower critical or cutoff frequencies, also degrade resolution (see Chapter 10). The loss of spatial resolution is, however, more than offset by the gain in *contrast resolution*, the ability to distinguish count differences in adjacent tissues. **Figure 11-3** illustrates the difference between the two types of resolution. The improved contrast resolution means that the degraded spatial resolution, while noticeable, does not impair our ability to detect lesions.

Sensitivity is generally not measured specifically for SPECT, but it is nonetheless the limiting factor for obtaining high-quality images. Many of the improvements in gamma cameras since about 1990 have been aimed at increasing system sensitivity. Advances include multihead cameras and collimators that maintain sensitivity while improving resolution, as well as Tc-99m-based radiopharmaceuticals

(a) Spatial resolution

Spatial resolution, measured in mm

Distance across image

(b) Contrast resolution

Contrast resolution, measured as a percentage of organ counts per voxel

Distance across image

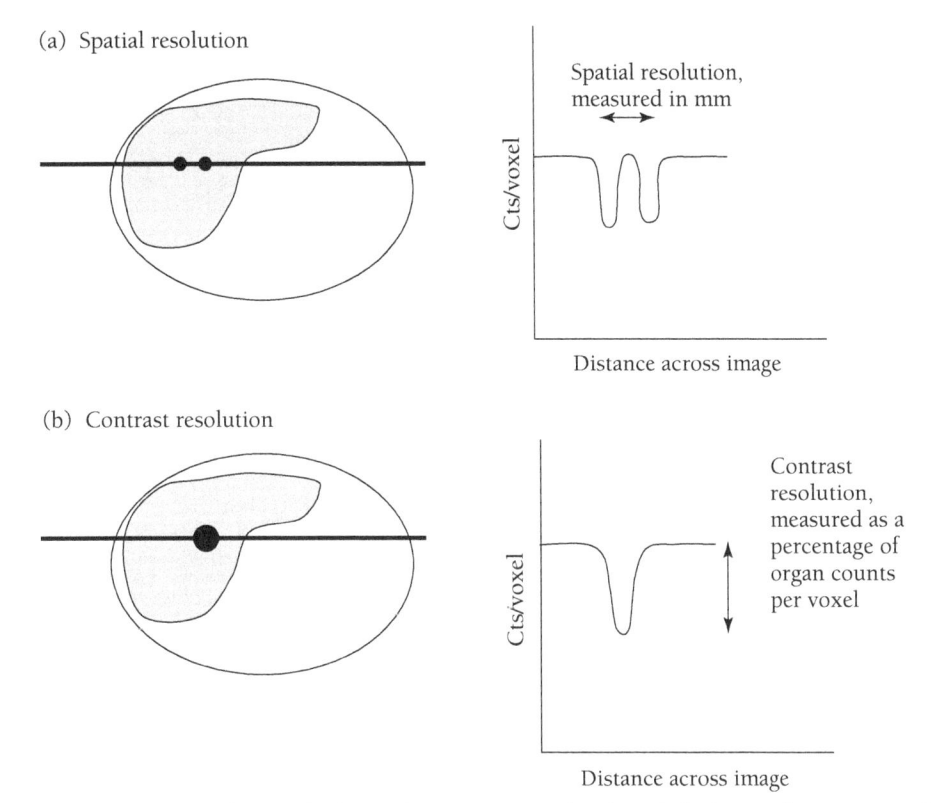

Figure 11-3 Spatial resolution vs contrast resolution. The figures show a transverse slice through the liver, with one or two cold lesions, and count profiles including those lesions. Spatial resolution (the horizontal double-headed arrow in Fig. 11-3a) is the ability to resolve two objects, and it is measured in distance units. Contrast resolution (the vertical double-headed arrow in Fig. 11-3b) is the ability to detect a lesion that has more or fewer counts than the surrounding tissues. It is measured as the relative count change from lesion to background. The power of SPECT lies in its ability to improve contrast resolution.

that have more gamma ray emissions and allow for higher radiopharmaceutical dosages. The goal of all these developments is to obtain adequate counts for the SPECT study within a time frame that is tolerable for most patients.

Effect of Acquisition Parameters

The quality of a SPECT study depends on factors that relate to acquisition, reconstruction, and display. Acquisition parameters are discussed in detail, because they have by far the greatest effect on image quality. Factors relating to reconstruction are covered in the next section. A summary of recommendations for improving image quality is provided in **Table 11-1**.

Choice of Collimator

Recall that the collimator is the limiting factor in planar imaging in terms of both resolution and sensitivity. SPECT further limits both total sensitivity (due to the limited imaging time) and resolution (which is degraded because the gamma camera must be farther away to clear the patient during the rotation). Therefore, the choice of collimator is crucial in maintaining both sensitivity and resolution in SPECT. Resolution is favored in this trade-off. In a phantom study using both high- and ultra-high-resolution collimators, a 2-mm improvement in resolution was found to be comparable, in terms of image quality, to an increase in counts by a factor of 2.5 to 3.4 (7).

One way to maintain resolution when imaging at a distance is to increase the hole length or bore of the collimator. In Appendix E, collimator resolution R_{coll} is shown to vary according to the formula

$$R_{coll} \approx \frac{d(L_e + b)}{L_e} \quad (11\text{-}2)$$

where d = hole diameter, L_e = effective hole length, and b = object–collimator distance. The most common way to improve collimator resolution is to decrease the hole diameter. But the effective hole length term L_e is in both the numerator and the denominator; its presence in the denominator indicates that resolution decreases (improves) as L_e increases (see Sample Calculation E-3). The net effect of a long-bore collimator is to diminish the degradation of resolution with depth, compared to a shorter-bore collimator. Many SPECT systems, particularly those with two or more detectors, have available "very high" or "ultrahigh" resolution collimators with long hole lengths for low-energy (Tc-99m) studies.

Slant-hole collimators represent a second option for minimizing the degrading effect of increased object–collimator distance. For example, a collimator with holes angled 30° from perpendicular can be used for brain SPECT, with the camera tilted 30° caudally (toward the feet), keeping the collimator holes perpendicular to the axis of rotation but avoiding the patient's shoulders (**Figure 11-4**).

Table 11-1

Improving Image Quality in SPECT

Desired Result	Ways to Bring About	Parameters to Change	Caveats/Trade-offs	References
Make image less grainy/noisy	Acquisition parameters	Fan-beam or cone-beam collimator	Smaller FOV	1, 4
		Longer time per frame	Patient motion	4
		Fewer stops (same total acquisition time)	Potential streak artifacts	4, 5
		Smaller matrix dimension (larger pixels)	Degraded resolution	6
	FBP reconstruction	Lower critical frequency or higher order	Loss of image sharpness/spatial resolution	1, 2, 3, 7
Make images less smooth	FBP reconstruction	Higher critical frequency or lower order	More noise/graininess in reconstructed images	1, 2, 3, 7
Improve spatial resolution	Acquisition parameters	Higher-resolution or long-bore collimator	Fewer counts; more noise in reconstructed images	1, 5
		Elliptical or body contour orbit	None	1, 5
		Larger matrix dimension (smaller pixels) or electronic zoom	Fewer counts per pixel on average	6
		More projections	Noise (if total acquisition time is not increased)	3
	FBP reconstruction	Higher critical frequency or lower order	More noise/graininess in reconstructed images	1

[1]Christian P, Waterstram-Rich K. *Nuclear Medicine Technology and PET/CT: Technology and Techniques.* 6th ed. St. Louis, MO: Saunders; 2007:276, 278, 285.
[2]Van Laere K, Koole M, Lemahieu I, Dierckx R. Image filtering in single-photon emission computed tomography: principles and applications. *Comput Med Imaging Graph.* 2001;25:127–133.
[3]Steves A, Wells P. *Review of Nuclear Medicine Technology.* 3rd ed. Reston, VA: Society of Nuclear Medicine; 2004:33.
[4]Ell PJ, Gambhir SS. *Nuclear Medicine in Clinical Diagnosis and Treatment.* Edinburgh, NY: Churchill Livingstone; 2004:1816.
[5]Wagner HN, Szabo Z, Buchanan JW, eds. *Principles of Nuclear Medicine.* 2nd ed. Philadelphia, PA: WB Saunders; 1995:332–338.
[6]Groch MW, Erwin WD. SPECT in the year 2000: basic principles. *J Nucl Med Technol.* 2000;28:233–244.
[7]Lee KH. *Computers in Nuclear Medicine: A Practical Approach.* 2nd ed. Reston, VA: Society of Nuclear Medicine; 2005:141–142.

The reduction in the radius of rotation leads to a significant improvement in resolution (8). The user must determine the exact detector angle that produces the best images (e.g., of a line source or a 3D phantom), because the actual slant angle may be different than the stated angle (1).

Focused collimators such as fan-beam and cone-beam collimators provide a third avenue to improved resolution in SPECT. They better utilize the large FOV of modern cameras for small organs such as the heart, thus increasing sensitivity, and they improve resolution by virtue of the magnification that they add. As with the long-bore collimator, they show less deterioration of resolution with increasing distance. The improvement with these collimators can be significant: for equal spatial resolution, sensitivity is increased as much as 50 to 100% over a parallel-hole collimator (9). Both fan-beam and cone-beam collimators require specific center-of-rotation corrections, careful evaluation of extrinsic field uniformity, and reconstruction algorithms specific to the individual collimator. For a fan-beam collimator, the focal length is used to correct for the collimator's varying magnification with depth, so it must be known precisely (10). Noncircular orbits are not allowed with fan-beam collimators (11).

Energy Window

The choice of energy window is a compromise between increasing total counts and not increasing the relative contribution of scatter. The usual best option is a 20% window centered on the photopeak of the radionuclide in question. When a radionuclide has multiple photopeaks, all should be used for SPECT studies to increase the total counts in the study. The use of an asymmetric energy window can produce significant nonuniformity, and are recommended for SPECT imaging only if all aspects of the system are tuned with the asymmetric window in mind.

Matrix Size

The options regarding matrix size are limited. A 32 × 32 matrix is too blocky to be acceptable, and a 256 × 256 matrix is unnecessarily fine. So we are left with only two choices: 64 × 64 or 128 × 128. But the decision of which to use is not trivial. Increasing the matrix dimension from

(a) Camera in anterior projection

(b) Camera in lateral projection

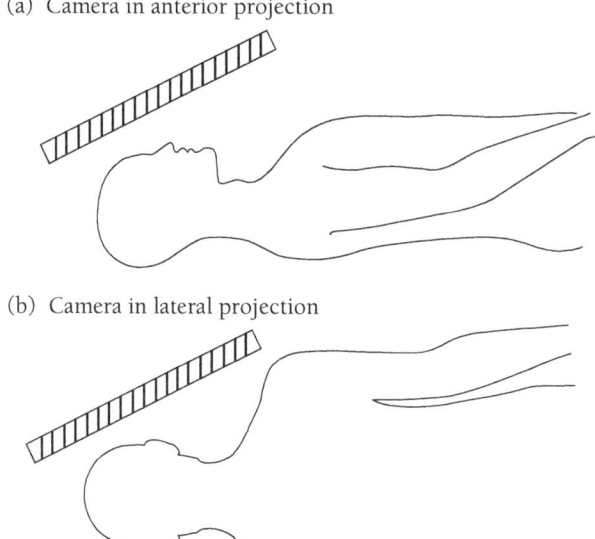

Figure 11-4 Use of a slant-hole collimator for brain SPECT. The slant-hole collimator allows for a tighter radius of rotation around the head by allowing the gamma camera to stay close to the brain while clearing the shoulders. Improvement in image quality is noticeable. However, the loss of spatial resolution is variable within tomographic slices, such that resolution is better at the superior aspect of the brain compared to the inferior aspect. This is so because the plane of equal resolution is parallel to the collimator face (see Chapter 7).

64 × 64 to 128 × 128 cuts the average count density in each projection by a factor of 4, and the percentage of noise in the reconstructed image matrix is estimated to increase by a factor of 3 (12). If a change from a 64 × 64 matrix to a 128 × 128 matrix is contemplated, either the acquisition time or the radiopharmaceutical dosage must be increased to compensate for the increased noise. In addition, the move from 64 × 64 to 128 × 128 quadruples computer space requirements.

Matrix dimension (also called *linear sampling*, referring to the number of ray-sums in a 2D count profile) is also closely related to spatial resolution. According to sampling theory, the sampling frequency must be at least twice the highest spatial frequency component in the image. In SPECT, we utilize only 64 × 64 or 128 × 128 matrix sizes. We must therefore turn the sampling theorem around to say that the sampling frequency (dictated by the matrix size) limits the spatial resolution achievable. If a gamma camera with a 38-cm field of view is used to image an object into a 64 × 64 matrix, the pixels are ostensibly 6 mm on a side. If, as the sampling theorem indicates, a minimum of 2 pixels is required to define an object, then the smallest object we can visualize is 12 mm. If we wish to see smaller lesions, we need to increase the sampling frequency, for example, by increasing the matrix dimension to 128 × 128, which allows us to visualize an object of 6 mm. One reference even suggests that 3 pixels rather than 2 are needed to define an object (12), but any pixel size smaller than one-third of the system FWHM is pointless and only serves to increase noise. The important point is to keep the matrix size consistent with the spatial resolution of the gamma camera and the size of the object(s) being imaged. Pixel size should never be the limiting factor in the system's spatial resolution.

Zoom

Electronic zoom factors may be used instead of focused collimators to improve resolution. The use of a zoom factor during acquisition effectively reduces the pixel size, such that a 64 × 64 matrix with a zoom factor of 2 is equivalent in terms of image resolution to a 128 × 128 matrix. In general, pixel dimension can be calculated based on the dimension of the FOV and the zoom factor (13):

$$\text{Pixel dimension} = \frac{\text{FOV dimension}}{zn} \quad (11\text{-}3)$$

where z is the zoom factor and n is the matrix dimension (64 or 128). Keep in mind, however, that the intrinsic resolution of the camera does not change, so electronic zoom will not have a significant impact on resolution beyond a zoom factor of about 2. Both the center of rotation and the flood field uniformity should be checked with the desired zoom factor applied. Before starting a zoomed acquisition, one must verify that all parts of the organ of interest are within the FOV at all angles.

Sample Calculation 11-1 Pixel Dimension of a Zoomed Image

A gamma camera is 45 cm in diameter, and a 1.25 zoom is applied to a set of images acquired in a 64 × 64 matrix. What is the size of the zoomed pixels?

Using Equation 11-3, we calculate the pixel dimension as

$$\text{Pixel dimension} = \frac{45 \text{ cm (FOV)}}{(1.25 \text{ zoom})(64 \text{ pixels})} = 0.56 \text{ cm}.$$

The zoom factor decreases the size of the pixels below the 0.70 cm they would be in this camera without the zoom.

Detector Orbit

This topic encompasses several subtopics. The first is the mode of rotation. SPECT systems usually offer two options: continuous and step-and-shoot. The step-and-shoot mode is easy to understand: With the gantry stationary, a projection is acquired into a single frame. When the acquisition of that projection ends, the gantry rotates to the next angle, and after it stops moving, a new projection is acquired. In continuous mode, as the name indicates, the gantry rotates continuously. The acquisition is set up as a dynamic planar study, in that counts are acquired into consecutive frames for a preset period of time. During that time, the gantry is moving, so some blurring occurs within each projection. This leads to a loss of resolution, particularly in the tangential direction (13). While this blurring in most cases is minimal, the step-and-shoot mode is more widely employed.

The second subtopic is the shape of the orbit. Early SPECT systems were only capable of circular orbits. A circular orbit by necessity has a larger object–collimator distance in the anterior and posterior projections compared to the lateral projections (**Figure 11-5**), because the body thickness is usually greater in the X direction than the Y direction. An elliptical orbit, in which the user specifies the long and short axes of the ellipse, brings the camera closer to the patient at many angles.

Even better is a body contour orbit, which follows the undulations of the patient's body. Early body contour orbits were generated by mapping the camera's orbit manually as the gamma camera made a quick pass around the patient prior to starting the acquisition. More recently, detection systems such as infrared sensors have been incorporated into collimators. Use of a body contour orbit can improve resolution by as much as 2.5 mm over a circular orbit (8). However, specific training in their proper use is necessary. For example, the corner of a bed sheet hanging off the imaging table is detected by an infrared system as an object to be avoided. When a zoom factor is used in conjunction with a noncircular orbit, some systems incorporate a roving image mask to keep a particular point in space at the center of each projection.

The third subtopic related to detector orbit is the total angle of rotation. Radon's original theory required views from angles all around the object, and most nuclear medicine studies adhere to this (**Figure 11-6** shows an example of why this is usually true). The lone exception is in imaging of the heart, specifically myocardial perfusion imaging, where there continues to be some controversy. Some argue that the heart lies so far to one side of the body that the information obtained from projections on the opposite side not only is unnecessary but may even be detrimental. Others suggest that the posterior wall of the myocardium is not adequately imaged in a 180° acquisition. The magnitude of these issues is different depending on the imaging radionuclide (Tl-201 vs Tc-99m). Phantom studies have shown quantifiable differences in uniformity and lesion detectability between the two orbits (14). Nonetheless, the most common choice for cardiac studies is a 180° orbit, because it allows for longer time per image (and thus less noisy images) within a tolerable imaging period. Virtually all other SPECT studies are done over 360°.

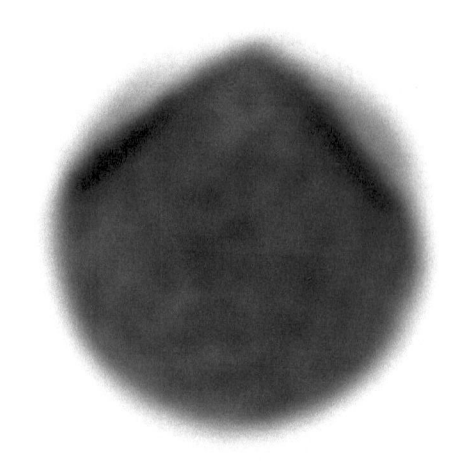

Figure 11-6 Acquisition through 180° of a cylindrical phantom. This is a single 2D slice through a 3D image matrix of a cylindrical phantom, following an acquisition over 180° using a gamma camera with two heads in a 90° configuration. The slice shows that the bottom half of the cylinder was imaged fully, but the top half clearly was not seen in one-half of the projections. Image courtesy of Virginia Mason Medical Center.

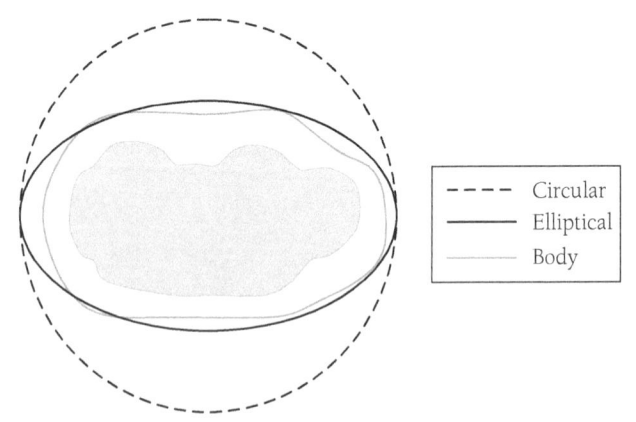

Figure 11-5 SPECT orbit choices. The figure shows a transaxial body slice at the level of the shoulders in a female patient whose left arm is raised over her head. A circular orbit that is large enough to clear the arms puts a significant distance between the collimator and the patient in the anterior and posterior projections. An elliptical orbit eliminates most of the distance, but a body contour orbit has the potential to do even better. Both the elliptical and contour orbits result in considerable improvement in image quality, because of the improved spatial resolution.

The final and most important subtopic of detector orbit is the number of projections, also called *angular sampling*. If we return to Radon's theory, an infinite number of projections are required to perfectly reproduce a 3D object. If time were not an issue, more projections would result in a better study. But in SPECT, time clearly is an issue. If more stops are acquired without increasing the total imaging time, then each stop has fewer total counts and therefore more noise. So trade-offs must be made.

On the other hand, using too few stops clearly decreases image quality (**Figure 11-7**). Not acquiring enough stops leads to reconstruction errors and streak artifacts, whether FBP or iterative reconstruction is used. In FBP in particular, the ramp filter removes excess counts around an area of increased activity. More projections mean more application of the ramp filter and therefore more subtraction of these backprojection rays. A good rule of thumb is that the angular sampling should at least equal the matrix size for these projections: 64 stops over 360° for a 64 × 64 matrix and 128 stops for a 128 × 128 matrix. If the count rate is high enough, a study with a 64 × 64 matrix may utilize 128 stops.

Time per Stop

It should be obvious by now that the time per stop must be chosen taking all of these factors into account. If counts

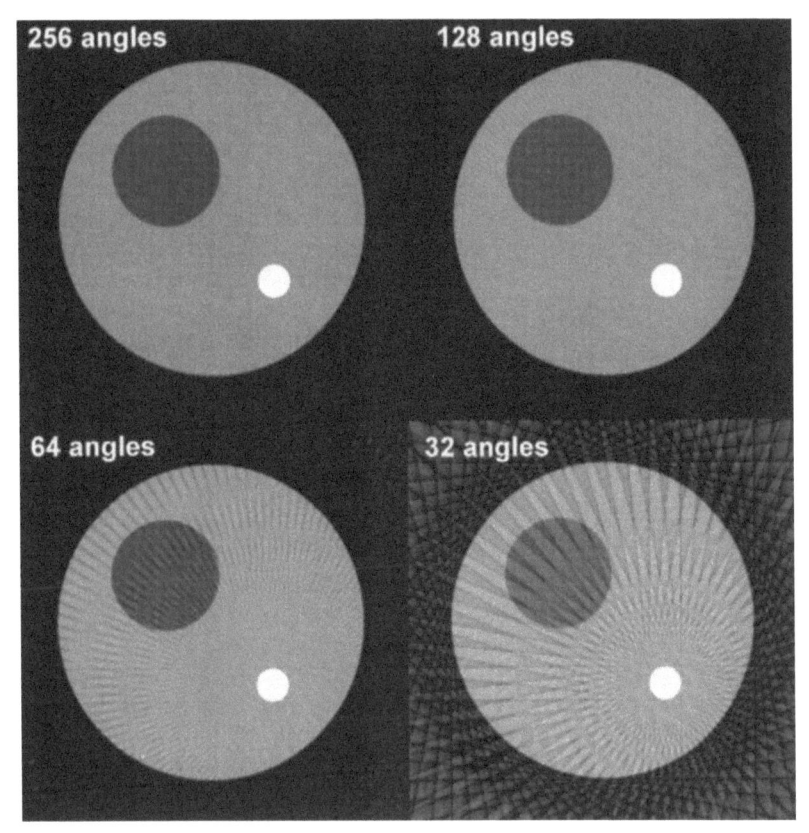

Figure 11-7 Effect of the number of projections on SPECT studies. These images are computer simulations showing how the number of projections acquired affects image quality. As the number of projections decreases, the cancellation effect of the filter in FBP is insufficient, so that the backprojection rays become more apparent. When iterative reconstruction is used, angular undersampling results in degradation of spatial resolution. Reprinted from: Cherry SR, Sorenson JA, Phelps ME. *Physics in Nuclear Medicine*. 3rd ed. Philadelphia, PA: Saunders; 2003:286. Used with permission from Elsevier Science.

are plentiful, the number of stops and the matrix size can be increased and the energy window narrowed to get better-quality information. But doing so is beneficial only if the patient can stay still. A practical maximum for most patients is 30 to 45 min; keep in mind that in step-and-shoot mode, the time the camera is rotating is added to the actual imaging time (time per stop times number of stops).

The difficulty of eliminating patient motion is made worse by the need to have one or both arms over the head in order to decrease the radius of rotation, as in cardiac studies. The technologist should make every effort to address issues of patient comfort prior to starting the study. Arm holders and pillows under the knees greatly increase patient comfort and thereby decrease motion. It is an instinctive reaction to turn one's head toward a person speaking, so when communicating with the patient during the study (e.g., to indicate the time remaining), one should first say, "Don't move." As mentioned previously, motion correction programs should be used when motion is evident.

Improving Image Quality after Acquisition

In planar imaging, improving image quality generally means repeating the acquisition. With SPECT, on the other hand, we have some ability to improve image appearance after acquisition, in the reconstruction process. Filtered backprojection in particular provides the option of altering the parameters of the filter and hence the resulting 3D image matrix. This puts greater importance on knowing the features of both normal and abnormal results for each SPECT study.

Filtered Backprojection

Recall the shape of the ramp filter multiplied by the roll-off filter (**Figure 11-8**). We can think of this graph as consisting of a graph of weighting factors. The Y value of the filter function in Figure 11-8 corresponds to the weight to be given to the image data with the corresponding frequency (the X value). Low-frequency components are given a low weight, because the backprojection process overrepresents them, leading to the $1/r$ blurring that impairs unfiltered backprojection. The weighting factors then increase with increasing frequency in the upsloping portion of the filter function. The highest weighting factors are ideally given to the middle-frequency region where the object detail lies. But image noise, which dominates the image power spectrum at high frequencies, must be given a low weighting factor to prevent it from making the 3D image matrix too grainy. So we use the roll-off filter to cause the filter function to decrease back to zero.

We can control the shape of the roll-off filter, and hence the overall shape of the filter function, by adjusting one or more variables in the mathematical function that

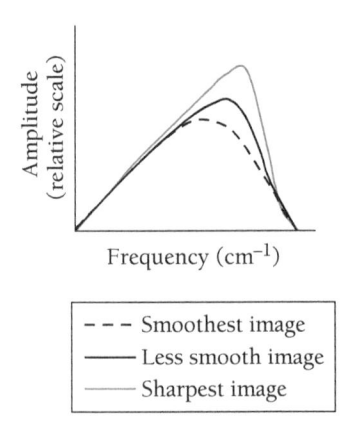

Figure 11-8 Filters for FBP reconstruction. The graph shows three filters. The one that peaks farthest to the right produces a 3D image matrix with more detail than the other two. The flattest of the three curves peaks farthest to the left, indicating that it keeps more low-frequency data and uses less high-frequency data, thus producing the smoothest 3D image matrix.

describes the roll-off filter. Such adjustments allow us to control where the filter returns to the X-axis and stops incorporating image data of high frequency. This in turn means that we can change the appearance of the resulting images from smooth to coarse and grainy. The Butterworth filter is used as the example, because it is the filter most commonly used in clinical practice.

For a given situation, count statistics are the primary determinant of the optimal filter (15). A grainy image has too much noise, either because the total counts are low or because the filter is not removing enough of the high-frequency part of the image data. We can only solve the problem of low counts by acquiring a new set of 2D projections for a longer time. But we can decrease the graininess by reducing the critical frequency of the Butterworth filter. This has the effect of reducing the contribution of high-frequency data, making the reconstructed 3D image matrix smoother. Conversely, reconstructed images that look too smooth can be made sharper by increasing the critical frequency, which leads to the inclusion of more high-frequency data, thus restoring some of the sharpness to the 3D image matrix.

The Butterworth filter has a second variable, the order (see Eq. 10-2 and Fig. 10-12), which controls the slope of the transition down to zero amplitude. We can adjust it as well: increasing the order makes the image less grainy, while decreasing the order increases the amount of detail seen. A change in order has much less effect on image appearance than a change in critical frequency; it is best used to "fine-tune" the filter after the critical frequency is optimized.

Artifacts Resulting from Filter Choices

All of the low-pass filters applied to SPECT images roll off smoothly to the X-axis of the amplitude–frequency graph. One might think that it would be better to define precisely the frequency at which the sharpness and noise are best balanced, and to use a filter with a value of 1 below that frequency and 0 above it. But this would create an oscillating artifact called *ringing*, also known as the Gibbs phenomenon (**Figure 11-9**). This artifact is attributable to the Fourier transformation process and cannot be eliminated; however, a more gradual roll-off of the low-pass filter minimizes it.

As we manipulate the roll-off filter to modify the 3D image matrix, we must be concerned about the Nyquist frequency. Recall that the Nyquist frequency represents an absolute maximum for incorporation of frequencies into the reconstruction process. The roll-off filter must therefore arrive at zero amplitude before the Nyquist frequency is reached. If a filter allows frequencies above the Nyquist to be used in the reconstruction, an artifact called *aliasing* results.

(a) Fourier transformation of a sharp edge

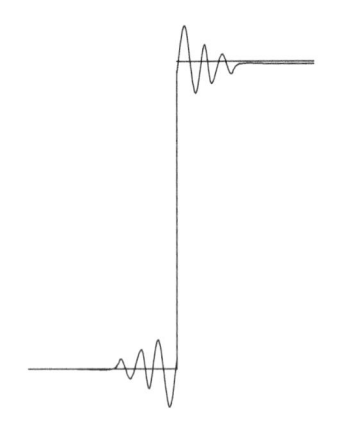

(b) Cylindrical phantom reconstructed using a Butterworth filter with low critical frequency and high order

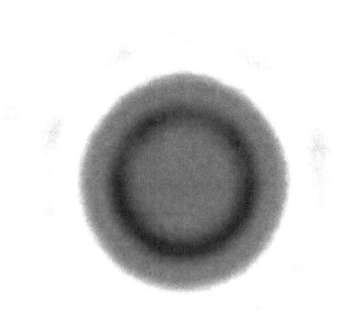

Figure 11-9 The ringing artifact or Gibbs phenomenon. Fourier transformation is inherently unable to perfectly represent sharp boundaries. Figure 11-9a shows a square wave, with the best possible Fourier transform superimposed on it. Very high-frequency sine waves are needed to accurately duplicate the square wave, but we are not allowed to use frequencies above the Nyquist limit. The result is an oscillating high–low pattern at the edge of the square wave. A similar effect is seen in the image of a uniform cylindrical phantom (Fig. 11-9b), reconstructed with a Butterworth filter using a combination of a low critical frequency and a high order. This effect is used to better show sharp boundaries in high-resolution modalities such as computed tomography; but in nuclear medicine, it is detrimental and should be avoided. Figure 11-9b courtesy of Virginia Mason Medical Center.

Aliasing occurs whenever a signal has a higher frequency than the highest sampling frequency. One commonly quoted example of aliasing occurs when bicycle spokes or a car's hubcaps appear to be rotating backward. In that situation, the brain preferentially visualizes the lowest frequency, preventing the eye from appreciating the higher frequency that is also present. **Figure 11-10** shows that in the imaging situation, aliasing is caused by a mismatch between the sampling frequency and the frequency of the data contained in the image. Because the sampling rate (the pixel size) is slower (larger) than the image frequency, an incorrect lower-frequency output signal is created, rather than the higher-frequency information that is actually present. The higher-frequency data are said to be aliased to the lower frequency, and the image is deprived of information at the higher frequency. Further, the false lower-frequency data are "folded back" into the reconstructed image, thus muddying the information at the lower frequency.

This artifact may be difficult or impossible to detect visually, so it is important to verify that the Nyquist frequency has not been exceeded by the low-pass filter. But this can be a challenge, because the X-axis of a filter graph can be given in several different units. True spatial frequencies are given in frequency units of cycles/cm or cycles/mm (usually given as cm^{-1} or mm^{-1}). Some computer programs express frequencies as cycles/pixel, in which case a mm/pixel conversion factor must be used to determine the actual spatial frequency. On this scale, the Nyquist frequency is always 0.5 cycle/pixel. Finally, the frequency axis may be expressed as a fraction of the Nyquist frequency. The variation in terminology makes understanding the graphical filter depiction that much more challenging.

The Nyquist frequency thus establishes an upper limit for frequencies that can be incorporated into an image in an FBP reconstruction. We need to ensure that the roll-off filter reaches zero amplitude below the Nyquist frequency, so that aliasing does not occur. Because the Nyquist frequency is inversely related to the pixel size, it is the pixel size that determines the maximum frequency that can be included in a SPECT reconstruction. Use of a smaller pixel size allows the incorporation of higher frequencies in the reconstruction.

Note that the interpreting physician usually makes the initial choice of filter for a given type of study, and the technologist may modify that choice, in order to obtain the best possible images of a particular patient. In some types of studies, filter parameters are kept the same for all patients. This is true of myocardial perfusion studies in which the patient's results are to be compared to a normal database. In other situations, the filter may be optimized on a patient-by-patient basis to generate the "best-looking" images. The latter situation requires close consultation between the nuclear medicine physician and the technologist, to ensure that both are using the same definition of "best-looking."

Iterative Reconstruction

The iterative reconstruction process does not provide nearly as much opportunity for manipulation as FBP. Most commercially available programs use the ordered-subsets expectation maximization (OSEM) algorithm to determine when convergence has been reached. It is possible to change the maximum number of iterations performed and to decide whether to apply a postreconstruction filter, but neither of these options is commonly employed to improve image appearance.

Image quality is affected in the forward-projection step of the iterative reconstruction process. Better corrections for attenuation, scatter, and depth-dependent resolution loss will generate a 3D image matrix that more accurately reflects the radiopharmaceutical biodistribution in the object being imaged. Concerted efforts have recently been made on this front, and impressive results have been reported. Experts in the field, as a general rule, believe that iterative algorithms employing these refined corrections have the potential to produce the best-quality SPECT images.

Summary

SPECT imaging provides significant improvement over planar imaging. Image contrast is up to six times better than planar images (13). Spatial resolution at depth (using FBP reconstruction) is about 8 to 15 mm, which, while not as good as planar images, when combined with the improved contrast resolution, yields much greater lesion detectability. This detection ability is further improved by the many additional display methods that can be applied to SPECT images. Since its arrival on the clinical scene in the early 1980s, SPECT has revolutionized the field of nuclear medicine.

But SPECT does not eliminate all of the liabilities of nuclear medicine imaging. The problem of resolution loss with distance is made worse by the need to rotate the gamma camera around the patient. Imaging times for each projection are shorter than would be used for equivalent

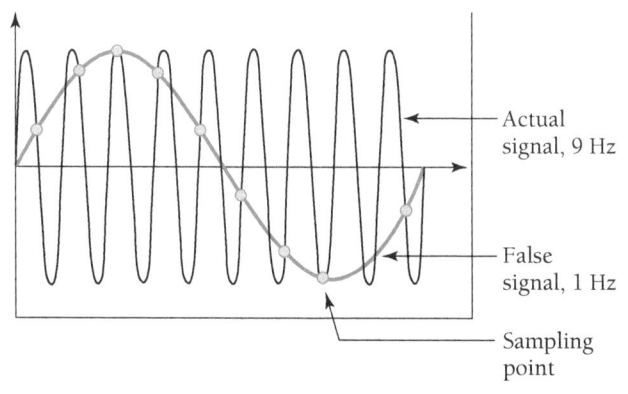

Figure 11-10 Illustration of aliasing. The thin line represents high-frequency data in the image, and the points represent the sampling information obtained by a system sampling at a lower frequency. The high-frequency data are lost because the system is not sampling at such a high frequency. The low-frequency sampling creates a false low-frequency signal (the thick line) that is not related to the high-frequency data being measured. Further, any good data in the output signal at the lower frequency are "muddied" by the addition of this aliased signal. Reprinted from: Lee K. *Computers in Nuclear Medicine: A Practical Approach*. 2nd ed. Reston, VA: Society of Nuclear Medicine; 2005:145, Fig. 11.21. Used with permission from the Society of Nuclear Medicine.

planar images, which increases the relative contribution of noise to each image and in turn leads to problems with reconstruction. And the partial volume effect, caused by the finite voxel size, interferes with our ability to see detail and to obtain quantitative information.

Moreover, all the advantages that SPECT brings can be destroyed by poor choices and inattention to detail. As can be seen from our discussion, every choice that can be made in terms of acquisition parameters will have multiple effects on the final images. Similarly, choices relating to reconstruction can cause significant detriment to the final result. Agreement between the technologist and the nuclear medicine physician on the desired result is vitally important. Many factors go into producing high-quality SPECT images. Ignoring any one of them could result in a subpar study, which in turn could lead to a critical misdiagnosis.

References

1. English RJ. *SPECT: A Primer*. 3rd ed. Reston, VA: Society of Nuclear Medicine; 1995:58, 160.
2. Soret M, Bacharach SL, Buvat I. Partial-volume effect in PET tumor imaging. *J Nucl Med*. 2007;48:932–945.
3. Jaszczak RJ, Whitehead FR, Lim CB, et al. Lesion detection with single-photon emission computed tomography (SPECT) compared to planar imaging. *J Nucl Med*. 1982;23:97–102.
4. Siegel JA, Benedetto AR, Jaszczak RJ, et al. AAPM Report No. 22: Rotating scintillation camera SPECT acceptance testing and quality control. New York, NY: American Association of Physicists in Medicine; 1987.
5. Graham LS, Fahey FH, Madsen MT, et al. AAPM Report No. 52: Quantitation of SPECT performance. Woodbury, NY: American Institute of Physics; 1995.
6. Miller TR. Emission tomography and image reconstruction. In: Fahey FH, Harkness BA, eds. *Basic Science of Nuclear Medicine* [CD-ROM]. Reston, VA: Society of Nuclear Medicine; 2001.
7. Fahey FH, Harkness BA, Keyes JW, et al. Sensitivity, resolution and image quality with a multi-head SPECT camera. *J Nucl Med*. 1992;33:1859–1863.
8. Heller SL, Goodwin PN. SPECT instrumentation: performance, lesion detection and recent innovations. *Semin Nucl Med*. 1987;17:154–199.
9. Tsui BMW, Zhao X, Frey EC, McCartney WH. Quantitative single-photon emission computed tomography: basics and clinical considerations. *Semin Nucl Med*. 1994;24:38–65.
10. Mahowald JL, Robins PD, O'Connor MK. The evaluation and calibration of fan-beam collimators. *Eur J Nucl Med*. 1999;26:314–319.
11. Wagner HN, Szabo Z, Buchanan JW, eds. *Principles of Nuclear Medicine*. 2nd ed. Philadelphia, PA: WB Saunders; 1995:337.
12. Cherry SR, Sorenson JA, Phelps ME. *Physics in Nuclear Medicine*. 3rd ed. Philadelphia, PA: Saunders. 2003:364.
13. Groch MW, Erwin WD. SPECT in the year 2000: basic principles. *J Nucl Med Technol*. 2000;28:233–244.
14. Liu YH, Lam PT, Sinusas AJ, Wackers FJTh. Differential effect of 180° and 360° acquisition orbits on the accuracy of SPECT imaging: quantitative evaluation in phantoms. *J Nucl Med*. 2002;43:1115–1124.
15. Lee KH. *Computers in Nuclear Medicine: A Practical Approach*. 2nd ed. Reston, VA: Society of Nuclear Medicine; 2005:141–142.

Additional Resources

Cherry SR, Sorenson JA, Phelps ME. *Physics in Nuclear Medicine*. 3rd ed. Philadelphia, PA: Saunders; 2003:Chapter 17.

English RJ. *SPECT: A Primer*. 3rd ed. Reston, VA: Society of Nuclear Medicine; 1995:Chapter 4.

Groch MW, Erwin WD. SPECT in the year 2000: basic principles. *J Nucl Med Technol*. 2000;28:233–244.

Heller SL, Goodwin PN. SPECT instrumentation: performance, lesion detection and recent innovations. *Semin Nucl Med*. 1987;17:154–199.

Lee KH. *Computers in Nuclear Medicine: A Practical Approach*. 2nd ed. Reston, VA: Society of Nuclear Medicine; 2005:Chapter 11.

Wagner HN, Szabo Z, Buchanan JW, eds. *Principles of Nuclear Medicine*. 2nd ed. Philadelphia, PA: WB Saunders; 1995:Chapter 18.

CHAPTER 12 — Improving SPECT Images

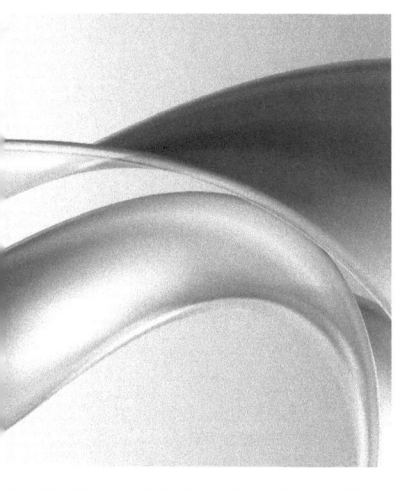

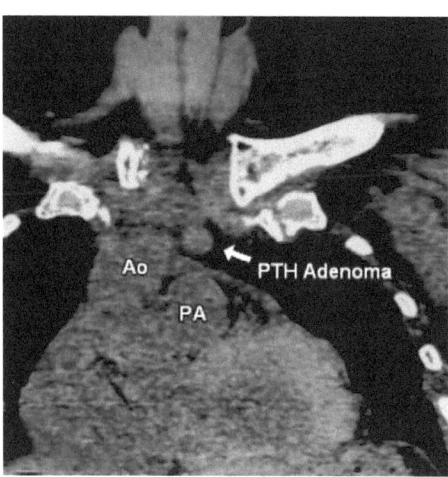

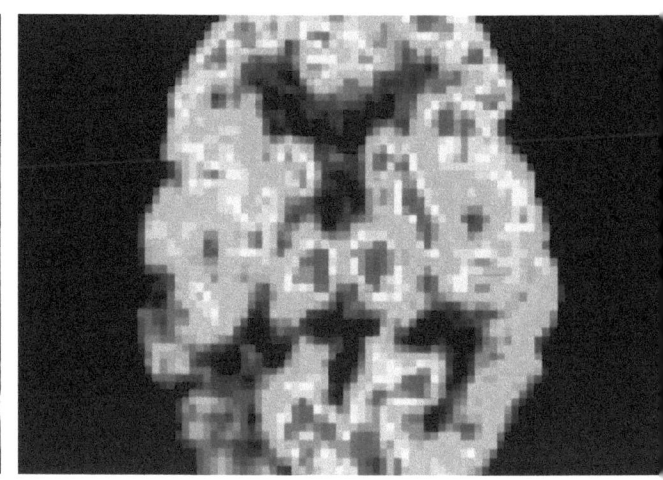

Learning Outcomes

1. Differentiate between narrow-beam and broad-beam geometries in photon attenuation, and discuss the effect on the measured linear attenuation coefficient.
2. Describe the process and limitations of Chang attenuation correction on reconstructed SPECT images.
3. Discuss the need for, methods used to obtain, and issues relating to patient-specific attenuation maps.
4. State why a daily reference scan is needed when transmission-based attenuation correction is used, and outline radiation safety aspects of Gd-153 rod sources.
5. Describe the concept behind image segmentation, and discuss the need for it in transmission-based attenuation correction.
6. Explain the importance of scatter compensation in the context of attenuation, and briefly describe methods used.
7. Discuss how resolution recovery and noise regularization can be addressed in iterative reconstruction.
8. Outline the clinical benefits of implementation of attenuation correction, scatter compensation, resolution recovery, and noise regularization.

Introduction

As myocardial perfusion studies have gained in popularity, the problem of gamma ray attenuation has become more of a concern. The objective of SPECT is to provide a 3D view of radiopharmaceutical distribution in the body. But if gamma rays coming from deep in the body are attenuated, they cannot contribute to the reconstructed image. The tomographic slices thus do not accurately represent the relative differences in activity between different parts of the body, which is the goal of the SPECT study.

Attenuation correction (AC) is therefore used to obtain a 3D image matrix that takes attenuation into account, thus more accurately reflecting the radioactivity distribution. Attenuation correction has been addressed in nuclear medicine in several ways. One possibility is to correct for attenuation mathematically, after reconstructing the 3D image matrix. Another method creates a patient-specific *attenuation map*, a separate 3D representation of the amount of attenuation occurring in each voxel. The end result of AC, whichever way it is accomplished, is to increase the count/voxel values relative to the amount of attenuation experienced by that voxel.

But if AC is done without consideration of scatter, we may simply be amplifying scatter counts rather than improving our images. Once we know how to correct for the effects of attenuation, we must also take into account scattered gamma rays and their effect on the image. So we will look at the methods used for *scatter compensation* (SC) and how they are applied.

We can also try to account for the degraded resolution that gamma cameras experience as the object–collimator distance increases. This is very important for SPECT imaging, because the rotating gamma camera must be at some distance from the patient's body. Internal organs are therefore even farther from the collimator in the SPECT situation than in planar imaging. *Resolution recovery* (RR) attempts to correct for the loss of resolution with distance.

Finally, the 2D projections used as the basis for SPECT studies are noisy, and noise interferes with image contrast in a significant way. *Noise regularization* (NR) can be incorporated into iterative reconstruction algorithms so that noise is suppressed, but without losing resolution (as happens in filtered backprojection). The camera vendors have put considerable effort into addressing the issues of AC, SC, RR, and NR, and all four are discussed in this chapter. In addition, we look briefly at some new cameras intended to optimize *myocardial perfusion imaging* (MPI).

Attenuation and Scatter

The physics definition of *attenuation* is "a phenomenon in which the amount of detected radiation is reduced by . . . scattering or absorption" (1, emphasis added). In other words, both photoelectric and Compton interactions cause attenuation of gamma rays, and in radiation detection (as opposed to imaging) situations, scattered gamma rays are usually excluded from measurement. **Figure 12-1a** illustrates this *narrow-beam geometry*, from which is derived the *attenuation equation*

$$I(x) = I(0)e^{-\mu_\ell x} \tag{12-1}$$

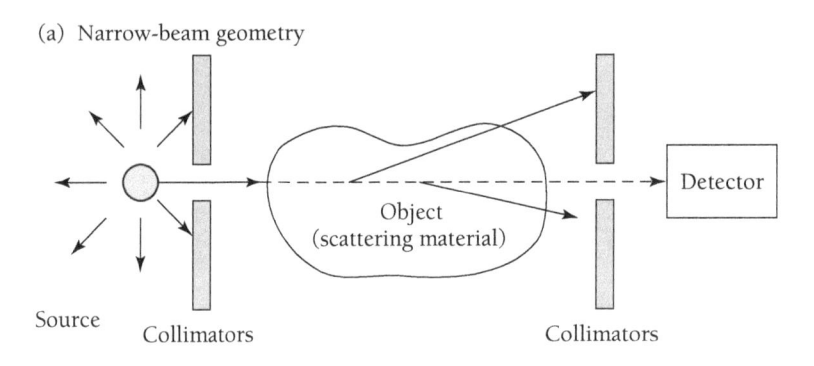

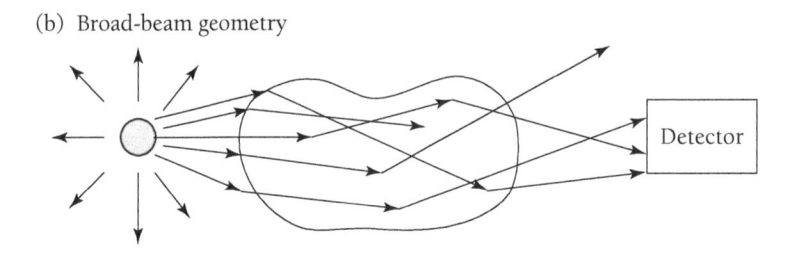

(a) Narrow-beam geometry

(b) Broad-beam geometry

(c) Photon transmission in narrow- and broad-beam situations

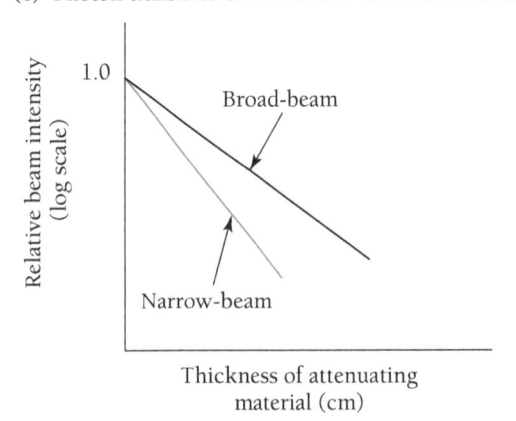

Figure 12-1 Narrow- vs broad-beam geometry. In the narrow-beam situation (Fig. 12-1a), solid collimators both before and after the attenuating object absorb photons traveling in directions other than directly toward the detector. The broad-beam situation (Fig. 12-1b) removes both sets of collimators, allowing measurement of all photons that reach the detector, not just those traveling in a direct path. The increase can be expressed with an effective attenuation coefficient (Eq. 12-2). Figure 12-1c shows the relative strength of the attenuated photon beam as the thickness of the attenuating material increases in the two situations.

Chapter 12: Improving SPECT Images

where *I* is the beam intensity (e.g., counts per unit time), measured either with no attenuating material present ($I(0)$) or with *x*-cm thickness of attenuating material present ($I(x)$). The value for the linear attenuation coefficient μ_ℓ depends on the energy of the photons in the beam, for the most part decreasing as energy increases. It varies also with the composition of the absorbing material. Tabulated μ_ℓ values are determined under conditions of narrow-beam geometry, such that scattered photons are not registered.

But this is not what happens in real life. Figure 12-1b shows the more realistic setting of *broad-beam geometry*. Typically, gamma rays in the energy range used in nuclear medicine are more likely to undergo Compton scattering interactions than photoelectric absorption in human tissue. These interactions produce secondary gamma rays whose direction of travel is different than that of the original gamma ray. We would ideally be able to identify and exclude scattered gamma rays based on their loss of energy. But Compton scattering most often results in small scattering angles, such that many scattered gamma rays still have energies that are within the energy window. Therefore, the actual radiation intensity in the broad-beam situation is greater than the attenuation equation predicts.

One way to account for this discrepancy would be to include a multiplicative build-up factor in the attenuation calculation to account for the scattered gamma rays. Alternatively, we can determine an effective value for the linear attenuation coefficient (μ_{eff}) that takes broad-beam geometry into consideration:

$$I(x) = I(0) e^{-\mu_{\text{eff}} x} \qquad (12\text{-}2)$$

The linear attenuation coefficient for 140-keV gamma rays in water decreases from 0.15/cm under narrow-beam conditions to about 0.12/cm when broad-beam conditions are assumed. Figure 12-1c shows graphically the relationship between attenuation and absorbing material thickness in narrow-beam and broad-beam geometries.

The situation in gamma camera imaging is more similar to broad-beam than narrow-beam geometry. Gamma rays absorbed in photoelectric interactions are lost to the image, decreasing the total number of counts. Scattered gamma rays are even worse than attenuated gamma rays from the imaging standpoint, because they are registered in a different location than they were emitted, and thus degrade spatial resolution and image contrast. Some 20 to 50% of total counts in a SPECT study are scattered gamma rays.

Note that the magnitudes of both absorption and scatter change with depth and with the composition of the scattering material (**Figure 12-2**). In addition, as gamma rays travel through an attenuating material, more low-energy gamma rays are absorbed than high-energy gamma rays (a phenomenon called *beam hardening*), so that the energy composition of the photon beam changes as it is attenuated. Thus, if we are to take attenuation and scatter into account in the context of SPECT imaging, we must consider

- the path length a photon must travel to reach the camera;
- the types of tissues that lie along the path;

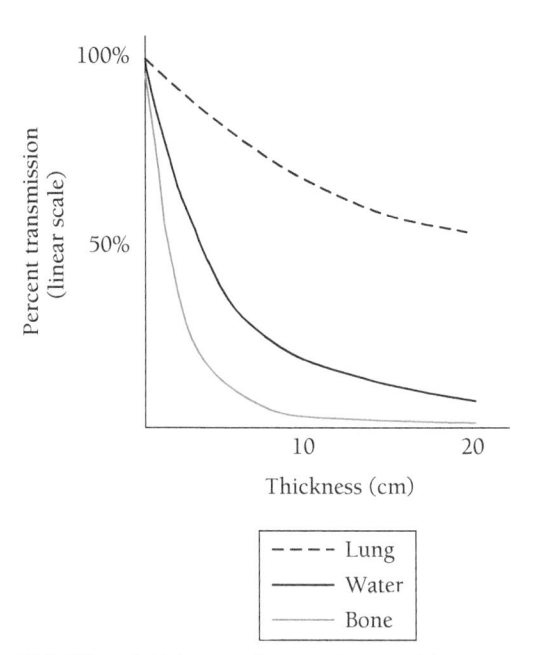

Figure 12-2 Effect of thickness and attenuating material on transmission of 140-keV gamma rays. The graph illustrates the different attenuation properties of several tissue types (with water standing in for soft tissue) under narrow-beam conditions. The large differences in attenuation between bone, soft tissue, and lung make the application of a single attenuation coefficient inappropriate in the thorax. Reprinted from: Zaidi H, Hasegawa B. Determination of the attenuation map in emission tomography. *J Nucl Med*. 2003;44:291–315, Fig. 2. With permission from the Society of Nuclear Medicine.

- the broad-beam attenuation properties of those tissues; and
- the change in beam hardness and the consequent changes in attenuation properties of the tissues.

Finally, consider that these values are not constant but variable (and considerably so) from patient to patient and from projection angle to projection angle (**Figure 12-3**).

The last aspect to touch on before discussing correction methods is the effect of distance. We already know that gamma cameras demonstrate degradation of spatial

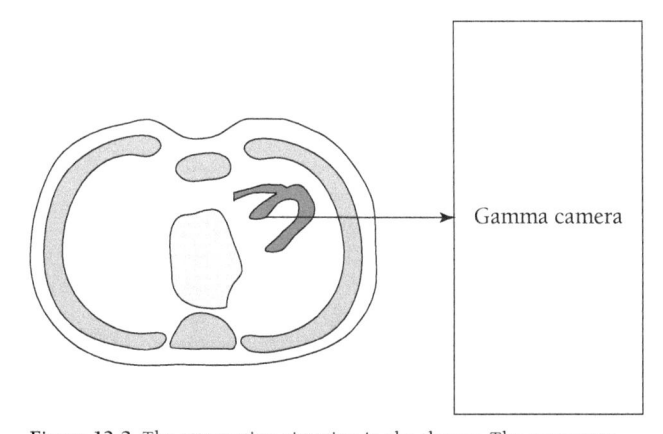

Figure 12-3 The attenuation situation in the thorax. The transverse cross section shows a slice through the body at the level of the heart. A gamma ray originating in the septal wall of the heart must pass through blood, myocardial muscle, lung, rib, soft tissue (potentially including both muscle and fat), and air before arriving at the gamma camera. The thickness of each type of tissue will differ from patient to patient.

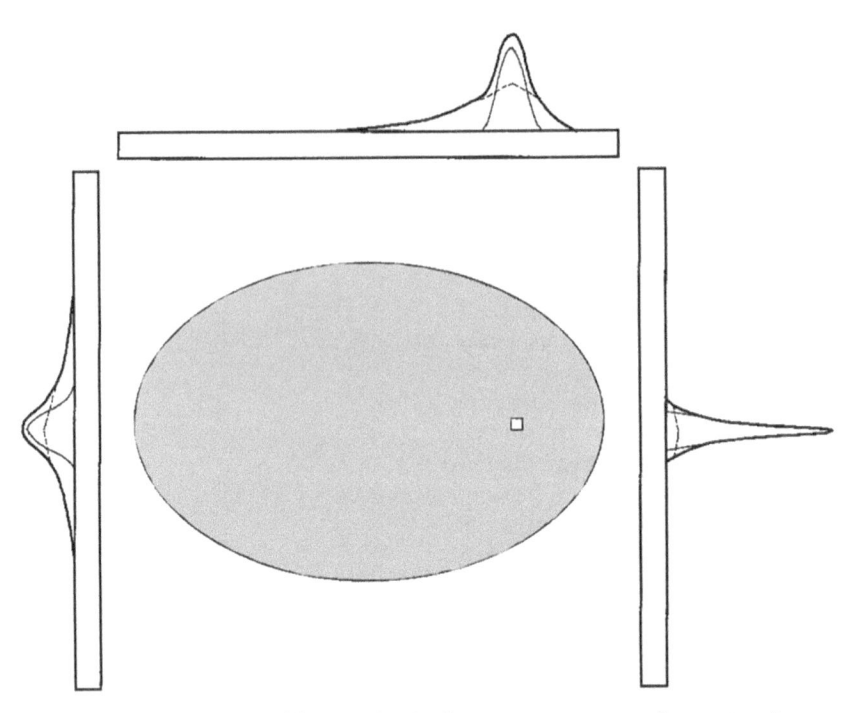

Figure 12-4 Effect of depth and scatter on the point-spread function (PSF) relative to an asymmetrically positioned point source within a scattering medium. The point source (the small square) is located on the left side of the transverse slice of the (nonradioactive) object. The geometric (thin solid line), scatter (dashed line), and total (thick solid line) PSFs at three acquisition angles are shown. The PSFs illustrate several important points: (1) the geometric PSF varies significantly with distance, (2) the contribution of scatter is highly variable, and (3) the scatter PSF is not symmetric. All three factors lead to significant degradation of resolution depending on the source's location in the object in SPECT studies. Reprinted from: Henkin RE, Boles MA, Dillehay GL, et al. *Nuclear Medicine*. St. Louis, MO: Mosby-Year Book; 1996: Fig. 22-3. Used with permission from Elsevier Science.

resolution with distance. In SPECT, each projection sees a given point of activity at a different depth, so that the width of the count profile (e.g., from a point source) varies from angle to angle (**Figure 12-4**). Scatter not only widens the response function further, but also makes it asymmetric (see, for example, the top count profile of Fig. 12-4). Of course, these response functions are not smooth curves as are shown, but rather digitized points with considerable noise fraction. Thus, correction methods would ideally correct for not only attenuation and scatter but also the variation in detector response with depth and the presence of noise, as all four are intertwined.

Chang Attenuation Correction

The method of AC most commonly applied to images reconstructed with filtered backprojection (FBP) is that proposed by Chang in 1978 (2). It only attempts to account for attenuation of gamma rays in a homogeneous medium and does not consider issues of scatter and detector response. In this method, the 2D projections are first reconstructed into a 3D image matrix. The operator then defines the body contour, usually by drawing a tight ellipse around one or more transverse slices. Count threshold methods may also be used to determine the body contour.

The computer then calculates an average *attenuation correction factor* (ACF) for each voxel, based on the voxel's average distance to the ellipse. (We do not need to include the distance from the ellipse to the camera face, because this is assumed to be air and have minimal attenuation.) Most Chang programs calculate the average ACF using about 15 evenly spaced projections and an effective attenuation coefficient value appropriate to soft tissue attenuation. Each voxel is then multiplied by its ACF to create the attenuation-corrected 3D image matrix. The mathematics of Chang-type attenuation correction is illustrated in **Figure 12-5**, and the results for a cylindrical phantom are illustrated in **Figure 12-6**.

As shown, and as usually applied, the Chang method utilizes only a single value for the attenuation coefficient. Thus, there is an underlying assumption that the attenuating tissue is of uniform (soft-tissue) composition. This assumption is reasonably true in some parts of the body, such as the brain and the abdomen. When the assumption of uniform attenuation is not met, the Chang method produces artifacts that are at least as objectionable as those caused by the attenuation in the first place. And attenuation is certainly not uniform in the region of the heart, where bone, lungs, airways, and soft tissues may all be found. It is this confluence of tissue types that has motivated the attempt to find ways to measure attenuation and to incorporate that information into image reconstruction.

Patient-Specific Attenuation Maps

The issue of attenuation in the chest in MPI, as illustrated in Figure 12-3, can be alternatively addressed by creating an attenuation map of the area being imaged. If we consider the attenuation equation as applied to the transmission of an external beam of photons through a large object

Projection t

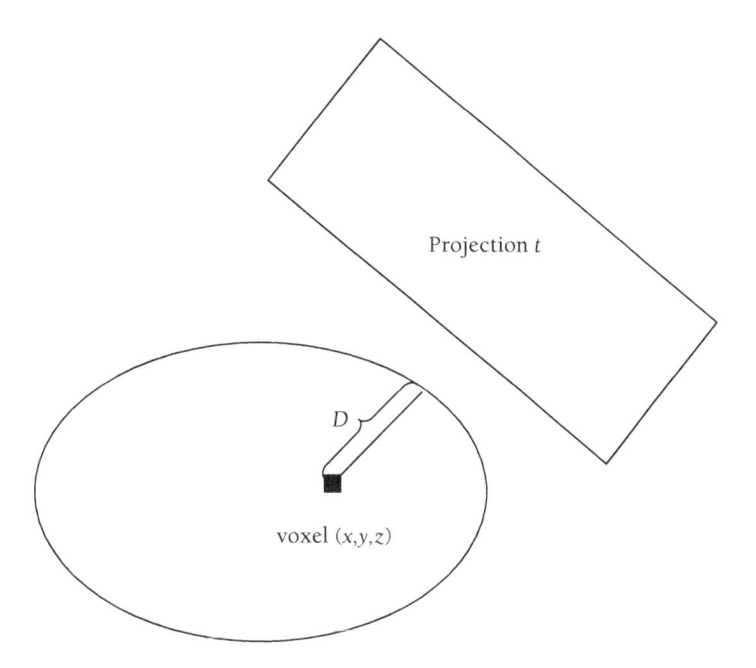

D = distance to edge of ellipse from voxel (x,y,z) at projection angle t.

D_{avg} = average distance from voxel (x,y,z) to edge of the ellipse, measured at 10 to 15 angles and converted to mm using the camera's pixel size calibration factor.

$$\text{Corrected counts in voxel } (x,y,z) \text{ for projection angle } t = \frac{\text{reconstructed cts in voxel } (x,y,z)}{e^{-\mu_{\text{eff}}D}}.$$

$$\text{Corrected counts in voxel } (x,y,z) = \frac{\text{reconstructed cts in voxel } (x,y,z)}{e^{-\mu_{\text{eff}}D_{avg}}}.$$

Figure 12-5 Mathematics of the Chang attenuation correction method. The correction factor for an individual voxel in a given projection angle t is equal to the effective attenuation of the tissue between the voxel and the edge of the ellipse, in a direction perpendicular to the projection t (with μ_{eff} defined as in Eq. 12-2). For each voxel, the average of the distance from the voxel to the ellipse is incorporated into the attenuation correction factor. An up-to-date pixel size calibration factor is required to convert from voxels to mm. The average distance may be calculated using all projection angles or only 10 to 15 equally spaced projections.

(Eq. 12-1), we can consider the attenuation factor $e^{-\mu x}$ as being composed of many small Δx segments, each with its own linear attenuation coefficient μ_ℓ:

$$I(x) = I(0) \sum_{\Delta x} e^{-\mu_\ell \Delta x}. \qquad (12\text{-}3)$$

If we measure $I(0)$ with no attenuating material present and $I(x)$ with attenuating material present, from a number of different angles, then we can reconstruct the linear attenuation coefficient of each small volume element. This is exactly what CT scanning depicts; in application to SPECT imaging this equation is used to create the attenuation map. If this map can then be applied to a SPECT emission data set, we can use it to correct for attenuation that the emission gamma rays would experience. The common term for this type of AC is *transmission-based AC* (TBAC).

Options

Transmission scanning requires an external radiation source, and both x-ray and radionuclide sources have been used. We concentrate for the moment on the latter. We must first decide whether the transmission (attenuation map) and emission (radiopharmaceutical biodistribution) scans are to be acquired simultaneously or sequentially. A sequential protocol (usually transmission followed by emission) allows use of the same radionuclide for both, thus eliminating an energy correction step. But sequential protocols have one very large drawback, in that they generally require the emission acquisition to follow immediately after the transmission acquisition. Because many nuclear medicine radiopharmaceuticals require some delay between injection and imaging, sequential protocols are not very practical. Simultaneous acquisition of both transmission and emission data is the more popular choice.

Radionuclide Choice

The use of a simultaneous acquisition process then dictates that the transmission radionuclide must be distinguishable from the emission radionuclide. A common choice is Gd-153 because it can be used as a transmission source for both Tc-99m (140 keV) and Tl-201 (80, 135, and 167 keV). To use the transmission data generated by Gd-153, one must correct its measured attenuation (usually in a window around 100 keV; its two photopeaks are at 99 and 103 keV) to the expected attenuation at the emission radionuclide energy or energies. One must also correct for cross talk between the transmission and emission windows. When Gd-153 is used as the transmission source and Tc-99m as the emission radionuclide, scattered Tc-99m gamma rays will be counted in the Gd-153 window.

(a) Not corrected

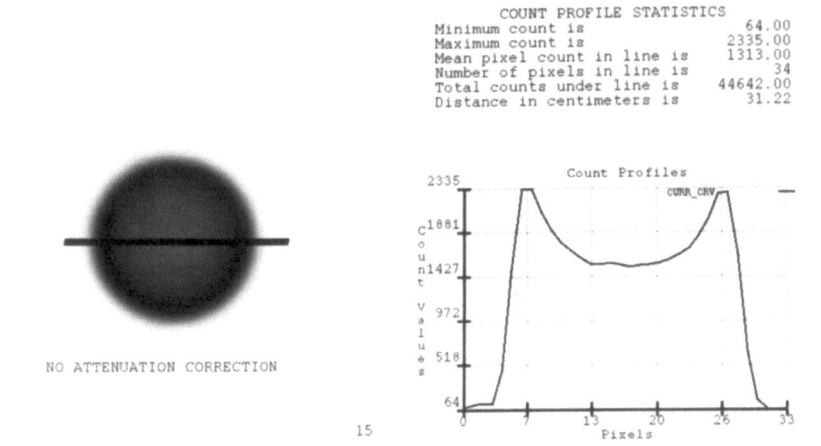

(b) Corrected with $\mu_\ell = 0.15/\text{cm}$

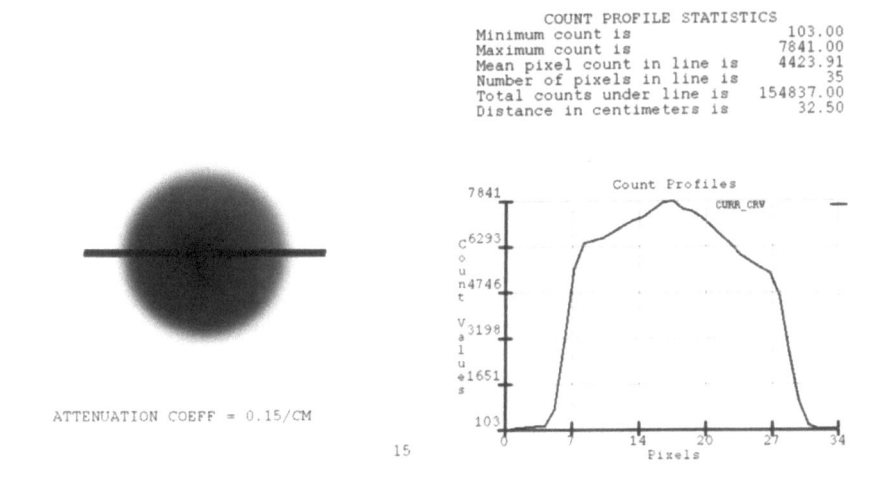

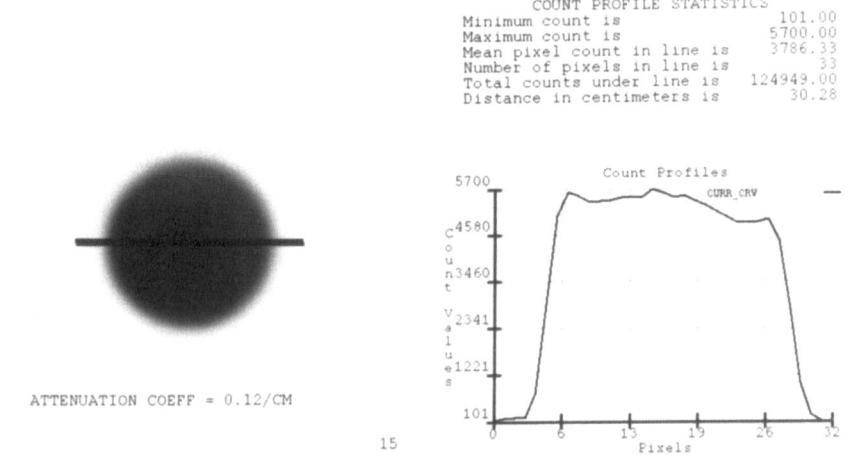

(c) Corrected with $\mu_{\text{eff}} = 0.12/\text{cm}$

Figure 12-6 Mathematical correction for attenuation in a uniform cylindrical phantom. A cylindrical phantom filled with radioactivity is reconstructed with (a) no attenuation correction, (b) Chang attenuation correction with $\mu_\ell = 0.15/\text{cm}$, and (c) Chang attenuation correction with $\mu_{\text{eff}} = 0.12/\text{cm}$. Accompanying count profiles through the center of the phantom are shown for each situation. Note the hot rim on the uncorrected slice and the overcorrection with $\mu_\ell = 0.15/\text{cm}$ (the narrow-beam attenuation coefficient for water at 140 keV). Use of 0.12/cm (the effective linear attenuation coefficient, taking broad-beam geometry into account) gives the flattest count profile, but it is still not completely flat. Images courtesy of Virginia Mason Medical Center.

These must be subtracted from the transmission window counts, or the measured attenuation will be less than the actual attenuation. A separate energy window set between the transmission and emission energies provides the raw data for this correction.

Source Geometry

We must then determine how the source will be placed relative to the patient and the camera head(s). Several different geometries have been proposed; two of the most common are illustrated in **Figure 12-7**. The geometry shown in Figure 12-7a has an inherent advantage, in that one camera head is devoted to the transmission image at all times; however, a triple-head camera is required and a 360° rotation must be performed to obtain a complete set of transmission and emission projections.

The arrangement shown in Figures 12-7b and 12-7c is the most popular at this time, specifically for myocardial perfusion imaging, which is commonly done with a 180° rotation. The line sources move across the FOV of the camera head on the opposite side of the patient. A sliding image window moves across the FOV in tandem with the line source, such that events falling in the Gd-153 energy window are registered only in this image window. The system uses the remainder of the FOV to acquire events in the emission energy window (and also in a scatter window positioned between the emission and transmission energies, in most acquisition programs). The line-source motion is timed to finish just before the emission image. Note that this geometric arrangement is possible only with two camera heads oriented at a 90° angle relative to each other.

The Reference Scan

When a radionuclide source for TBAC is used, a *reference scan* must be obtained. The reference scan is simply an image made using the transmission source (as it moves across the face of the camera for the arrangement in Fig. 12-7b), with nothing in the FOV, not even the imaging bed. The reference scan is acquired using the energy window(s) of the emission radionuclide. If more than one emission radionuclide is to be used, as in dual-isotope myocardial perfusion imaging, there must be a reference scan for each radionuclide's energy window.

The reference scan serves several important purposes. First, it verifies the proper operation of the transmission scanning system. Second, it corrects for attenuation of the source housing. Transmission-source housing usually has several struts supporting the line source itself; these should not be counted as attenuation in patient studies. Third and most important, the reference scan provides $I(0)$ for Equation 12-3. As the radionuclide source decays, $I(0)$ must reflect the decrease in activity, or the calculated attenuation will be falsely high. The reference scan must therefore be acquired each day and archived along with the day's clinical studies employing TBAC. **Figure 12-8** shows an example reference scan.

Characteristics of Attenuation Maps

The transmission projections obtained in a patient study are converted to attenuation coefficient values using Equation 12-3 and then reconstructed into the *attenuation map*, a 3D image matrix in which the intensity of each voxel reflects the degree of attenuation in that part of the body. **Figure 12-9** shows transverse slices of attenuation maps from several patients. As described previously, lungs attenuate only slightly, so they are given a very low intensity. Soft tissue attenuates more, and bone still more, so they are given higher intensities. Note also how noisy these reconstructed images are. Noise depends in part on patient size, and diversity of size (and hence diversity in amount of noise) is apparent even in this small group of six patients.

Noise in transmission images is also related to the strength of the transmission source. Radionuclide sources decay over time; Gd-153 has a half-life of 242 days. To maximize the source's useful life, it may start at a higher activity than the camera can handle because of dead time. It may therefore initially require shielding of some kind. As the source decays, the shielding is removed to maintain the photon flux at an adequate level. Eventually, the source will need to be replaced.

At all times, the amount of noise in the attenuation map is driven by the transmission projections with the lowest counts. A low-count, too noisy attenuation map will introduce errors into the attenuation-corrected emission images. One way to address the adequacy of the transmission scan for a given patient is to use the camera's information density parameter. The system estimates the transmission count density through the patient and reports the time per stop needed to achieve a minimally acceptable transmission scan. When the time exceeds a maximum, indicating that the count density generated by the source is no longer adequate, it is time to install a new transmission source. The department's budget needs to include funding for source replacement, so that the count density in the transmission projections will be adequate at all times.

The issue of noise in the attenuation map can be managed using a technique called *image segmentation*. Rather than trying to define a specific attenuation coefficient for each voxel, the attenuation map is segmented into a few different types of tissues, and known attenuation coefficients are applied to these regions. In the thorax, the different tissues include bone, soft tissue, and lungs. Rather than a detailed attenuation map, all we really need is a patient-specific delineation of these three types of tissues. This approach has been shown to greatly reduce the error due to the noise characteristics of radionuclide-generated attenuation maps (3).

Radiation Safety Aspects of Transmission Imaging

The radiation safety considerations for TBAC are not insignificant. The use of line sources results in patient exposure of 0.4 to 25 millirem (mrem) (4–250 microsieverts [μSv]) depending on the type of study (3). This

(a) Stationary line source

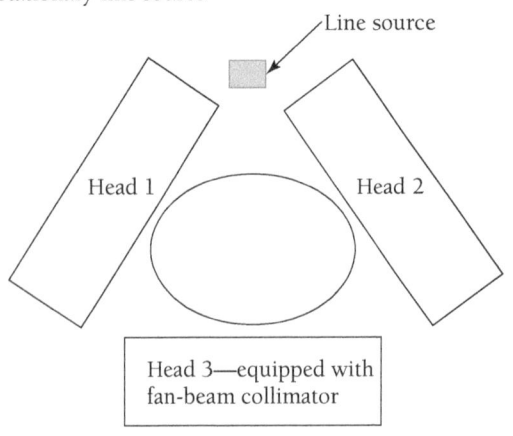

(b) Moving line source

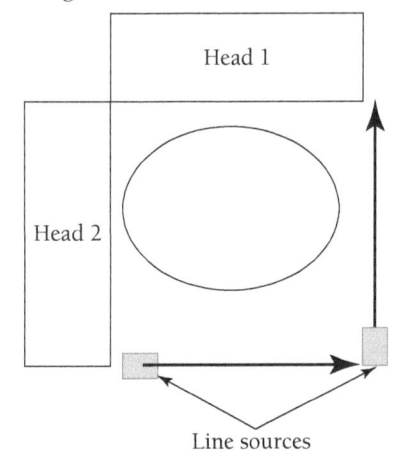

(c) Commercially available system using moving line sources

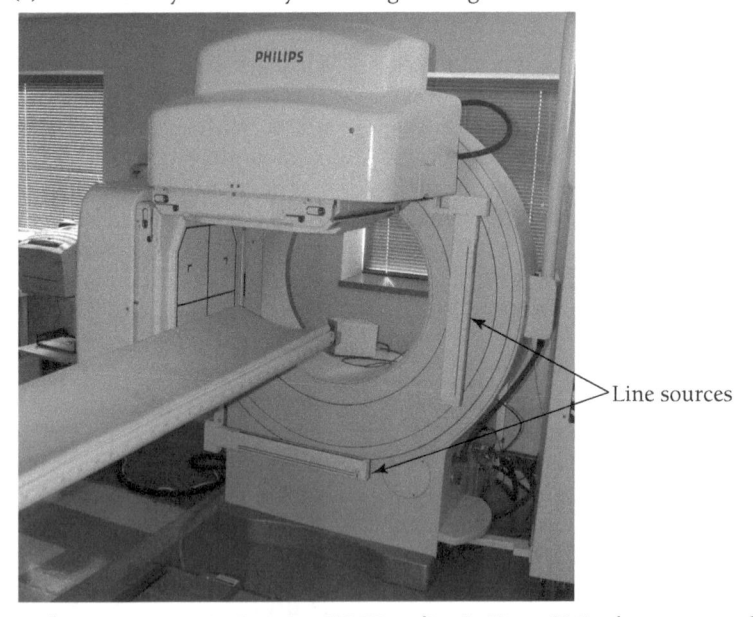

Figure 12-7 Geometries used for simultaneous transmission/emission SPECT studies. In Figure 12-7a, the two camera heads on either side of the line source collect emission images, while the camera head opposite the line source collects the transmission image. This third head must be equipped with a fan-beam collimator in order to register counts through the entire side-to-side width of the object. In the geometry shown in Figure 12-7b, each line source moves across the FOV of the camera head opposite it, crossing it one time during each projection (heavy arrows). An electronic image window moves in tandem with the line source and collects counts at the transmission radionuclide energy. The remainder of the FOV collects counts at the emission energy and in a scatter window between the emission and transmission energies. An example of this implementation of TBAC is shown in Figure. 12-7c. The geometry of Figure 12-7a requires a three-head camera and a 360° orbit, whereas that of Figure 12-7b is employed with a two-head camera and a 180° orbit. Figure 12-7c courtesy of Philips Healthcare.

Figure 12-8 Gadolinium-153 reference scan. A reference scan for each line source must be acquired each day the line sources are used for clinical studies and for each radionuclide energy window used. The reference scan supplies the $I(0)$ value for measuring attenuation in patients. It also verifies that the line-source system is working properly and corrects for attenuation of the source housing and supporting struts. The struts can be seen as slightly photopenic, widely spaced vertical "bars" in the reference scan. Image courtesy of Swedish Medical Center.

is small in relation to the dose equivalent received from the emission radiopharmaceutical, which is on the order of 10 to 15 mSv.

Gd-153 line sources have activity in the neighborhood of 200 to 250 mCi (7.4–9.2 GBq) when new. This radionuclide has K-shell characteristic x-rays of 40 to 50 keV, which do not contribute to the transmission projections, so the line sources are shielded with copper to absorb them. Even so, the exposure rate from the shielded line source may be as high as 0.2 mR/hr, which is an order of magnitude greater than background radiation levels in most areas. The personnel operating the transmission-source-equipped tomograph should therefore be aware of the increased potential for radiation exposure. The department's radioactive materials license may require changes to accommodate the high source activity, and sealed-source inventory and wipe testing are required.

CT-Generated Attenuation Maps

Several manufacturers have incorporated CT tomographs in tandem with SPECT tomographs. The transmission scan must be acquired separately from the emission scan (i.e., sequential rather than simultaneous acquisition), but in most configurations, the imaging table simply slides from one tomograph to the other, limiting the misregistration problems of sequential protocols. The linear attenuation coefficients obtained by CT scanning must be corrected to match the energy of the emission radionuclide; this correction will vary with the CT acquisition protocol. The CT image may then be segmented into a few tissue types. A high-quality CT system has spatial resolution far greater than that of a gamma camera, so the matrix is downsampled (e.g., from 512 × 512 to 128 × 128). The radiation dose to the patient from a low-level CT scan (obtained only

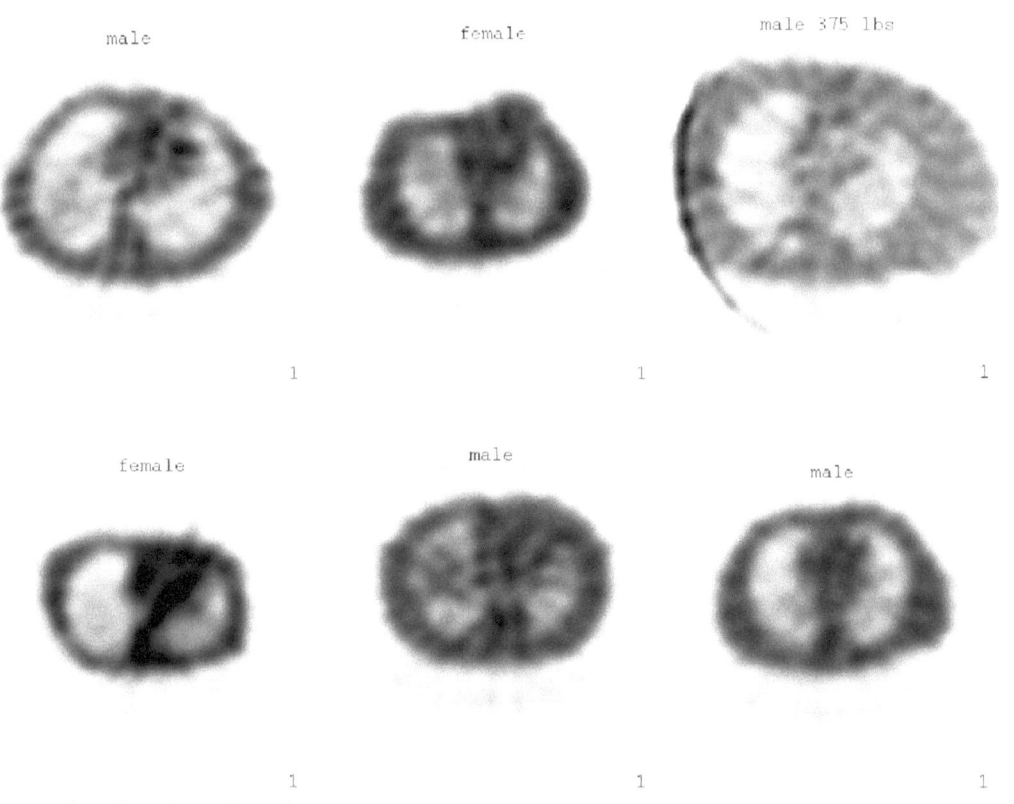

Figure 12-9 Transverse slices through the thorax from 3D attenuation maps of several patients, obtained using a Gd-153 line source. Note the noisiness of the transmission slices as well as the variability from patient to patient. The transmission scan in the upper right image demonstrates a truncation artifact on the left side of the image (the right side of the patient's body). See Chapter 13 for more information about truncation artifacts. Images courtesy of St. Joseph Medical Center.

Patient-Specific Attenuation Maps

for purposes of AC) is about 5 mSv, significantly higher than that for a radionuclide transmission source (3) but lower than that from a diagnostic CT scan (4).

Even if we factor in these additional issues, however, CT-based attenuation maps have several attractive qualities. The photon flux is much higher for a CT scanner than a radionuclide source, so noise is a nonissue. There is no decaying source to be replaced. The radiation exposure of the technologist may decrease, because there is radiation coming from the CT scanner only when it is turned on. And there is the added benefit of being able to correlate the nuclear medicine functional information with the anatomic details seen in the CT slices.

Incorporation of the Attenuation Map into Iterative Reconstruction

Now that we know how to generate a patient-specific attenuation map, we need to put it to use. Incorporating the attenuation map into FBP is complicated and generally not done. In iterative reconstruction, the attenuation map is incorporated into the forward-projection step as shown in Figure 10-13. The attenuation coefficients for each voxel are used to estimate the likelihood of attenuation in that voxel, and the forward-projection step takes that into account in generating the estimated 2D projections. They can also be used to aid in the estimation of scatter.

Compensation for Scatter, Resolution Loss, and Noise

Scatter Compensation

Correction for the effects of attenuation is accomplished in a multiplicative way (i.e., count densities are increased relative to what they would be without AC). If many of these counts are scatter, which they generally are, we may be multiplying bad information into significance. The number and energy of scattered photons also vary with the depth and density of body tissues, similar to attenuation. Hence, SC needs to go hand in hand with AC.

Early scatter correction methods were subtractive. In this technique, a second (and sometimes a third) energy window below the photopeak is used to determine the *scatter fraction* (the proportion of counts in an acquisition that is attributed to scatter), based on either the whole-image energy spectrum or a pixel-by-pixel evaluation of the energy spectrum. The scatter fraction is then subtracted from the counts in each pixel of the 2D projection, prior to reconstruction. This is simple to accomplish and is applicable to FBP reconstruction. But because subtraction decreases total counts, this method results in a concomitant increase in noise. In addition, in any given projection, the scattered gamma rays are mostly coming from a different depth than the unscattered gamma rays, so their estimation based on a 2D energy spectrum is not necessarily reflective of the 3D situation.

Newer SC methods model scatter and incorporate the results of the modeling as additional information in the forward-projection step of iterative reconstruction. Scatter is measured at different depths in air and in phantoms, using acquisition parameters similar to those of patient imaging situations. This information is used to create a picture of how gamma rays are scattered in tissue. Patient-specific attenuation maps may also be incorporated to estimate the effects of different body structures in the scatter model. The model is then applied to the forward-projection step, so that the estimated 2D projections include the assumed effects of scatter in the patient. Model-based SC results in a 10 to 20% improvement in contrast over subtraction-based methods (5).

Resolution Recovery

One of the most important contributors to the relatively poor spatial resolution of gamma cameras is the collimator. Intrinsic camera resolution of 3 to 4 mm is degraded to 10 to 12 mm (or worse) by the addition of the collimator. But just as we use the geometry of a collimator to describe this degradation, we can turn the geometry around to try to recover some of that resolution. The next sections discuss resolution recovery in both FBP and iterative reconstruction.

Resolution Recovery Filters

The filtering done in FBP offers a way to compensate for degraded resolution at high spatial frequencies, using a different kind of low-pass filter than the standard Butterworth filter. The gamma camera itself can be thought of as a kind of low-pass filter, because it blurs the information contained in the object due to its finite resolution capabilities. That is, the shape of the modulation transfer function (MTF) curve in Figure 8-12 is similar to the shape of the low-pass filter in Figure 10-11a. We should be able to recover some of that information detail by deconvolution of the MTF, which represents the blurring function of the gamma camera. The inverse of the MTF can thus be used as a resolution recovery filter. The filter (also called an *adaptive* or *restorative* filter) multiplies the middle-frequency data by a value greater than 1, thus increasing the contribution of those data to the reconstruction process above what would happen with just FBP. A resolution recovery filter must be combined with a roll-off filter to prevent noise from becoming amplified (**Figure 12-10**).

Two resolution recovery filters that have been applied to nuclear medicine are the Wiener and Metz filters. The Metz filter is based on the measured MTF of the gamma camera–collimator system, and the Wiener filter on the signal-to-noise ratio (SNR) of the specific imaging situation. Unfortunately, the mathematical models used to optimize these filters are uncertain, and neither the MTF nor the SNR can be known exactly in every imaging situation, so these filters are somewhat subjective (6).

Modeling of Resolution Loss

Here again iterative reconstruction offers a new and better approach. The effects of collimator-based loss of resolution can be modeled in iterative reconstruction similarly to the effects of scatter. Resolution loss can be visualized by recognizing that activity at a specific location projects

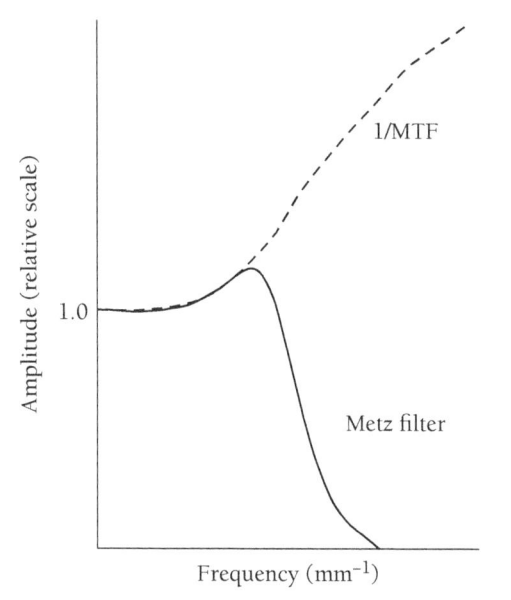

Figure 12-10 Resolution recovery filter. To avoid incorporation of excess noise in the resolution recovery process, the inverse MTF (dashed line) must be modified by a roll-off filter at high frequencies. Resolution recovery occurs up to the frequency at which the filter leaves the dashed line to roll off to zero. The Metz filter is used here as an example.

as a circle of photons at the scintillation crystal, rather than as a single point. The farther the location of the source from the camera, the larger the circle. The specific algorithms used by commercial vendors to correct for this resolution loss are proprietary, but their approaches can be outlined in a broad sense. One method treats resolution loss at depth as an average value that is based on the camera's full width at half-maximum (FWHM), measured at 10 cm. This overcorrects for objects nearer to the camera and undercorrects for those farther away. Another method uses the FWHM as measured at different distances from the collimator surface to determine the incremental amount of blurring that can be expected with each successive slice of the 3D image matrix. A more complex approach attempts to untangle the information on resolution from the projection data by using a deconvolution technique. Depending on the specifics of implementation, the resolution recovery model may be applied in two or three dimensions, and it may be included in the backprojection step as well as the forward-projection step of the iterative cycle.

Noise Regularization

One of the drawbacks of standard gamma cameras is the need for absorptive collimation, which drastically decreases the number of photons available to create each image. Nuclear medicine images are noisy, and noise interferes in a significant way with contrast, which is our ability to identify abnormalities. During acquisition, we can only decrease noise by using a more sensitive collimator (with concomitant loss of resolution), using a longer acquisition time (increasing the potential for patient discomfort and motion), or increasing the administered dose (leading to concerns about excessive radiation exposure). We can decrease noise after acquisition by smoothing, which again degrades resolution and contrast (because filtering always involves the loss of information). One of the major advantages of the resolution recovery methods described above is that they reduce noise while at the same time improving spatial resolution (7).

But noise is nonetheless an important limiting factor in SPECT imaging. In comparison to filtered backprojection, iterative reconstruction has additional ways to improve the noise characteristics of the reconstructed 3D image matrix. These techniques utilize a process known as the *Bayesian inference method*, in which fresh evidence is applied to a starting assumption. In this methodology, the starting point for an iteration is called the *prior probability*, or just *the prior*, meaning it is what we know before adding the new evidence. The modified belief is called the *posterior probability*, because it is what we believe to be true after the new evidence has been considered.

The essence of the Bayesian method in SPECT is to apply identified constraints (i.e., the "fresh evidence") to the prior radiopharmaceutical distribution, to obtain the posterior distribution. Bayesian inference considers each new assumption in a step-wise fashion, with each posterior distribution serving as the prior distribution for the next set of evidence. The maximum-likelihood expectation maximization (MLEM) algorithm then attempts to maximize the posterior distribution's congruence with the acquired data, so the algorithm is sometimes referred to as a *maximum a posteriori* (MAP) algorithm. The term *regularization* refers to the fact that inclusion of the priors causes the MLEM algorithm to converge more quickly.

What kinds of assumptions are included in the prior? The expectation maximization algorithm in itself provides the first one, namely, that the count/pixel values have statistical variability. Additional prior assumptions incorporated into most algorithms include the following (3, 7):

- The statistical variability in nuclear medicine images obeys the Poisson statistical model.
- Areas with high count densities will have less noise.
- Voxels cannot have negative values.
- Local collections of voxels should be reasonably similar.

An attenuation map, if available, provides an important prior assumption. The map shows where anatomic boundaries are, allowing the reconstruction process to permit greater count/pixel variation in these areas.

According to experts in the field (8), the use of iterative reconstruction, in and of itself, leads to significant improvement in SPECT images compared to FBP. Noise regularization and resolution recovery are considered to be second in importance for improving image quality. According to one editorial (9), "The resolution recovery aspects of these algorithms can be emphasized to provide significant improvements in spatial resolution and image quality of SPECT sets, and the noise suppression aspects can be emphasized to permit decreased imaging times for SPECT acquisitions." Attenuation correction and scatter compensation are felt to be helpful but less essential (8).

Implementation

Each of the previous advances is individually beneficial in providing higher-quality SPECT images (10). The use of iterative reconstruction accomplishes a level of NR even without additional algorithms incorporating prior assumptions. Resolution recovery serves as the foundational correction on which AC and SC rely. Only when we can accurately predict the relationship between activity at depth in an object and counts in a 2D projection can we determine the likelihood of attenuation or scatter. This has benefits not only for the specific improvements that each correction intends, but also for the reconstruction process itself. According to one researcher, "If the correct physical model is used in estimating the projections, then the feedback of the iterative process drives the convergence [of the iterative cycle] with implicit recovery of resolution" (11).

Application of these correction methods puts greater stress on both the engineering and the quality control of the camera systems that use them. Angular and radial positioning mechanisms, for example, must have tighter tolerances, because their information about detector location must be known more exactly. Greater attention to camera maintenance is needed to maintain these tighter tolerances. And stricter adherence to routine quality control is essential to prevent artifacts from being introduced into the reconstruction process. All of the corrections are designed for use on an optimally performing system; if the system is not performing at a high level, then the corrections may not work as intended.

Software Methods

Attenuation correction requires either the addition of a transmission source (either a radionuclide or an x-ray tube for CT imaging) to the gamma camera gantry or else a fused anatomic image set. But SC, RR, and NR can all be implemented without requiring new hardware. Major gamma camera vendors have worked to include RR and NR in their reconstruction algorithms, and most have the ability to incorporate SC and AC as well. The results are impressive. Spatial resolution shows improvement by a factor of about 2 (from ~10–12 mm FWHM without these improvements to ~4–5 mm FWHM with RR/NR/SC) (12). Addition of a transmission scan and attenuation correction allows for additional improvement of contrast. These processing programs take into account collimator characteristics, rotational orbit shape and radius, and scatter window counts, all of which are specific to the acquisition protocol used. Some require input of patient weight and dosage as well.

But we are not limited to vendor proprietary systems. One third-party vendor, Ultra-SPECT, offers a program that includes RR and NR and can be used with any camera system, provided that the collimator being used is included in the program's database. This program estimates the patient–collimator distance based on the silhouette seen on the projection images, and it chooses an optimal noise model to meet the operator's desired balance between resolution and smoothness (13). It can incorporate CT-based AC if available. The company supplies a hardware platform that sits between the acquisition terminal and the processing station, and it promotes half-time or even quarter-time cardiac studies.

The improvements in image quality with AC/SC/RR/NR so far have been aimed primarily at myocardial perfusion imaging, and the clinical implications of their utilization in this arena are further addressed in the section Clinical Benefits. But all types of nuclear medicine images stand to benefit. In particular, combining SPECT with CT anatomic registration is not helpful if the SPECT study shows a hot

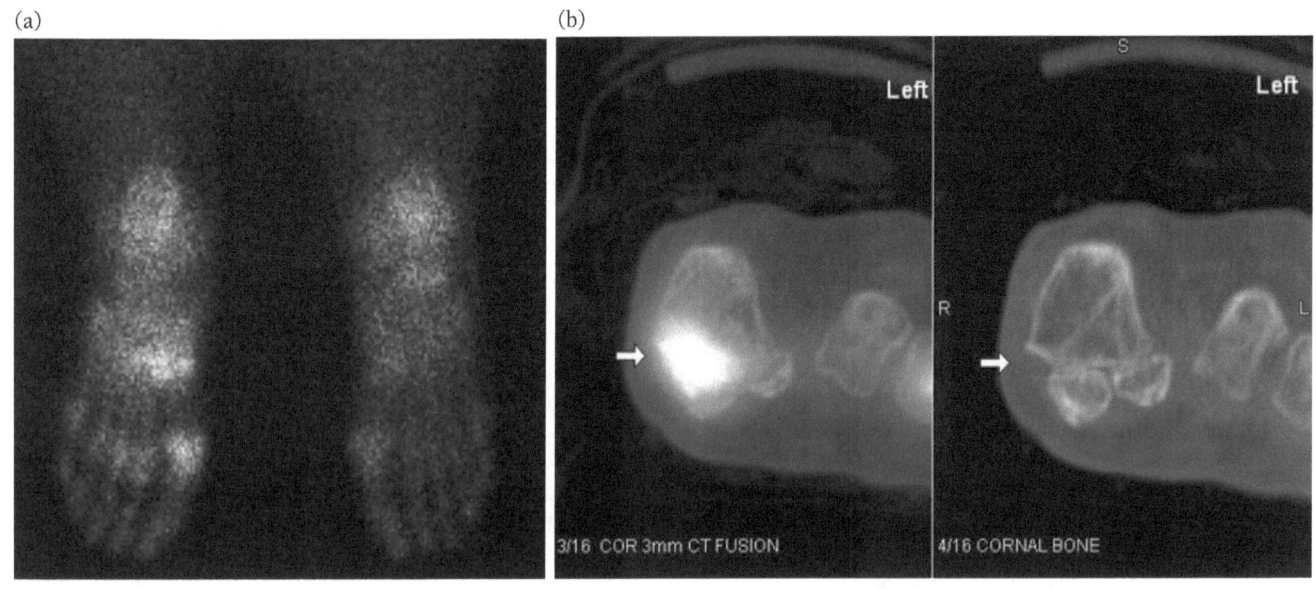

Figure 12-11 Planar bone scan image vs SPECT using Philips Astonish software. The left-hand image shows a plantar view of the feet in a patient being imaged for evaluation of arthritic changes. Increased activity is seen in the area of the first metatarsophalangeal joint of the left foot, but cannot be localized any more precisely. The right-hand image is a transverse CT slice through the metatarsophalangeal joint space, showing the head of the first metatarsal and tibial and fibular sesamoid bones. The middle image, in which the SPECT study processed with SC/RR/NR is overlaid on the CT slice, shows that the increased activity is localized to the joint space between the first metatarsal and the tibial sesamoid. The fibular sesamoid is not involved. (See color plate.) Images courtesy of Valley Medical Center and Valley Radiologists.

spot that is much larger than any specific structure on the co-registered CT image. Application of these reconstruction programs allows the SPECT image to be much more meaningful, as is shown in **Figure 12-11**.

New Imaging Devices

Part of the problem with using a standard gamma camera to image the heart is that most of the FOV is registering gamma rays coming from other parts of the body. We could get better information if we could limit the FOV to focus on the heart itself. One way to accomplish this, in the context of an Anger gamma camera, is to use a cone-beam collimator. But several vendors have introduced non-Anger-based imaging systems to address this issue. Four that are commercially available are discussed here (7) and shown in **Figure 12-12**.

Digirad Cardius 3 XPO

This system uses three heads, each with 768 pixelated CsI(Tl) detectors (a camera with two heads is also available). The heads are fixed, while the patient rotates in a specially designed chair, with the arms supported

(a) Digirad Cardius 3 XPO

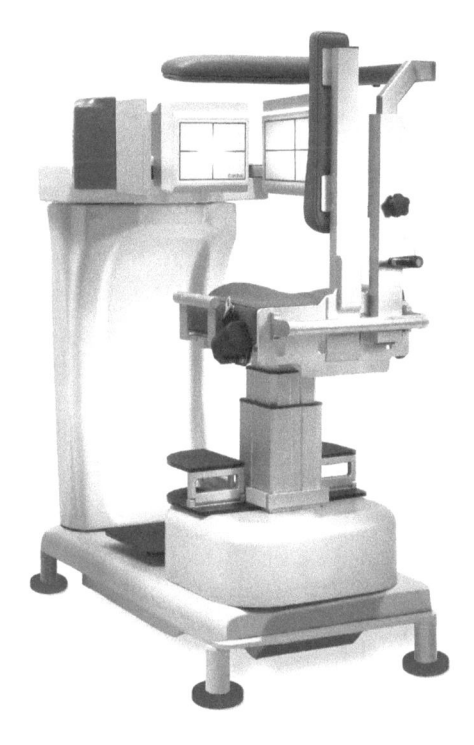

(b) GE NM 530c

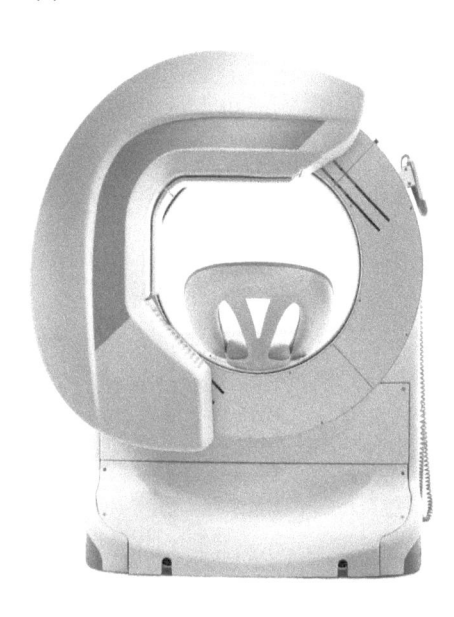

(c) CardiArc

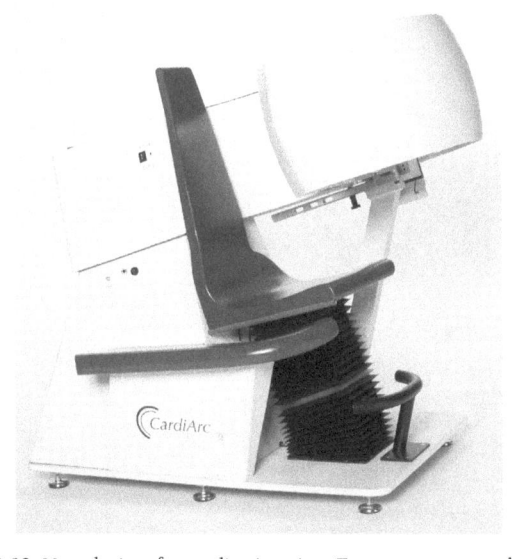

(d) Spectrum Dynamics D-SPECT

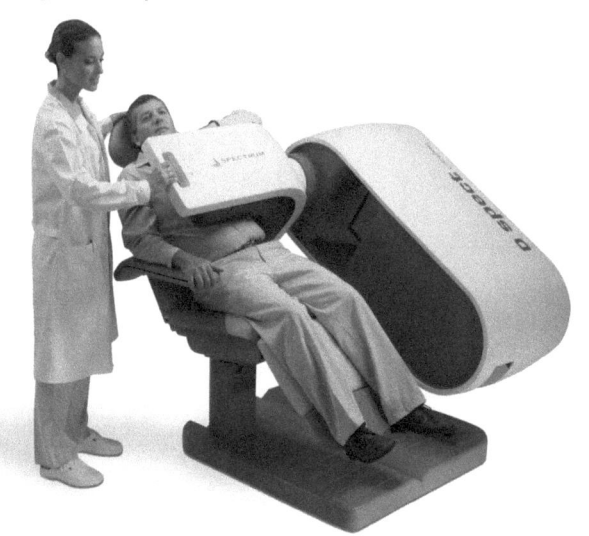

Figure 12-12 New devices for cardiac imaging. Four new cameras designed for myocardial perfusion imaging are shown. All incorporate a focused field of view, and all provide high-quality myocardial images with shorter acquisition times than generally used for MPI studies on a standard gamma camera. All incorporate the image improvement techniques discussed in this chapter. Figure 12-12a courtesy of Digirad Corporation. Figure 12-12b courtesy of GE Healthcare. Figure 12-12c courtesy of CardiArc Corp. Figure 12-12d courtesy of Spectrum Dynamics, Inc.

above the imaging area. Acquisition times of 7.5 min are routinely used, and the accompanying software package can further decrease the imaging time to 4 to 5 min for a cardiac study (7). A version of this system includes a fan-beam x-ray source for AC, using the camera heads as the transmission detectors.

GE Discovery NM 530c

This camera uses 19 cadmium–zinc–tellurium (CZT) detector arrays, each of which sees the heart through a pinhole collimator. Nine of the pinholes are oriented perpendicularly to the patient's longitudinal axis, while the other 10 have angled views of the heart from above or below the row of 9; all reside in a stationary gantry with a right-angle bend in it. The gantry does not move during acquisition, which decreases acquisition time and for the most part eliminates motion artifacts. The 3D image matrix is reconstructed from the 19 views using an iterative reconstruction program that incorporates the detector efficiency of each CZT crystal. This system can also be purchased with CT, allowing for MPI with attenuation correction, calcium scoring, and CT angiography, all in a 5-min acquisition period (7).

CardiArc

This system consists of three curved NaI(Tl) crystals backed by photomultiplier tubes (PMTs), in a 180° arc. Horizontal lead vanes create collimation in the axial direction, and a lead "aperture arc" with six narrow slits provides the transaxial collimation (**Figure 12-13**). In effect, the combination of vanes and slits creates a long-bore parallel-hole collimator in the axial direction and multiple pinholes in the transaxial direction. The aperture arc rotates to create many "lines of sight" through the slits, thus providing a total of 1,280 sampling angles (compared to 30 to 64 in cardiac studies on standard gamma cameras). Proprietary digital logic combines these views into a 3D image matrix. The system's strengths are high spatial resolution and high scan speed. The company's web page, http://www.cardiarc.com, has a good animation showing how the system works.

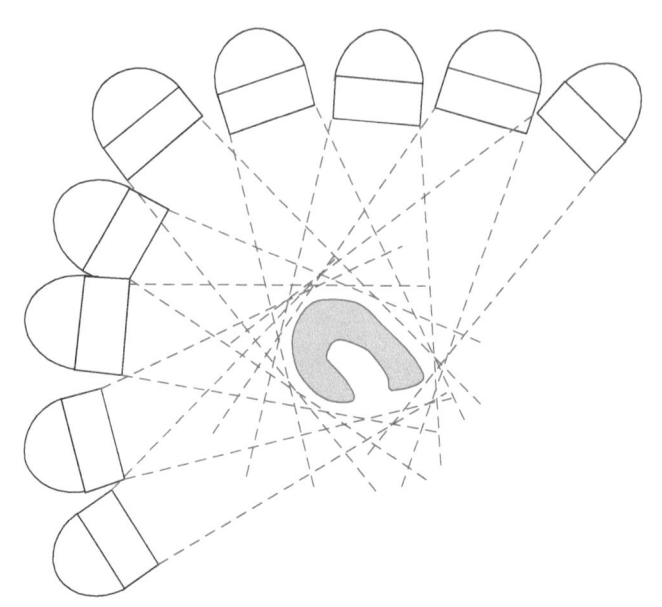

Figure 12-14 Spectrum Dynamics D-SPECT system. The figure shows (in cross section) the nine detector columns around the heart. All detectors are centered on the myocardium, and the columns rotate individually over a maximum angle of 110° to detect photons coming from different angles.

Spectrum Dynamics D-SPECT

In this system, nine columns of pixelated CZT crystals (1,024 per column, in a 64 × 16 arrangement) swivel through individual limited angles to provide optimal views of the heart (**Figure 12-14**). The columns are set in a 90° gantry and use registered collimators, in which each collimator hole is aligned with and the same size as the CZT crystals. Following a 20-sec scan to verify positioning, the columns rotate to optimally visualize the myocardium. A list-mode acquisition includes ECG R waves, allowing for gated studies. The improved sensitivity of this system

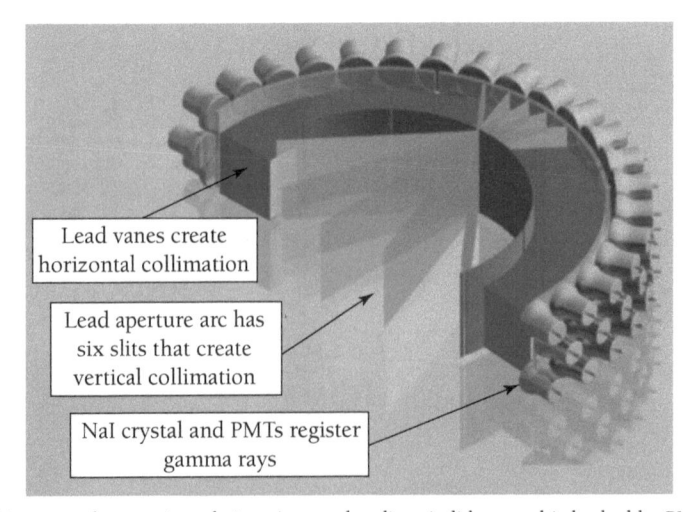

Figure 12-13 CardiArc camera. This camera has a unique design. A curved sodium iodide crystal is backed by PMTs. In front of the crystal, a set of thin lead vanes creates horizontal collimation. On the other surface of the vanes is the aperture arc, which has six narrow vertical slits that provide vertical collimation. Through each slit the camera registers a different view of the myocardium. The aperture arc rotates to generate 1,280 different views of the myocardium, which are combined to create a tomographic data set. Courtesy of CardiArc Corp.

(8 to 10 times that of a standard gamma camera) allows for very short acquisitions: 2-min scans with the D-SPECT system were shown to be comparable to 11-min scans with a conventional camera (14). This company also offers an animated description of image acquisition on its website, http://www.spectrum-dynamics.com.

Each of these systems aims to improve image quality by focusing on gamma rays coming from the myocardium. They also offer other benefits, including increased patient comfort, ability to effectively image large patients, and decreased space requirements. All incorporate (to a greater or lesser extent) AC, SC, RR, and NR. They are not (in most instances) usable for other imaging situations, but they have distinct advantages when a department can afford to have a dedicated cardiac camera, as well as in a cardiology office with high volumes of MPI patients.

Clinical Benefits

All of the developments discussed in this chapter, both software-based reconstruction methods and innovative new imaging devices, show improvement in spatial resolution and SNR. But these are not necessarily the point of their development. Instead, the goal is to "trade" these improvements for a decrease in either acquisition time or radiopharmaceutical dosage. Particularly in the cardiac imaging arena, improved spatial resolution is not required, because the coronary artery territories are relatively large, making perfusion defects easy to identify. But the long acquisition times are difficult for many patients, and the high effective dose of myocardial perfusion studies is being questioned in this era of increasing concerns about radiation exposure. So improvement in the quality of the images can, in turn, improve efficiency, allowing for greater patient throughput while at the same time reducing the radiation burden to patients. Much of the image quality needed to decrease imaging time and/or dose can be garnered through NR and RR.

Attenuation correction has an additional role to play. Currently most nuclear medicine departments obtain both stress and rest MPI scans, the latter mainly to provide a view of the patient's "normal" (nonstressed) myocardial perfusion. We cannot simply use the stress data from a database of normal patients, because there is too much patient-to-patient variability due to attenuation. With AC, it may be possible to identify myocardial ischemia with only a stress scan (15, 16). Use of AC for MPI increases the sensitivity, specificity, and normalcy of myocardial perfusion imaging (17) (**Figure 12-15**).

The incorporation of CT into SPECT opens up even more possibilities. When SPECT images are co-registered with CT slices, areas of abnormal radiopharmaceutical uptake can be correlated with anatomic structures. The image improvements outlined in this chapter have shown that they can improve resolution to the extent that anatomic correlation is meaningful. The marriage of anatomy and physiology that first reached prominence with PET/CT is now equally appealing in the SPECT world.

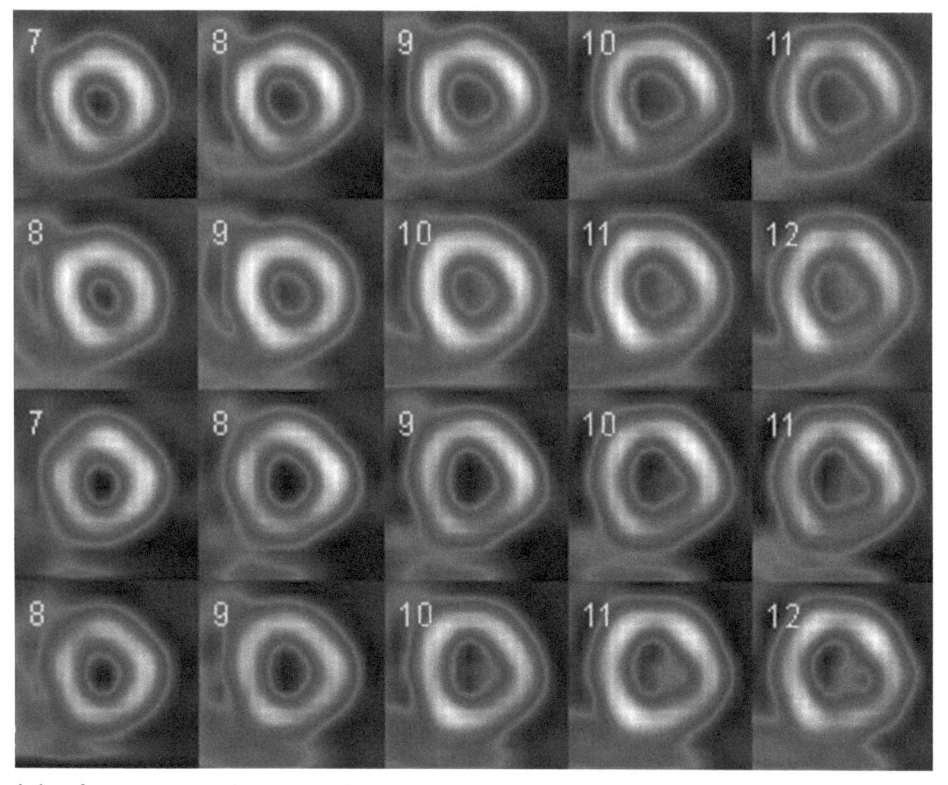

Figure 12-15 Myocardial perfusion SPECT without and with attenuation correction. The top two rows of this image show stress and rest short-axis views of a patient's myocardium. A significant inferolateral defect is seen, which is larger at stress but also apparent at rest. This could be interpreted as evidence of a prior infarction. Application of attenuation correction using Gd-153 rod sources (bottom two rows) causes the inferolateral wall to appear more normally perfused at rest, increasing the likelihood that the stress defect represents ischemia. (See color plate.) Courtesy of Philips Healthcare.

Summary

The incorporation of NR, RR, AC, and SC is finally addressing one of the major negatives of gamma camera imaging, namely, the conflict between sensitivity and spatial resolution that is inherent in a standard collimator. Concentrated effort by a number of researchers and industry scientists has resulted in a significant improvement in image quality. And patients benefit not only from superior images, but also from decreased radiation exposure and imaging times. We can expect to see increasing adoption of these technological advances (in the form of software upgrades) in general nuclear medicine departments. And as time goes on, we may see more and more departments investing in both cardiac-specific imaging systems and SPECT/CT tomographs.

References

1. Henkin RE, Boles MA, Dillehay GA, et al., eds. *Nuclear Medicine*. St. Louis, MO: Mosby-Year Book; 1996:216.
2. Chang LT. A method for attenuation correction in radionuclide computed tomography. *IEEE Trans Nucl Sci*. 1978;NS-25:638–643.
3. Zaidi H, Hasegawa B. Determination of the attenuation map in emission tomography. *J Nucl Med*. 2003;44:291–315.
4. Keidar Z, Israel O, Krausz Y. SPECT/CT in tumor imaging: technical aspects and clinical applications. *Semin Nucl Med*. 2003;33:205–218.
5. Madsen MT. Recent advances in SPECT imaging. *J Nucl Med*. 2007;48:661–673.
6. Van Laere K, Koole M, Lemahieu I, Dierckx R. Image filtering in single-photon emission computed tomography: principles and applications. *Comput Med Imaging Graph*. 2001;25:127–133.
7. Garcia EV, Faber TL, Esteves FP. Cardiac dedicated ultrafast SPECT cameras: new designs and clinical implications. *J Nucl Med*. 2011;52:210–217.
8. Technical Advances in MPI Imaging. SNM Society of Nuclear Medicine 58th Annual Meeting, San Antonio, TX; 2011.
9. Patton JA, Slomka PJ, Germano G, Berman DS. Recent technologic advances in nuclear cardiology. *J Nucl Cardiol*. 2007;14:501–513.
10. Narayanan MV, King MA, Pretorius PH, et al. Human-observer receiver-operating-characteristic evaluation of attenuation, scatter, and resolution compensation strategies for Jc-99m myocardial perfusion imaging. *J Nucl Med*. 2003; 44:1725–1734.
11. Vija AH. Flash 3D, CT attenuation and scatter compensation. Presented at the 53rd Annual Meeting of the Society of Nuclear Medicine, San Diego, CA; 2006.
12. Janowitz WR. Initial clinical experience with philips precedence SPECT/CT system. Presented at the 53rd Annual Meeting of the Society of Nuclear Medicine, San Diego, CA; 2006.
13. Borges-Neves S, Pagnanelli RA, Shaw LK, et al. Clinical results of a novel wide-beam reconstruction method for shortening scan times of Tc-99m cardiac SPECT perfusion studies. *J Nucl Cardiol*. 2007;14:555–565.
14. Gambhir SS, Berman DS, Ziffer J, et al. A novel high-sensitivity rapid-acquisition single-photon cardiac imaging camera. *J Nucl Med*. 2009;50:635–643.
15. Miles J, Cullom SJ, Case JA. An introduction to attenuation correction. *J Nucl Cardiol*. 1999;6:449–457.
16. Chang SM, Nabi F, Xu J, et al. Normal stress-only versus standard stress/rest myocardial perfusion imaging: similar patient mortality with reduced radiation exposure. *J Am Coll Cardiol*. 2010;55:221–230.
17. Travin MI. Cardiac cameras. *Semin Nucl Med*. 2011;41:182–201.

Additional Resources

Bailey DL. Transmission scanning in emission tomography. *Eur J Nucl Med*. 1998; 25:774–787.
Bateman TM, Cullom SJ. Attenuation correction single-photon emission computed tomography myocardial perfusion imaging. *Semin Nucl Med*. 2005;35:37–51.
Cherry SR, Sorenson JA, Phelps ME. *Physics in Nuclear Medicine*. 3rd ed. Philadelphia, PA: Saunders; 2003:Chapters 16, 17.
Galt JR, Cullom SJ, Garcia EV. Attenuation and scatter compensation in myocardial perfusion SPECT. *Semin Nucl Med*. 1999;29:204–220.
Garcia EV, Faber TL, Esteves FP. Cardiac dedicated ultrafast SPECT cameras: new designs and clinical implications. *J Nucl Med*. 2011; 52:210–217.
Henkin RE, Boles MA, Dillehay GA, et al., eds. *Nuclear Medicine*. St. Louis, MO: Mosby-Year Book; 1996:Chapters 17, 22.
King MA, Tsui BMW, Pan T-S. Attenuation compensation for cardiac single-photon emission computed tomographic imaging: part 1. Impact of attenuation and methods of estimating attenuation maps. *J Nucl Cardiol*. 1995;2:513–524.
Lee KH. *Computers in Nuclear Medicine: A Practical Approach*. 2nd ed. Reston, VA: Society of Nuclear Medicine; 2005:Chapter 11.
Madsen MT. Recent advances in SPECT imaging. *J Nucl Med*. 2007; 48:661–673.
Travin MI. Cardiac cameras. *Semin Nucl Med*. 2011; 41:182–201.
Zaidi H, Hasegawa B. Determination of the attenuation map in emission tomography. *J Nucl Med*. 2003;44:291–315.

CHAPTER 13

Quality Control and Artifacts in SPECT

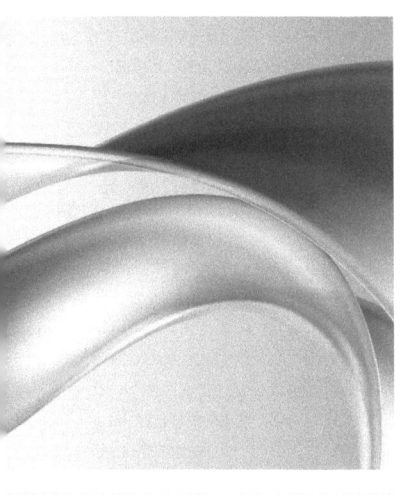

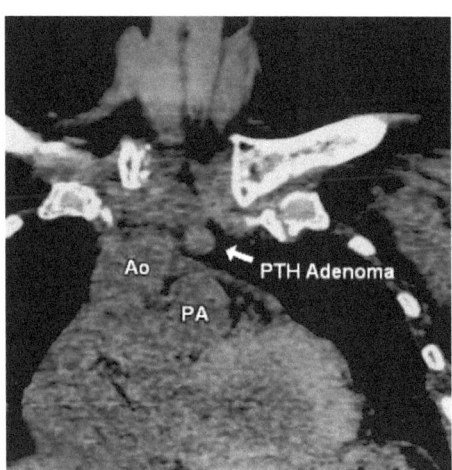

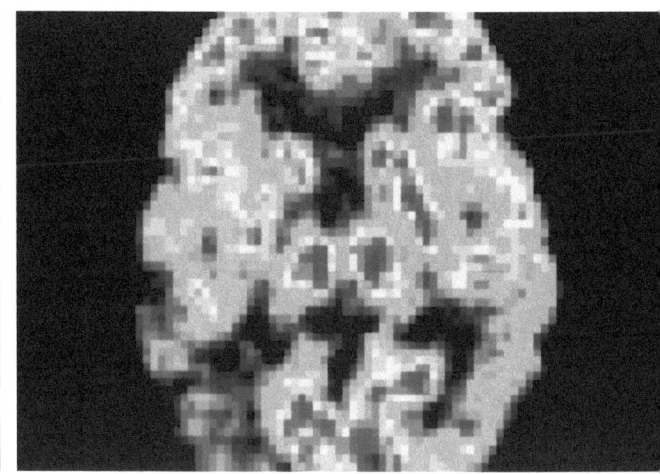

Learning Outcomes

1. Identify several reasons for performing acceptance testing on SPECT systems.
2. Discuss the importance of planar uniformity for SPECT imaging, including desirable values for uniformity and the types of artifacts that can be produced in a SPECT system without good uniformity.
3. Outline the center-of-rotation quality control test, and discuss the meaning of the *X*-axis offset and the types of artifacts produced in a SPECT system without good center-of-rotation corrections.
4. Describe the need and procedure for the following quality control tests:
   a. The reference scan for transmission-based attenuation correction
   b. Rotational stability test
   c. Pixel size determination
5. Convert filter frequency values from a fraction of the Nyquist frequency to cycles/pixel and absolute frequency units.
6. Diagram the three orthogonal directions in which spatial resolution is measured, using a line source of radioactivity.
7. Discuss the uses of cylindrical phantoms and the Jaszczak phantom in evaluating system performance.
8. Describe the appearance and origin of ray artifacts, ring artifacts, motion artifacts, and truncation artifacts.

Introduction

Single-photon emission computed tomography (SPECT) has become a mainstay of nuclear medicine. But it requires more careful attention to detail than planar imaging. Acceptance testing is considerably more rigorous for SPECT than for planar imaging. Quality control must be scrutinized closely, including both planar and rotational tests as well as the transmission-based attenuation correction (TBAC) system, if one is used. Three-dimensional phantoms must be imaged to truly assess SPECT system performance. The operator must be able to recognize the artifacts that occur in SPECT imaging and take steps to uncover and correct their causes. Quality control (QC), patient preparation, acquisition quality, and processing choices significantly impact image quality (and therefore diagnostic results).

One way to think about quality control and artifacts in SPECT is to note the assumptions of Radon's original theory. These include the following (1):

- A complete set of projections is obtained.
- The internal distribution does not change during the time needed to acquire the projections.
- The detectors have uniform sensitivity throughout the acquisition.
- The center of rotation is accurately known.

The detector uniformity and center of rotation are quality control tests that are essential to obtaining high-quality

SPECT images. The projections must be sufficiently numerous and (with the exception of cardiac imaging) need to completely encircle the object being imaged (as discussed in Chapter 11). Movement of activity within the patient and motion by the patient produce identifiable artifacts. Thus each assumption must be met; it is when one or more is not met that artifacts appear.

Acceptance Testing

Because SPECT uses gamma camera images to create a 3D image, acceptance testing on a SPECT system must include all the planar gamma camera tests and then some. An experienced medical physicist performs both planar tests and SPECT-specific acceptance tests (Table 13-1), according to the National Electrical Manufacturers Association (NEMA) protocols. Some of the tests listed in Table 13-1 are not in the NEMA protocols but are recommended by experts (2). In addition, software should be tested and the results of image reconstruction examined closely.

Most SPECT tomographs currently sold are of the multihead variety. This leads to additional requirements in acceptance testing, because the various calibration factors should be no more than 0.5% different (3) and the acceptance test results no more than 10% different (4) between the camera heads. One recommendation is first to perform acceptance tests on each head separately and then add the data sets together and look for evidence of mismatch or interference patterns. Finally, repeat the tests with all heads combined in one study (4).

The importance of acceptance testing for SPECT tomographs cannot be overemphasized. Artifacts can be hard to recognize on reconstructed images, as we see in this chapter. Further, many systems do not meet all of the vendor specifications (2). Acceptance testing is the last opportunity to verify the quality of the system before the purchase is finalized.

SPECT Quality Control

SPECT imaging places a high premium on planar image quality. Any aberration in the 2D projections will be carried into the SPECT reconstruction and may be further amplified if filtered backprojection (FBP) is used as the reconstruction method. Any inaccuracy in the rotation of the camera will also be propagated through the study. Routine quality control is therefore related to planar uniformity and mechanical/rotational precision, which are required to ensure that the SPECT images are of good quality. Table 13-2 provides a summary of recommended procedures and their frequencies.

Uniformity

The first requirement for a high-quality SPECT study is excellent planar uniformity. According to acceptance testing guidelines promulgated by the American Association of Physicists in Medicine (AAPM), camera uniformity should be corrected to 3% or better, using the formula for uniformity determination given in Equation 9-1 (5), although studies have shown that 1% planar nonuniformity can generate as much as 20% nonuniformity in reconstructed images (6). The improvements in gamma camera uniformity made during the 1980s were driven primarily by this requirement. To produce high-quality SPECT images, a gamma camera must be properly tuned and employ up-to-date energy and linearity corrections. The isotope-specific uniformity correction map should be reacquired on a regular basis to ensure the best possible uniformity. The flood image used to create the correction map should have statistical variability of 1% or less (i.e., at least 10,000 cts/pixel) in the same matrix size as for clinical studies. This calculates to about 30 million total cts for a 64 × 64 matrix and about 120 million cts for a 128 × 128 matrix. Uniformity of the planar gamma camera (with all corrections operating) should be checked daily.

The push for high-quality SPECT studies has also driven quality improvements of uniformity phantoms. Obviously, the uniformity of the flood image cannot be any better than the uniformity of the source used to obtain it. Thus, the flood source should have less than 1% variation in activity concentration from point to point (6, 7). Prior to the advent of SPECT, a fillable Plexiglas phantom was commonly used. A suitable radionuclide (usually Tc-99m) was added to the liquid in the phantom; then it was mixed well and imaged extrinsically. However,

---

Table 13-1

Additional Acceptance Tests for Tomographic Gamma Camera Systems

- Rotational capabilities and limits
  - Angle indicators
  - Step-size accuracy
  - Timing
  - Radial motion
  - Gantry controls
  - Safety features (especially emergency stops and pressure-sensitive collimator covers)
- Pixel calibration
- Center-of-rotation performance
- Rotational uniformity stability
- Collimator-hole angulation
- Patient-contour positioning
- Tomographic slice uniformity
- Tomographic spatial resolution
  - Transverse without scatter
  - Transverse with scatter
- Axial slice thickness
- System volume sensitivity
- System performance (Jaszczak phantom)
  - Lesion contrast
  - Rod resolution

National Electrical Manufacturers Association. *Performance Measurements of Scintillation Cameras*. Publication NU 1-2001. Rosslyn, VA: 2001.
Siegel JA, Benedetto AR, Jaszczak RJ, et al. AAPM Report No. 22: Rotating scintillation camera SPECT acceptance testing and quality control. New York, NY: American Association of Physicists in Medicine; 1987.

Table 13-2

Recommended Quality Control Tests for SPECT Tomographs

Test	Recommended Frequency
Uniformity	Daily[1,2,3,4,6]
Collimator visual inspection	Daily[3,4]
Center of rotation	Weekly–biweekly[2,3,4,5,6]
Spatial resolution/linearity (bar phantom)	Weekly–biweekly[2,3,4,6]
High-count flood/ uniformity correction map	Weekly–biweekly[2,3,4,5]
Tomographic spatial resolution	Quarterly–annually[1,3,4,6]
Jaszczak phantom	Quarterly–annually[1,2,3,4]
Pixel size	Quarterly–semiannually[2,3,4,5]
Tilt-angle check	Quarterly[3]
Collimator-hole angulation	Annually[1]

[1]Siegel JA, Benedetto AR, Jaszczak RJ, et al. AAPM Report No. 22: Rotating scintillation camera SPECT acceptance testing and quality control. New York, NY: American Association of Physicists in Medicine; 1987.
[2]Graham LS, Fahey FH, Madsen MT, et al. AAPM Report No. 52: Quantitation of SPECT performance. Woodbury, NY: American Institute of Physics; 1995.
[3]Hines H, Kayayan R, Colsher J, et al. National Electrical Manufacturers Association recommendations for implementing SPECT instrumentation quality control. *J Nucl Med.* 2000;41:383–389.
[4]English RJ. *Single-Photon Emission Computed Tomography: A Primer.* 3rd ed. Reston, VA: Society of Nuclear Medicine; 1995:116–117, 195.
[5]Greer K, Jaszczak R, Harris C, Coleman RE. Quality control in SPECT. *J Nucl Med Technol.* 1985;13:76–85.
[6]Zanzonico P. Routine quality control of clinical nuclear medicine instrumentation: a brief review. *J Nucl Med.* 2008;49:1114–1131.

sufficient mixing was hard to accomplish; in addition, Plexiglas tends to bulge at the center due to the weight of the water, causing the phantom itself to be nonuniform (although manufacturers of these phantoms are working to alleviate this problem).

The need for a more uniform extrinsic flood source was addressed by the development of Co-57 sheet sources manufactured with a high degree of consistency (in terms of photon flux/cm^2). Co-57 flood sources have a few drawbacks, including a limited life span and impurities that impact uniformity correction maps (6), but they are generally better than fillable phantoms that are hand-mixed. Some camera manufacturers still recommend intrinsic floods, based on the assumptions that (1) when properly positioned, a point source produces a uniform photon flux and (2) the collimator usually doesn't contribute to flood nonuniformity unless it has been damaged. The importance of the latter point was recently addressed, and collection of an extrinsic uniformity correction map was recommended (8).

If SPECT imaging with radionuclides other than Tc-99m is routinely done, the gamma camera's uniformity needs to be tested regularly with those radionuclides as well.

These floods may be either intrinsic or extrinsic; the latter should use the same collimator as is used for imaging. Uniformity may very well be worse with other radionuclides compared to Tc-99m or Co-57, but still should not exceed approximately 5% if artifacts in clinical studies are to be avoided (5).

Center of Rotation

One of the assumptions inherent to SPECT reconstruction is that the line in space about which the gamma camera rotates—the *axis of rotation* (AOR)—maps to the center of the 3D image matrix—the *center of rotation* (COR). In multihead cameras, the reconstruction process assumes that a focus of activity will be registered in the same 3D location by all detectors. The COR quality control test either confirms these assumptions or adjusts the acquired projections within the reconstruction process to make them true. If these assumptions are not true, the SPECT images will not reflect the actual distribution of the radiopharmaceutical in the object, no matter how good the other aspects of the study are.

Figure 13-1 illustrates the situation. The camera rotates around the AOR, which is parallel to the Z-axis. When a line source of radioactivity is imaged using SPECT acquisition techniques, the location of the line source in each pair of 180°-opposed 2D projections from a single camera head establishes the AOR (Fig. 13-1a), which must then be correlated to the COR of the 3D image matrix (Fig. 13-1b). Figure 13-1c shows the source from two views and the line representing the midpoint between them. In a rotationally sound system, the midpoint lines from different angles all cross at the same point, which is the AOR. The difference between the AOR and the COR is measured by the COR analysis program, and the correction, called an *offset*, is applied to patient studies.

A COR measurement is obtained using a point source or line source of radioactivity; a capillary tube filled with Tc-99m is ideal, but a hypodermic needle works as well. The source is put on the imaging table, preferably in a holder of some kind, and in line with but not at the exact location of the AOR. The source–collimator distance does not affect the measured COR offsets. Some systems, particularly those that employ a roving field-of-view (FOV) mask, require multiple point sources and may provide a phantom to locate them spatially. The source must be in the FOV from all angles, and no other radioactive sources should be seen in the FOV from any angle. The number of projections used for the acquisition is not crucial (32 stops over 360° is usually adequate), but the matrix size is critical. The finest matrix size routinely used for SPECT acquisitions (usually 128 × 128) should be used in the COR measurement. Time per stop should be gauged to produce 5,000 to 20,000 cts per 2D projection. Each camera head needs its own COR study obtained from a complete 360° rotation. The manufacturer's recommended protocol should be reviewed to ensure that its conditions are met.

After acquisition, a COR analysis program is used to determine the values of the X-axis offset, which is measured in units of pixels. The *X-offset* is the difference between the COR and the average matrix column that

(a) Axis of rotation

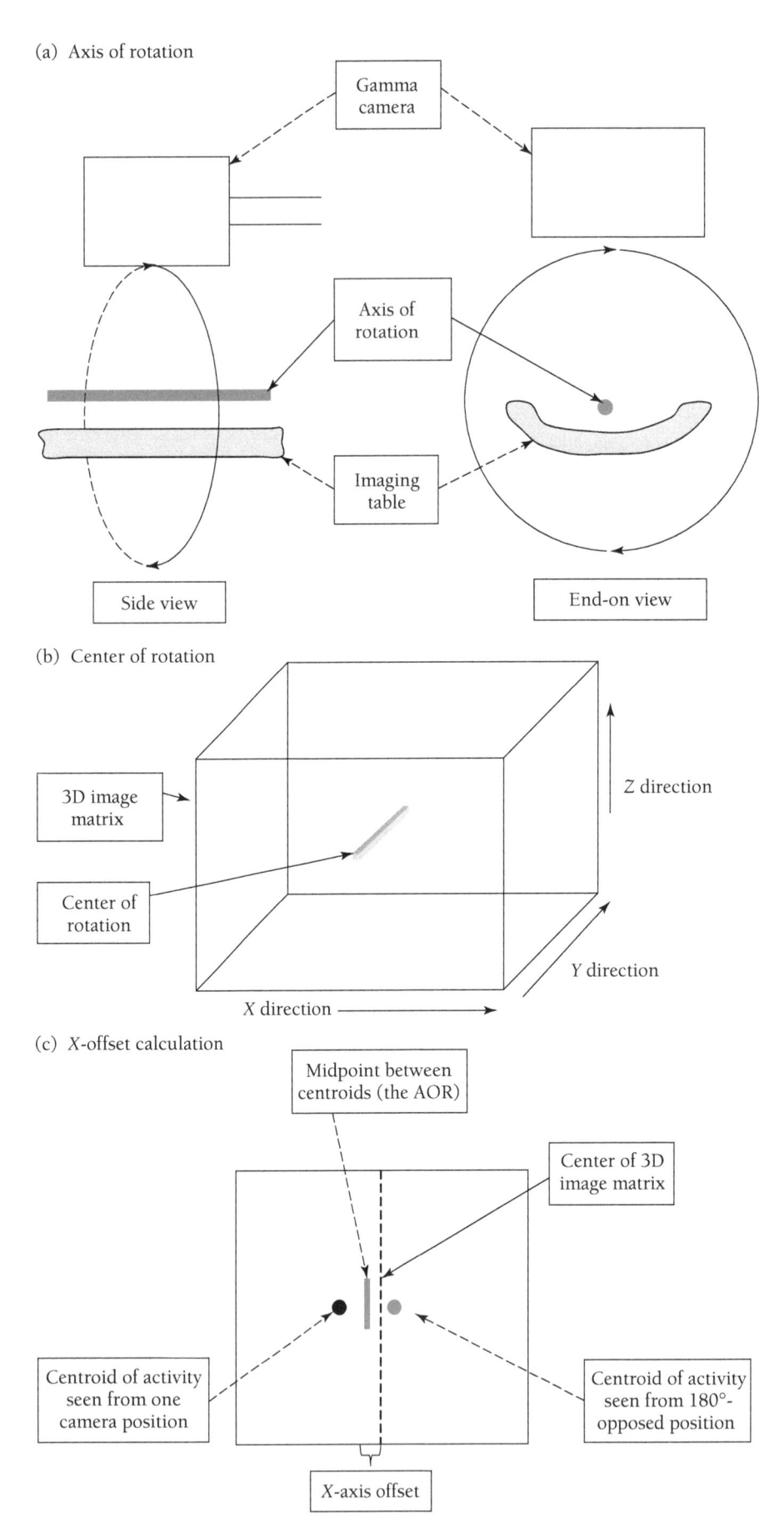

(b) Center of rotation

(c) X-offset calculation

Figure 13-1 Center of rotation. The purpose of the COR quality control test is to determine the relationship between the axis of rotation (Fig. 13-1a) and the center of rotation (the middle column of pixels) of the 3D image matrix (Fig. 13-1b). It is not necessary that the two be perfectly aligned, but rather that a correction, called the X-offset, be made so that they are in alignment (Fig. 13-1c).

collects data from the system's AOR. The essence of this determination is that the program identifies the centroid of the line source in two 180°-opposed projections (called a *conjugate pair*), averages their position, and compares the centroid average (which is the location of the AOR) to the center of a transverse image slice (Fig. 13-1c). In a 128 × 128 matrix, the center of a transverse slice is at pixel column 64.5, so an *X*-offset of +0.5 pixel indicates that the centroid average for that pair of detector positions was found in pixel column 65. Because the gamma camera cannot resolve to less than 1 pixel, an *X*-offset of less than 0.5 pixel is considered acceptable. The *X*-offset is then applied to all 2D projections, shifting their positions in the *X* direction so that the opposing views line up exactly.

If the COR test produces an *X*-offset greater than 0.5 pixel, the stored values should be cleared and new values determined. Following this procedure, a new COR measurement should produce an *X*-offset of less than 0.25 pixel. An *X*-offset value greater than 3 pixels should prompt a service call (although larger deviations are mathematically correctable). Systems utilizing multiple point sources often automate the COR analysis and directly implement any corrections needed. Depending on the system, an offset may be applied on an angle-by-angle basis, or an average value may be applied to all projections.

Figure 13-2a shows a printout of a COR analysis program from one manufacturer. Values given include the mean *X*-offset, the minimum and maximum *X*-offset values, the error range in the *X*-offset (the difference between the highest and lowest individual values), and the standard deviation of the *X*-offset. A large value for the *X*-offset error range can indicate a problem even when the *X*-offset value itself is less than 0.5 pixel. Similar values are given for the *Y*-axis; the *Y*-offset error range is reflective of camera head tilt (9). Note also that in many programs, the *Y*-axis values given by the program are now considered to apply to the *Z*-axis, according to Figure 10-1. In the early years of SPECT, the *Y*-axis was defined as the patient head-to-toe direction, similar to planar images.

A graph called a *sineogram* shows either the location of the centroid or the *X*-offset value, graphed vs the conjugate view number. The sineogram showing the centroid location should look like a sine wave (Fig. 13-2b); that showing the *X*-offset should be a straight line (Fig. 13-2a). Some systems also display a *Y*-offset or an axial location graph, both of which should produce a straight line. Deviation from flatness will also be evident in the error range and standard deviation values, which will be larger than usual. The error ranges of both the *X*- and *Y*-offsets should be examined and should not exceed 1 pixel. Figure 13-2c shows an example of an unacceptable COR sineogram. A second, extraneous source of radioactivity in the room caused the program to locate the centroid of activity between the two sources at some angles, producing an incorrect *X*-offset value for several conjugate pairs as well as unacceptable *X*-offset and error range values and an *X*-offset sineogram that is not a flat line.

(a) Acceptable COR *X*-axis offset

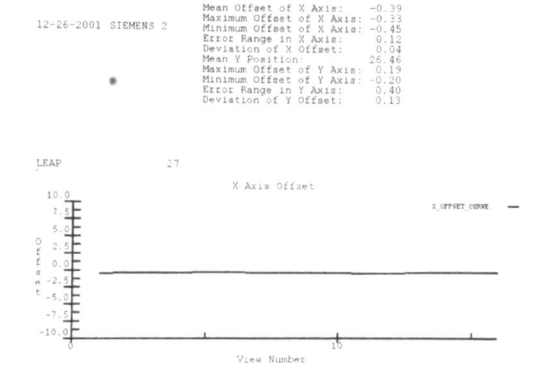

(b) COR plot of source *X*-centroid vs view number

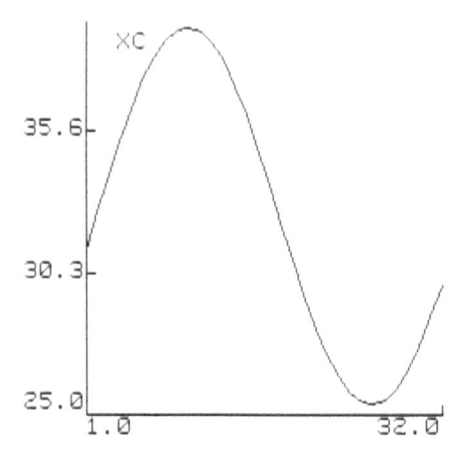

(c) Unacceptable COR *X*-axis offset; extraneous source in room

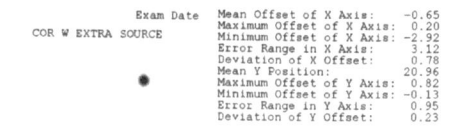

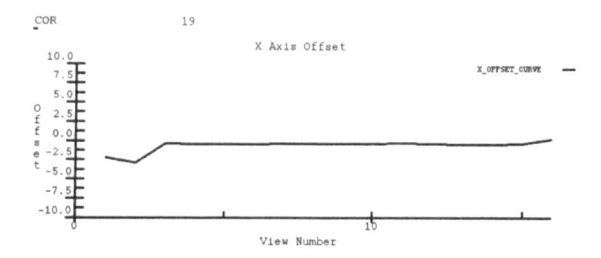

Figure 13-2 Examples of COR analysis programs. Figure 13-2a shows a program that graphs the offset vs projection pair. The "ideal" value for the offset is 0 pixels, and there should be little variation from angle to angle (i.e., the flat line in the sineogram). Figure 13-2b shows a graph of a sine wave curve fit to the centroid location, demonstrating the sinusoidal location change of the centroid point. Figure 13-2c shows a COR analysis in which an extraneous source was present in the room, which was seen by the gamma camera from several angles. This causes the centroid of activity to be located between the two sources, thus leading to a different offset value in the projection angles that see the extraneous activity. Images courtesy of Virginia Mason Medical Center.

(a) 360° acquisition with an artificially added COR error

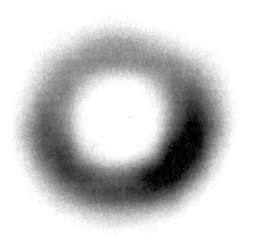

(b) 180° acquisition with the same error as in Figure 13-3a

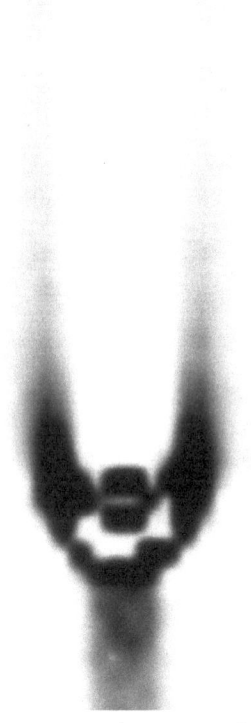

Figure 13-3 Visual appearance of reconstructed COR artifacts. Figure 13-3a is a reconstructed line source on a camera with an artificial 3-pixel COR offset. The incorrect offset causes activity from opposed projections to be seen in two different locations, resulting in the donut appearance. When a scan is only done over 180°, the donut becomes a pitchfork or tuning fork (Fig. 13-3b). There is a pixel-overflow artifact at the crux of the pitchfork. Images courtesy of Virginia Mason Medical Center.

If a COR line source is reconstructed, it should appear as a single point of activity in the transverse slices. If the COR offset is not correct, the line source will reconstruct to a donut pattern (**Figure 13-3a**). If the line source is exactly at the AOR, the donut will shrink to a dot, hence the recommendation to put the line source off-center for a COR measurement. In a 180° study, the donut shape appears as a pitchfork or tuning fork (Fig. 13-3b).

An incorrect center of rotation in a clinical study often produces a very subtle artifact. COR artifacts are generally not recognizable as such, even though they can wreak havoc with clinical images. With a 0.5-pixel offset error (uncorrected), a line source will show a 30% degradation of spatial resolution and a 40% loss of contrast (10). These values demonstrate that even a small error can result in a significant decline in the reconstructed image quality. It is therefore vitally important that the COR be checked and corrected according to the manufacturer's directions.

Misalignment of the COR can be caused by a number of factors. Given that each camera head is quite heavy, gravity and friction are bound to cause wear and tear to the mechanical parts over time. The heaviness of the collimator affects the measured COR in some systems, potentially requiring each collimator to have a separate COR correction. A related problem is camera head tilt. If the gamma camera heads are tilted relative to the AOR, a specific point in space will be seen at different positions from different angles (**Figure 13-4**). The tilt-angle check referenced in Table 13-2 verifies the head angle that is reported by the system. The COR can also be affected by changes in the function of PMTs, amplifiers, and analog-to-digital converters (ADCs) as the camera rotates, although considerable effort has minimized these sources of COR error.

The frequency of COR testing and the number of combinations to be tested depend in large part on the mechanical stability of the system. Some tomographs, because of their construction, essentially cannot have a COR error, while others require separate corrections for each combination of variables used clinically (i.e., collimator, matrix size, zoom factor). The current standard of

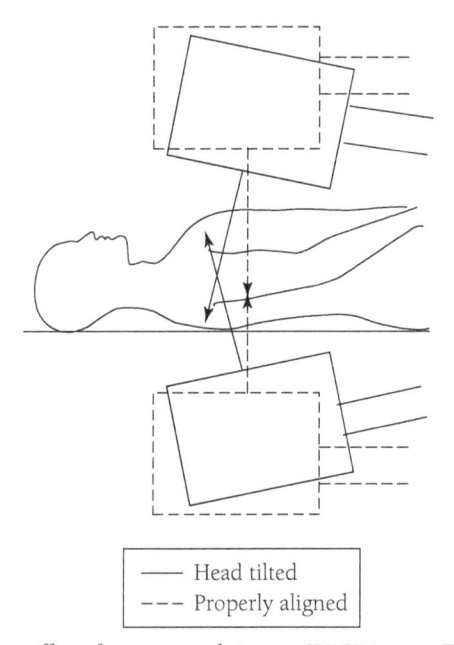

—— Head tilted
--- Properly aligned

Figure 13-4 Effect of camera angulation on SPECT images. The dashed-line boxes represent a gamma camera head (shown in two 180°-opposed positions) aligned parallel to the axis of rotation, and the solid-line boxes show an (exaggerated) head tilt. The solid arrows show the alignment of information as seen from the two opposing projections, demonstrating that different columns of tissue activity are seen at the two opposing angles when the camera head is tilted. This is contrary to the assumptions of the reconstruction and will create errors in clinical studies. In a COR test, head tilt looks like a COR error, and can potentially be "corrected," causing inappropriate offsets to be applied to subsequent clinical studies.

practice is to check the COR weekly, at least until the system can be shown to be stable over a period of at least several months. Likewise, one should check the COR using each collimator, matrix size, zoom factor, and relative head orientation (e.g., 180° vs 90°), until it is verified that the COR is stable from one choice to the next as well as from week to week for each combination of variables. Again, the manufacturer's recommendations should be followed. Accrediting bodies such as the American College of Radiology (ACR) require weekly COR testing as a condition of accreditation.

Reference Scan

In systems utilizing TBAC, a reference scan needs to be performed daily. This scan must be archived, as it will be needed for any reprocessing of the day's studies. In addition, it is used as a quality control evaluation for the performance of the TBAC system. The reference scan is performed according to the manufacturer's protocol. In many systems it is a short (2-min) scan of the line source across the camera's FOV with nothing, including the imaging table, between the line source and the camera face. The energy windows are those of the radionuclide being used for emission imaging, a window centered on the transmission source photopeak, and possibly a scatter window located between the two. If dual-isotope imaging is being performed (e.g., Tl-201 and Tc-99m for myocardial perfusion studies), reference scans for both radionuclide windows must be acquired. A separate reference scan for each detector is required in multihead systems.

The reference scan is analyzed for uniformity and total counts. The number of counts in the reference scan is commonly used as a gauge of the adequacy of source activity. For example, one vendor recommends replacing attenuation correction sources (or removing shielding) when a 2-min reference scan has less than 1.8 million cts. Uniformity values for the reference scan may be quite large (30% or greater), but this is acceptable, because the $I(0)$ values are applied on a pixel-by-pixel basis. Examples of unacceptable reference scans are shown in **Figure 13-5**.

Quality control of the transmission images is equal in importance to QC of the reference scan and the emission study. Total counts and count density are the crucial factors for getting an adequate attenuation map. Both values should be checked at the end of every patient study, as they depend on the patient's body habitus as well as the strength of the radionuclide source. The TBAC analysis program should report whether a minimum count density

(a) Unacceptable reference image

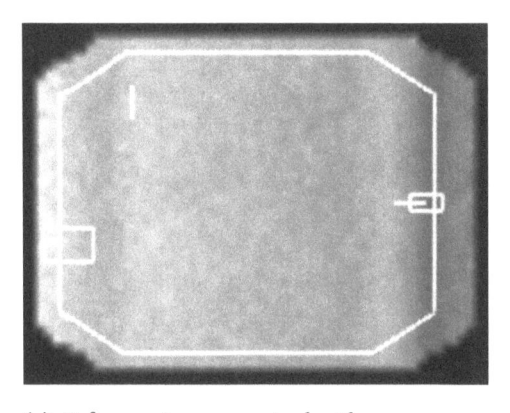

(b) Image of rod source producing the artifact in Figure 13-5a

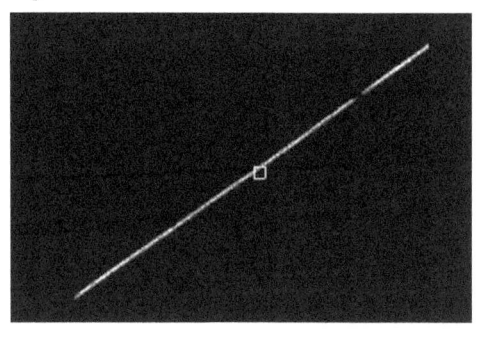

(c) Reference image acquired with poor uniformity correction map

(d) Same reference image after storing a new uniformity correction map

Figure 13-5 Unacceptable reference scans. Figure 13-5a shows a reference image demonstrating a loss of counts along the right edge of the image. The rod source was removed from its housing and laid on the gamma camera collimator (Fig. 13-5b); the defect in the rod source is clearly seen and explains the reference image. Figure 13-5c shows a reference image acquired on a Tl-201 energy setting, on a camera with an old uniformity correction map for Tl-201. After acquisition of a new Tl-201 uniformity correction map, the reference scan looks much more acceptable (Fig. 13-5d). The acceptability limits for uniformity of reference images are so high that this abnormality would not have been caught by quantitative analysis, but is apparent on visual inspection. Figures 13-5a and 13-5b courtesy of Philips Healthcare. Figures 13-5c and 13-5d courtesy of St. Joseph Medical Center.

has been achieved in the study. Some programs also provide additional quality control checks, for example, for truncation (see later in this chapter).

The use of TBAC is intended to address artifacts in clinical images, but in itself it can be a source of artifact. Both insufficient counts and inadequate correction for down-scatter have been shown to lead to artifacts in attenuation maps, which in turn may cause, for example, the myocardial defect size to appear larger than expected (11). Attenuation maps with truncation artifacts can also produce false defects in the emission images. The authors of this study emphasize the importance of viewing the reconstructed attenuation map for each patient before incorporating it into the attenuation correction process.

Rotational Stability

Given that SPECT requires the gamma camera to rotate, it is wise to verify system performance at several angles. To measure the stability of the camera's uniformity during rotation, a sheet source is taped securely to the collimator and imaged with the camera at 0°, 90°, 180°, and 270° angles. The images are each in turn subtracted from the 0° image (**Figure 13-6**). The subtraction images should have the appearance of noise only; any noticeable increase or deficit in count density may be due to a problem that occurs only with rotation (4). A recent study showed that the transmission-scanning system may also have variability related to rotational angle that would not be uncovered in a stationary reference scan and that can potentially have significant effects on clinical images (12).

Pixel Size Determination

The measurement of pixel size is a planar quality control test and was discussed in Chapter 9. But its primary importance relates to SPECT imaging, so it is mentioned again here. Reconstruction assumes that the pixel size is equal in both the X and Y directions of the camera face (this is actually an issue of the relative gains applied to the X and Y signals). Further, knowledge of pixel size to within 0.5 mm is required for Chang attenuation correction (6). Determination of pixel size can be done infrequently (i.e., quarterly); variation greater than a few percent of pixel size between the X and Y directions, variation between heads in a multidetector system, or change from previous values will require the attention of service personnel.

Collimator-Hole Angulation

Similarly, the angulation of collimator holes is a planar QC measure, but variations in hole angulation have their greatest consequence in SPECT imaging. When a particular channel or region of the collimator is angled differently than the rest of the collimator, the gamma rays seen through that channel or region are placed in the 3D image matrix, assuming no difference from the remainder of the collimator. The effect is similar to that of a COR error, but it may be even harder to perceive. A 1° hole angulation error can result in as much as a 3.5-mm offset error (10). Collimator defects cause much more prominent artifacts on reconstructed SPECT images than on planar images (13). Collimator-hole angulation should be checked on new collimators and whenever collimator damage is suspected.

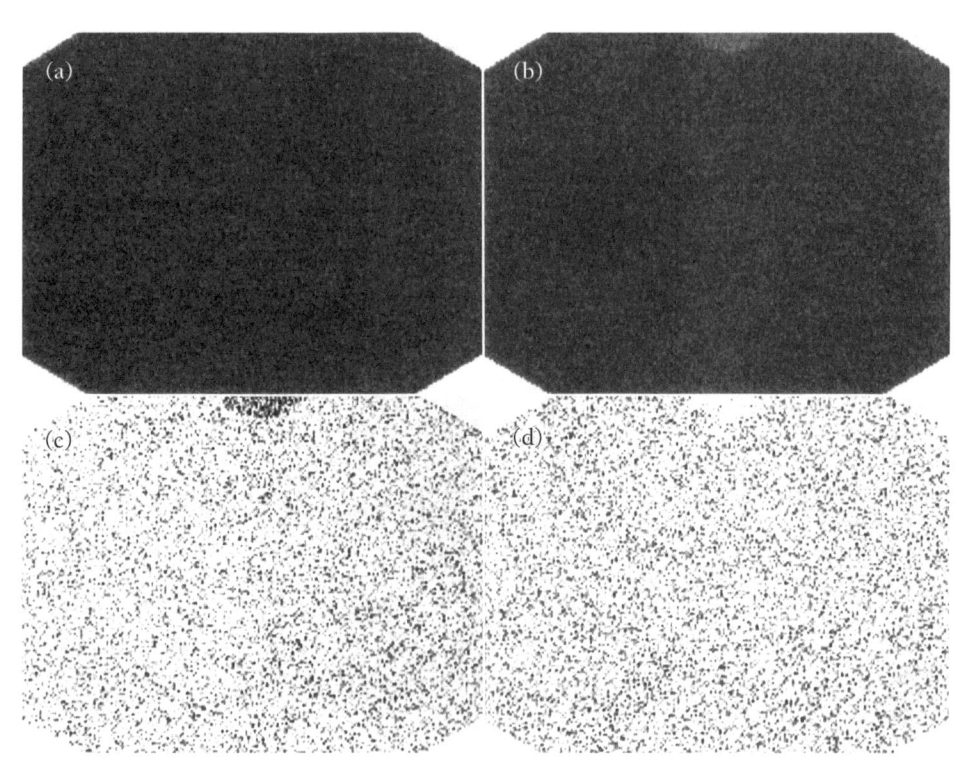

Figure 13-6 Rotational nonuniformity. The top two images are flood sources acquired with the flood source taped securely to the collimator face and imaged with the camera at (a) 0° and (b) 90°. The lower two images show the results of subtraction (c = a − b and d = b − a). A photomultiplier tube at the top margin of the camera head is not functional in the 90° orientation; the abnormality is much more visible on subtraction images than on the floods themselves. Reprinted from: Early PJ, Sodee DB. *Principles and Practice of Nuclear Medicine*. 2nd ed. St. Louis, MO: Mosby-Year Book; 1995:305. With permission from Elsevier Science.

Tomographic Measures of SPECT Performance

The QC tests discussed so far in this chapter determine a gamma camera's ability to produce satisfactory SPECT studies, but they do not measure the quality of the resulting images. We can apply the concepts of spatial resolution, uniformity, sensitivity, and image quality, as defined for planar imaging, to the reconstructed SPECT images. Several options for quantitative testing of these parameters are described below.

The reader should realize by now that reconstruction methods and parameters significantly affect not only image appearance but also quantitative values. One should attempt to duplicate both acquisition and reconstruction methodology as much as possible when measuring SPECT camera performance using NEMA, AAPM, or other published protocols. To date, most such protocols have used FBP as the reconstruction method of choice, with a specific filter indicated. One must be very careful in converting the specified filter to one's particular camera system (see, for example, Reference 2). Both the units used for the Nyquist frequency and the particular formula used for the low-pass filter may vary from system to system. Only when filter parameters are stated in absolute frequency units of per cm or per mm can the same filter be applied independent of the pixel size.

Sample Calculation 13-1 Conversion of Filter Cutoff Frequency

A NEMA protocol for a SPECT phantom test uses a Hann filter with a cutoff frequency of 0.8 × Nyquist frequency. The camera has a 52-cm field of view, and a 128 × 128 image matrix is to be used. Determine the camera's Nyquist frequency and the value of the recommended cutoff frequency in cycles/pixel and frequency (per-cm) units.

The pixel dimension for this camera and image matrix is

$$\text{Pixel dimension} = \frac{52\,\text{cm}}{128\,\text{pixels}} = \frac{4.1\,\text{mm}}{\text{pixel}}.$$

The Nyquist frequency is therefore

$$\text{Nyquist frequency} = \frac{1}{(2)(\text{pixel dimension})}$$
$$= \frac{1}{(2)(4.1\,\text{mm})} = \frac{0.12}{\text{mm}}.$$

The cutoff frequency is

$$0.8 \times \text{Nyquist} = 0.8\left(\frac{0.12}{\text{mm}}\right) = \frac{0.096}{\text{mm}} \cong \frac{0.1}{\text{mm}}.$$

We can also express the Nyquist frequency as 0.5 cycle/pixel, so the cutoff frequency is equivalent to 0.4 cycle/pixel.

Spatial Resolution Measurement

The full width at half-maximum (FWHM) and full width at tenth-maximum (FWTM) can be measured using a line source of radioactivity, much as in planar imaging but with a SPECT acquisition technique. The NEMA procedure (14) uses three 1-mm-diameter line sources (containing either Tc-99m or Co-57) inside a cylinder filled with water. One of the line sources is positioned in the center of the cylinder, and the other two are positioned near the edge of the cylinder so that the three are in a right-angle orientation (**Figure 13-7**). The cylinder is positioned so it is aligned with the AOR. The protocol calls for a 360° rotation, a matrix that produces pixels no larger than 2.5 mm, at least 100,000 cts per projection, and a 15-cm radius of rotation. After reconstruction with a ramp filter, count profiles through each line source are generated in directions perpendicular to the long axis of the line source. The actual count profiles are not smooth, so the data points may be used to interpolate a parabolic function. The FWHM and FWTM are measured (down to 0.1 pixel, based on the interpolation) and converted from pixels to mm using the system's pixel size calibration. Count pro files should be generated in at least three transverse slices and the FWHM and FWTM values averaged.

With the three line sources, we can quantify multiple components of in-plane resolution. The central line source tells us the resolution at the center of the 3D field of view, which is ideally where structures of greatest interest are located. For this central line source, the FWHM and FWTM values in the X and Y directions should be within 1 mm of each other. The two peripheral line sources provide FWHM values in the radial and tangential directions, with *radial* being along a line connected to the center of the FOV and *tangential* being perpendicular to the radial line. Figure 13-7a shows the radial and tangential directions for the lateral line source; in the inferior line source the radial axis is the Y-axis count profile and the tangential axis is the X-axis count profile.

The AAPM guidelines (3) also suggest a measurement of the axial FWHM (also referred to as slice thickness) (15). A line source is aligned in the X direction (i.e., perpendicular to the AOR, as in Fig. 13-7b). Acquire at least 20,000 cts per projection over 360°. Generate a 1-pixel count profile, and use this to produce a plot of counts vs transverse slice number. Use the count profile to determine the FWHM and FWTM; these values should be within 1 mm of those measured for the line source aligned with the AOR.

Uniformity Measurement

Acceptance testing requires a 20-cm-diameter cylindrical phantom that can be filled with water. In the context of acceptance testing, a phantom made for this specific purpose is preferred. But for routine evaluation of tomographic slice uniformity, a gallon-size bleach bottle (cleaned of its bleach, of course) works nicely. Ten to 15 mCi (370–550 MBq) of Tc-99m is diluted

(a) In-plane resolution

Cross section of cylindrical phantom with three line sources

Count profile in tangential direction

Count profile in radial direction

(b) Axial resolution

X-axis

Z-axis

Cts/pixel in slice

Slice number

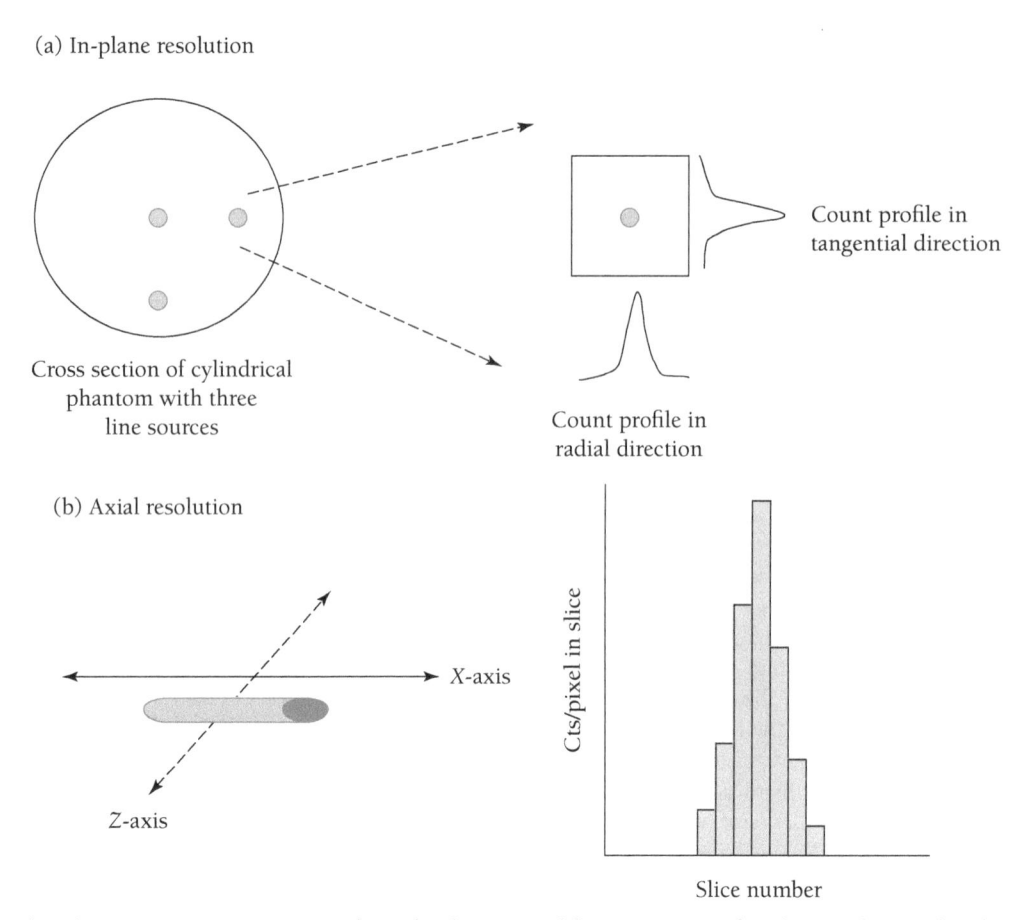

Figure 13-7 Spatial resolution in SPECT. Figure 13-7a shows the phantom used for measurement of in-plane resolution. Three line sources are aligned with the Z-axis, and count profiles of each source are generated in several different transverse planes. The centrally located line source is evaluated for FWHM and FWTM in both the X and Y directions. The peripherally located line sources are evaluated for FWHM and FWTM in the radial and tangential directions, as described in the text. The count profiles shown in Figure 13-7a (right) are for the lateral line source of the phantom; the axes that describe radial vs tangential direction are swapped for the inferior line source. Axial resolution is measured by orienting the line source in the X direction (perpendicular to the camera's AOR) and evaluating a count profile generated from successive transverse slices (Fig 13-7b).

with a sufficient volume of water to fill the bottle, with good mixing at several points during the filling process to ensure a truly uniform radioactivity distribution. If the phantom is to be used for sensitivity measurement (3), the activity concentration must be precisely known.

The AAPM test for tomographic slice uniformity images the phantom using a 128 × 128 matrix, the finest angular sampling available (usually 128 stops), and a circular orbit with a radius of 15 cm. At least 500,000 cts should be acquired in each 2D projection. A uniformity image with a thickness of four slices is reconstructed, using a ramp filter (or other routinely used filter) and Chang attenuation correction. It is then analyzed for integral and differential uniformity, using commercially available uniformity analysis programs. The limits of analysis are set to be the center 15-cm × 15-cm part of the slice. The AAPM recommends that this test be repeated with a noncircular orbit and with each collimator routinely used for SPECT imaging. All images should be evaluated visually for ring artifacts (see later in this chapter). The root–mean–square noise, a measure of statistical quality similar to the coefficient of variation, can also be calculated according to the formula

$$\text{Root–mean–square noise} = \frac{\text{standard deviation of ct/pixel values}}{\text{mean ct/pixel}} \times 100\%.$$

(13-1)

With all corrections operating, integral uniformity on modern systems measures 10 to 29%, and the root–mean–square noise is 3 to 9% (2).

System Volume Sensitivity

The concept of sensitivity is most important in SPECT from the standpoint of the compromise between total counts and patient tolerance for the long imaging time. Measurement of sensitivity using a planar image of a cylindrical phantom is included in the AAPM acceptance testing protocol (3) but is not discussed here. The NEMA test for volume sensitivity (14) requires a SPECT acquisition of a cylindrical phantom with accurately known activity concentration. The radionuclide is chosen to be appropriate for the collimator being tested. The test is performed on a system in which flood corrections of the count skimming/adding variety (i.e., the uniformity correction map) are turned off, so as not to alter the number of counts detected in any way. The total time of the acquisition and the summed counts from all projections are determined and inserted into the equation

$$\text{System volume sensitivity} = \frac{\text{total cts}/\text{total time (sec)}}{\text{activity concentration }(\mu\text{Ci}/\text{ml})}. \quad (13\text{-}2)$$

The activity concentration of the phantom is decay-corrected to the halfway point of the SPECT acquisition. The sensitivity per axial centimeter can then be determined by dividing the system volume sensitivity by the length of the cylindrical phantom. Results should specify both the radionuclide utilized and the method of acquisition (continuous vs step-and-shoot).

Jaszczak Phantom

This phantom (named after its inventor, Ronald Jaszczak; also called a *performance phantom*) provides excellent information about SPECT performance. It consists of a 20-cm-diameter Plexiglas cylinder with both rod and sphere inserts (**Figure 13-8**). The rods are made of Lucite® and are of varying sizes in a six-sector format, providing a 3D "bar phantom." The spheres are made of solid Lucite (fillable spheres for creating hot lesions can be purchased) and sit on Lucite stems that are threaded at the opposite end. The rod insert is placed in the cylinder, and the sphere stems fit through it and into the threaded holes in the bottom of the cylinder, holding the rod insert in place. The top section of the phantom has neither rods nor spheres and is used to measure uniformity.

The phantom with its rod and sphere inserts is filled with water and 10 to 20 mCi (370–740 MBq) Tc-99m. It must be mixed well at several points in the filling process to ensure uniformity of radionuclide distribution. The lid of the Plexiglas cylinder is held in place by plastic screws (metal is not used in order to avoid attenuation). These screws break easily, so care must be taken as they are tightened or loosened. A SPECT acquisition is then done using a 64 × 64 matrix, 64 stops over a 360° rotation, and about 200,000 cts per projection.

After acquisition, the study may be reconstructed using a Hann or Hamming filter with a cutoff frequency of 1 Nyquist (**Figure 13-9**) (2, 10). Uniformity is measured

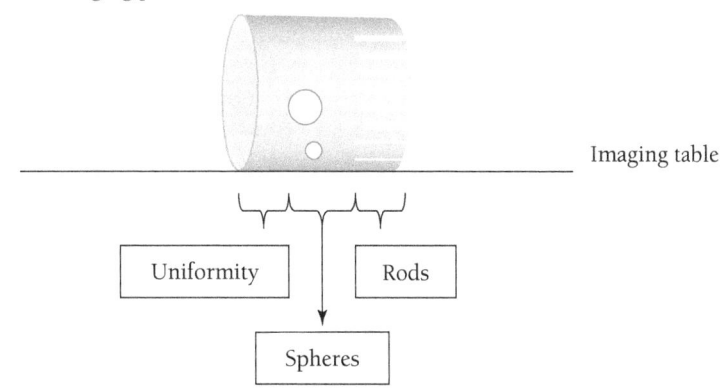

Figure 13-8 Jaszczak phantom. The Jaszczak phantom and its successors allow for measurement of uniformity, semiquantitative spatial resolution (the rods), and real-life spatial resolution (the spheres). Figure 13-8a courtesy of Biodex Medical Systems.

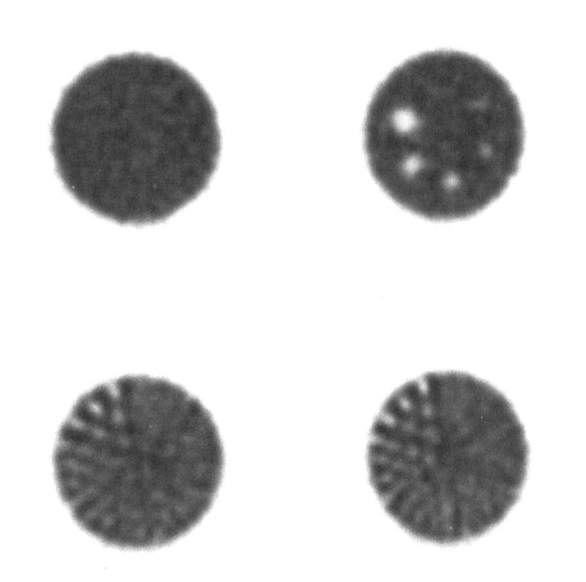

Figure 13-9 Reconstructed slices of a Jaszczak phantom. The top left slice shows the uniformity section of the phantom; the top right, the cold spheres; and the bottom two slices, the rod section of the phantom. Image courtesy of Virginia Mason Medical Center.

on a transverse slice through the uppermost portion of the cylinder, similarly to what was described for the cylindrical phantom. In the lower part of the phantom, about 15 transverse slices containing the rods are summed to provide a semiquantitative measure of spatial resolution (16). Lesion detectability is evaluated in two ways: semiquantitatively, based on the smallest sphere seen, and quantitatively, in the form of lesion contrast:

$$\text{Contrast} = \frac{(\text{avg. cts/pixel in uniform section}) - (\text{minimum cts/pixel in cold sphere})}{\text{avg. cts/pixel in uniform section}} \times 100\%.$$

(13-3)

Calculated values for contrast in one study ranged from about 63% in the largest sphere to about 20% in the smallest sphere (2).

Sample Calculation 13-2   Lesion Contrast in a Jaszczak Phantom

A Jaszczak phantom study yields count densities of 105 cts/voxel in the center of a cold sphere and an average of 285 cts/pixel in the surrounding cylinder. What is the lesion contrast?

Per Equation 13-3, the contrast is

$$\text{Contrast} = \frac{285 \text{ cts/pixel} - 105 \text{ cts/pixel}}{285 \text{ cts/pixel}} \times 100\% = 63\%.$$

The implication of this number is that the apparent activity concentration in the cold sphere is almost two-thirds that of the cylinder, as a result of scatter.

If time for quality control studies is limited, the Jaszczak phantom offers the best overall evaluation of SPECT image quality. Agencies that accredit nuclear medicine laboratories require a phantom study on SPECT cameras at least annually.

SPECT Artifacts

SPECT artifacts are more problematic than those of planar images, because reconstruction amplifies small errors in the individual projections into significance. The different types of artifacts can be attributed to various aspects of the SPECT imaging and reconstruction process. Ray artifacts come specifically from the process of backprojection. Ring artifacts are a consequence of the rotational, multiview nature of SPECT imaging. Motion artifacts stem from the time-consuming nature of the studies. And truncation artifacts result from the addition of attenuation correction to the procedure. All are recognizable to some extent, especially on phantom images and when they are severe. But they can be difficult to spot on clinical images. The operator needs to look carefully for evidence of these artifacts and, if possible, correct them so that they do not affect clinical results.

Ray Artifacts

Ray artifacts result specifically from the use of FBP as the reconstruction. In particular, a very hot or very cold lesion may be insufficiently corrected by the applied filter, and the ray will be apparent even in the final slices (**Figure 13-10** shows an extreme example). Rays created by backprojection are two-dimensional, because the backprojection process is two-dimensional. Ray artifacts do not cross from one transverse slice to the next unless the amount of reorientation is significant (as in Fig. 13-10d).

Ray artifacts become particularly noticeable when the activity causing the ray artifact is significantly more intense than the surrounding tissue. An extreme example of this phenomenon can occur in gated SPECT imaging (17). In a gated study, if a long R-R interval is chosen relative to the patient's actual heart rate, then the next R wave may occur before the acquisition into the final gated frame is finished. If this occurs often in the course of the study, the final frame of the gated cine may be quite count-poor. But gated SPECT processing programs generally normalize the frames of the gated study, such that the few counts in the final frame are multiplied into significance. Backprojection then spreads these statistical "hot spots" across the 3D image matrix. This "flashing artifact" results in an uninterpretable gated SPECT study.

If a ray artifact will interfere with visualization of the organ of interest, it should, if possible, be removed. In some situations, such as a hot injection site in the arm, this is easily done. In other cases, the area creating the ray artifact is internal, and one may need to use other means to cause it to shift positions. Ray artifacts emanating from the urinary bladder may be decreased to some extent by voiding. Increased uptake in the intestines may be caused to move by administration of cathartics. Time can also be a helpful factor in some situations. Note that it is usually

(a) Raw projections

(b) Ray artifacts seen in the reconstruction process

(c) Short-axis views including the artifact

(d) Horizontal long-axis views including the artifact

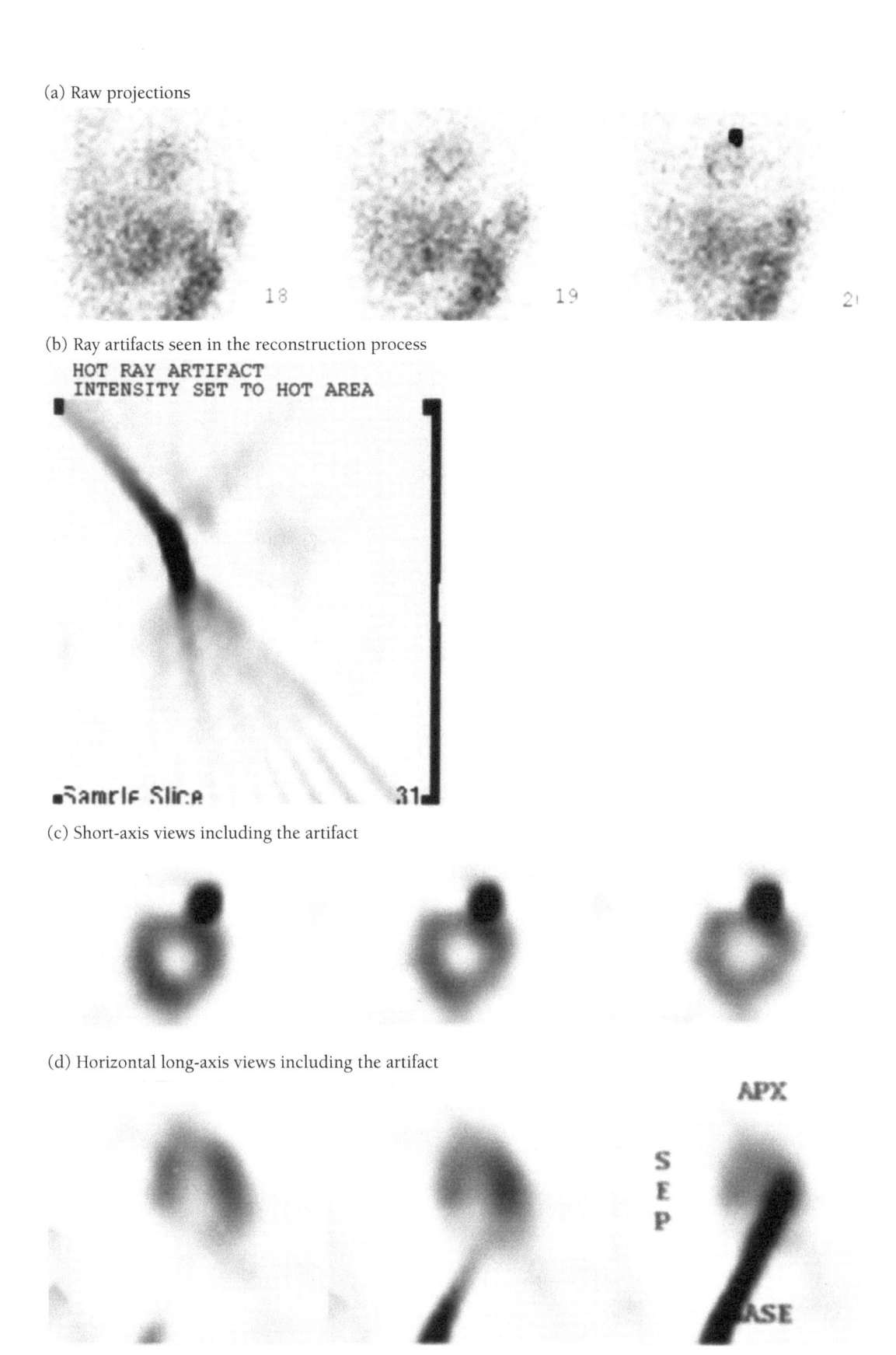

Figure 13-10 Ray artifact. The images show several projections of a cardiac study, including one frame in which a very intense source of activity is imaged. The identity of this source of activity was never determined; it was seen in only the one projection. Figure 13-10b shows the rays generated by the reconstruction process; because the source is not seen in all frames, the rays are not appropriately subtracted by filtering in other projections. Figures 13-10c and 13-10d illustrate the reconstructed short-axis and horizontal long-axis images and the effect of this ray artifact. Images courtesy of Virginia Mason Medical Center.

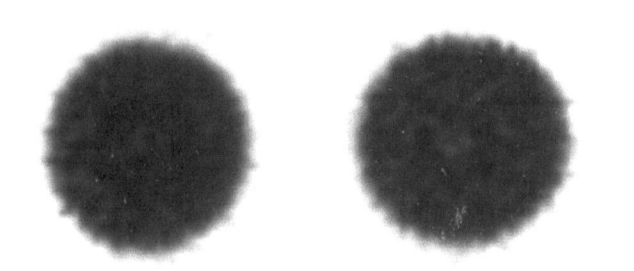

Figure 13-11 Ring artifact. The image shows evidence of a subtle ring artifact resulting from a flood nonuniformity. Ring artifacts often have alternating dark and light rings. Image courtesy of Virginia Mason Medical Center.

difficult to judge before the acquisition whether a ray artifact may be created that will interfere with image interpretation. Given the speed of modern computer systems, it behooves the technologist to process the study at least partially before releasing the patient, to determine whether a modified acquisition is needed.

Ring Artifacts

Because SPECT imaging requires a rotating gamma camera, any abnormalities inherent to the detector or the rotational mechanics will be carried through every projection, leading to a ring artifact (**Figure 13-11**; in the literature, these are sometimes referred to as "bull's-eye artifacts"). Abnormalities that will be seen as ring artifacts include flood nonuniformities and collimator defects. An integral or differential uniformity value of 5%, imperceptible to the eye, can cause significant ring artifacts (5). Ring artifacts can also result from COR errors and head-tilt errors, because both cause the apparent AOR to be different from the actual AOR. Thus the classic COR error, in which a line or point source appears as a donut, is actually a ring artifact. Ring artifacts are only corrected by addressing the underlying problem.

(a) Horizontal long-axis images of the heart at stress (top row) and rest (bottom row), with duplication of the lateral wall in the stress images due to significant motion

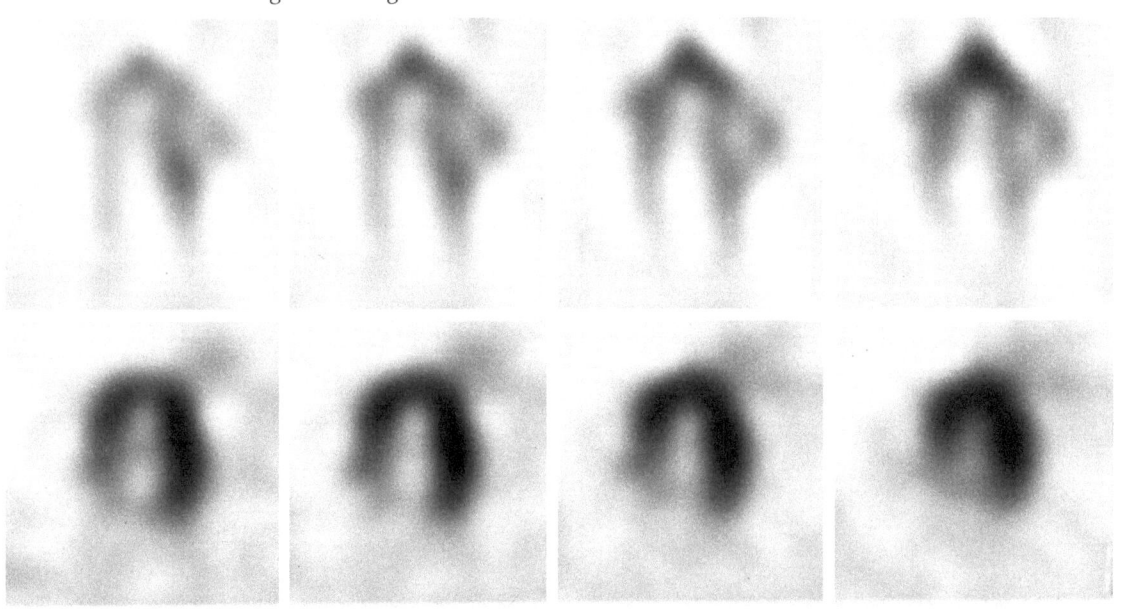

(b) Short-axis images of the same study, showing the same wall duplication

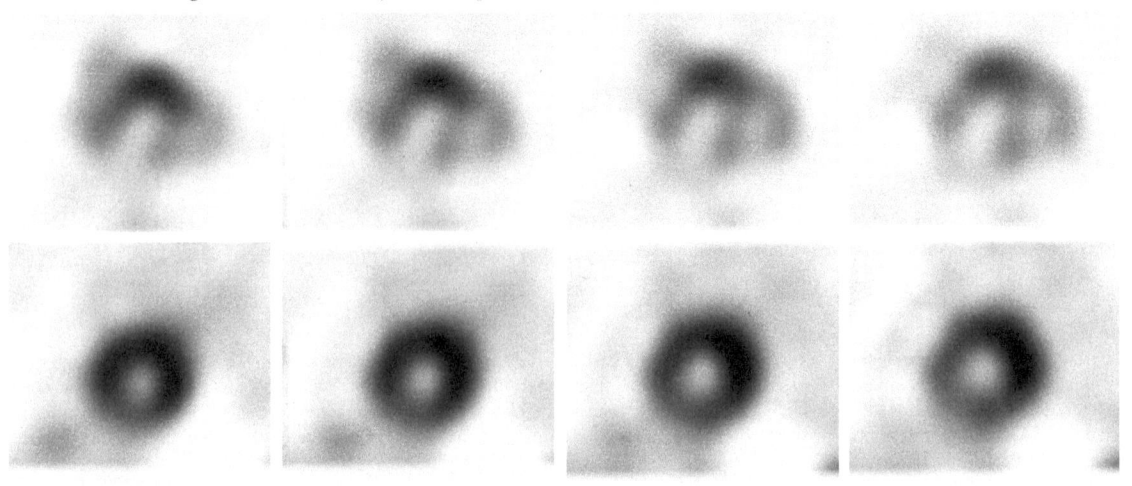

Figure 13-12 Motion artifact. When motion occurs in the process of acquiring a SPECT study, the same anatomic area is seen in two different places. This study illustrates a drastic example of a motion artifact, with apparent duplication of the lateral heart wall, because the motion occurred about halfway through the study. Images courtesy of Virginia Mason Medical Center.

Camera nonuniformities are the most common source of ring artifacts. While planar images can be interpreted with uniformity as high as 5%, SPECT images suffer degradation when planar uniformity exceeds 2 to 3%. Ring artifacts will be most noticeable when the nonuniformity is small in size and/or centrally located. They are easily masked by poor statistics or excessive filtering. Technologists should therefore be aware that nonuniformities that are invisible on planar images can produce distortions that make SPECT images difficult to interpret.

Motion Artifacts

The theory of 3D image reconstruction assumes that the radiopharmaceutical distribution is the same from the beginning to the end of the acquisition period. If a localized area of increased activity moves, it will be seen in two different locations in the 3D image matrix. Motion of 2 or more pixels results in clinically significant artifacts (18). **Figure 13-12** shows an extreme example of motion on a myocardial perfusion study. The visibility of a motion artifact depends on not only the magnitude of the movement, but also the time when it occurs during the course of the acquisition. Motion artifacts can be subtle and difficult to detect on clinical studies, so it is vital that (1) the patient understand the importance of not moving and (2) the technologist evaluate the study for motion before allowing the patient to leave.

There are multiple ways to evaluate for motion. A cine viewing of the raw data may be the quickest method. Other techniques for detection of patient motion include the sinogram (see Fig. 11-1) and a summed image of all the projections. The sinogram is best suited for detecting horizontal motion, whereas the summed image works better for vertical motion (16). Many computers offer motion correction programs. These should be utilized as needed, but the results should always be examined to ensure the program has not made matters worse rather than better.

A phenomenon that combines elements of ray artifact and motion is seen when an area of increased activity moves or fills during the study. Take, for example, the filling bladder on a bone SPECT study (**Figure 13-13**). At the beginning of the study, the bladder is (ideally) small,

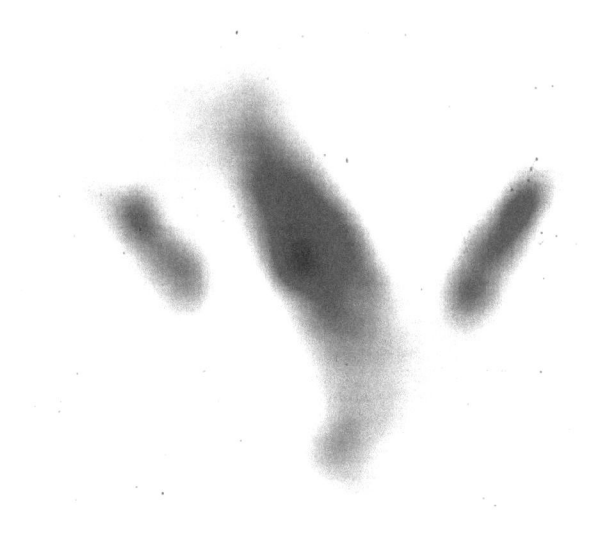

Figure 13-13 Filling bladder artifact. When an organ such as the bladder changes size during a SPECT acquisition, the backprojection filter does not cancel out the extra activity. The rays are seen to be "pointing" in the direction of the projections that saw the larger bladder, and their intensity increases as the intensity of the bladder increases. Image courtesy of Virginia Mason Medical Center.

but as the projections are being acquired, it fills, occupying a greater volume within the pelvis. The hot bladder produces ray artifacts, but only in directions corresponding to the projections that saw the excess activity. A similar effect can be seen with moving intestinal activity on a Tc-99m sestamibi study. Iterative reconstruction may deal with changing activity locations better than FBP (19).

Truncation Artifacts

A *truncation artifact* occurs in transmission scanning (using either a radionuclide source or CT) when a part of the body is not seen in all projections. Transmission image reconstruction assumes that the entire object is in the FOV from all angles. If this condition is not met, reconstruction algorithms incorrectly place counts and/or count boundaries where they should not be. Two examples of truncation artifacts are shown in **Figure 13-14**. Truncation is more likely to occur with a limited-FOV collimator, such

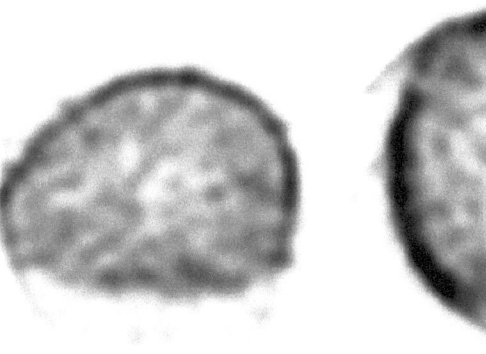

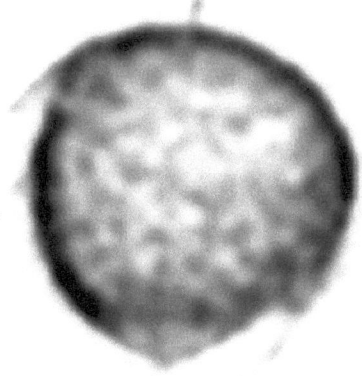

Figure 13-14 Two examples of truncation of transmission images. If the entire body is not included in the transmission projections, a cupping artifact results. This artifact shows high-count densities along the edge of the body from the angle(s) where truncation occurred. These high-count densities often extend beyond the body contour (especially prominent in the attenuation map on the right). The transmission images shown here are in the lower part of the abdomen. Truncation artifacts in the region of the heart, if used to correct emission images, may result in unidentifiable artifacts in the corrected 3D image matrix. Image courtesy of St. Joseph Medical Center.

as a cone-beam or fan-beam collimator, and with large patients. Even moderate truncation artifacts can cause problems with reconstructed images (11). In iterative reconstruction, it is possible to correct for truncation artifacts by extrapolating the truncated image data from the untruncated part of the transmission map and/or the scattered photons registered in a secondary energy window. One can also reduce the effect of a truncation error by constraining the volume to be reconstructed to untruncated areas. Because of problems created by truncation, the transmission images should be evaluated after acquisition but before the patient leaves, just as the emission images are.

Summary

By now it should be apparent to the reader that generation of high-quality SPECT images requires significantly greater vigilance than does planar imaging. Artifacts of the imaging process are hard to spot, even in the ideal situation of a line source or uniform phantom. They may not be detectable as artifacts on clinical images, and they can be hidden by one's choice of filter, if FBP reconstruction is used. The development of iterative reconstruction methodology has the potential to limit ray artifacts, but not ring artifacts or motion artifacts. Therefore, SPECT will always require meticulous attention to the details of quality control and quality assurance.

References

1. Madsen MT. Recent advances in SPECT imaging. *J Nucl Med.* 2007;48: 661–673.
2. Graham LS, Fahey FH, Madsen MT, et al. AAPM Report No. 52: Quantitation of SPECT performance. Woodbury, NY: American Institute of Physics; 1995.
3. Siegel JA, Benedetto AR, Jaszczak RJ, et al. AAPM Report No. 22: Rotating scintillation camera SPECT acceptance testing and quality control. New York, NY: American Association of Physicists in Medicine; 1987.
4. Henkin RE, Boles MA, Dillehay GL, et al., eds. *Nuclear Medicine.* St. Louis, MO: Mosby-Year Book; 1996:241–243.
5. Zanzonico P. Routine quality control of clinical nuclear medicine instrumentation: a brief review. *J Nucl Med.* 2008;49:1114–1131.
6. Lee KH. *Computers in Nuclear Medicine: A Practical Approach.* 2nd ed. Reston, VA: Society of Nuclear Medicine; 2005:151, 152, 154.
7. Rogers WL, Clinthorne NH, Harkness BA, et al. Field-flood requirements for emission computed tomography with an Anger camera. *J Nucl Med.* 1982;23: 162–168.
8. Bolstad R, Brown J, Grantham V. Extrinsic versus intrinsic uniformity correction for gamma cameras. *J Nucl Med Technol.* 2011;39:208–212.
9. Hines H, Kayayan R, Colsher J. et al. National Electrical Manufacturers Association recommendations for implementing SPECT instrumentation quality control. *J Nucl Med.* 2000;41:383–389.
10. Graham LS. A rational quality assurance program for SPECT instrumentation. *Nuclear Medicine Annual 1989.* New York, NY: Raven Press; 1989.
11. Celler A, Dixon KL, Chang Z, et al. Problems created in attenuation-corrected SPECT images by artifacts in attenuation maps: a simulation study. *J Nucl Med.* 2005;46:335–343.
12. Evans SG, Hutton BF. Variation in scanning line source sensitivity: a significant source of error in simultaneous emission-transmission tomography. *Eur J Nucl Med Mol Imaging.* 2004;31:703–709.
13. Blend MJ, Patel BA, Byrom E. Collimator-induced defects in planar and SPECT gamma camera images: a multicenter study. *J Nucl Med Technol.* 1995;23: 167–172.
14. National Electrical Manufacturers Association. *Performance Measurements of Scintillation Cameras.* Publication NU 1-2001. Rosslyn, VA; NEMA Publications; 2001.
15. Cherry SR, Sorenson JA, Phelps ME. *Physics in Nuclear Medicine.* 3rd ed. Philadelphia, PA: Saunders; 2002; 319.
16. Graham LS. SPECT data acquisition and quality control. In: Fahey FH, Harkness BA, eds. *Basic Science of Nuclear Medicine* [CD-ROM]. Reston, VA: Society of Nuclear Medicine; 2001.
17. DePuey EG, Garcia EV, Berman DS. *Cardiac SPECT Imaging.* Philadelphia, PA: Lippincott Williams & Wilkins; 2001:109, 260–261.
18. Germano G. Technical aspects of myocardial SPECT imaging. *J Nucl Med.* 2001;42:1499–1507.
19. Miller TR. Emission tomography and image reconstruction. In: Fahey FH, Harkness BA, eds. *Basic Science of Nuclear Medicine* [CD-ROM]. Reston, VA: Society of Nuclear Medicine; 2001.

Additional Resources

Eisner RL. Principles of instrumentation in SPECT. *J Nucl Med Technol.* 1985;13: 23–31.
English RJ. *SPECT: A Primer.* 3rd ed. Reston, VA: Society of Nuclear Medicine; 1995:Chapters 3, 8.
Graham LS. A rational quality assurance program for SPECT instrumentation. *Nuclear Medicine Annual 1989.* New York: Raven Press; 1989.
Graham LS. The AAPM/RSNA physics tutorial for residents: quality control for SPECT systems. *Radiographics.* 1995;15:1471–1481.
Henkin RE, Boles MA, Dillehay GL, et al., eds. *Nuclear Medicine.* St. Louis, MO: Mosby-Year Book; 1996:Chapter 19.
Hines H, Kayayan R, Colsher J, et al. National Electrical Manufacturers Association recommendations for implementing SPECT instrumentation quality control. *J Nucl Med.* 2000;41:383–389.
Lee KH. *Computers in Nuclear Medicine: A Practical Approach.* 2nd ed. Reston, VA: Society of Nuclear Medicine; 2005:Chapter 11.
Zanzonico P. Routine quality control of clinical nuclear medicine instrumentation: a brief review. *J Nucl Med.* 2008;49:1114–1131.

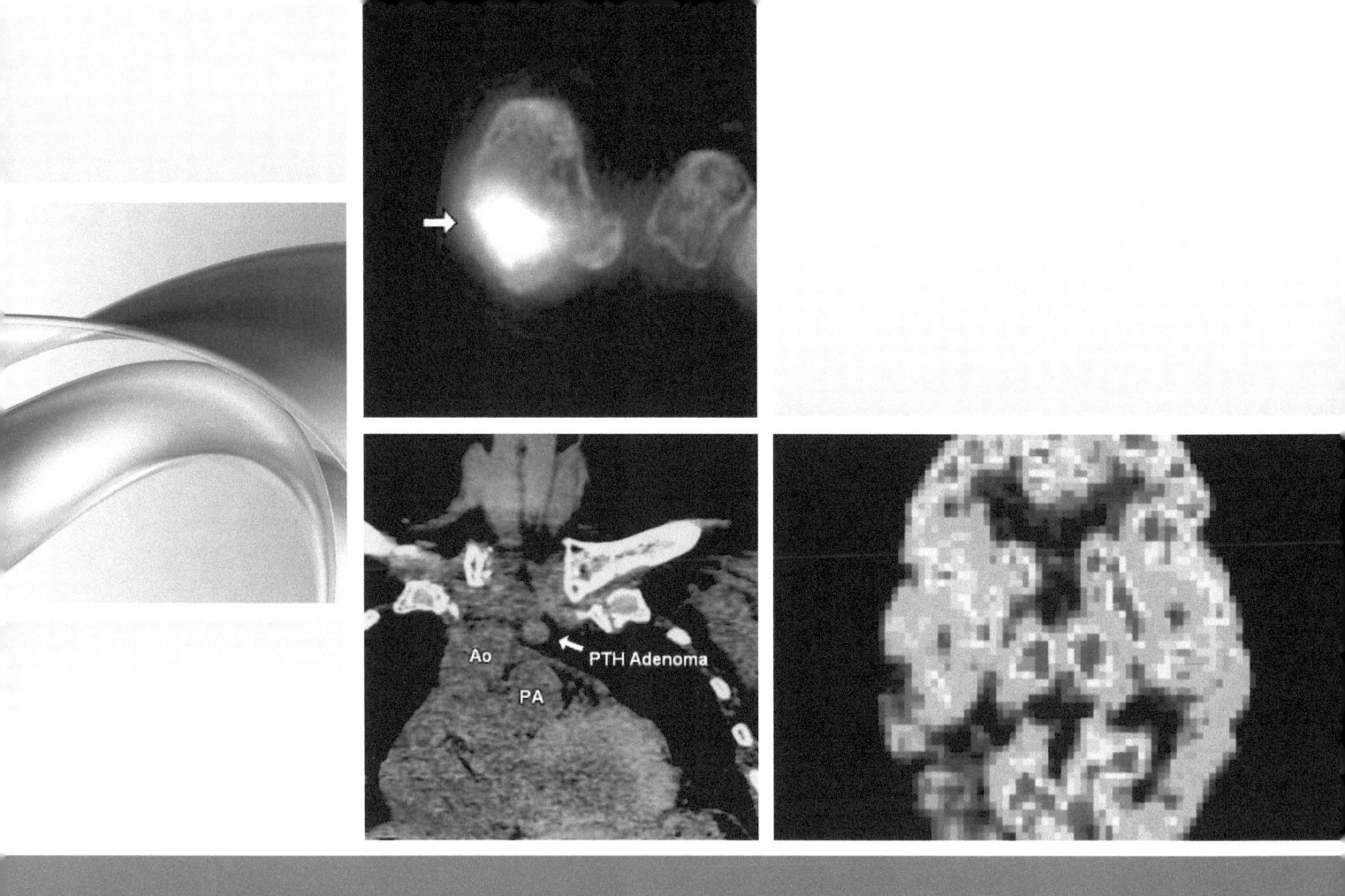

PART IV
Positron Emission Tomography (PET)

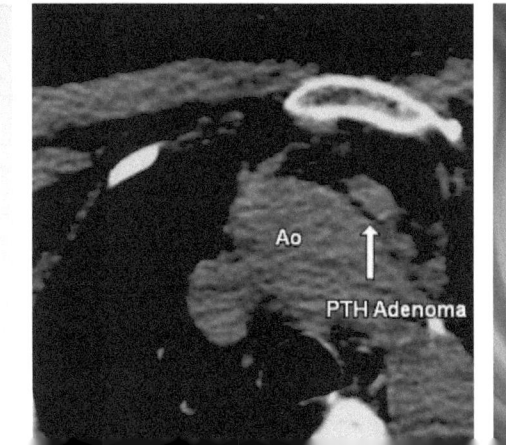

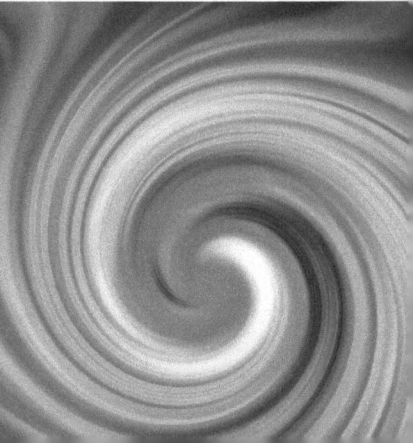

CHAPTER 14
Principles of Positron Emission Tomography (PET)

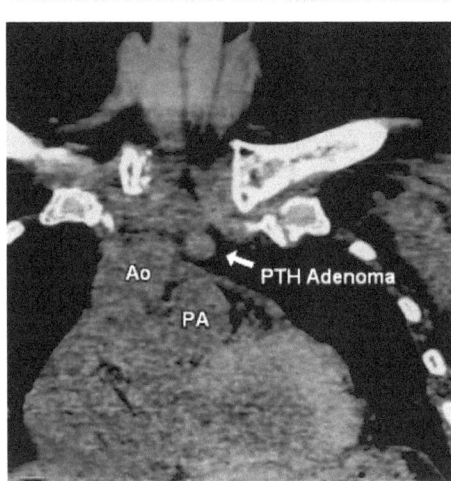

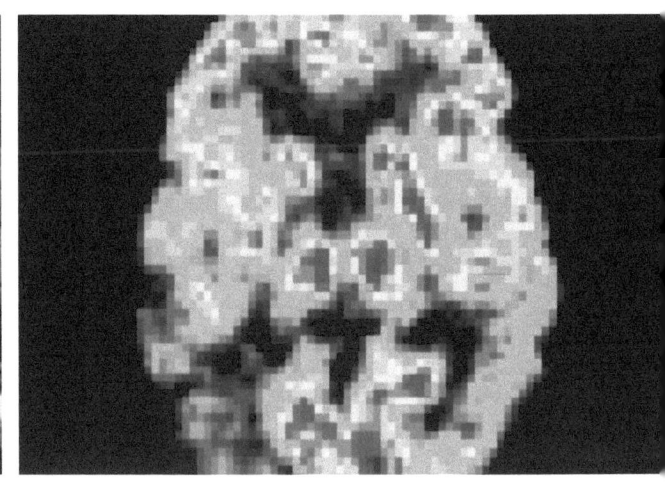

Learning Outcomes

1. Describe, in both words and diagrams, the essential concepts of coincidence imaging.
2. Describe positron-emitting radionuclides and annihilation photons and the important characteristics of the scintillation materials used for coincidence imaging.
3. Define *line of response*, and describe the layout of a sinogram.
4. Distinguish between trues, singles, randoms, and scatters in coincidence imaging.
5. Describe how attenuation is measured in PET, and contrast it with attenuation correction in SPECT.
6. Discuss the basic concepts behind time-of-flight PET.
7. Briefly discuss why PET is considered more quantitative than SPECT.

Introduction

The modality of *positron emission tomography*, commonly called *PET*, has contributed greatly both to our basic understanding of living systems and to the clinical diagnosis of a variety of diseases. It offers a number of advantages over single-photon imaging, the most significant of which are the use of actual biological molecules and the ability to perform absolute quantitation, allowing the measurement of physiologically meaningful quantities. These qualities make it highly likely that PET will continue to make important contributions to both the research and clinical arenas.

PET requires that we think differently about both the imaging process (discussed in this chapter) and the imaging systems or *tomographs* (discussed in Chapter 15). (As noted in Chapter 10, this term is not in common use, but it is employed here to avoid confusion that can arise when other terms such as *scanner* are used.) PET imaging has significant dissimilarities compared to single-photon imaging with a gamma camera, so much so that the major thread that links the two types of imaging is the administration of a radiopharmaceutical that illuminates a physiologic process. Thus the reader may wish to start with a "clean slate," as it were, in order to comprehend the complexities of PET instrumentation.

The essence of PET is the administration of a positron-emitting radiopharmaceutical, followed by detection of the two 511-keV annihilation photons resulting from the annihilation interaction of the positron with an electron. This process is outlined in **Figure 14-1**. The annihilation photons are simultaneously released in 180°-opposed directions. They travel at the speed of light (approaching 3×10^{10} cm/sec), such that it takes only 3 nanoseconds (nsec) for an annihilation photon to traverse a 90-cm-wide PET tomograph. To be considered a valid event, the two annihilation photons must both be detected within a very short *coincidence timing window* (CTW) of 5 to 12 nsec. When this condition is met, the two photons are said to be *in coincidence* with each other. The phrase *coincidence*

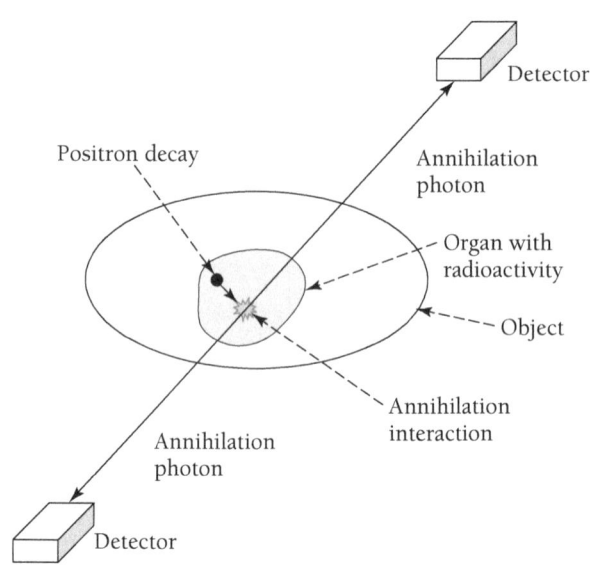

Figure 14-1 Detection of annihilation photons from a positron-emitting radionuclide. The figure shows an object containing an area of radiopharmaceutical uptake. When a radionuclide atom decays, it emits a positron, which travels a short distance, losing kinetic energy via ionization and excitation interactions. When it has lost all (or almost all) of its energy, it annihilates with an electron, producing two annihilation photons emitted at a 180° angle, each with 511 keV of energy. These annihilation photons, if both are detected by the two 180°-opposed detectors within a very short coincidence timing window, are assumed to be a "good" event, and a count is registered in the line connecting the two detectors. The figure is shown with exaggerated distances for clarity; in real life, the positron travels a distance of only a few millimeters or less before annihilating.

imaging is used to describe any imaging technique that relies on the coincident detection of annihilation photons.

A Brief History of PET

Coincidence imaging has a long history (1), but it has been slow to enter clinical practice, for a variety of reasons that are outlined in this section. In 1951, Brownell and Sweet used two sodium iodide crystals to detect Cu-64 phthalocyanime in the brain, and in 1953 rectilinear scanners were used to image positron-emitting radiopharmaceuticals. Dr. Hal Anger developed the first positron camera based on coincident detection of annihilation photons in 1959 (2). The first ring-type detector system for annihilation photon imaging was created by Rankowitz et al. in 1962. An early prototype PET tomograph used a hexagonal array of sodium iodide detectors mounted on a horizontal support. The object to be examined was placed on a turntable that rotated within the plane of the hexagonal array. The first commercial PET tomograph reached the market in 1974.

In the 1980s, PET was seen primarily as a research tool, for several reasons. One was that the positron-emitting radionuclides were primarily produced on site, in a cyclotron. Another was that the tomographs were quite labor-intensive, requiring the daily attention of a physicist. Both the cyclotron and the physics support were more commonly found in university settings. Moreover, the imaging being performed at that time was elucidating biochemical and physiological processes, many for the first time. The feeling of the research community in the middle to late 1980s was that PET should not be moved too quickly into clinical practice, because there was still so much it could clarify about the function of the human body.

In 1991, the Society of Nuclear Medicine (SNM) published a special supplement entitled "Clinical PET: Its Time Has Come." At that point, the PET tomograph had reached a relatively mature state, the clinical use of F-18 fluorodeoxyglucose (FDG) for detection of malignancies was well documented, and the time seemed right for PET to come into its own as a clinical imaging modality. But this transition did not come about for 10 years. A major reason for the delay was that PET radionuclides were not readily available. An additional hurdle was the regulatory approval of PET radiopharmaceuticals, which are not compounded as other nuclear medicine radiopharmaceuticals are, but are actually manufactured on site. The passage of the Food and Drug Administration (FDA) Modernization Act in 1997 eased some of these restrictions.

A third reason that PET did not become a clinical tool was that reimbursement for PET exams was nonexistent. Medicare (the U.S. government's federally funded health insurance plan for the elderly) had realized by the early 1980s that it was slowly but surely going broke, a situation that was attributed in part to the increasing use of new diagnostic technologies, including computed tomography (CT) and magnetic resonance imaging (MRI). So Medicare worked slowly to approve PET exams, and it did so only on an indication-by-indication basis. Without a source of radiopharmaceuticals or a guarantee of payment, an institution would have been foolhardy to make a large capital investment in a PET tomograph. In the mid-1990s, Medicare finally approved PET scans for a small number of clinical indications.

The technology that finally gave PET the push it needed was the gamma camera, specifically dual-head SPECT tomographs modified to do coincidence imaging. As nuclear medicine departments began to do PET imaging with these systems, the first distribution network for PET radiopharmaceuticals was created by PETNet, Inc. Ultimately, gamma cameras, even with modifications, produce suboptimal PET images, and most nuclear medicine facilities have moved to dedicated PET or PET/CT tomographs. But the hybrid systems provided the bridge that moved PET fully into the clinical setting. Thus, it took a confluence of events to make PET imaging a viable clinical modality.

The majority of Medicare-approved indications involve the use of FDG, and the majority of PET centers are doing primarily FDG oncology imaging (imagine the field of nuclear medicine consisting of only bone scans for metastases). Fortunately, the benefits of FDG imaging are sufficient to justify the expense of PET. An FDG scan can show not only a primary malignancy, but also all the places to which it has spread. Posttherapy FDG scans provide significant information about the success of the therapeutic regimen, and this appears to be true even when the FDG scan is done early in the course of treatment. A number of other PET radiopharmaceuticals have been created, and over time some will move into clinical use. The placement of PET and CT tomographs on one gantry has further strengthened this modality by providing an anatomic framework to complement the physiologic information provided by PET. PET has proved its utility in the research setting, and it is now doing the same in the clinic.

Physics of Positron Emitters and Annihilation Photons

Positron-Emitting Radionuclides

Annihilation photons are produced by the annihilation interaction of a positron with an electron. So to understand PET, we need first to consider positrons. Radionuclides that emit positrons are neutron-deficient. Positron decay competes with electron capture as the decay mode, with positron decay being favored in lighter elements and electron capture in heavier elements. **Table 14-1** lists some clinically useful positron-emitting radionuclides. Many of these radionuclides are produced in a cyclotron, although two are daughters of other radionuclides and can be obtained from generator systems.

Note in particular the first four radionuclides. Carbon, oxygen, and nitrogen are common constituents of biologically significant molecules. Because these radionuclides do not affect in any way the behavior of the molecules into which they are incorporated, they perfectly match the ideal of a radioactive "tracer." Most radiopharmaceuticals used in single-photon imaging do not approach this ideal so closely. Fluorine-18 is substituted for a hydrogen atom or hydroxyl (–OH) group, which does affect behavior in the body to a certain extent, making F-18-labeled radiopharmaceuticals somewhat less ideal as tracers for biologic processes. On the other hand, of these four radionuclides only F-18 has a long enough half-life to be shipped any distance.

Annihilation Photons

We commonly speak of imaging a positron-emitting radionuclide in PET, but in actuality we are imaging the annihilation photons that result when the positron combines with an electron in an annihilation interaction. An important limitation of PET is the fact that the positron travels some distance before annihilating. Recall from nuclear physics that when a radionuclide decays via positron emission, the transition energy is shared between the positron and a neutrino. The positron must lose its share of that transition energy through interactions with other atoms before it annihilates with a nearby electron. The kinetic energy given to the positron determines how far it may travel before coming to rest. Positrons from a single transition have a range of energies and therefore travel a range of distances before annihilating. This range varies from radionuclide to radionuclide; the average and maximum ranges for different positron emitters in water are given in Table 14-1.

What this means for imaging is that the point of annihilation is not the same as the location of radionuclide decay. It violates the basic assumption of radionuclide imaging, namely, that the radiation emission accurately represents the location of the radiopharmaceutical. Further, the higher the positron energy, the more significant the difference becomes. A radionuclide such as Rb-82 that emits high-energy positrons will show significant image degradation compared to a radionuclide that emits lower-energy positrons, such as F-18. Thus, the choice of radionuclide directly affects image quality.

The process of annihilation also adds a degree of uncertainty. If the positron loses all of its kinetic energy before annihilating, the two annihilation photons are exactly 180° opposed. If the positron still has a small amount of kinetic energy remaining at the moment of annihilation,

Table 14-1

Positron-Emitting Radionuclides Commonly Used in PET

Radionuclide	Half-life	β+ Energy (max)	β+ Range (max)[a]	β+ Range (average)[a]	Production Method
C-11	20.4 min	0.96 MeV	3.8 mm	1.1 mm	Cyclotron
N-13	9.96 min	1.19 MeV	5.0 mm	1.5 mm	Cyclotron
O-15	123 sec	1.72 MeV	8.0 mm	2.5 mm	Cyclotron
F-18	110 min	0.635 MeV	2.2 mm	0.6 mm	Cyclotron
Ga-68	68 min	1.9 MeV	9.0 mm	2.9 mm	Generator (from Ge-68)
Rb-82	76 sec	2.6, 3.4 MeV	15.5 mm	5.9 mm	Generator (from Sr-82)

[a]Range is given for the positrons traveling through water. The term *range* refers to the linear distance traveled by the positrons. Both maximum and average values are given, corresponding to positrons of maximum or average energy, from each radioactive transition.

Cherry SR, Sorenson JA, Phelps ME. *Physics in Nuclear Medicine*. 3rd ed. Philadelphia, PA: Saunders; 2003:331.
Zanzonico P. Positron emission tomography: a review of basic principles, scanner design and performance, and current systems. *Semin Nucl Med.* 2004;34:87–111.
Valk PE, Bailey DL, Townsend DW, Maisey MN. *Positron Emission Tomography: Basic Science and Clinical Practice*. London: Springer; 2002:50.
Wahl RL. *Principles and Practice of Positron Emission Tomography*. Philadelphia, PA: Lippincott Williams & Wilkins; 2002:5.
Phelps ME, ed. *PET: Physics, Instrumentation, and Scanners*. New York, NY: Springer; 2006:4.

Table 14-2

Scintillation Crystals Used for PET

Property	NaI(Tl)	BGO	LSO	LYSO	GSO	BaF$_2$	LaBr$_3$
Linear attenuation coefficient at 511 keV (cm^{-1})	0.34	0.92	0.87	0.86	0.62	0.44	0.47
Attenuation length (1/μ, cm)[a]	2.88	1.05	1.16	1.20	1.43	2.2	2.12
Energy resolution at 511 keV (%)	6.6	10.2	10	14	8.5	11.4	N/A
Relative light yield[b] (%)	100	15	75	80	30	5	160
Decay time (nsec)	230	300	40	41	65	0.8	25
Hygroscopic?	Yes	No	No	No	No	Slightly	No
Chemical composition[c]	NaI:Tl	Bi$_4$Ge$_3$O$_{12}$	Lu$_2$SiO$_5$:Ce	Lu$_{1.9}$Y$_{0.5}$SiO$_5$:Ce	Gd$_2$SiO$_5$:Ce	BaF$_2$	LaBr$_3$

[a]Attenuation length is the average crystal thickness needed to stop 511-keV photons.
[b]Relative light yield is stated relative to NaI(Tl) at 100%.
[c]The elements listed after the colon are impurities that contribute to more efficient scintillation.

Lewellen TK. Recent developments in PET detector technology. *Phys Med Biol.* 2008;53:R287–R317.
Bailey DL, Townsend DW, Valk PE, Maisey MN. *Positron Emission Tomography: Basic Sciences.* London: Springer; 2005.

the two annihilation photons are no longer exactly 180° opposed, in order to conserve momentum. This noncolinearity results in variability of ±0.5° relative to the expected 180° relationship (3). The detection system will by necessity assume exact colinearity, leading to a slight mispositioning of some events. The two effects of positron range and noncolinearity imply that spatial resolution in PET has a lower limit that cannot be further reduced.

The approximate colineariry of the annihilation photons, coupled with their near coincidence in arriving at two opposed detectors, renders absorptive collimation unnecessary. As long as the two photons are detected on opposite sides of the tomograph and within the CTW, they are considered to be the result of an annihilation interaction that occurred along the line connecting the two detectors. So rather than being at the correct angle to pass through a collimator hole, as happens in a gamma camera, a good event in PET is determined by the coincident detection of two 511-keV photons. This is called *electronic collimation*. PET tomographs are more sensitive than gamma cameras because they have no collimators. This is a significant advantage of PET over single-photon imaging and is one of the reasons that PET can yield quantitative results.

Scintillation Crystals for Annihilation Photon Detection

Annihilation photons are detected by scintillation crystals, but several additional considerations are necessary beyond those pertaining to single-photon scintillation crystals. First and foremost, the scintillation crystal should have high efficiency for interaction with 511-keV photons. Second, and also very important, the scintillation crystal should have a short decay constant and high scintillation light output. A fast, bright scintillator will generate a signal with less timing variation than a slow and/or dim scintillator. The scintillators used for PET have timing resolution (uncertainty in the determination of the time of photon detection) of 2 to 6 nsec (4), allowing for a CTW in the range of 5 to 12 nsec. A short decay constant is also desirable because the count rates in PET are quite high. But we would still like to have decent energy resolution (in order to separate scattered photons from unscattered photons), which requires a lot of scintillation photons (see Chapter 2). **Table 14-2** lists seven scintillation crystals that have been used as PET detectors, along with several pertinent properties of each.

NaI(Tl)

Sodium iodide has been used with great success in single-photon imaging, and it has excellent energy resolution and very high light yield. But its low efficiency for interaction with annihilation photons means that its utility for PET is limited. One manufacturer produced a PET system in the 1990s that used six large sodium iodide crystals, but the recent trend has been to make PET tomographs with many small crystals. If the individual crystals are to be small (a common set of dimensions is 4 × 4 × 30 mm), then sodium iodide cannot do the job. In Table 14-2, the attenuation length is the mean distance traveled by an annihilation photon before having an interaction. Sodium iodide's mean attenuation length of 28.8 mm implies that only slightly more than one-half of annihilation photons entering a 30-mm-long crystal will interact in the crystal.

BGO

Bismuth germanate, or BGO, was first employed in PET tomographs in the late 1970s (the O refers to oxide, as the compound is formed by mixing molten bismuth oxide and germinate oxide). It represented a quantum leap over sodium iodide in terms of efficiency for interaction with 511-keV photons. It has the highest linear attenuation coefficient of all of the scintillators in Table 14-2. This allows for smaller crystals, which in turn improves spatial resolution. It is rugged and nonhygroscopic (5). However, the decay time and light yield of BGO are limiting factors. The long decay time limits the maximum count rate, while the low light yield limits the possibility of pulse clipping (which would otherwise be a work-around for the long decay time). BGO was the scintillation crystal of choice in PET tomographs throughout the 1990s, and it continues to be employed today.

Newer Scintillators

Currently three new materials—gadolinium oxyorthosilicate (GSO), lutetium oxyorthosilicate (LSO), and lutetium yttrium oxyorthosilicate (LYSO)—are gaining in popularity. All three are doped with cerium (Ce) to improve their scintillation efficiency. These scintillators have higher light yields and shorter decay times than BGO while maintaining reasonably good efficiency for 511-keV photon interactions. The shorter decay times in particular allow a shorter CTW to be used and a higher counting rate to be registered. In fact, the decay time for GSO can be manipulated by changing the amount of Ce included, such that an increase in the Ce content from 0.5 to 1% decreases the decay time from 85 to 55 nsec (6). GSO has energy resolution second only to sodium iodide, giving it an advantage from that standpoint. However, it is not as rugged as BGO or LSO and requires careful handling in the manufacturing process. LSO is rugged and nonhygroscopic, but has some natural radioactivity (Lu-176, 2.6% abundance, 3.75×10^{10} year half-life, and E_γs at 306 and 202 keV; [7]) that complicates the determination of some performance measures (8).

Sample Calculation 14-1 Maximum Count Rates for PET Scintillators

Calculate the maximum possible count rates for BGO and LSO, assuming that scintillation light is collected for the entire pulse time for each event (i.e., pulse clipping is not employed).
Decay time of BGO = 300 nsec:

$$\text{Maximum count rate} = \frac{1 \text{ ct}}{300 \times 10^{-9} \text{ sec}}$$

$$= \frac{3.3 \times 10^6 \text{ cts}}{\text{sec}} = 3.3 \text{ Mcps}.$$

Decay time of LSO = 40 nsec:

$$\text{Maximum count rate} = \frac{1 \text{ ct}}{40 \times 10^{-9} \text{ sec}}$$

$$= \frac{2.5 \times 10^7 \text{ cts}}{\text{sec}} = 25 \text{ Mcps}.$$

The shorter decay time of LSO makes a very large difference in the maximum allowable count rate.

Scintillators for Time-of-Flight PET

Finally, in Table 14-2, barium fluoride (BaF_2) and lanthanum bromide ($LaBr_3$) are included because of their possible application in *time-of-flight* (TOF) PET. Note their short decay constants. The principle of TOF-PET is that if events can be detected with very fine timing, then an annihilation event can be localized not just to the line between the two crystals, but to a small portion of that line. This requires measuring the difference in arrival times of the two annihilation photons, which can be done only with a very fast scintillator. This topic is discussed further in a later section of this chapter.

Data Collection

Coincidence Detection

The essence of a PET system, then, is two opposed crystals made of appropriate scintillation material, both connected to a coincidence circuit (**Figure 14-2**). When an object containing a positron-emitting radiopharmaceutical is placed between them, positron annihilation results in the release of pairs of annihilation photons. The two detectors must register two annihilation photons within the CTW in order to count a coincidence. The identification of a coincidence tells us that an annihilation interaction has occurred somewhere in the column of space connecting the two detectors.

Clearly we need more efficiency than just a single pair of crystals, and current PET tomographs consist of multiple rings of tiny scintillation crystals around a narrow imaging table (**Figure 14-3**). Each crystal acts as a separate detector. Each scintillation crystal is allowed to be in coincidence with many scintillation crystals on the opposite side of the ring. It is not allowed to be in coincidence with crystals on its own side of the ring, because an event between two closely spaced crystals could not have originated from an object in the middle of the ring. Each pair of crystals for which coincidence is allowed designates one *line of response* (LOR). Similar to the ray-sum in SPECT imaging, the LOR designates the column of tissue connecting the two crystals, thus indicating the location of the annihilation. Once a coincidence is determined to have occurred, the tomograph identifies the two crystals that registered it, and a count is added to the appropriate memory location for that LOR. The LOR is therefore the functional equivalent of the pixel in a frame-mode acquisition in single-photon imaging.

Sinograms

The raw data "matrix" of a PET scan is a plot of counts per second registered in each LOR, called a *sinogram* (an example is shown in **Figure 14-4**). One point of confusion is that the LOR (which represents the volume between two crystals in the ring tomograph) is not a line but rather a point on the sinogram. In the multi-ring PET tomograph, each ring of crystals (which identify a *direct plane*) has its own sinogram, with memory locations for all possible LORs. In addition, the acquisition parameters may allow

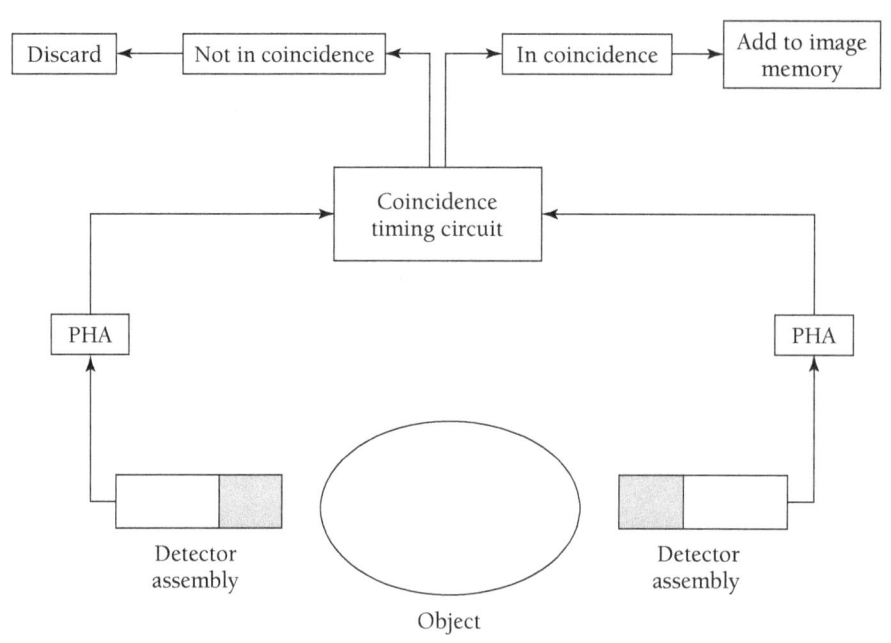

Figure 14-2 Schematic of coincidence imaging. The essential components of a PET imaging system are two opposed scintillation crystals as detectors, a pulse height analyzer (PHA) for each detector, a coincidence timing circuit with timing capabilities in the 10-nsec range, and an image memory space.

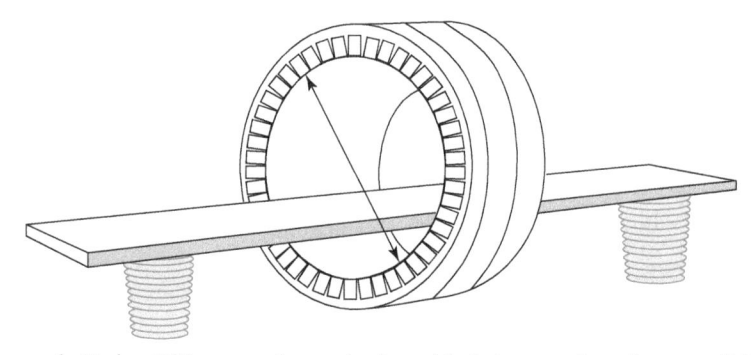

Figure 14-3 Ring-type PET tomograph. Modern PET tomographs are circular and include many rings of very small detectors (20 or more rings are common). The imaging table and its supporting structures on each end are included to provide a 3D perspective. A single line of response between two crystals on opposite sides of the imaging table is shown.

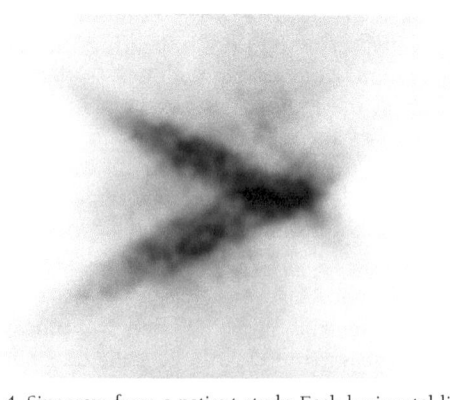

Figure 14-4 Sinogram from a patient study. Each horizontal line of the sinogram represents LORs at a particular angle. Each area of increased radioactivity is seen in a different location when we view it from different angles, so these areas appear to move in a sine wave pattern from the top to the bottom of the sinogram. Unlike the raw data from a SPECT study, PET sinograms do not look like images. See Figure 14-5 for a more complete explanation of sinograms. Image courtesy of Puget Sound Cancer Center.

interactions to be registered between crystals in different rings (called *cross planes*). Each allowed cross plane has its own sinogram as well.

Unlike projections acquired into frames in single-photon imaging, a PET sinogram does not provide a 2D representation of radiopharmaceutical distribution. **Figure 14-5** shows several ways to conceptualize the PET sinogram. Figure 14-5a shows how a hot spot in the object moves sinusoidally across the sinogram as the angle of the view changes. Figure 14-5b shows the sinogram as the polar coordinate (r, θ) representation of a line in Cartesian coordinate (x, y) space. In this view, adjacent points on any one horizontal line represent parallel LORs with different r values. All of the LORs at a given angle (i.e., a horizontal line across the sinogram) are called a *projection*, analogous to a 2D projection in SPECT imaging (Fig. 14-5c). Figure 14-5d may be the easiest to grasp. Each diagonal line on the sinogram represents one crystal's possible LORs. Each point in the sinogram is the intersection of diagonal lines representing

Chapter 14: Principles of Positron Emission Tomography (PET)

two crystals that are allowed to be in coincidence. When an annihilation event is detected, the computer identifies the two crystals involved and adds a count to the memory location where the diagonal lines for those two crystals cross.

Once the acquisition and therefore the sinogram are complete, 3D images are obtained by reconstruction of the sinograms. Reconstruction is usually iterative. Ultimately, transverse, sagittal, and coronal images are displayed, and dynamic triangulation, rotating cine, maximum-intensity projections, and other techniques are used, very similar to those employed in SPECT.

Types of Events in PET

Figure 14-6 illustrates the different kinds of events that can occur in a PET tomograph. So far we have considered only *true* events (often just called *trues*), in which the two annihilation photons from a single annihilation interaction are detected within the CTW (Fig. 14-6a). But several other possibilities exist. One possibility is that only one of the two annihilation photons interacts in a scintillation crystal (Fig. 14-6b). Each annihilation photon surpassing a low-energy threshold is called a *single event*, or a *single*. Singles are not ultimately counted unless a coincident photon is detected, but each single must be held until its CTW closes. Depending on the study, the dosage, and the particulars of the tomograph, the singles event rate may be 10 to 100 times the true coincidence rate (3, 4). The singles rate increases relative to the square of the dosage, because each radioactive disintegration potentially produces two singles.

Random Coincidences

Random coincidences (or just *randoms*) occur when two singles from two separate annihilations are detected within the CTW (Fig. 14-6c). The system will by necessity assume that both came from a single annihilation interaction, and that the annihilation interaction occurred in the LOR connecting the two detectors. Because they can occur between any two detectors, random coincidences add a featureless

(a) LORs through a single focus of radioactivity

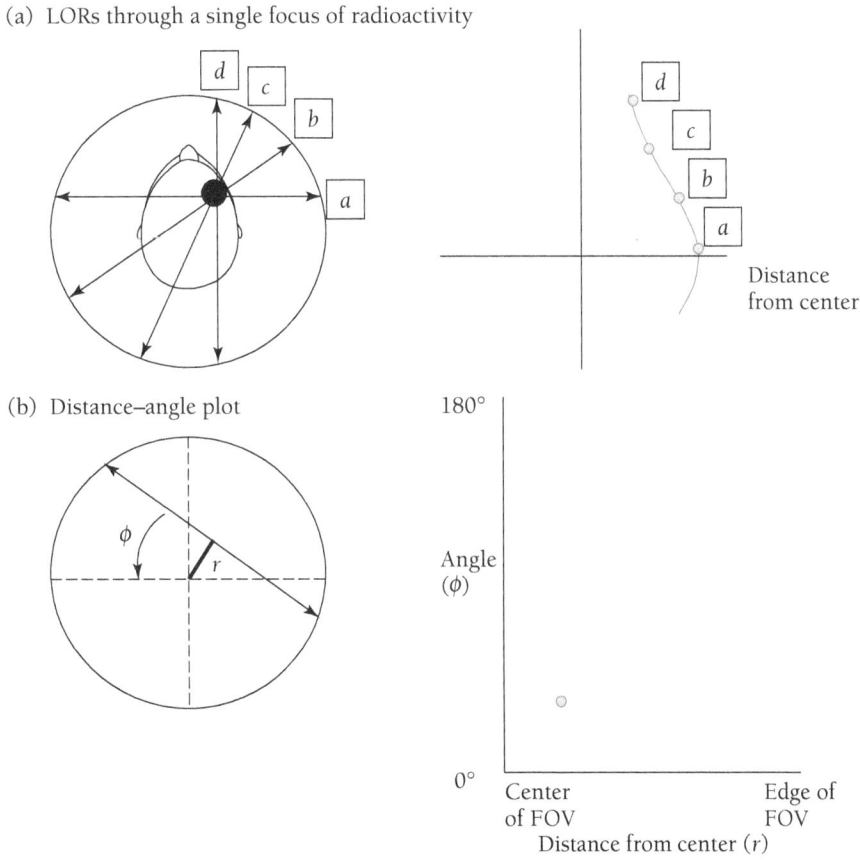

(b) Distance–angle plot

Figure 14-5 Conceptualizations of the PET sinogram. The left-hand side of Figure 14-5a shows a cross-sectional view of the head with a single focus of radiopharmaceutical accumulation, and the ring tomograph around it. Four LORs labeled *a* to *d* are also shown. The plot on the right side shows the sinogram, including the four LORs labeled *a* to *d*. As the head is viewed from different angles, the area of increased activity is seen to move in a sine wave fashion (hence the name *sinogram*). In Figure 14-5b, only a single LOR is shown, along with its polar coordinates. The distance *r* measures the radial distance between the LOR and the center of the ring, and the angle ϕ is relative to the X-axis, according to an equation of the form $r = x \cos \phi + y \sin \phi$. It thus converts the LOR's location from Cartesian (*x*, *y*) coordinates to a polar (*r*, ϕ) coordinate system. All coincidences measured in this LOR are included in the sinogram at the point shown. Figure 14-5c illustrates the projection concept, in which a set of parallel LORs constitutes a single horizontal line of the sinogram. Figure 14-5d shows how sinograms can be understood as LORs between pairs of detectors. Each diagonal line represents a single detector, and each point along that line represents the detectors that it is allowed to be in coincidence with. In the diagram, diagonals for detectors A and B are shown. A coincidence between these two detectors will result in a count being added at the point of intersection of the two diagonals. Each memory location in the sinogram collects data from one LOR.

(c) Parallel LORs

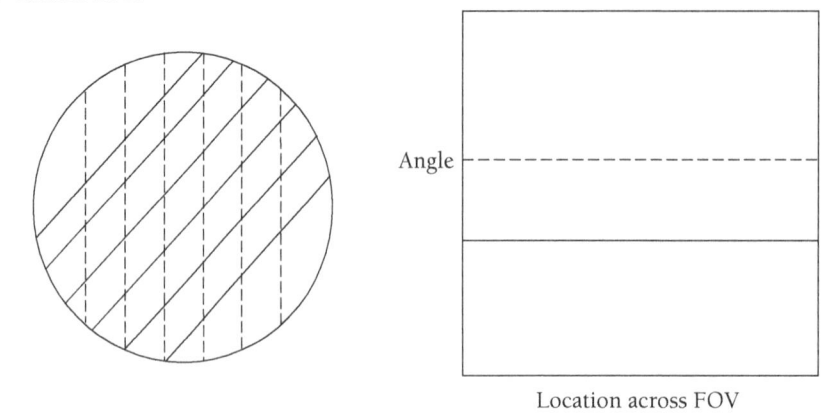

Angle

Location across FOV

(d) Intersection of two detector response lines

Detector A

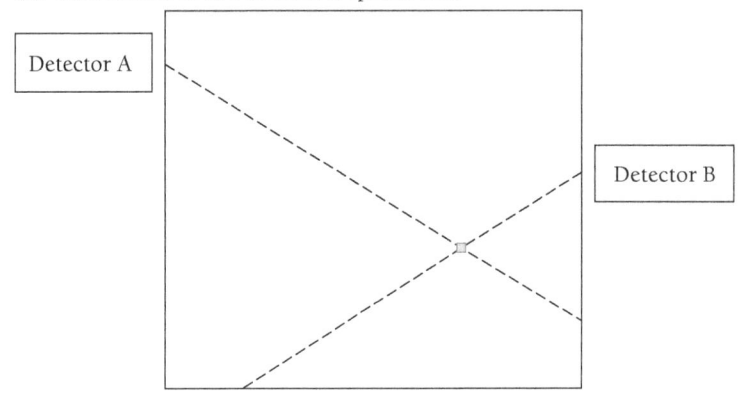

Detector B

Figure 14-5 (continued)

background to the image. The randoms rate also increases relative to the square of the dosage, because a random consists of two singles. The graph in Figure 14-6e shows that at some point, the number of randoms is equal to the number of trues; working in an activity range beyond this point is not recommended (9). By reducing the CTW, a fast scintillator like LSO also decreases the number of random coincidences (according to Reference 10, by a factor of 2 compared to BGO).

Scatter Coincidences

A *scatter* event (Fig. 14-6d) originates from a single annihilation interaction, and hence it represents a true coincidence. But because one or both of the annihilation photons undergoes Compton scattering within the object, the LOR is incorrect. The effect is similar to that for random coincidences, in that scatter adds a featureless background that extends beyond the boundary of the object. Scatter can also contribute significantly to the total counts in an acquisition, depending not on activity but on the specifics of the object being imaged and the acquisition mode.

In this and the following chapters, an *event* is assumed to mean any photon interaction whose energy exceeds a low-energy threshold, whereas a *count* is an accepted coincidence. Counts may thus be trues, randoms, or scatters.

A minimum of approximately 10^6 to 10^9 true coincidences is required to be able to reconstruct a statistically meaningful image (4). Random and scatter counts are ultimately subtracted from the total number of coincidences registered within the CTW. Both scatters and randoms vary to some extent with the local environment and may therefore be corrected for on an LOR-by-LOR basis. Corrections are essential if quantitative results are to be obtained.

Correction for Attenuation

Attenuation correction is also required for the ct/sec values in the reconstructed image to have quantitative meaning. As in SPECT, attenuation causes a decrease in true events, and the decrease gets larger with the depth of the annihilation interaction within the object. But attenuation is more of a problem in PET than in SPECT, because of the requirement that *both* annihilation photons be detected. For example, if each annihilation photon has a 25% chance of reaching a scintillation crystal without undergoing a Compton interaction, then the likelihood that both will do so is 25% times 25%, or only 6.25%. Given that the 511-keV half-value layer of tissue is approximately 7.2 cm, a head-sized object attenuates more than 85% and a body-sized object more than 95% of available photons (11).

(a) True coincidence (b) Single

(c) Random coincidence (d) Scatter coincidence

(e) Count rate vs activity

— Singles
— Randoms
--- Trues
-- Scatters

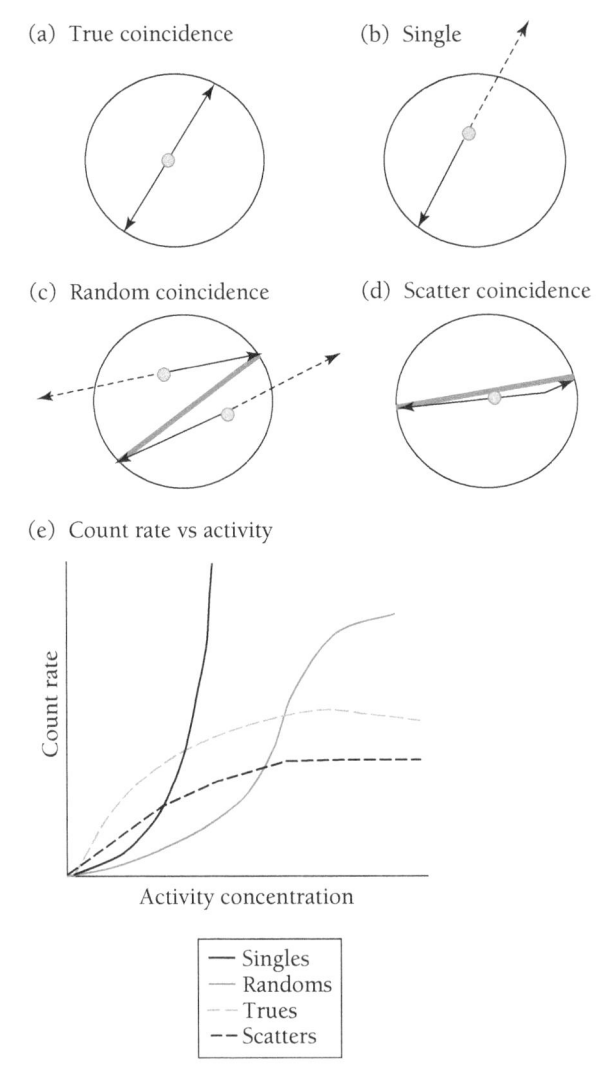

Figure 14-6 Types of events in PET. In these diagrams, the arrows indicate annihilation photons, dashed arrows indicate annihilation photons that pass through the tomograph (represented by the circle) without interacting in a detector, and thick solid lines show the assumed LOR in Figures 14-6c and 14-6d. In a true coincidence (Fig. 14-6a), both annihilation photons from one annihilation interact in detectors, without any scatter interactions in the object being imaged. A single occurs when one of the two annihilation photons is absorbed in a detector, while the other is not; no coincidence is detected (Fig. 14-6b). A random coincidence (Fig. 14-6c) occurs when two annihilation interactions (the two dots) occur simultaneously and one annihilation photon from each interaction is detected. The tomograph assigns a count to the LOR indicated by the thick line. In a scatter coincidence (Fig. 14-6d), both annihilation photons originate from the same annihilation reaction, and are thus in coincidence, but one has undergone a Compton scattering interaction. Again, the assumed LOR (the thick line) is incorrect. In Figure 14-6e, the effect of increasing activity concentration on the count rates of trues, randoms, and singles is shown. Singles increase geometrically, because each annihilation reaction produces two annihilation photons. Randoms result from singles, so the randoms rate also increases in an exponential fashion, up to a point at which dead time becomes significant. Trues, on the other hand, plateau because the dead time incurred by the singles and randoms limits the maximum detectable trues rate. The exact shape and the crossing points of the various curves depend on both the acquisition mode used and the activity distribution in the object, but the graph gives the general trend for the different types of events.

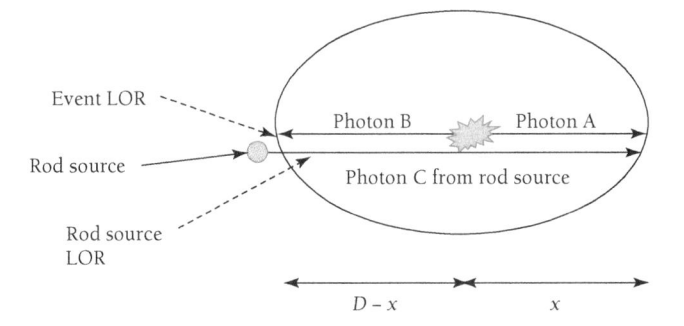

D = object thickness along the LOR
x = distance traveled by photon A in the object
μ = linear attenuation coefficient of the object

Probability that photon A will escape the object = $e^{-\mu x}$
Probability that photon B will escape the object = $e^{-\mu(D-x)}$
Probability that both photons will escape the object = $e^{-\mu x}e^{-\mu(D-x)}$
  = $e^{-\mu D}$
Probability that annihilation photon C from the rod source will pass through the object without interacting = $e^{-\mu D}$

Figure 14-7 Attenuation correction in PET. In this illustration, the object is assumed to have a uniform composition and therefore a single linear attenuation coefficient. An annihilation interaction occurs, resulting in photons A and B, each of which has a finite likelihood of passing through the object without undergoing a photoelectric or Compton interaction. The likelihood that both will do so is the product of the individual likelihoods, because each is an independent event. When photon C from the external rod source passes through the same LOR, it must travel the same distance D through the object as photons A and B combined, and thus it provides a measurement of attenuation at that angle.

Images that are not attenuation-corrected show significant differences when compared to attenuation-corrected images.

In contrast to SPECT, however, the problem of attenuation correction in PET can be solved exactly, because the amount of attenuation does not depend on the location of the radiopharmaceutical within the object. The likelihood that both photons will escape the object without interacting is dependent only on the total thickness of the object (**Figure 14-7**). Thus, the count rate from a radioactive source within the object depends only on the object's thickness, and not on the source's location within the object. The total attenuation can therefore be directly measured using an external source of photons, which may be either a radionuclide or a CT x-ray tube. A transmission-based attenuation map is acquired and applied to the emission data in PET as it is in SPECT. The details of attenuation correction are discussed in Chapters 15 (radionuclide source-based attenuation correction) and 18 (CT-based attenuation correction).

Time-of-Flight PET

Like SPECT, the basic information about an event in PET is that it occurred in a particular columnar volume within the object. Specifically for PET, that volume is defined by the two crystals registering the two coincident annihilation photons, called the LOR. But we have no further

Dot = location of annihilation interaction

Shaded area = range of location of annihilation interaction, as determined by TOF

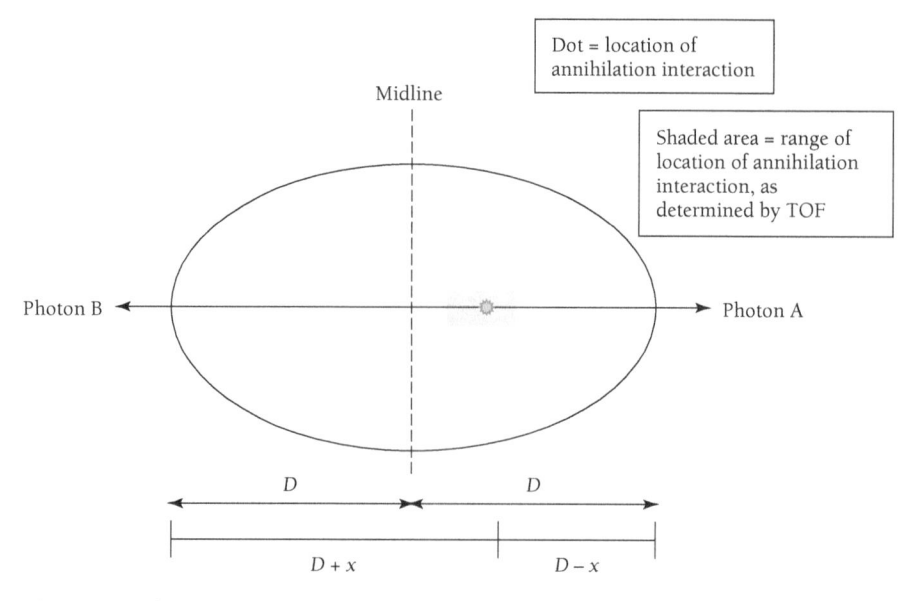

Photon A travels $D - x$, arrives at $(D - x)/c$
Photon B travels $D + x$, arrives at $(D + x)/c$

$$\Delta t = \frac{(D + \Delta x) - (D - \Delta x)}{c} = \frac{2\Delta x}{c}$$

where c is the speed of light, x is the distance from the annihilation to the midline, and t is the difference in time of the arrival of the two photons.

Figure 14-8 Time-of-flight mathematics. In this figure, because the point of annihilation is in the right side of the object, photon A will be detected before photon B. We can determine mathematically that the timing difference (Δt) between arrivals is proportional to the annihilation event's distance from the midline (Δx). The size of Δx, indicated by the shaded box, is dependent on the accuracy of the measurement of Δt. Timing electronics do not currently allow Δt to be known exactly. But even the ability to localize the annihilation event to a portion of the LOR, as shown, improves the signal-to-noise ratio and the quality of the image.

information about where along the LOR the annihilation might have occurred. Reconstruction, whether by FBP or iterative methods, includes this basic limitation. One important source of noise in PET scans is incorrectly positioned true counts.

Time-of-flight PET (sometimes abbreviated TOF-PET) allows the tomograph to more closely identify the part of the LOR where an event originated. If an event occurs at any point other than the midline of the LOR, the crystal closer to the annihilation will detect its photon first, while the other crystal will detect its photon somewhat later (**Figure 14-8**). If we can measure the time difference between the arrival of the two photons (Δt), we can then determine a limited range for the annihilation event within the LOR (Δx) according to the equation

$$\Delta x = \frac{c \Delta t}{2}. \quad (14\text{-}1)$$

This in turn greatly clarifies the location of areas of increased activity (**Figure 14-9**).

This is not a new idea, of course; physicists have been aware of the concepts of TOF-PET from the earliest days of coincidence imaging. In the 1980s, PET tomographs using BaF$_2$ or CsF as the scintillation crystals were manufactured (13). The intent was to image radiopharmaceuticals labeled with O-15, which has a 2-min half-life. Very quick studies can be performed with O-15, but the scintillator must be very fast to accommodate the high count rates generated. As noted in Table 14-2, BaF$_2$ has such a short decay time that it could manage the O-15 studies, and also allowed for time-of-flight event positioning. But BaF$_2$ has poor efficiency for stopping annihilation photons, and so most commercial tomographs through the first decade of the 21st century were non-TOF systems. However, newer scintillators such as LaBr$_3$ and LYSO have revived interest in TOF-PET. In addition, advances in electronics have improved the ability to measure small (<1 nsec) timing differences, and have been shown to be stable over time (14). So tomographs with TOF capabilities are again on the market.

Quantitative Abilities

One of the major attributes of PET is its ability to provide quantitatively meaningful results. In other words, we can measure a physiologic process such as oxygen metabolism or glucose utilization, and the cps/voxel can be translated into activity concentration, which in turn can be related to the physiologic process being monitored, in real terms (e.g., mg/ml). This ability stems from several aspects in which PET differs from other types of imaging, including single-photon nuclear medicine techniques.

The first reason that PET can be quantitative has to do with the nature of the radionuclides employed. Oxygen, nitrogen, and carbon are all real constituents of biologic

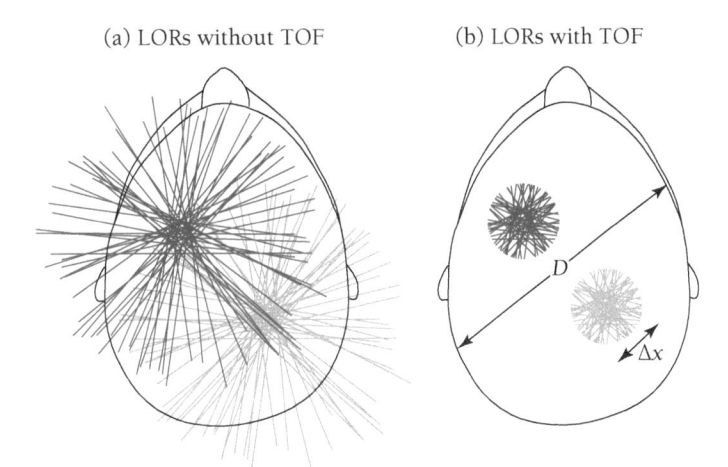

Figure 14-9 Effect of TOF-PET on image contrast and noise. Time of flight limits the range of each annihilation's location to something less than an entire LOR. This simple representation of the effect of TOF-PET shows a brain scan with two areas of increased activity. While the location of the two areas can be appreciated without TOF in Figure 14-9a, the use of TOF in Figure 14-9b makes them much more obvious. In iterative reconstruction, the limiting of the LOR for each event results in much quicker convergence. Figure courtesy of Dr. Thomas Budinger (12).

molecules; the presence of the radionuclide does not alter the biologic treatment of these molecules in any way. We are thus imaging and measuring actual physiologic functions in PET studies using these radionuclides.

Additionally, several aspects of the imaging process allow measurements to be quantitatively meaningful. There is no need for absorptive collimators, which is a major (and variable) source of photon loss in gamma camera imaging. We can account for attenuation exactly in PET, so variability in body habitus from patient to patient can be accommodated. We can correct for other variables, such as scatter and dead time, with reasonably good accuracy. And finally, with our data expressed as the count rate per voxel, we can determine a calibration factor that converts the raw information (count rate in a voxel) to activity concentration, in a form that is accurate from one study to the next.

The benefits of this ability to be quantitative are immense. For years, PET was part of a major research effort used to delineate physiologic processes that could not be examined directly using other methodologies. More recently, with the development of small-animal tomographs, PET is becoming an important tool in drug research and development. The ability to image drug biodistribution and physiology in vivo, in a quantitatively accurate way, is expected to speed drug development significantly. And PET is also increasingly used as a surrogate biomarker for measuring the effectiveness of newly developed medications. Thus we can expect that utilization of PET will continue to extend beyond clinical imaging.

Summary

As can be seen from this chapter, PET has both similarities and differences compared to single-photon imaging. The basic principles are the same: a radiopharmaceutical is used to delineate a physiologic process, and the resulting radiation emissions are detected with a scintillation crystal. But the fact that the radiation emission in PET consists of a pair of coincident annihilation photons requires different types of scintillation crystals, more sophisticated electronics, and consideration of different types of coincident events. In addition, as technology has continued to improve, new techniques such as TOF-PET add to the information that can be extracted from the tomograph.

Positron emission tomography requires a different set of thought processes on the part of the technologist. The ability to perform absolute quantitation places additional burdens on the PET tomograph, the applied corrections, and the performance of the study. In Chapter 15, we discuss further application of corrections for randoms, singles, scatters, and attenuation, as well as corrections related to PET tomograph operation. PET offers significant advantages over single-photon imaging, but these advantages can only be realized if the underlying physics is understood and correctly accounted for, both by the tomograph and by the operator.

References

1. Rich DA. A brief history of positron emission tomography. *J Nucl Med Technol.* 1997;25:4–11.
2. Tapscott E. First scintillation camera is foundation for modern imaging systems. *J Nucl Med.* 1998;39:15N–27N.
3. Valk PE, Bailey DL, Townsend DW, Maisey MN. *Positron Emission Tomography: Basic Science and Clinical Practice.* London: Springer; 2002:51, 58, 69.
4. Phelps ME, ed. *PET: Physics, Instrumentation, and Scanners.* New York, NY: Springer; 2006:8, 17, 35.
5. Melcher CL. Scintillation crystals for PET. *J Nucl Med.* 2000;41:1051–1055.
6. Surti S, Karp JS. Imaging characteristics of a three-dimensional GSO whole-body PET camera. *J Nucl Med.* 2004;45:1040–1049.
7. Knolls Atomic Power Laboratory. *The Chart of the Nuclides.* 16th ed. Schenectady, NY: Lockheed Martin; 2003.
8. Brambilla M, Secco C, Dominietto M, et al. Performance characteristics obtained for a new 3-dimensional lutetium oxyorthosilicate-based whole-body PET/CT scanner with the National Electrical Manufacturers Association NU 2-2001 standard. *J Nucl Med.* 2005;46:2083–2091.
9. Wagner HN, Szabo Z, Buchanan BS. *Principles of Nuclear Medicine.* 2nd ed. Philadelphia, PA: Saunders; 1995:354.
10. Bacharach SL. The new-generation positron emission tomography/computed tomography scanners: implications for cardiac imaging. *J Nucl Cardiol.* 2004;11:388–392.

11. Henkin RE, Boles MA, Dillehay GL, et al., eds. *Nuclear Medicine*. St. Louis, MO: Mosby-Year Book; 1996:287.
12. Budinger, TF. Hal Anger memorial lecture: Radionuclide enhancements above and beyond signal to noise: losing the background. Society of Nuclear Medicine 57th Annual meeting, Salt Lake City, UT, 2010.
13. Lewellen TR. Time-of-flight PET. *Semin Nucl Med.* 1998;28:268–275.
14. Karp JS, Surti S, Daube-Witherspoon ME, Muehllehner G. Benefit of time-of-flight in PET: experimental and clinical results. *J Nucl Med.* 2008;49:462–470.

Additional Resources

Budinger TF. PET instrumentation: what are the limits? *Semin Nucl Med.* 1998;28: 247–267.

Cherry SR, Sorenson JA, Phelps ME. *Physics in Nuclear Medicine*. 3rd ed. Philadelphia, PA: Saunders; 2003:Chapter 18.

Henkin RE, Boles MA, Dillehay GL, et al., eds. *Nuclear Medicine*. St. Louis, MO: Mosby-Year Book; 1996:Chapter 23.

Lewellen TR. Time-of-flight PET. *Semin Nucl Med.* 1998;28:268–275.

Melcher CL. Scintillation crystals for PET. *J Nucl Med.* 2000;41:1051–1055.

Phelps ME, ed. *PET: Physics, Instrumentation, and Scanners*. New York, NY: Springer; 2006.

Turkington TG. Introduction to PET instrumentation. *J Nucl Med Technol.* 2001;29: 1–8.

Valk PE, Bailey DL, Townsend DW, Maisey MN. *Positron Emission Tomography: Basic Science and Clinical Practice*. London: Springer; 2002:Chapters 2, 5, 11.

Wahl RL. *Principles and Practice of Positron Emission Tomography*. Philadelphia, PA: Lippincott Williams & Wilkins; 2002:Chapters 1, 3.

Zanzonico P. Positron emission tomography: a review of basic principles, scanner design and performance, and current systems. *Semin Nucl Med.* 2004;34: 87–111.

CHAPTER 15 — PET Instrumentation

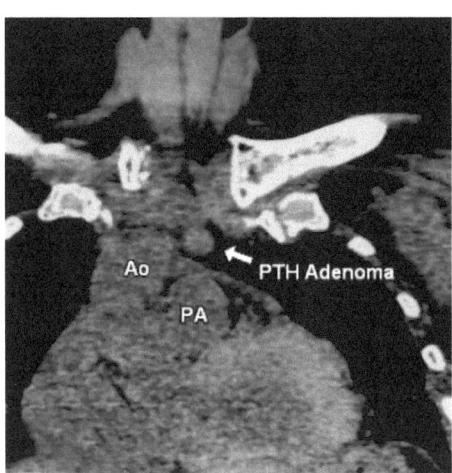

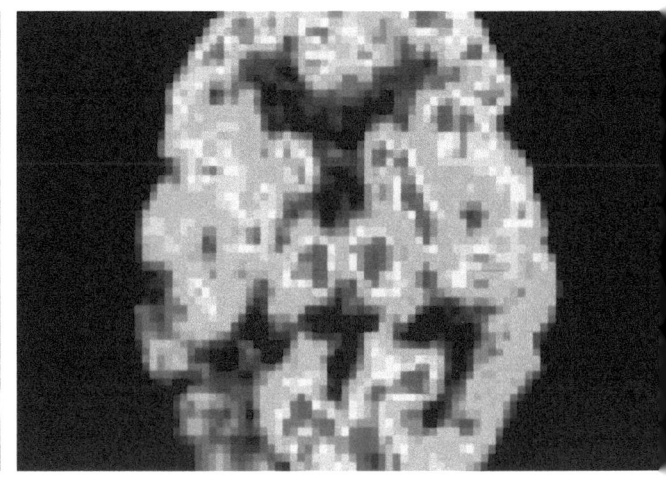

Learning Outcomes

1. Outline the components of a PET tomograph, the essential steps in event detection, and the process of image acquisition.
2. Describe the operation of detector blocks in a PET tomograph, and discuss variations on the most common design.
3. Discuss the electronic detection of coincidence events and the delayed-coincidence and estimation-from-singles methods of randoms estimation.
4. Compare and contrast the measurement of attenuation using a positron-emitting vs a single-photon-emitting radionuclide source.
5. State the reasons for each of the following corrections:
   a. Normalization
   b. Dead time
   c. Scatter
   d. Attenuation
   e. Decay
6. Differentiate between 2D and 3D PET imaging in terms of the physical differences in the tomograph and of the effect on sensitivity, scatter, and reconstruction.
7. Discuss additional acquisition choices and PET imaging devices.

Introduction

The basic concepts of PET imaging were discussed previously; this chapter shows how those concepts are utilized to acquire images. Our consideration will include the physical construction of a standard PET tomograph, including several variations on detector block design; the electronics needed to register prompt and random coincidences; radionuclide transmission sources and geometries; and corrections that must be applied to the raw data to obtain meaningful images. An overview of the image acquisition process will hopefully present enough of a picture that a nuclear medicine technologist unfamiliar with PET will understand the tomograph's operation.

In addition to the "standard" tomograph design, we will consider several options. The choice of 2D or 3D was for some time a major consideration when preparing acquisition protocols, but has lessened in importance as electronics have advanced and faster scintillators have become available, and some manufacturers have stopped marketing PET scanners with 2D capability altogether. We will encounter time-of-flight (TOF) technology in some of the latest-model tomographs. And we will look at systems used to image specific body parts. The availability of new and evolving options is an indication of the maturation of the field of PET imaging.

Overview of PET Tomograph Composition

Figure 15-1 shows the essential composition of a PET tomograph, and **Figure 15-2** provides some photographs of the inside of an actual PET tomograph. **Figure 15-3** defines the imaging planes of a PET tomograph. The photon-detecting portion of the tomograph consists of multiple rings of scintillation crystals. The scintillation crystals are small, rectangular prisms (about 4–6 mm square × 20–30 mm long, about the size of an adult's little finger), each with the long axis of each crystal oriented in the radial direction. There are 18 to 32 rings of these small detectors in the gantry, for a total of approximately 10,000 to 30,000 separate detectors. The diameter of the rings is 80 to 90 cm, but the tomograph's housing limits the gantry bore (through which the patient and the imaging table must pass) to 50 to 60 cm. The axial field of view (FOV), that is, the length of the gantry bore in the axial direction, is 15 to 22 cm. Two thick (1+ cm) *axial shields* made of lead are found on the axial front and back of the gantry. Their purpose is to block photons that originate outside of the axial FOV.

Electronically, the scintillation crystals are organized into detector blocks. A "typical" detector block consists of an 8 × 8 array of scintillation crystals, coupled to four photomultiplier tubes (PMTs) (**Figure 15-4**). Detector blocks are further grouped into buckets or cassettes, which may be treated as a unit when allowed coincidences are considered. As shown in **Figure 15-5**, each detector bucket is only allowed to be in coincidence with a limited number of other detector buckets in the ring. The angle of allowed coincidences in turn determines the transaxial FOV. Both detector blocks and allowed coincidences will be discussed in greater detail.

Figure 15-1b shows *septa* between the rings of scintillation crystals. These are long (7–10 cm), thin (1–5 mm) tungsten slats that can be retracted. When the septa are in place as shown in the figure, the tomograph is in *2D imaging mode*. If the septa are retracted from the ring, the tomograph is in *3D imaging mode*. The main effect of the septa is to decrease the number of coincidences detected between two different rings of the detector (called *cross-plane coincidences*). The choice of 2D vs 3D mode entails many considerations that are discussed later in this chapter. Some tomographs, particularly those utilizing faster scintillators, do not have septa and thus allow only 3D imaging.

Three *rod sources*, each indicated by a dot, are shown in Figure 15-1a. Each is made of positron-emitting material, and they are in the form of rods oriented in the axial direction. They provide an external source of annihilation photons, to be used for attenuation correction and normalization. They retract into a shielded housing when not in use. Figure 15-2d shows a rod source next to a human hand for size comparison. PET/CT tomographs currently on the market may or may not have rod sources for quality control purposes, but they are routinely used in older PET-only systems.

Figure 15-1c illustrates the basic electronics of a PET tomograph. Any signal generated in a detector, after passing a low-energy discriminator, is assigned a timing signal. This signal is sent to a coincidence circuit, which has a narrow (5–12 nanosecond [nsec]) coincidence timing window (CTW). If two events are recorded by the coincidence timing circuit within the CTW, from detectors allowed to be in coincidence, then the two events are evaluated relative to the energy window, and the two specific detectors recording the two events identify the line of response (LOR). Accepted counts are added to the prompt sinogram. The delay sinogram is discussed in "Coincidences and Random Events."

Overview of Acquisition, Reconstruction, and Image Display

Figure 15-1d shows a typical commercially available PET tomograph. The patient lies on the imaging table and passes through the gantry bore. As noted, the tomograph is only 15 to 22 cm long in the axial (head-to-toe) direction, so many studies require multiple acquisitions to

(a) Ring tomograph showing detectors and detector blocks (transaxial view)

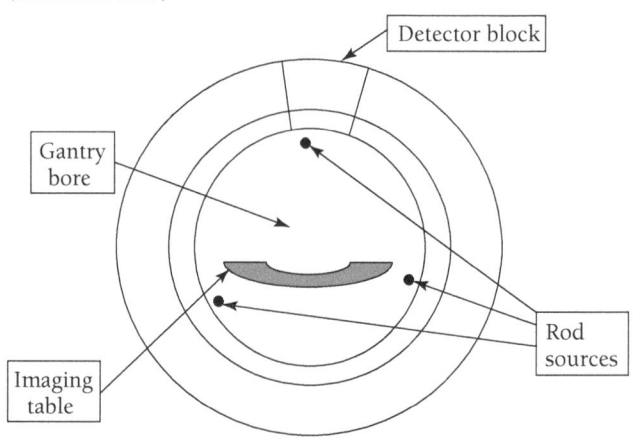

(b) Two detector blocks (shown in axial view)

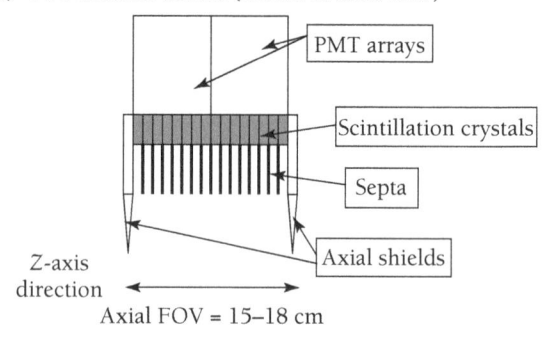

Figure 15-1 PET tomograph design. Figure 15-1a shows the PET tomograph in transaxial view, while Figure 15-1b illustrates a detector block in an axial orientation (i.e., going into the plane of the page of Fig. 15-1a). The axial shields block annihilation photons originating outside of the tomograph's FOV, while the septa block off-angle photons in 2D imaging, which is discussed later in this chapter. Figure 15-1c shows a block diagram of prompts and randoms acquisitions. Figure 15-1d shows a commercial system (photo courtesy of Siemens Medical Systems).

(c) Block diagram of electronics

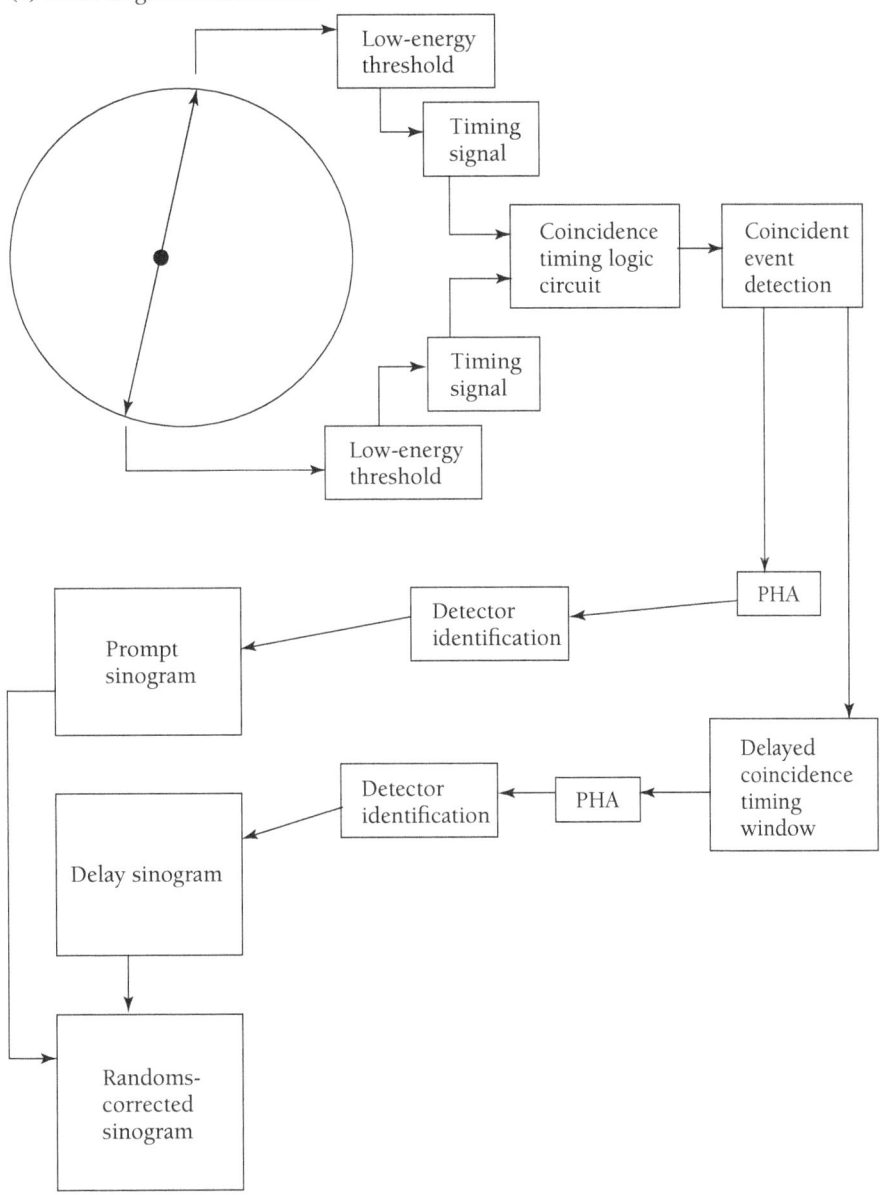

(d) Commercially available system

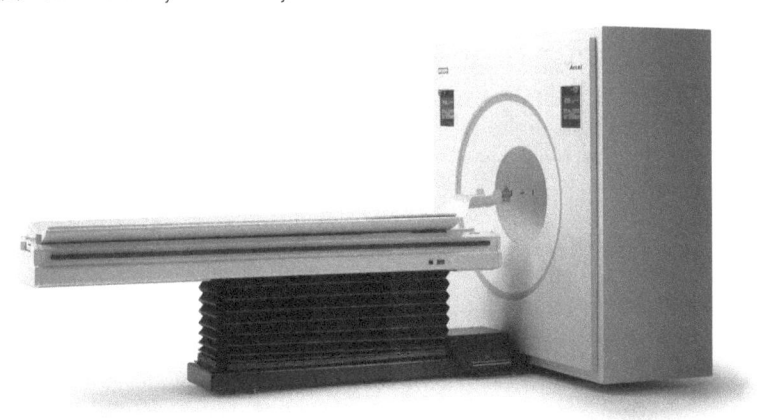

Figure 15-1 (continued)

Overview of Acquisition, Reconstruction, and Image Display 211

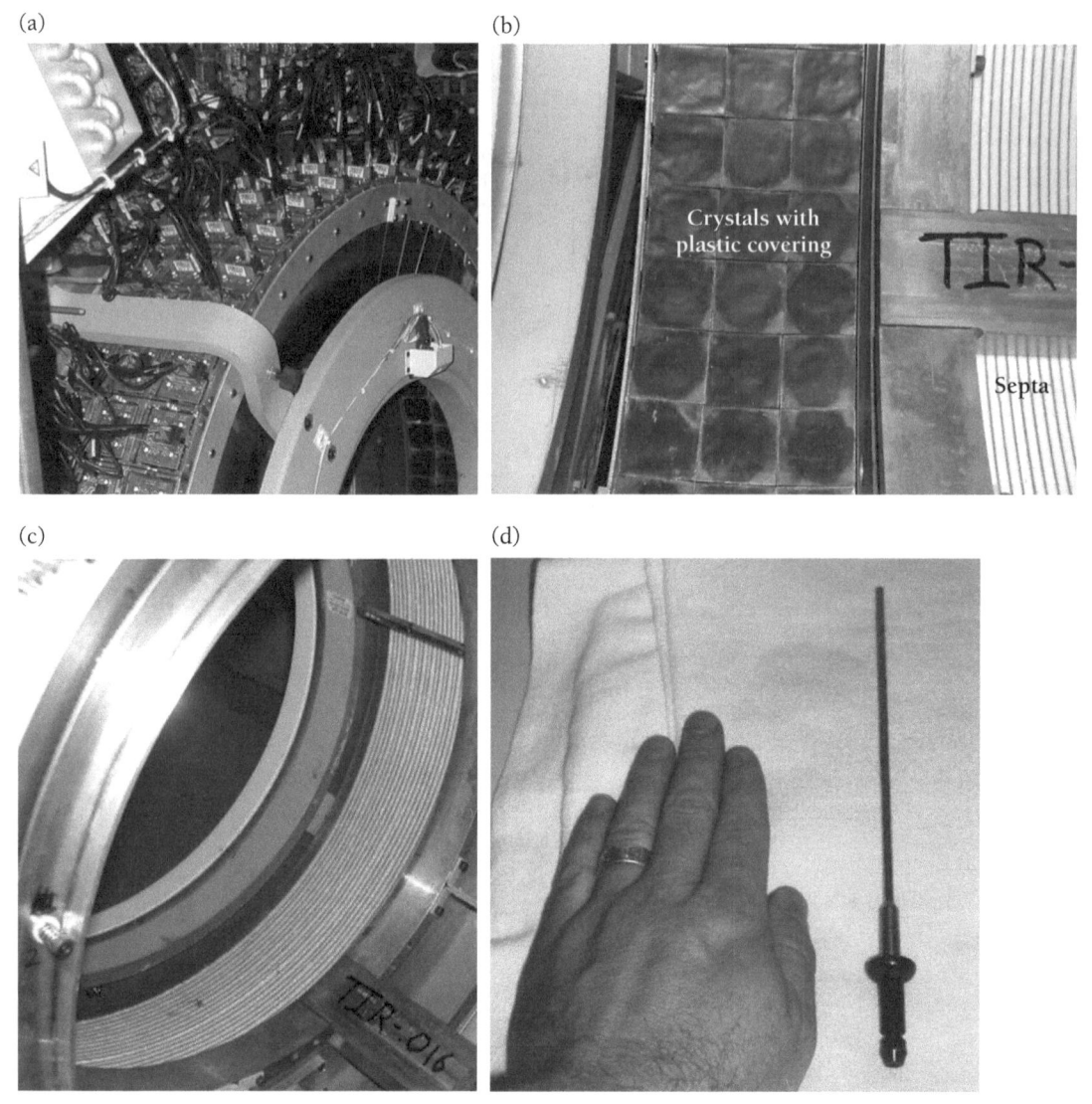

Figure 15-2 Internal photos of a PET tomograph. These photographs provide some additional views of a non-CT PET tomograph from about the year 2000. The block detector construction common to PET tomographs includes both the electronics (Figure 15-2a) and the detector blocks (Fig. 15-2b). Each square in Figure 15-2b is a 2-inch-square detector block of 8 × 8 BGO crystals. The septa are seen to the right of the detector blocks, in their retracted position (a low-atomic-number material fills the spaces between septa, to keep them aligned). Figure 15-2c shows the septa in place between rings of crystals. Figure 15-2d shows a rod source used for attenuation correction and quality control. Photos courtesy of Puget Sound Cancer Center.

include the entire area of interest. These individual locations of the tomograph relative to the patient's body are called *bed positions*. All bed positions for a particular study are acquired for the same length of time, and then they are appended together in the reconstruction process to create a continuous 3D image matrix.

The different types of PET acquisitions are set up as protocols within the acquisition computer, much as they are in modern gamma cameras. The protocols are usually identified according to the part of the body being imaged (e.g., brain, heart, whole body), with specific parameters for each. But in terms of bed positions, we are really looking at only a few situations. Some organs, such as the heart, can be imaged in a single bed position. The brain is usually imaged over two bed positions. Oncologic imaging has been characterized by the phrase "eyes to thighs," which requires 5 to 8 bed positions, although with the advent of PET/CT the upper limit has been moved to the base of the skull to avoid excessive radiation exposure to the eyes. Dynamic and gated imaging at a single bed position can also be performed.

Data acquisition can be in a list-mode format (see Chapter 6) or more commonly in *histogram mode* (analogous to frame mode in gamma camera imaging). Recall from Chapter 14 that the tomograph can accept events that occur within a single ring of crystals (*direct planes*) and coincidences that are registered in two different rings (*cross planes*). Events from the cross planes are assigned to a transaxial plane that is located at the midpoint of the cross plane. If the rings contributing to the cross plane are separated by an even number of rings, the transaxial plane is located between two rings and is called a *virtual plane*

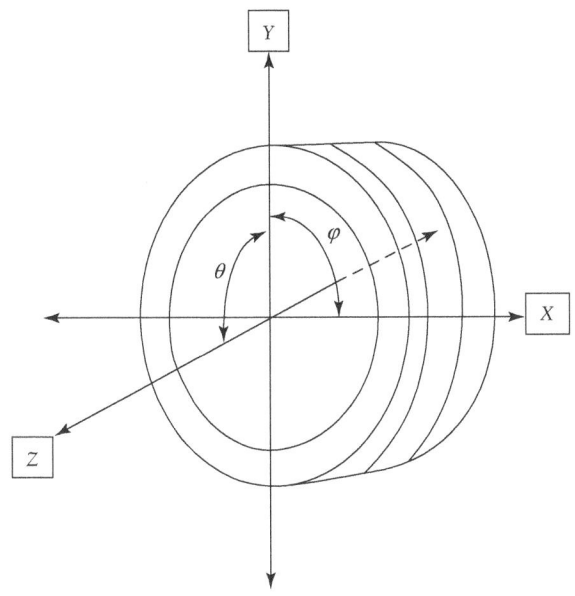

Transaxial plane = X–Y plane
Axial direction = Z direction
Radial direction = all lines in the transaxial plane that
    intersect the center point
Azimuthal angle = φ = angle in the X–Y plane
Polar angle = θ = angle in the Y–Z plane

Figure 15-3 Imaging planes in PET (5). The X- and Y-axes lie within a single ring of detectors and define the transaxial plane (perpendicular to the axial direction, shown by the Z-axis). The imaging table (and therefore the long axis of the patient) lies along the axial direction. The terms *front* and *back* refer to the tomograph's axial direction, where the axial shields of Figure 15-1b are located.

(**Figure 15-6**). The acquisition protocol specifies which cross-plane coincidences are allowed (direct plane coincidences are allowed in all acquisition modes). In histogram mode, two sinogram matrices are created for each direct plane and each allowed cross plane. These are the *prompt sinogram* and the *delay sinogram* shown in Figure 15-1c. Within each sinogram, each allowed LOR is assigned a memory location.

During acquisition, a coincidence detected in a given LOR increments the corresponding memory location in the prompt sinogram by 1. *Prompt events* (all those accepted by the CTW) include not only true coincidences but also random and scatter events. In addition, Figure 15-1c shows a second delayed circuit that acquires counts into a delay sinogram as a way of estimating the number of random coincidences per second. This method of subtracting randoms is used on several commercial systems and is discussed in greater detail in the section Coincidences and Random Events, along with an alternate method for estimating randoms. The values in each LOR are stored as count rates, to facilitate conversion to activity units (which will be needed for quantitative results such as the standardized uptake value [SUV]).

Attenuation correction is vital for both visual and quantitative accuracy of PET images. A PET-only tomograph, using rod sources for transmission acquisitions, acquires emission and transmission acquisitions at each bed position. The most common protocol is to acquire an emission image (E) followed by a transmission image (T), then move to the next bed position and acquire T followed by E. (Note that this is different than the simultaneous acquisition technique often used in SPECT. In PET, the positron-emitting rod sources are shielded while emission data are being obtained.) *Interleaving* the emission and transmission acquisitions in this alternating manner (ET/TE/ET/TE …) shortens the time of the study by a few minutes, because the rod sources are only extended and retracted half as often. Each transmission acquisition requires an additional sinogram for each direct plane and each allowed cross plane. With PET/CT, the CT study is typically acquired in its entirety before the emission acquisition is started.

Sample Calculation 15-1 Acquisition Time for a PET Whole-Body Scan

A patient is to have a PET scan using a protocol that acquires emission information for 5 min and transmission information for 2 min at each bed position. The axial FOV is 15 cm, and the scan length for the eyes-to-thighs scan is 92 cm. What is the total exam time?

$$\text{Number of bed positions} = \frac{92\text{-cm scan length}}{15\text{ cm/bed position}}$$
$$= 6.1333 \text{ bed positions.}$$

To get complete coverage of the area of interest, we need to round up to 7 bed positions.

$$\text{Exam time} = 7 \text{ bed positions} \times \frac{7 \text{ min}}{\text{bed position}} = 49 \text{ min.}$$

This does not include the time required for extension and retraction of the rod sources. Nor does it allow for any overlap of bed positions, which might be required to account for front-to-back variation in sensitivity depending on the imaging mode (see "2D vs 3D Imaging Modes").

The prompt sinogram must be corrected for several factors in addition to the subtraction of random coincidences, including attenuation, scatter, dead time, and radioactive decay. A normalization correction accounts for the fact that the individual detectors do not respond equally to a uniform source of annihilation photons. After all corrections have been applied, the sinogram is reconstructed into a 3D image matrix, using similar algorithms as for SPECT imaging. Iterative reconstruction using ordered-subsets expectation maximization (OSEM) is commonly used in PET, although one manufacturer utilizes a different algorithm called the *row action maximum likelihood algorithm* (abbreviated RAMLA) that produces

(a) Detector block cutting

PMT C
PMT D
PMT A
PMT B
Scintillation crystal scored to create individual detectors

(b) Anger positioning logic in detector block

Axial direction
Z
C D
A B
X
Circumferential direction

$$X = \frac{(B - A) + (D - C)}{A + B + C + D}$$

$$Z = \frac{(C - A) + (D - B)}{A + B + C + D}$$

Energy $= A + B + C + D$

(c) Quadrant sharing

(d) Panel detectors

Optical coupling grease

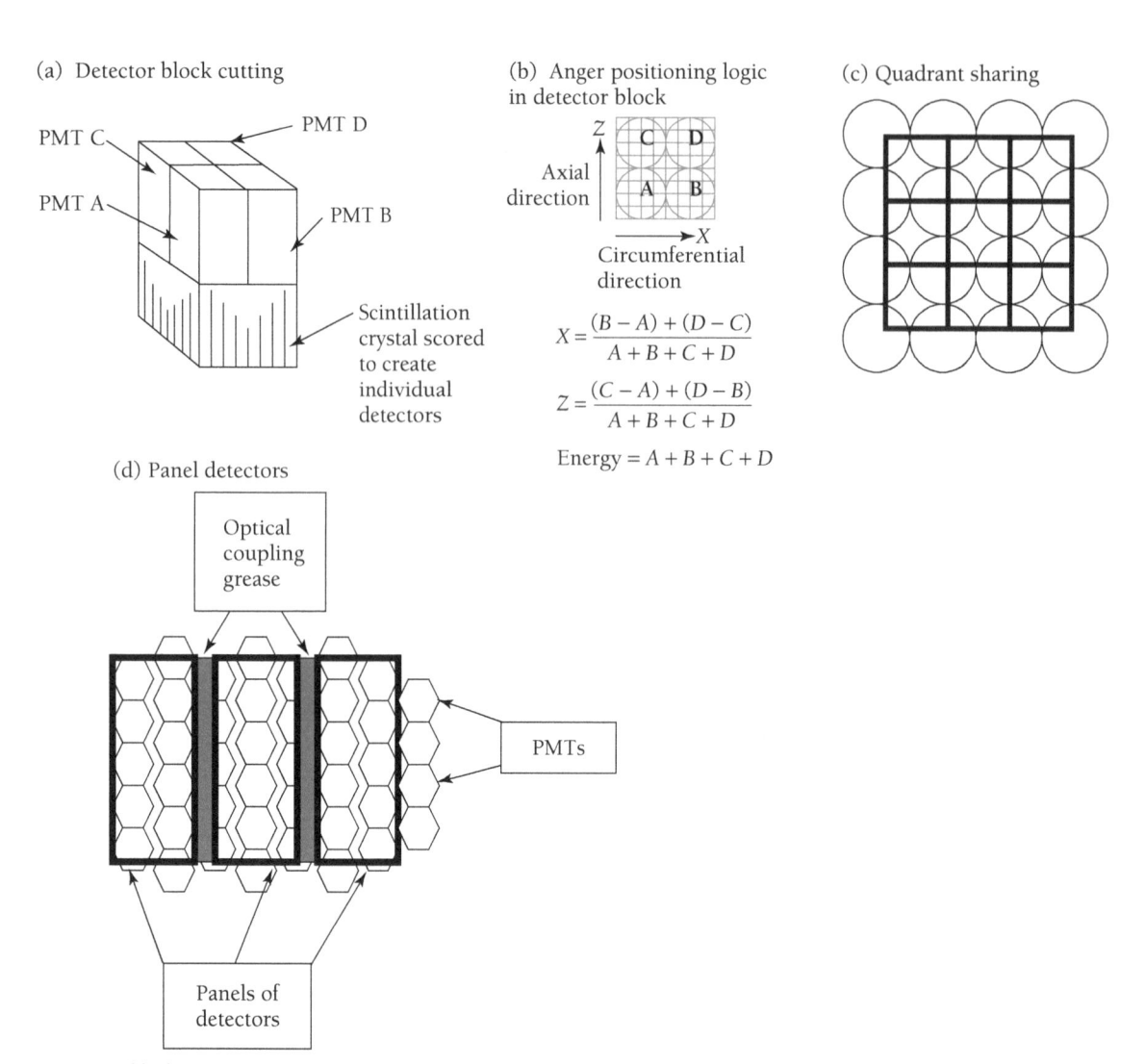

PMTs

Panels of detectors

Figure 15-4 Detector block arrangements. Figure 15-4a illustrates a common block-cutting method. A large block of scintillation material is cut into smaller detector elements that function as individual crystals. The scoring permits different amounts of scintillation light to reach the 4 PMTs, allowing the identification of the individual detector element detecting an annihilation photon. Figure 15-4b depicts Anger positioning logic in a detector block; because each of the 64 detectors produces a characteristic amount of light in each of the 4 PMTs, localization of an event to a specific detector is easily accomplished. The calculations of X and Z shown are used along with a detector identification map to determine the detector where the interaction occurred. In Figure 15-4c, the concept of quadrant sharing is illustrated. Instead of each of the 4 PMTs being assigned to 1 detector block, the (round) PMTs are shared across 4 (rectangular) detector blocks. Figure 15-4d depicts a modular detector, in which the space between detector blocks (called panels) is filled with optical coupling grease, and a row of PMTs is coupled over this space. In this detector, events are localized to an exact position, rather than to an individual scintillation crystal.

similar results (1). Voxel values in the reconstructed image matrix are expressed in terms of count rates or SUVs.

The concept of *image matrix* is applied in PET in a different sense than it is in planar and SPECT imaging. A gamma camera acquiring a planar image in digital form requires an image matrix in which to store counts. Because the raw data of a SPECT study are a series of planar images, the image matrix and therefore the voxel size carry through from the 2D projection images to the reconstructed 3D image matrix. In PET, data are stored in sinogram matrices, but the size of the sinogram matrix relates only to the number of detectors allowed to be in coincidence. The image matrix that defines the size of the pixels in a transaxial plane is created at the beginning of the reconstruction process; it is specified in the acquisition or processing protocol. The matrix is not directly related to the quality of the acquired data, as in SPECT.

The most common choices of matrix size for reconstructed clinical PET images are 128×128, 144×144, and 168×168. A 256×256 matrix is often used for quality control acquisitions. The matrix refers to the transaxial slices of the 3D image matrix; the third dimension (the Z or axial direction) of the study depends on the number of bed positions acquired. The choice of matrix dimension is based on the sampling theorem, the FOV size, and the spatial resolution of the tomograph. The chosen matrix should produce small enough voxels that image resolution is limited by the system parameters and not voxel size.

The same techniques used to display SPECT data are utilized with PET. Studies with multiple bed positions are fused into a large 3D image matrix; coronal slices provide the best overall visualization of these data. Dynamic triangulation is often combined with a maximum intensity

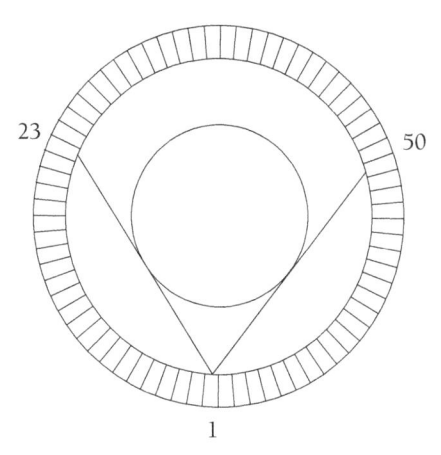

Figure 15-5 Allowed coincidences and field of view. Each detector bucket in a ring is allowed to be in coincidence with only a subset of the other detector buckets in the ring; namely those within a specified angle on the opposite side of the ring. In the diagram, all of the detector buckets between bucket 23 and bucket 50 are allowed to be in coincidence with the single detector bucket 1. Buckets 2 through 22 and 51 through 72 are not allowed to have coincidences with bucket 1. The angle of allowed coincidences, in turn, determines the FOV of the acquisition, represented by the circle in the middle.

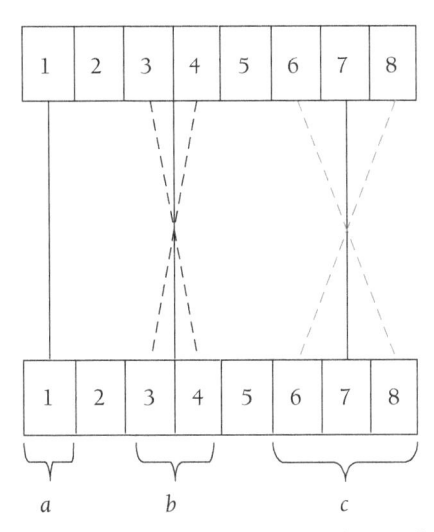

Figure 15-6 Direct and cross planes. Situation *a* shows a direct plane resulting from a coincidence detected within ring 1 of this 8-ring tomograph. Situation *b* shows a coincidence involving both ring 3 and ring 4. Events in this cross plane are assigned to a virtual plane (the solid line) that lies exactly between rings 3 and 4. Situation *c* illustrates a cross plane between rings that are separated by another ring of crystals. In this case, the midpoint of the cross plane lies at ring 7, so the events from the 6–8 cross plane are assigned to the ring 7 direct plane. In the cross-plane situations, an annihilation event can be located at any point on a dashed line, but is placed in the corresponding plane. Thus, there is some loss of resolution when cross planes are utilized.

projection (MIP) image, using only the anterior projection rather than a rotating cine display. When the operator clicks on a hot spot in the MIP image, the three orthogonal slices containing that hot spot are displayed. When PET images are fused with anatomic images (usually CT images), the PET images are generally shown in color and the anatomic images in a gray scale.

Detector Blocks

PET system design has moved in a direction opposite that of most single-photon cameras, in that many small scintillation crystals are employed in place of a single large crystal. Commercial PET tomographs have scintillation crystals composed of BGO, LSO, or GSO. Very recently, tomographs have become available that utilize lutetium-based scintillators and time-of-flight methodology. Most use some variation on the concept of detector blocks originally proposed by Casey and Nutt (2), each block consisting of a large number of small crystals and coupled to only a few PMTs. (The expense of the PMTs, in terms of both manufacturing and electricity, has led to the decision to limit their number. The overall cost of a PET tomograph is directly related to the number of detector blocks and the amount of associated electronics required [3].) Most PET systems (with the exception of the modular system described below) only identify the crystal interacting with an annihilation photon, rather than trying to determine an exact location, as is done in single-photon imaging. The detector block design accomplishes this task easily.

Basic Detector Block Operation

A *detector block* consists of 36 or 64 individual detectors, each 4 to 6 mm square by 20 to 30 mm in length. These may be created by gluing crystals together or by scoring a large block of scintillator material to various depths to create individual detectors (Fig. 15-4a) (4, 5). Reflective material may be inserted between crystals or into the scored spaces to prevent scintillation photons from crossing over into a neighboring detector. Four PMTs (in the most common arrangement) are coupled to the faces of the crystals opposite the center of the gantry. Each detector block requires a single high-voltage input of 900 to 1200 volts (V) and has an output signal cable for each PMT.

Both Anger positioning logic and electronic means are used to identify the detectors within a block. Figure 15-4b shows the mathematics of determining the X (circumferential) and Z (axial) coordinates of an event. The correlation between a given (X, Z) location and the identity of a particular crystal is then determined from a lookup table called a *detector identification map* that is generated from a *flood histogram*. The flood histogram is created by uniformly irradiating a detector block with annihilation photons and plotting the resulting X and Z values into an image matrix. The flood histogram shows some spatial distortion, but the lookup table allows each detected photon to be localized to a particular detector.

When an annihilation photon interacts in the block, it thus produces a light intensity pattern in the four PMTs that is characteristic of a specific crystal. The PMT output signals are amplified, filtered, and then totaled to generate the energy signal. The energy signal, after passing a low-energy threshold, triggers a timing signal, which is sent to the coincidence timing circuit. Once a coincidence is verified, the four PMT output signals are passed along for pulse height analysis and (X, Z) position. The lookup table identifies the specific crystal registering the interaction. Finally, the two crystals determined to be in coincidence for this event identify its LOR.

Detector blocks may be further organized into larger units called *cassettes* or *buckets*. Buckets are allowed to be in coincidence only with buckets on the opposite side of the ring. Referring to Figure 15-5, each of the divisions shown on the ring is a bucket. Bucket 1 is allowed to be in coincidence with buckets 23 through 50, but not buckets 2 through 22 or 51 through 72. This restriction simplifies the electronics of coincidence determination and allows for simultaneous evaluation of multiple events. It also determines the transaxial FOV, in that coincidence events originating outside of the allowable angle will not be registered. An additional advantage of the bucket architecture is that individual buckets are easily changed out for servicing.

Alternative Detector Block Configurations

A different detector block configuration, called *quadrant sharing*, uses larger PMTs that cover one corner each of four different detector blocks (Fig. 15-4c). Tomographs employing quadrant sharing have fewer PMTs by a factor of four compared to the arrangement described above, thus saving manufacturing and electricity costs. However, it increases the dead time, as the 4 PMTs servicing a given detector block are also involved in detecting events in 8 other blocks. It also requires detector blocks to be assembled into larger planar panels, with gaps between panels, and a hexagonal or octagonal rather than a circular ring (3). With this arrangement, replacement of detector blocks is a more complex operation.

One PET tomograph model uses detector panels that have greater similarity to a gamma camera. Instead of detector blocks, this system employs flat modules composed of 22×29 crystal arrays of $4 \times 6 \times 20$ mm GSO crystals (Fig. 15-4d) (6). The modules are optically coupled together side by side, and hexagonally shaped PMTs are positioned between modules as well as beyond the individual modules. Each event is seen by seven PMTs in this system, compared to only four in a standard PET block. Rather than being localized just to an individual detector, each count is assigned an exact position. This means that each LOR may be distinct from all others, thus requiring the more complex RAMLA reconstruction algorithm. The system includes a position-based energy correction table and an algorithm that corrects event position, similar to energy and linearity corrections in a gamma camera. The manufacturer holds that this configuration generates better position information than a block detector, while achieving high sensitivity and high count-rate capability (6).

Avalanche Photodiodes

An alternative to PMTs that is currently being explored is the avalanche photodiode (see Appendix B). These have higher quantum efficiency than PMTs (60–80% likelihood of producing an electron following absorption of a scintillation light photon vs 15–25% for PMTs). The gain factor, however, is only 2 to 3 orders of magnitude, compared to 6 to 8 orders of magnitude for a PMT. An avalanche photodiode thus produces a smaller output signal than a PMT, but the expense and operational electricity needs are considerably lower. The smaller size of avalanche photodiodes and their incorporation into multielement arrays also allow for a more compact design of the PET tomograph. In addition, they are unaffected by magnetic fields, making them ideal for tomographs combining PET with magnetic resonance imaging (MRI). Some PET/MRI units that are commercially available utilize avalanche photodiodes instead of PMTs. Their stability and long-term reliability are being examined, and they may someday replace PMTs in commercial PET tomographs (3). At this time, PMTs are still utilized in most tomographs because they are reliable and perform well with respect to timing and electronic noise (7).

Energy Discrimination

PET tomographs use pulse height analyzers (PHAs) to determine photon energy; these are similar to those found in other radiation detection instruments, so the concept and technology are familiar to us. However, the setting of the energy window is a point of greater discussion in PET than in single-photon applications, especially as the new scintillation materials are incorporated into commercial models. So even though this is not a parameter that is changed on a study-by-study basis, a short discussion of the issues is appropriate.

Recall that the purpose of an energy window is to eliminate scattered photons from the prompt sinogram, thus improving image quality. This represents a trade-off: as we remove photons based on energy, we decrease the number of counts registered and therefore reduce the signal-to-noise ratio (SNR) of the final image. The statistical variability in photon energy determination depends on how much scintillation light is generated following absorption of a photon. Thus, the ability to evaluate energy (and thereby eliminate scatter) improves with the newer scintillators compared to BGO. Commercial tomographs using GSO employ an energy window of 435 to 590 keV (4) and LSO- and LYSO-based tomographs a window of 425 to 650 keV (8, 9), compared to a window of 350 to 650 keV for BGO.

The choice of energy window also determines the scatter fraction (the percentage of all prompts that are scatter events) and therefore the degree of scatter correction needed. Because scatter correction is a subtraction operation, removing more scatter will decrease the SNR. Further, the spatial distribution of scatter changes as the energy window width is changed (10). Scatter compensation methods (discussed later) need to take the energy window setting into account.

Energy resolution is hindered by the high counting rates encountered in PET. The absence of a collimator means that the number of events per second is considerably greater than in single-photon imaging. One way to accommodate the fast event rate is to cut short the time allowed for registering scintillation photons from any one photon interaction (this pulse-clipping technique is illustrated in Fig. 8-5). While pulse integration time in single-photon imaging can be several μsec, in PET it is typically cut to only a few hundred nsec (11). Thus effective energy resolution is worse than what might be achieved in low-count situations, in the neighborhood of 10 to 25% in commercial PET tomographs.

Coincidences and Random Events

Coincidence Circuit

The essence of PET imaging is the determination that two annihilation photons have been detected at virtually the same time. This is accomplished by a coincidence circuit, as illustrated in **Figure 15-7**. Each detected event is assigned a timing signal, which is a logic pulse the width of the CTW. If a second event occurs before the logic pulse terminates, and its location is in an allowable bucket, then the coincidence logic circuit detects the overlap of the two timing signals and sends the energy and position information on to be evaluated.

The length of the CTW is therefore an important determinant of system performance. First, it must accommodate the 3- to 4-nsec time required for a photon (e.g., one generated by an annihilation near the edge of the ring) to cross the gantry bore. Second, it must be matched to the choice of scintillation material, in that a scintillator with a long decay time will require a longer period for collection of scintillation light. The newer scintillators LSO, LYSO, and GSO, with their shorter decay times, allow for a shorter CTW, while BGO has a longer scintillation light decay time and therefore requires a longer CTW. Current

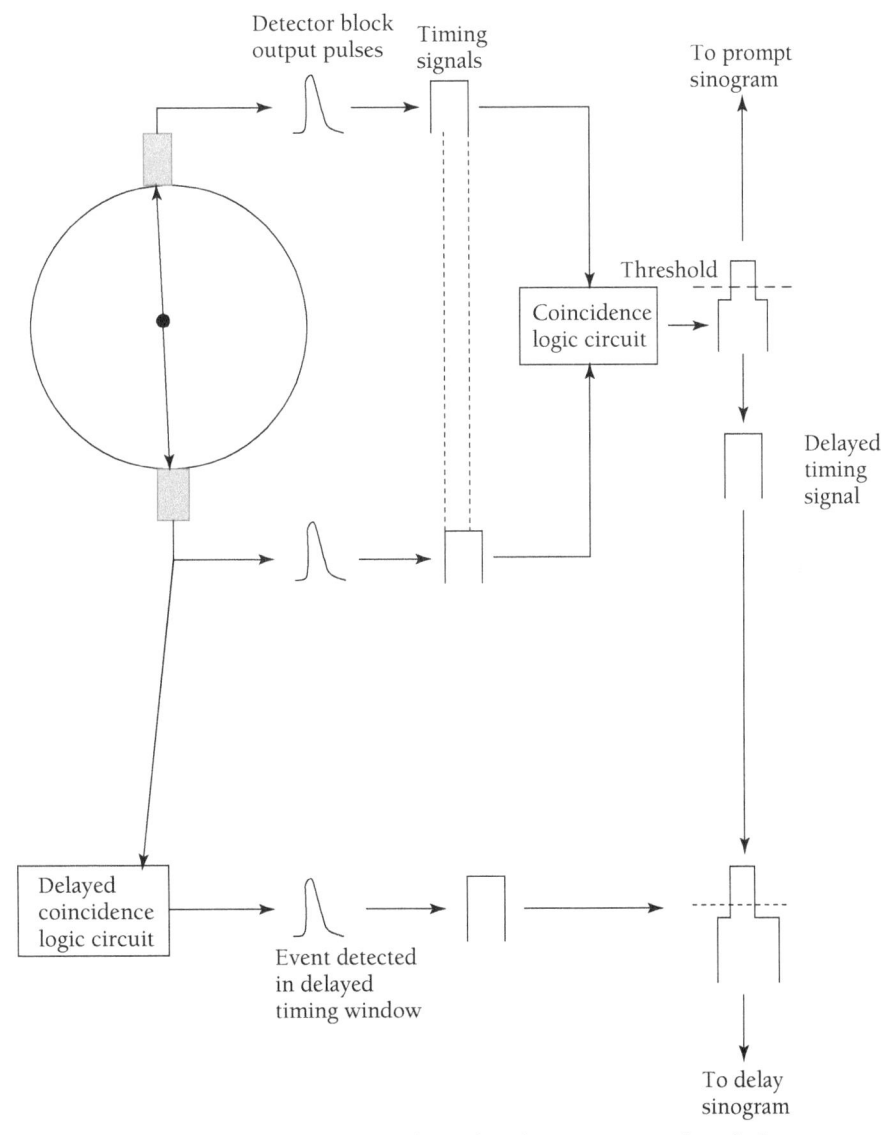

Figure 15-7 Coincidence and random detection circuitry. Each event detected produces an output pulse, which in turn generates a timing signal. One type of coincidence logic circuit sums the two timing signals; if they overlap (as shown by the pair of vertical dashed lines), the sum crosses a threshold value and the two events are deemed a coincidence. The determination that a coincidence has occurred then generates a delayed timing signal, which is summed with any events detected in the same detector pair in the delayed timing window. If an overlap of this delayed timing signal with another event is detected, a count in the corresponding LOR is added to the delay sinogram.

commercial tomographs employing LSO and LYSO utilize a coincidence timing window of 6 nsec, GSO tomographs use 8 nsec, and BGO tomographs use 11 to 13 nsec (12). Last, we should recognize that coincidence timing also represents a trade-off between the acceptance of true coincidences and the rejection of random coincidences. If the CTW is lengthened, more randoms as well as more trues will be detected, with the randoms rate increasing faster than the true coincidence rate.

Randoms Determination

Randoms are essentially accidental coincidences, but there is no direct way to distinguish them from true coincidences. The LOR of a random, arising as it does from two unrelated annihilation interactions, bears no relationship to either of the actual annihilation events that give rise to it (see Fig. 14-6c). For both image quality and quantitative purposes, therefore, we must subtract randoms. There are two ways to accomplish this: the *estimation-from-singles method* and the *delayed-coincidence method*. Neither method identifies randoms directly; instead they both identify LORs with high singles rates, and we use that information to estimate where more randoms are likely to occur.

Estimation from Singles

The number of random counts in each LOR can be estimated by some simple mathematics. If we know the rate at which single events are being detected in each of the two crystals defining an LOR, then the random coincidence rate is the likelihood that both detectors would detect a single event at the same time:

$$R = 2\tau S_i S_j \quad (15\text{-}1)$$

where R is the randoms count rate, τ is the CTW width, and S_i and S_j are the singles rates of the two crystals determining the LOR. The factor of 2 in Equation 15-1 comes from the fact that any amount of overlap between the two timing signals is considered in coincidence. The equation is given as $R = \tau S_i S_j$ in some references, incorporating the factor of 2 into the value of τ.

The singles-by-estimation technique measures the single event rate at each detector and uses Equation 15-1

directly to estimate the random coincidence rate. The main advantage of this method is that the randoms estimate is relatively noiseless, because of the high singles rate in PET studies. But it needs accurate knowledge of the timing offset between each pair of detectors as well as an additional layer of electronics. These requirements allow a greater opportunity for systematic error (3).

Delayed-Coincidence Window

In the delayed-coincidence method, one of the timing signals is held for several timing window widths (usually 60–100 nsec) and then is regenerated. If a single event is registered in the same LOR during the time of the regenerated signal, the two events are processed in the same way as the prompt event. Because of the delay, there are no true coincidences in this delayed window, but the probability of a random coincidence is the same as in the prompt window. Thus, the delay circuit can be used as an estimate of the singles rate in the LOR, and hence the randoms rate that might be occurring within the prompt timing window. Randoms are either subtracted from the prompt sinogram on the fly or stored in a delay sinogram, to be subtracted from the prompt sinogram at a later point in the reconstruction process.

The delayed-coincidence method thus measures the singles rate most precisely in the LORs that have prompt coincidences (whereas the estimation-from-singles method calculates the randoms rate in all LORs). The delayed-coincidence method has a significant drawback, in that it includes Poisson fluctuations that are propagated into the prompt sinogram when the delay sinogram is subtracted. This in turn may compromise some of the assumptions underlying the maximum-likelihood iterative reconstruction algorithm (5) and force modification of the Poisson model used in its implementation. It may be beneficial to smooth the delay sinogram prior to subtraction to reduce the magnitude of this problem. The estimation-from-singles method, on the other hand, does not have this problem because the single event rate at an individual crystal is considerably higher than the true coincidence rate. A second drawback of the delayed-coincidence method is that it keeps the detector blocks busy for considerably longer than the time needed to register the prompt coincidence. They are not able to detect another event until the time for the delayed coincidence has passed.

Transmission Sources and Geometries

Attenuation correction is required to obtain quantitatively accurate results in PET. Prior to the advent of hybrid PET/CT machines, attenuation correction was most commonly accomplished using rod or pin sources to produce a transmission scan, which was then reconstructed into an attenuation map. The transmission scan is either acquired before the injection of the radiopharmaceutical or is interleaved with the emission scan, a choice that is predicated primarily on the length of the uptake phase of the radiopharmaceutical being imaged. The great majority of clinical studies to date use FDG, which requires a 30- to

---

Sample Calculation 15-2 Estimation of Random Coincidences from Single Count Rates

Two scintillation crystals in a PET tomograph are each detecting singles at a rate of 50,000 per second. The system has a CTW of 6 nsec. What is the estimate of the randoms rate between these two crystals?

Equation 15-1 gives a random rate of

$$R = (2)(6 \times 10^{-9}\,\text{sec})\left(5 \times 10^4\,\frac{\text{cts}}{\text{sec}}\right)\left(5 \times 10^4\,\frac{\text{cts}}{\text{sec}}\right)$$

$$= 30\ \text{randoms/sec}.$$

90-minute uptake phase, so interleaved transmission/emission imaging is performed.

Positron-Emitting Attenuation Radionuclide

While many technologists will never work with a PET tomograph that has rod sources for attenuation correction, some of the older systems will be around for a while, so brief attention to radionuclide-based transmission imaging is in order. The most commonly used radionuclide source for transmission imaging is Ge-68, which decays to Ga-68, a positron-emitting radionuclide. The Ge-68 is generally fashioned into rods with activity of 3 to 10 mCi (110–370 MBq) and a tomograph may have one, two, or three rods (12). The use of a positron-emitting transmission source requires that we have a way to distinguish between emission coincidences and transmission coincidences. In PET, this is accomplished by *rod windowing*. To be included in the transmission scan, a coincidence must be detected within a narrow range of detector blocks that are in line with the rod source location (**Figure 15-8a**). Counts registered in the colinear detectors are assumed to come from the rod and not the patient; counts measured outside of the rod window are excluded from the transmission sinogram. In addition, emission counts within the rod window will contribute to the transmission data. It is therefore necessary to subtract an equivalent count rate (based on the emission LOR count rate) from each transmission LOR.

Single-Photon-Emitting Attenuation Radionuclide

Another choice is to use a radionuclide with a different energy. One manufacturer has employed Cs-137 for this purpose (Fig. 15-8b). This approach, called singles transmission scanning, has several advantages. First, rather than annihilation photons, a Cs-137 decay produces a single 662-keV photon, making it more easily identifiable in the mix of events found in a PET study. Second, Cs-137 has a 30-year half-life and thus needs replacement much less often than the Ge-68 source (which has a 271-day half-life). Third, because a coincidence is not required, the data acquisition rate is higher. The Cs-137 source (activity of 5–20 mCi [185–740 MBq] in the form of one or two point sources [4]) is well shielded from the near detectors, thus reducing dead-time effects in these detectors. On the negative side, the use of Cs-137 changes the attenuation situation from narrow-beam to broad-beam geometry, leading to a significant scatter component in the transmission data set that must be corrected. The attenuation coefficients at 662 keV are scaled to 511 keV before the attenuation map is applied to the emission data set.

A PET-only tomograph using rod sources requires a considerable amount of time for the transmission scan, often as much as one-third to one-half of the total imaging time. Even so, the transmission study is quite noisy, because only 2 to 5% of the photons from the transmission source actually pass through the body without being attenuated. One way to decrease the noise level of the

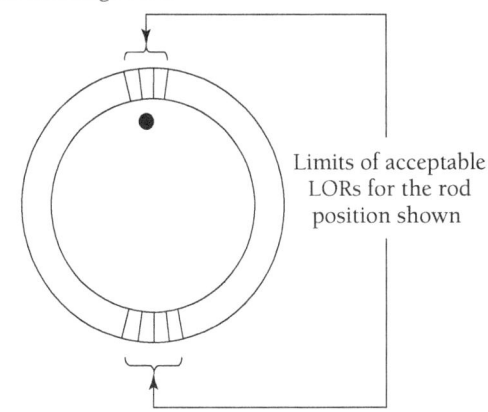

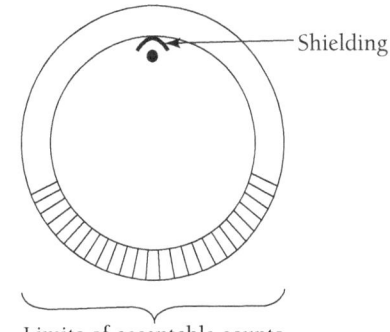

Figure 15-8 Transmission source configurations for PET. When a positron-emitting rod source is used, a three-point colinearity between the rod and the two responding scintillation detectors is required. This effectively limits the acceptable events to a narrow-beam geometry (see Fig. 12-1). If a single-photon source such as Cs-137 is used, a broad-beam situation is encountered (Fig. 15-8b). So the difference in measured linear attenuation coefficients is larger than would be expected from the energy difference alone. The Cs-137 source must be shielded from the nearby detectors.

transmission scan would be to increase the source activity, but this approach runs the risk of an unacceptably high singles detection rate in the detectors closest to the source, leading to excessive dead time. The high counting rate experienced by the detectors nearest the rod source is the primary limitation on the rods' activity (3). It also decreases the noise-equivalent count rate (NECR, a PET tomograph performance measure; see Chapter 16), due to the increased number of random and scatter coincidences. A more acceptable solution is to incorporate 2 to 4 rods of moderate activity, decreasing the imaging time while maintaining reasonable count statistics.

CT-Generated Attenuation Map

Ultimately, the "best" attenuation correction method for PET may be to add a CT scanner to the tomograph. (This topic is discussed in greater depth in Chapter 18.) Several of the advantages of this arrangement over radionuclide-based transmission images should be mentioned:

- Many thousands of photons are available, leading to an essentially noiseless attenuation map.
- Total acquisition time is greatly reduced.

- The CT scan provides the anatomic information that is sometimes lacking in PET studies.

There are issues related to the combining of the two modalities (these are also addressed in Chapter 18). But the benefits of combined PET/CT appear to far outweigh the concerns, as evidenced by the fact that PET-only tomographs have in large part been withdrawn from the market.

Corrections

In addition to corrections for random coincidences, a number of additional corrections must be made after the acquisition is completed. All of the corrections discussed in this section are incorporated in all modern PET tomographs, but the order in which they are applied may vary from system to system. The details of determining the values of the various correction factors are discussed in Chapter 17.

Normalization

In gamma cameras, we must compensate for nonuniformities in photon detection in order to create a usable image; the nonuniformities are due to the electronics involved in event detection. In PET, we have the additional complexity of multiple detectors instead of just one large scintillation crystal. Without normalization, the LOR-to-LOR variation in response to a uniform source of annihilation photons can be as high as a factor of 4 to 5 (13). To obtain a meaningful 3D image, this variability must be corrected. A normalization factor is thus determined for each LOR, such that after normalization all LORs have equal responses, and the variability in the image is due only to the radionuclide distribution within the object being imaged.

Normalization also corrects for variability across the volume of the tomograph. As we see later in this chapter, any acquisition mode other than direct planes only leads to a variation in the number of LORs contributing to each sinogram. For example, in 3D mode with all detector rings allowed to be in coincidence, there are fewer LORs contributing to the imaging planes at the axial front and back of the tomograph, compared to imaging planes in the middle of the tomograph. Correction of this variation by normalization is particularly important when multiple bed positions are to be appended together into a whole-body scan. The normalization scan also compensates for the variability of LOR densities within one imaging plane.

Normalization is accomplished through the acquisition of a high-count *normalization scan*, analogous to the high-count flood used to determine the uniformity correction map of a gamma camera. Either rod sources or a solid cylinder of positron-emitting radionuclide is used for this acquisition, which requires an acquisition time of 6 hr or more. Due to the inherent LOR-to-LOR variability, the sinogram resulting from this process is not uniform in any way (**Figure 15-9**). But we can easily create a uniform image, simply by multiplying each LOR's value by a correction factor to make it equal to the average. Once the average number of coincidences per LOR (N_{AVG}) is calculated, the correction factor for the LOR between detectors i and j on opposite sides of the ring is

$$\text{NORM}_{ij} = \frac{N_{AVG}}{N_{ij}} \quad (15\text{-}2)$$

where N_{ij} is the number of measured coincidences in LOR_{ij} in the normalization scan. Normalization of a clinical study is then accomplished by multiplying the measured counts in LOR_{ij} by its normalization factor NORM_{ij}.

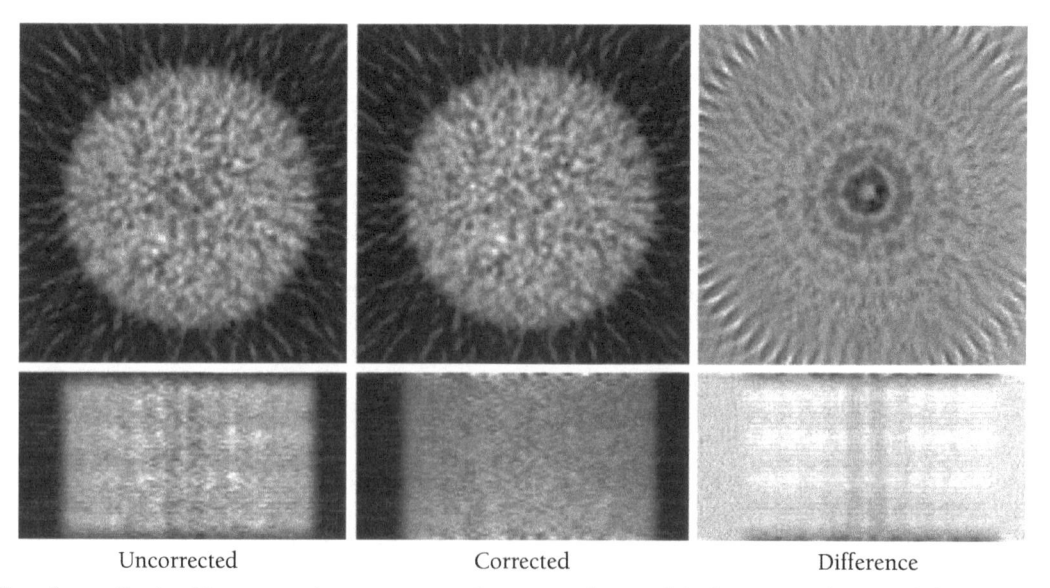

Figure 15-9 Effect of normalization. The top row shows reconstructed transverse slices, and the bottom row shows axial slices. The leftmost two are of a uniform cylindrical phantom, reconstructed without application of normalization factors. The middle two are the same acquisition, but reconstructed with the normalization factors applied. The rightmost two are the difference between the first two sets, indicating the relative size of the normalization factors. The difference transverse slice has dark rings, indicating a pattern of smaller and larger normalization factors in concentric circles. This corresponds to the spatial distribution of LORs shown in Figure 16-5a. Reprinted from: Phelps ME, ed. *PET: Physics, Instrumentation, and Scanners*, New York, NY: Springer; 2006:54, Fig. 33. With permission from Springer Science + Business Media, LLC.

Dead Time Correction

Two causes of dead time in PET are the same as in single-photon detection, namely, scintillation decay time and signal-processing time. PET has an additional source of dead time, in that it is possible for more than two events to be detected within one CTW. All events in such a "multiple" coincidence must be rejected, thus increasing dead time. To get quantitatively correct information in a PET study, a dead time correction is required.

Dead time correction may involve a model for the paralyzable and nonparalyzable factors contributing to overall dead time, and it may require the input of the average single event rate and the coincidence rate for each detector (3). These models are complex, because of the block detector design and the random coincidence circuitry. Dead time corrections (modeled or empirical) are usually supplied by the manufacturer. It makes sense that a high event rate in a particular LOR increases the dead time in that LOR, but not all systems apply dead time corrections on an LOR-by-LOR basis.

Scatter Correction

Correction for scatter is even more important for PET than for SPECT, because of the emphasis on quantitation. We can demonstrate the significant contribution of scatter by considering count profiles of line and cylindrical sources (**Figure 15-10**). Scatter is the most difficult correction to determine, because a scatter coincidence is a

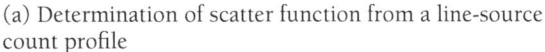

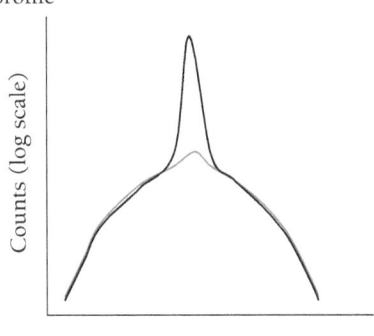

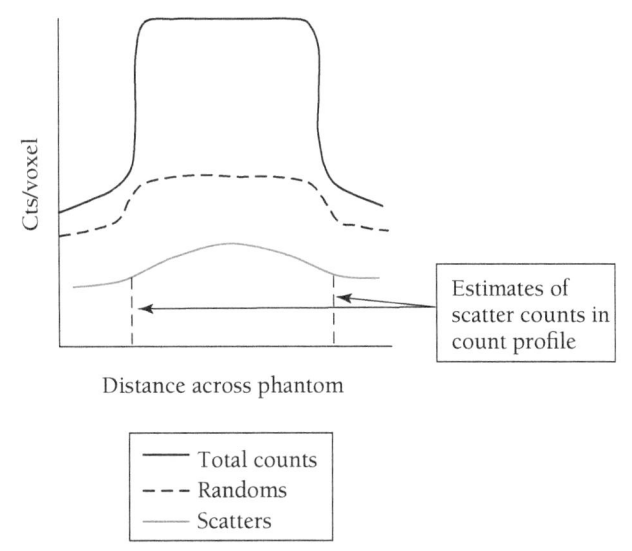

Figure 15-10 Scatter correction using count profiles. Figure 15-10a shows count profiles across a reconstructed line source of radioactivity. True coincidences can only come from the line source itself, while scatters may be detected beyond the boundaries of the line source. By putting the line source at several locations within the FOV, a location-specific estimate of the distribution of scatter events can be made. In Figure 15-10b, a count profile through a cylindrical phantom is shown. Scatter is estimated from the remaining counts in the "tails" of the count profile, beyond the boundaries of the phantom (the vertical dashed lines). This technique for scatter estimation is used in 2D PET.

true coincidence (because both annihilation photons arise from a single annihilation interaction); it is only identifiable by the loss of energy by one of the annihilation photons. The majority of Compton scattering interactions of 511-keV photons result in shallow scattering angles of 30° or less and therefore only a small loss of energy (3). And as was noted above, PET tomographs use wide energy windows, in order to maximize the acceptance of true coincidences, thus also accepting many scatter coincidences.

So rather than try to identify scatter coincidences in a particular acquisition, PET systems use various models of scatter and apply them to acquired studies. This aspect of PET continues to evolve. But there is universal agreement that any form of scatter correction is better than none (10). In addition, scatter correction should be performed before attenuation correction, so that the latter does not simply multiply scattered counts into significance (3).

Attenuation Correction

When a radionuclide is used as the transmission source, a *blank scan* (comparable to the reference scan needed for transmission-based attenuation correction in SPECT) must be acquired every day. The attenuation along each transmission LOR is normalized to the blank scan, to determine an attenuation correction factor (ACF):

$$\text{ACF}_j = \frac{\text{blank scan counts in LOR}_{ij}}{\text{transmission scan counts in LOR}_{ij}}. \quad (15\text{-}3)$$

This value is used as a correction factor for each LOR, in that multiplying by the ACF will increase the count rate in the LOR to what it would be with no attenuation. In PET, ACFs are typically around 20 and can exceed 100 (14). The ACF values will exhibit considerable noise when they are determined using radionuclide rod or point sources. In most systems, the measured values are used to identify tissue types, and the actual attenuation map is generated from known attenuation coefficients of these tissue types (i.e., it is a segmented map).

Sample Calculation 15-3 Attenuation Correction Factor

A blank scan registers 50,000 cts/sec in a particular LOR, and in the post-injection transmission scan the same LOR has 5,000 cts/sec. The LOR in the emission scan has 2,000 cts/sec. What is the count rate in the emission LOR after attenuation correction?

The emission counts need to be subtracted from the transmission counts before determining the attenuation correction factor. The attenuation correction factor for this LOR is:

$$\text{ACF} = \frac{50{,}000 \text{ cps}}{5{,}000 - 2{,}000 \text{ cps}} = 16.7.$$

Therefore, the emission LOR count rate should be increased by a factor of 16.7, to approximately 33,000 cts/sec, to account for attenuation.

Decay Correction

Positron-emitting radionuclides have very short half-lives, and PET scans often require multiple bed positions of several minutes each. In order for the coronal and sagittal images (which contain data from all bed positions) to be meaningful, the data set from each bed position must be decay-corrected. A common practice is to apply decay-correction factors from the midtime point of each bed position back to the time of injection (15). Another option is to decay-correct back to the start time for the image acquisition.

Summary

The corrections to an individual LOR can be summarized in the following equation:

$$N_{\text{final}} = \left(N_{\text{prompt}} \times \text{DT} - N_{\text{delay}} - N_{\text{scatter}}\right) \\ \times \text{NORM} \times \text{ACF} \times \text{DC} \quad (15\text{-}4)$$

Sample Calculation 15-4 Corrections for PET Raw Data

A voxel in a PET scan has a raw count rate of 1,500 cps. The following corrections are to be applied:

- Normalization factor = 1.8
- Dead time loss of 15%
- Randoms = 150 cps
- Scatter = 30%
- Attenuation correction factor = 6 (i.e., five-sixths of annihilation events are lost due to attenuation)
- Decay correction = 1.40

What is the corrected value for the voxel?

Working from Equation 15-4, we need first to correct for dead time. A 15% dead time loss implies that the actual prompts rate is 115% of the measured rate, so 1,500 cps × 1.15 = 1,725 cps. We then subtract the random coincidence rate: 1,725 cps − 150 cps = 1,575 cps. We will apply the 30% scatter fraction to the randoms-corrected count rate and get a scatter count rate of 472 cps, which brings the scatter-corrected count rate down to 1,103 cps. Finally, we apply the multiplicative correction factors: 1,103 cps × 1.8 × 6 × 1.40 = 16,677 cps.

where N refers to a count rate in each case and DT, NORM, ACF, and DC stand for the (unitless) dead time correction, normalization, attenuation correction factor, and decay-correction values, respectively (15). Last, for absolute quantitation, a cross-calibration with the dose calibrator or well counter is required. The calibration factor has the form of (cps/voxel) ÷ (μCi/ml) and is divided into the corrected voxel count rate.

Acquisition Options

Any new technology evolves from an initial or prototype design to include an increasing number of variations and applications. This has happened in PET over the last decade or so, as new products have provided additional options for acquisition. Most involve changes at the level of the tomograph rather than the acquisition protocol, and hence require purchase of a new system for implementation.

2D vs 3D Imaging Modes

The first acquisition option is actually not new at all. Figure 15-1b shows septa between the rings of crystals. Annular septa are thin rings made of lead or tungsten, extending from the crystals into the bore of the gantry (envision them as very large, very thin washers that extend from the crystal rings several inches into the gantry bore). They are used to define direct planes and to absorb many off-angle photons.

Septa can be compared to a Venetian blind. When the blind is drawn up (the septa are retracted out of the FOV), light can pass through the window at all angles. When the blind is let down (the septa are extended—in place between crystal rings), light only passes through the spaces between the slats of the blind. (The analogy does not include the ability to turn the septa as slats in a blind can be turned to completely block the light; they are always oriented in a transaxial direction.)

A tomograph that has extended septa is operating in *2D mode* (Fig. 15-2c). The septa absorb off-angle annihilation photons, decreasing the number of random and scatter coincidences. When the septa are retracted (Fig. 15-2b), the scanner is in *3D mode*. More scattered and random events are registered, but so are many true events that involve different tomograph rings. Tomographs using BGO as the scintillator use 2D imaging in part to decrease the overall count rate; systems utilizing new, faster scintillators do not have significant count-rate issues, and many do not even offer septa as an option.

The 2D/3D Continuum

The determination of the imaging planes allowed to contribute to the acquisition is both physical and electronic (16). **Figure 15-11** shows five options for an eight-ring tomograph. The most restrictive option is to only allow direct plane coincidences (strict 2D). The sensitivity in this mode is the least of any option, but accepted events are more likely to be trues and less likely to be scatters or randoms.

The septa are not long enough to block all cross-plane events, and so we can electronically allow some of these to be accepted (2D acquisitions with *spans* of 3 and 7). Resolution is somewhat degraded when cross-plane events are accepted, because the coincidences are all assigned to a single transaxial plane, even though their origins span several rings of crystals. But sensitivity is greatly increased. The span of 3 is sometimes referred to as "high resolution" and the span of 7 as "high sensitivity," in an (imperfect) analogy to gamma camera collimators.

In 3D imaging, the septa are retracted out of the FOV, so all crystals are potentially "live" to all events. Once again, we can limit the allowable LORs electronically. Figure 15-11 shows a strict 3D acquisition, with all LORs allowed, and a situation in which the maximum spread of allowable LORs is limited to 5 rings. This *ring difference* excludes coincidences that cross a wide portion of the FOV and hence are most likely to have originated far from the virtual plane to which they are assigned. (Some references use the terms *span* and *ring difference* interchangeably.)

Axial Sensitivity

Figure 15-11b emphasizes the relative sensitivities of the different 2D and 3D acquisition modes. In a 3D acquisition, the planes at the axial front and back of the gantry have far fewer LORs contributing to them compared to the middle planes. This has an important implication in acquisitions involving multiple bed positions. We must account for these axially dependent sensitivity differences either by normalizing to equalize the counts per plane or by overlapping the bed positions (**Fig. 15-12**). The latter technique is more commonly employed, with an overlap of several cm between bed positions (17). The sensitivity profile of each acquisition mode is determined as part of the normalization scan and it can be included in reconstruction when needed.

Sample Calculation 15-5 Bed Positions with Overlap

A PET tomograph is operated in 2D mode with a span of 7, and requires 3 cm of overlap between bed positions. The length to be imaged in a particular patient is 78 cm. The axial length of the tomograph is 15 cm. How many bed positions are needed?

In this situation, the axial length is effectively reduced from 15 to 12 cm by the need for 3-cm overlap. So we can calculate the number of bed positions as in Sample Calculation 15-1:

$$\text{Number of bed positions} = \frac{78\text{-cm scan length}}{12\text{ cm/bed position}}$$
$$= 6.5 \text{ bed positions.}$$

We would round up to 7 bed positions to ensure that the desired length is covered.

(a) LORs

Strict 2D 2D span of 3 2D span of 7 Strict 3D 3D ring difference of 5

(b) Relative sensitivities in the axial direction

Strict 2D 2D span of 3 2D span of 7 Strict 3D 3D ring difference of 5

Relative sensitivity

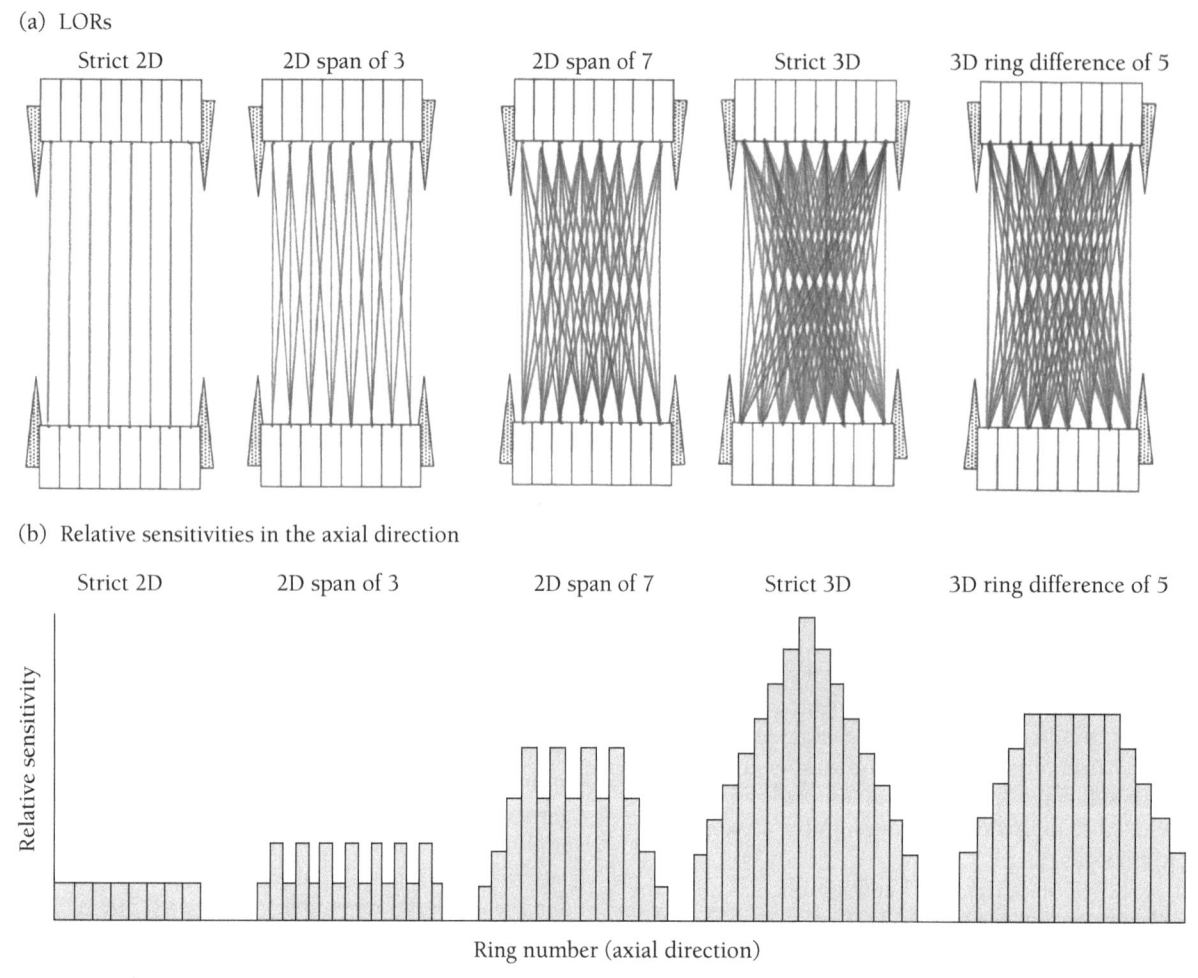

Ring number (axial direction)

Figure 15-11 2D and 3D options. Several possible imaging modes in 2D and 3D are shown (septa are not shown for the sake of clarity). The removal of septa, thus allowing cross-plane events to be registered, increases the sensitivity of the tomograph, as shown in Figure 15-11b. But this has a detrimental effect in terms of resolution, because cross-plane events do not necessarily originate in the plane to which they are assigned. The choice of imaging mode is set within the study protocol, so it is not necessary to be cognizant of the choice being made in a given situation.

(a) Strict 3D, no overlap

Normalization required

(b) 3D with limited ring difference, no overlap

Normalization required

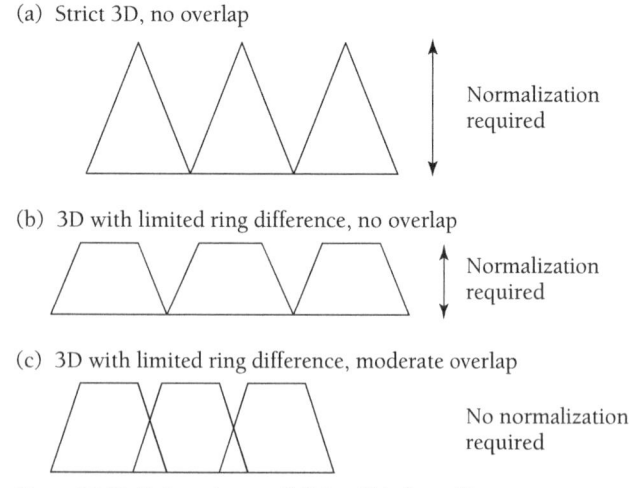

(c) 3D with limited ring difference, moderate overlap

No normalization required

Figure 15-12 Bed overlap possibilities. This figure illustrates sensitivity in the axial direction for a variety of choices for overlap between bed positions. Each triangle or trapezoid represents one bed position, similar in shape to the graphs shown in Figure 15-11. The double-headed arrow to the right of Figures 15-12a and 15-12b shows the relative amount of normalization that must occur to create readable coronal and sagittal images. Greater overlap requires less normalization but a longer total imaging time.

Other Considerations

The 3D acquisition mode requires that we treat scattered photons, random events, and even attenuation correction differently. When rod sources are used to measure attenuation, the activity needs to be less for 3D than for 2D. Randoms are generated from a larger volume of the object being imaged in 3D compared to 2D imaging (**Figure 15-13**) and must be dealt with more carefully (18). Scatter correction using the "tails" method of Bergstrom (Fig. 15-10b) is commonly used in 2D mode (12), while 3D employs simulation of scatter (19, 20), often utilizing the transmission map. A tomograph capable of both 2D and 3D acquisitions will need to have separate normalization and dead time corrections for each mode.

In 3D, the total number of LORs increases dramatically: a system containing 10,000 crystals has about 100 million LORs in 3D mode (12). Before reconstruction of a 3D acquisition, it is common to translate the many LORs into 2D projections, a process called *rebinning*. Several complicated algorithms are used; a common one, called *Fourier rebinning* (FORE), utilizes Fourier transformation of the data, resulting in more accurate localization to a 2D

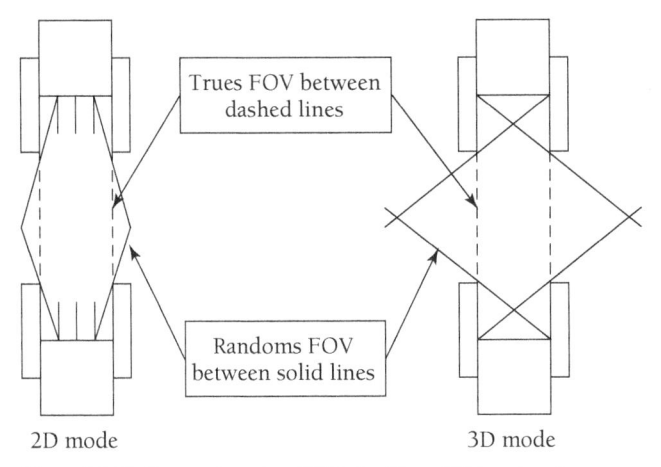

Figure 15-13 True and random FOVs for 2D vs 3D imaging. In a cross-sectional view of PET geometry, it can be seen that the FOV for true coincidences is the same width in 2D and 3D situations. The removal of septa in the 3D situation, on the other hand, allows random coincidences from a much larger volume of the object to be registered in the acquisition. Reprinted from: Brasse D, Kinahan PE, Laritzien C, et al. Correction methods for random coincidences in fully 3D whole-body PET: impact on data and image quality. *J Nucl Med.* 2005;46:859–867. With permission of the Society of Nuclear Medicine.

slice (17). Rebinning greatly decreases the time required for reconstruction.

Dynamic and Gated Modes

Dynamic and gated imaging are two well-used techniques in single-photon imaging that are also applicable to PET. While neither is widely used in clinical imaging at this time, dynamic imaging is a common technique in research PET, where many studies follow the movement of radiolabeled biomolecules or drugs over time. Gated cardiac imaging is a primary tool with SPECT, and it is becoming more available in PET as Tc-99m production has experienced difficulties. Respiratory gating, including correlation with CT images, is another area of active investigation.

These timed studies do not require a new tomograph, but will need some different techniques compared to static PET studies (i.e., those in which the radiopharmaceutical location is not changing). A single bed position is acquired, data are in list-mode format, and decay correction is very important. Noise will be a greater concern, given that these studies will likely have low per-frame count rates, and this will in turn require special considerations for randoms subtraction and scatter correction. Expect to see increasing utilization of these acquisition modes as time goes on.

Time-of-Flight Tomographs

The concept of TOF-PET was introduced in Chapter 14, and TOF tomographs based on lutetium scintillators first came into the market in 2006. Even faster scintillators may be incorporated in the future, as the electronic components are developed to match them. From the technologist's standpoint, TOF-PET tomographs will function very much like their non-TOF predecessors. One notable difference is that the data points will be stored in list mode rather than histogram mode, because list mode is a more efficient storage mechanism for large image data sets. Information about the difference in arrival times between two photons is incorporated into the forward-projection step of the iterative reconstruction process. This in turn drives the iterative process to converge more quickly, because of the enhanced knowledge of event locations (21). Time-of-flight information can also be applied to filtered backprojection (FBP) reconstruction, where its incorporation is referred to as *confidence-weighted backprojection*.

With TOF-PET coming so close on the heels of PET/CT, many nuclear medicine departments will be hard pressed to consider purchasing a TOF system. But the benefit is significant enough to warrant strong consideration. The improvement is a several-fold increase in the SNR, which in turn improves sensitivity and lesion detectability. This has the greatest impact in whole-body imaging and the effect increases with the size of the patient (22). The extra level of detail may in turn allow a decrease in dosage and hence in patient radiation exposure. Less of a gain in localization and resolution is seen in smaller patients due to the fact that TOF only limits, but cannot exactly pinpoint, the location of an annihilation event, given the current instrumentation.

Organ-Specific Systems

A final set of acquisition options becoming available is systems designed to image particular organs. The current situation mirrors what we have already observed in general nuclear medicine, in that the first wave of organ-specific PET devices are designed for the heart and the breast. Each may find additional uses over time.

The Naviscan high-resolution organ-specific PET scanner consists of two detector heads, each with an array of 2,028 LYSO crystals. The detectors scan within a larger frame to produce an FOV of 16.4 × 24 cm. Data are stored in list-mode fashion, and iterative reconstruction produces 12 or 24 image planes. Imaging of the breast follows mammography technique, using the two detector frames as the support and compression paddles. Spatial resolution down to 1.8 mm can be achieved with this system.

The Positron Attrius® cardiac PET scanner is optimized for cardiac imaging. It uses BGO as its scintillator, with crystal faces that are 8.5 × 9.8 mm. The crystals are in axially oriented modules of 2 × 16 crystals, with neighboring modules offset by one-half the crystal width. The staggered arrangement increases the number of cross planes, thereby improving spatial resolution and sensitivity. In addition, the tomograph incorporates a "wobble," a continuous back-and-forth motion of the gantry around the Z-axis. This increases the number of LORs that can be registered, further improving both resolution and sensitivity. A rotary encoder maps events to the proper LOR based on gantry position at the time of the coincidence detection. The system acquires in list mode and has both dynamic (time-mode) and gated (phase-mode) protocols. It uses relatively short septa and includes Ge-68 rods for segmented attenuation correction. It incorporates a high-quality motion correction system and proprietary cardiac analysis software. It is designed to maximize sensitivity without sacrificing resolution.

Summary

This chapter illustrates the complexity found in PET tomographs. The many individual detectors, the need for coincident detection of two annihilation photons, and the great number and different types of events being detected make this technology more complicated to understand than single-photon imaging. The need to correct for random, scatter, and attenuation events and the multiplicity of ways to do so increase the intricacy of the system. A PET tomograph goes through many steps to produce images, and most of those steps are not visible to the user.

These systems can in fact be operated in a "black box" fashion, with the operator making only a few key choices in regard to acquisition and reconstruction and leaving other decisions hidden within a specific protocol. As clinical study options are developed, however, it will become necessary to understand and evaluate the choices available. In addition, we can expect that the technology applied to PET tomographs will continue to evolve. We are already seeing the need for different types of image acquisitions, improved electronics, and even organ-specific instruments. In addition, the number of PET radiopharmaceuticals will proliferate over time, broadening the repertoire of the instruments and the technologists who operate them. Thus, the black box approach will eventually give way to a more in-depth application of both the tomograph mechanics and the reconstruction methods.

References

1. Bailey DL, Townsend DW, Valk PE, Maisey MN. *Positron Emission Tomography: Basic Science*. London: Springer; 2003;77.
2. Casey ME, Nutt R. A multicrystal two-dimensional BGO detector system for positron emission tomography. *IEEE Trans Nucl Sci*. 1986;33:460–463.
3. Phelps ME, ed. *PET: Physics, Instrumentation, and Scanners*. New York, NY: Springer; 2006:15, 22, 24, 37, 50, 62, 64, 66, 69, 90, 110.
4. Tarantola G, Zito F, Gerundini P. PET instrumentation and reconstruction algorithms in whole-body applications. *J Nucl Med*. 2003;44:756–769.
5. Wahl RL, Buchanan JW. *Principles and Practice of Positron Emission Tomography*. Philadelphia, PA: Lippincott Williams & Wilkins; 2002:51, 62, 70–73, 75.
6. Surti S, Karp JS. Imaging characteristics of a three-dimensional GSO whole-body PET camera. *J Nucl Med*. 2004;45:1040–1049.
7. Pichler BJ, Wehrl HF, Judenhofer MS. Latest advances in molecular imaging instrumentation. *J Nucl Med*. 2008;49:5S–23S.
8. Brambilla M, Secco C, Dominietto M, et al. Performance characteristics for a new 3-dimensional lutetium oxyorthosilicate-based whole-body PET/CT scanner with the National Electrical Manufacturers Association NU 2-2001 standard. *J Nucl Med*. 2005;46:2083–2091.
9. Kemp BJ, Kim C, Williams JJ, Ganin A, Lowe VA. NEMA NU 2-2001 performance measurements of an LYSO-based PET/CT system in 2D and 3D acquisition modes. *J Nucl Med*. 2006;47:1960–1967.
10. Zaidi H, Koral KF. Scatter modeling and compensation in emission tomography. *Eur J Nucl Med Mol Imaging*. 2004;31:761–782.
11. Saha GB. *Basics of PET Imaging Physics, Chemistry, and Regulations*. New York, NY: Springer Science + Business Media; 2005:21.
12. Zanzonico P. Positron-emission tomography: a review of basic principles, scanner design and performance, and current systems. *Semin Nucl Med*. 2004;34:87–111.
13. Wagner HN, Szabo Z, Buchanan BS. *Principles of Nuclear Medicine*. 2nd ed. Philadelphia, PA: Saunders; 1995:359.
14. Zaidi H, Hasegawa B. Determination of the attenuation map in emission tomography. *J Nucl Med*. 2003;44:291–315.
15. Henkin RE, Boles MA, Dillehay GL, et al. *Nuclear Medicine*, St. Louis, MO: Mosby-Year Book; 1996:287, 289.
16. Fahey FH. Data acquisition in PET imaging. *J Nucl Med Technol*. 2002;30:39–49.
17. Christian PE, Waterstram-Rich KM. *Nuclear Medicine and PET/CT: Technology and Techniques*. 6th ed. St. Louis, MO: Mosby-Year Book; 2007:326, 332, 335.
18. Brasse D, Kinahan PE, Laritzien C, et al. Correction methods for random coincidences in fully 3D whole-body PET: impact on data and image quality. *J Nucl Med*. 2005;46:859–867.
19. Ollinger JM. Model-based scatter correction for fully 3D PET. *Phys Med Biol*. 1996;41:153–176.
20. Watson CC, Newport D, Casey ME. A single scatter simulation technique for scatter correction in 3D PET. In: Grangeat P, Amans JL, eds. *Three-Dimensional Image Reconstruction in Radiology and Nuclear Medicine*. Dordrecht, The Netherlands: Kluwer; 1996:255–268.
21. Lois C, Jakoby BW, Long MJ, et al. An assessment of the impact of incorporating time-of-flight information into clinical PET/CT imaging. *J Nucl Med*. 2010;51:237–245.
22. Karp J, Surti S, Daube-Witherspoon ME, Muehllehner G. Benefit of time-of-flight in PET: experimental and clinical results. *J Nucl Med*. 2008;49:462–470.

Additional Resources

Bailey DL, Townsend DW, Valk PE, Maisey MN. *Positron Emission Tomography: Basic Science*. London: Springer; 2003; Chapters 2–5.

Cherry SR, Sorenson JA, Phelps ME. *Physics in Nuclear Medicine*. 3rd ed. Philadelphia, PA: Saunders; 2003:Chapter 18.

Fahey FH. Data acquisition in PET imaging. *J Nucl Med Technol*. 2002;30:39–49.

Henkin RE, Boles MA, Dillehay GL, et al. *Nuclear Medicine*. St. Louis, MO: Mosby-Year Book; 1996:Chapter 23.

Phelps ME, ed. *PET: Physics, Instrumentation, and Scanners*. New York, NY: Springer; 2006.

Tarantola G, Zito F, Gerundini P. PET instrumentation and reconstruction algorithms in whole-body applications. *J Nucl Med*. 2003;44:756–769.

Wagner HN, Szabo Z, Buchanan BS. *Principles of Nuclear Medicine*. 2nd ed. Philadelphia, PA: Saunders; 1995:Chapter 19, Sec. 2.

Wahl RL, Buchanan JW. *Principles and Practice of Positron Emission Tomography*. Philadelphia, PA: Lippincott Williams & Wilkins; 2002:Chapters 3, 4.

Zaidi H. Comparative evaluation of scatter correction techniques in 3D positron emission tomography. *Eur J Nucl Med*. 2000;27:1813–1826.

Zaidi H, Koral KF. Scatter modeling and compensation in emission tomography. *Eur J Nucl Med Mol Imaging*. 2004;31:761–782.

Zanzonico P. Positron-emission tomography: a review of basic principles, scanner design and performance, and current systems. *Semin Nucl Med*. 2004;34:87–111.

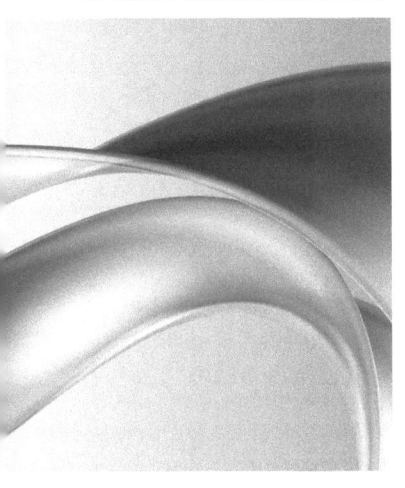

CHAPTER 16 — Image Characteristics, Performance Measures, and Quantitation in PET

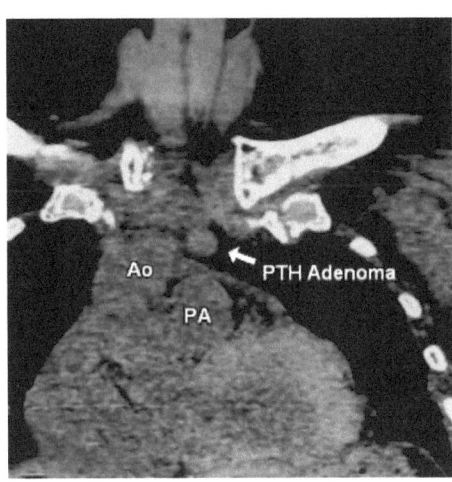

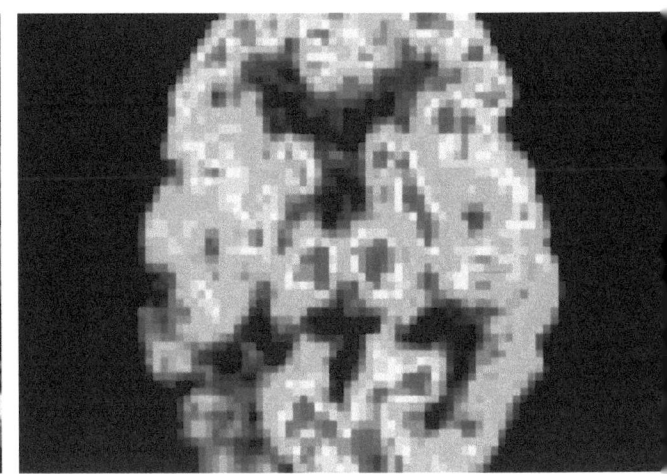

Learning Outcomes

1. Describe each of the following image characteristics as they relate to PET images:
   a. Noise
   b. Dead time
   c. Attenuation
   d. Scatter
   e. Partial volume effect
2. Explain how the recovery coefficient corrects quantitative information in small volumes.
3. Discuss parameters that affect spatial resolution, sensitivity, scatter fraction, and count rate, and define the noise-equivalent count rate.
4. Discuss factors affecting image quality in PET, including:
   a. Inherent limitations of annihilation photon imaging
   b. Impact of ring geometry
   c. Count rate issues
   d. 2D vs 3D acquisition mode
   e. Incorporation of time-of-flight (TOF) technology
5. Describe the standardized uptake (SUV) value as a semiquantitative measure of radiopharmaceutical uptake, and discuss its uses and limitations.

Introduction

As we did with planar and SPECT imaging, we now consider characteristics of PET images. In some ways, there will be congruence with prior chapters, because all types of nuclear medicine imaging must deal with the same underlying issues. But PET requires that some of these characteristics be addressed more specifically. In particular, the absence of a collimator makes considerations of scatter fraction, dead time, and count rate performance much more important in PET than in single-photon imaging. The ring geometry and detector size issues are unique to PET and pose limitations that must be considered. Finally, because of PET's quantitative properties, questions specific to the accuracy of quantitative results must be taken into account. We therefore encounter several new performance measures in this chapter.

Image Characteristics in PET

The list of image characteristics for PET mirrors the previous discussions of these issues. But for each image characteristic, PET will require a different set of considerations. These considerations will in turn play into the factors affecting performance measures. In particular, the ring geometry of the PET tomograph, the variety of scintillation materials employed as detectors, the high count rates experienced, and the distinctive properties of PET radiopharmaceuticals all impact the capabilities and limitations of PET.

Background

As always, the first component of background is nonspecific radiopharmaceutical distribution. It is likely that PET imaging in general will consist of hot-spot imaging rather than cold-spot imaging, as occurs in other nuclear medicine tests such as myocardial perfusion imaging. It is easier to spot a hot lesion than a cold lesion, even in the presence of background. But the level of background can still impact the ability to identify an area of increased activity. An analogy courtesy of Dr. Thomas Budinger: the stars are just as bright in the daytime as at night, but we can't see them during the day due to the brightness of the sunlight (1).

Lack of background is for the most part a positive image characteristic, but not always. For F-18 Fluorodeoxyglucose (FDG), the major PET radiopharmaceutical to date, the relative paucity of background activity is somewhat problematic. The absence of activity around a hot lesion can make its location difficult to pinpoint. It is this problem that makes the colocation of PET with an anatomic imaging device so attractive. Also with FDG, incorrect patient preparation can greatly increase background and by doing so may hide important pathology.

Two other potential components of background are random and scatter events. Randoms are accounted for in a straightforward manner. But scatter is generally modeled rather than measured, such that the quality of scatter subtraction depends on the model used.

A third source of background is the fact that (in a conventional PET tomograph) we localize each coincidence only to its line of response (LOR). The reconstruction process puts each event in its place, but may not do so with 100% accuracy. Incorrectly located events become part of the overall background. A major benefit of TOF-PET is that it more correctly positions events, thereby increasing the count rate in areas of higher counts and decreasing the number of extraneous counts in other areas. An improvement in the tumor/background ratio was demonstrated for TOF vs non-TOF acquisitions in a small series (2).

Noise

PET images contain noise, as do planar and SPECT images with gamma cameras. We might think that PET images would have less noise than single-photon images, because of the higher count rates achieved in the absence of absorptive collimators. But the noise situation is much more complex in PET. Noise results not only from the inherent variability of radioactive decay and from the reconstruction process, but also from random and scatter count rates and attenuation effects. All of these are corrected for, but the correction methods (especially those involving subtraction) may in fact increase the overall noise level.

In tomographic imaging, noise must be considered from a per-voxel viewpoint. In general, tomographic images require more counts than planar images to give statistically valid results (3). But in PET, each voxel can have events from many LORs, and each LOR has its own statistical uncertainty. So the uncertainty in voxel count rate is much greater than might be assumed based on just the total number of counts (4). This is much more the case in 3D imaging compared to 2D imaging, because the number of possible LORs increases geometrically (5). Its ability to deal with noise is one of the reasons iterative reconstruction is favored for PET.

Random coincidences are particularly problematic. They arise not only from annihilation events occurring within the area being imaged, but also from annihilation photons originating outside of the field of view (FOV) and even outside of the object. The randoms fraction (the percentage of all prompts that are randoms) is ideally less than 20%, but in areas of high radioactivity it can approach 50%. If random coincidences are not subtracted, they lead to an overestimation of the activity concentration that is more or less uniformly distributed across the reconstructed 3D image matrix, with extra randoms in the center of the FOV (6). All PET tomographs allow for subtraction of random coincidences, but the methods currently employed either require an extra layer of electronics or create a noisy map of the randoms fraction.

Dead Time

In PET, we must also be concerned about dead time. Recall that dead time is a function of the time required to process an event, and that the dead time of a complex system is determined by the dead time of the slowest component. In a PET tomograph with modern electronics, the slowest component is the pulse integration time, which in turn is dependent on the decay time of the scintillation crystal. Bismuth germanate (BGO), the scintillator of choice for PET through the 1990s, has a very long decay time, and as a result, BGO-based tomographs can have significant dead time (50% or even higher). This was a major factor driving the development of new scintillation materials. Tomographs utilizing these newer scintillators have less dead time, registering more counts per second per unit of activity concentration. This in turn allows the patient dosage to be decreased and/or the scan time to be shortened.

In terms of event types, single events are the largest contributor to dead time, because the detector block must process each one until the lack of a coincidence is verified (6). The single-event rate is very high, often 100 times the trues rate. Two other sources of dead time should also be noted. First, three or more annihilation photons may be detected within the coincidence timing window. These *multiple coincidences* must be discarded, thus potentially losing a true event. Second, the detector block architecture necessitates that a block is unavailable during the time of pulse integration. While processing one event, it cannot accept another. A quadrant-sharing design (see Fig. 15-4c) increases this source of dead time by a factor of 4, because PMTs are shared among four blocks.

Dead time has two important consequences. The first consequence is the loss of true coincidences. In most clinical situations, the dead time correction factor is much

Figure 16-1 Effect of attenuation correction. Without attenuation correction (Fig. 16-1a), the surface outline and the lungs both appear hot, because photons originating in these areas experience much less attenuation than do photons arising from other areas of the body. The structures that are more internal have apparently decreased activity compared to more superficial structures; this can be seen in the liver activity in the non-attenuation-corrected image. The attenuation-corrected image in Figure 16-1b more accurately reflects the distribution of the positron-emitting radionuclide in the body. However, attenuation correction can produce artifacts, so many nuclear medicine laboratories generate images both with and without attenuation correction. An area that has increased counts on the non-attenuation-corrected images is truly an area of increased activity in the patient. Images courtesy of Puget Sound Cancer Center.

(a) Non-attenuation corrected coronal slice

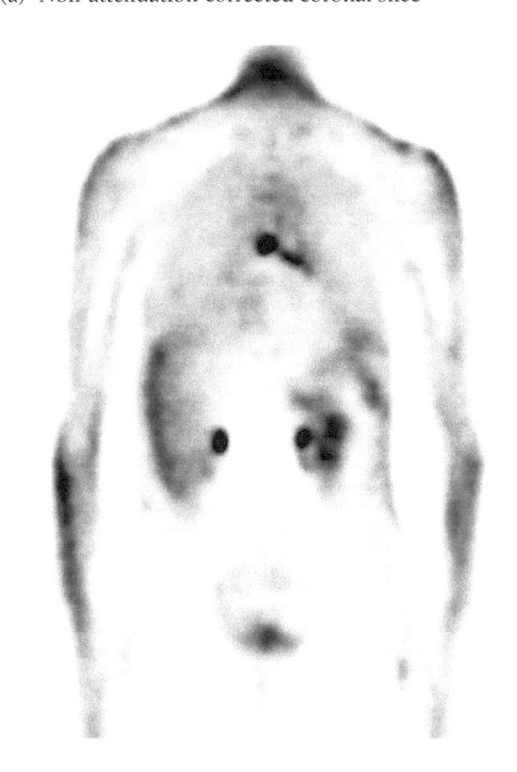

(b) The same slice as in Fig. 16-1a, but with attenuation correction

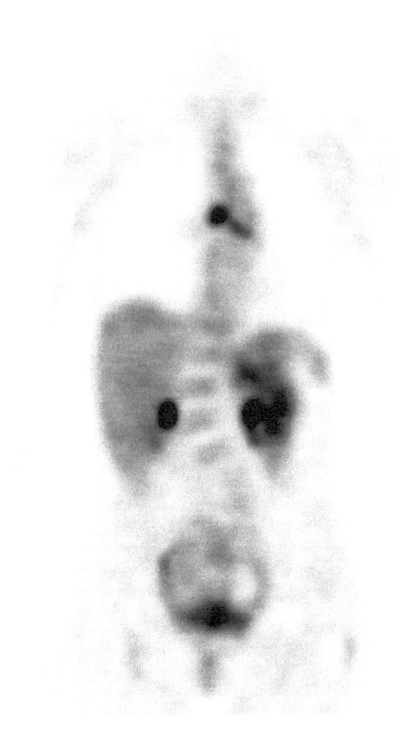

smaller than the corrections for scatter and attenuation. But if accurate quantitation is to be performed, a factor accounting for dead time losses must be included along with other corrections applied to the acquisition data (see Eq. 15-4). The second consequence of dead time is the mispositioning of events as a result of pulse pileup, the likelihood of which increases linearly with activity (7). Mispositioning degrades spatial resolution, thus impacting both image quality and quantitation (5), and complicates the identification of regions of interest. It can be significant even if the global dead time correction factor is small.

Attenuation

Coincidence imaging is affected to a much greater extent by attenuation compared to single-photon imaging, simply because of the requirement that both annihilation photons must escape the object in order to be counted. Attenuation correction factors can vary from 3 to 6 in the head and can be as high as 100 in the torso of a large patient (8). **Figure 16-1** shows PET images without and with attenuation correction. Note the significant difference in appearance between the two, particularly the outline of the body in the non-attenuation-corrected images. This is due to the fact that annihilation photons arising from the surface of the body are much less likely to be attenuated than those originating at any depth. The non-attenuation-corrected images are sometimes called "India ink" images, because they look as if ink was allowed to bleed around the edges of the body. Attenuation can be corrected accurately in PET, and all PET tomographs incorporate attenuation correction (although non-attenuation-corrected images are also often created and used in image interpretation).

When a rod source is used for attenuation correction, the resulting attenuation map may be very noisy, and this contributes significantly to the noise in the attenuation-corrected emission images. The operator needs to be aware of the noise level in the attenuation map; it may need to be smoothed before application to the emission data set (9). As the source activity decreases, the noise level in the attenuation map increases, and at some point the rod source must be replaced. The use of a CT-generated attenuation map removes this source of noise.

The most common solution to the high noise level in radionuclide-generated attenuation maps is to *segment* the data into a few tissue types and to assign either a predefined or a patient-determined attenuation coefficient to each type. The emission image is then corrected based on these assigned attenuation coefficients rather than the measured attenuation values in each voxel. Segmentation is generally a successful approach, although patient-to-patient variability in terms of attenuation coefficients has been noted (10).

Scatter

Scatter and attenuation are two parts of the same phenomenon. A scatter interaction by an annihilation photon removes a potential true event from one LOR and adds an event in an incorrect LOR. Thus, both attenuation and scatter can occur simultaneously.

Scatter is a major degrading factor in PET imaging. When 511-keV photons undergo Compton scattering interactions, they generally scatter at shallow angles of 30° or less, with small energy loss (5). Further, many annihilation photons not scattered in the object deposit energy in more than one crystal, thus appearing to be scattered photons even though they aren't. The relatively poor energy resolution of the scintillators used in PET makes it impossible to eliminate most scatter events based on the loss of energy that accompanies a Compton interaction. But the result of including scatter coincidences is mispositioning of annihilation events, which degrades spatial resolution and contrast and, therefore, image quality. Scatter correction must be applied before attenuation correction if the PET image is to represent the radiopharmaceutical distribution accurately (5). The techniques used for scatter correction vary depending on the situation, but it is absolutely necessary that scatter be subtracted.

Patient Motion

As with all types of nuclear medicine imaging, the blurring effect of patient motion can significantly degrade PET image quality. But attenuation correction adds an additional concern, because the transmission and emission data sets are often acquired sequentially and may not be properly coregistered if the patient has moved between them. Motion may thus result in undercorrection for attenuation in some areas and overcorrection in other areas. An area that is undercorrected for attenuation will be artifactually photopenic, while an area that is overcorrected will appear as a hot spot. One reason to generate and view non-attenuation-corrected images is to identify these artifacts. An area that has increased counts on non-attenuation-corrected images is a real hot spot. And of course, the quantitative accuracy of the PET data is certainly compromised by patient motion.

Partial Volume Effect

The partial volume effect is a function of the voxel size in a reconstructed 3D image matrix. Voxel size in PET is based on pixel size in a transaxial slice, which in turn depends on the system's FOV and the image matrix used for reconstruction. A 50-cm FOV with a 128 × 128 matrix produces a pixel size of 4 mm and a 256 × 256 matrix a 2-mm pixel size; other matrix sizes have also been used. As in SPECT, we would want the pixel size to be less than one-half of the system full width at half-maximum (FWHM), but making the pixels smaller than one-third of the FWHM does not gain any additional resolution. The slice thickness is approximately one-half of the thickness of an individual scintillation crystal.

The partial volume effect (PVE) in PET results both from the spillover of counts into neighboring voxels due to the finite resolution of the PET tomograph and from the within-voxel averaging that occurs in all forms of 3D imaging (11). The result of the PVE is that counts from a small volume are spread out over a larger volume (i.e., throughout several voxels) in the reconstructed image, such that the measured activity concentration is decreased relative to its actual value. These effects have significant consequences because of the quantitative aims of PET. In tumor imaging, for example, a tumor that has decreased in size between two PET scans will appear to have decreased activity concentration, just due to PVE. When PET is used to quantify biologic functions using tracer kinetic modeling, PVE can produce errors as great as 50% (12). So it is worth the effort to explicitly account for PVE.

As with SPECT, we have three choices for trying to correct PVE: resolution recovery filters (for use with filtered backprojection (FBP)), modeling of the physics of resolution loss (for use with iterative reconstruction), and application of empirically determined correction factors after reconstruction. The *recovery coefficient* is an example of the third option:

$$\text{Recovery coefficient} = \frac{\text{observed activity concentration}}{\text{true activity concentration}}$$

(16-1)

where both the observed activity concentration and recovery coefficient depend on the size of the object in question. Recovery coefficients are generated from phantom studies of known activity concentration and size (**Figure 16-2**) and are then applied to clinical studies as correction factors. For a cylindrical object, the recovery coefficient does not approach 1 (i.e., observed cps = actual cps) until the cylinder diameter is at least twice that of the system FWHM (12).

The accuracy of corrections made with the recovery coefficient depends on the object's shape, its orientation relative to the transverse plane of the tomograph, its location within the gantry bore, the degree of heterogeneity within the object, and the relative difference in activity concentration between the object and its surrounding tissue. The ability to reliably quantify the activity concentration in a complex, highly irregular organ such as the brain is compromised by these aspects of the PVE. Partial volume correction is dealt with in a less rigorous fashion in clinical imaging, in that the interpreting physician may provide the computer-determined quantity and state that the true value is probably larger because of the PVE.

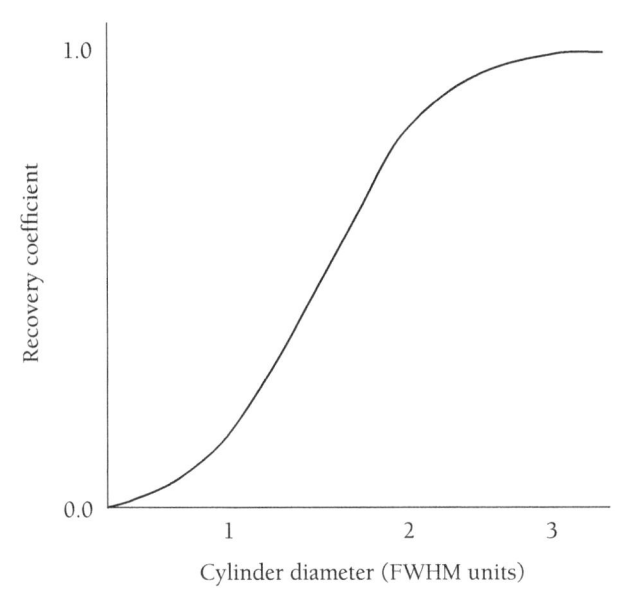

Figure 16-2 Recovery coefficient vs object size. The graph illustrates the partial volume effect. Although the recovery coefficient is commonly used to correct the activity concentration, which is clearly most important in PET, PVE also affects the object volume, such that small objects appear larger than they really are. Application of a recovery coefficient correction depends on the system resolution and lesion size, and it should be used cautiously with lesions less than the system FWHM. Modified from: Rousset OG, Ma Y, Evans AC. Correction for partial volume effects in PET: principle and validation. *J Nucl Med*. 1998;39:908, Fig. 3C. Used with permission from the Society of Nuclear Medicine.

Sample Calculation 16-1 Application of Recovery Coefficients

A brain lesion of 7.5 mm in diameter (as determined by MRI) is imaged with a PET tomograph with an FWHM of 6.0 mm. Its activity concentration is measured at 2,500 kBq/ml. Use Figure 16-2 to estimate the recovery coefficient, and apply it to obtain the corrected activity concentration.

The lesion is approximately 1.25 times the FWHM, corresponding to a recovery coefficient of about 0.3. The corrected activity concentration is then

$$\text{Corrected activity concentration} = \frac{2,500 \text{ kBq/ml}}{0.3}$$
$$= 8,333 \text{ kBq/ml}.$$

The actual counts are more than three times the measured counts, due to the lesion's small size and the significance of the partial volume effect.

Contrast

The end result of all the above factors is the contrast of the resulting images. Decreased dead time losses and improved signal-to-noise ratio (SNR) improve contrast, as do appropriate corrections for random coincidences, attenuation, and scatter events. Any statistical or systematic error in the determination of these corrections will in turn affect the quantitative information (counts per second [cps] per voxel). Patient motion and elevated background decrease contrast. And as discussed below, TOF-PET increases contrast to a significant degree.

Performance Measures in PET

The characteristics that affect image quality determine the measures used to evaluate the performance of PET tomographs. Two of the performance measures for planar and SPECT systems, namely, spatial resolution and sensitivity, are used also in PET, and once again there is a trade-off between them. But two other performance measures are new to us. The scatter fraction and noise-equivalent count rate (NECR) are very important to evaluation of image quality in PET. Uniformity, on the other hand, is a much less critical issue in PET, primarily because the inherent differences in efficiency between detectors are corrected by the normalization factors. **Table 16-1** gives some typical values for resolution, sensitivity, NECR, scatter fraction, and energy resolution for commercial tomographs. (While the references cited for this table are dated, the values for the various performance measures have not changed a great deal, according to company estimates and industry tabulations.)

Spatial Resolution

Spatial resolution is dependent on several factors, one of which is detector size. Given that the LOR volume is defined by the size of the detectors, employing smaller detectors should lead to improved resolution, at least up to the point of decreased efficiency for interaction with annihilation photons. Much effort in recent years has gone toward improving spatial resolution, in part to facilitate the use of PET with small animals in research and drug development applications. Small-animal PET tomographs have reached a spatial resolution of about 1 mm FWHM (13).

The components of spatial resolution in PET are the same as those in SPECT (see Fig. 13-7). Spatial resolution in the transaxial plane (radial and tangential values) is generally the same in 2D and 3D, but is somewhat degraded in the axial direction for 3D compared to 2D imaging (13). Resolution also degrades somewhat as the object moves from the center to the periphery of the FOV; the reasons for this are discussed below. Note that this characteristic of PET is quite different from gamma camera imaging, where the collimator–patient distance is a key determinant of resolution.

Sensitivity

Sensitivity (counts per sec per µCi or kBq) is of primary importance in PET, both from the standpoint of the tomograph's ability to accumulate true coincidences in the presence of singles, randoms, and scatters and from the standpoint of making quantitative measurements. Sensitivity is dependent on the choice of scintillation material, detector geometry, quality of applied corrections, and

Table 16-1
Typical Values for Performance Measures in Modern PET Tomographs

Performance Measure	Direction and Location	Range of Values
Resolution (FWHM)	Transaxial—1 cm from center	4.6–6.2 mm (2D)
		4.5–6.3 mm (3D)
	Transaxial—10 cm from center	5.4–7.0 mm (2D)
		5.4–7.4 mm (3D)
	Axial—0 cm from center	4.2–5.0 mm (2D)
		3.5–6.2 mm (3D)
	Axial—10 cm from center	5.0–6.5 mm (2D)
		5.3–7.1 mm (3D)
Sensitivity (cps net trues/(Bq/ml))		4.9–5.4 (2D)
		21.1–31.0 (3D)
Peak noise-equivalent count rate		25–60 kcps (3D)
Scatter fraction		10–17% (2D)
		25–36% (3D)
Energy resolution at 511 keV		10–25%

Tarantola G, Zito F, Gerundini P. PET instrumentation and reconstruction algorithms in whole-body applications. *J Nucl Med.* 2003;44:756–769. Zanzonico P. Positron-emission tomography: a review of basic principles, scanner design and performance, and current systems. *Semin Nucl Med.* 2004;34:87–111.

choice of acquisition mode. A 3D mode acquisition allows detection of up to 10 times the true event rate as 2D mode, but the concomitant increases in random and scatter events result in an effective increase of about 5 times (14). The system must have detector and electronics performance to match the increased prompt event rate in 3D imaging.

The efficiency of the scintillation material for 511-keV photons is especially crucial because of the requirement that both annihilation photons be detected: if a single scintillation crystal has a 75% probability of interacting with an annihilation photon, then the likelihood of two scintillation crystals interacting with two annihilation photons is only 56%. The size of the detectors is also a factor, because a larger detector (in any dimension) will be more efficient at stopping annihilation photons. The goal is to have small but highly efficient detectors.

Scatter Fraction

This performance measure indicates a tomograph's sensitivity to scatter coincidences. It is defined as the ratio of scatter coincidences to total counts:

$$\text{Scatter fraction} = \frac{N_{\text{scatter}}}{N_{\text{total}}} \quad (16\text{-}2)$$

in which N_{total} is the total number of coincidences (trues plus scatters, after correction for randoms), measured in a situation of low random coincidence rate and low dead time, and N_{scatter} is the estimated or calculated number of scatter events. A cold-sphere phantom allows estimation of the scatter fraction as the ratio of cps in a voxel in the center of the cold sphere to the average cps/voxel in the phantom around the sphere. A low scatter fraction is always desirable, because less scatter subtraction means less noise in the final emission image.

Sample Calculation 16-2 Scatter Fraction

A PET scan of a phantom with cold spheres yields the following (randoms-subtracted) results:

- Phantom count rate = 40,000 cps/voxel
- Center of cold sphere = 7,500 cps/voxel

What is the scatter fraction?

We assume that all of the counts in the cold sphere are scatter events:

$$\frac{N_{\text{scatter}}}{N_{\text{total}}} \times 100\% = \frac{7{,}500 \text{ cps}}{40{,}000 \text{ cps}} \times 100\% = 19\%.$$

The size of the cold sphere used for this calculation should be at least three times the tomograph's FWHM, to avoid PVE.

The scatter fraction depends not only on the radionuclide distribution but also on the tomograph design, the presence or absence of septa, and the lower-level discriminator setting of the pulse height analyzer (PHA) window. The latter parameter significantly affects the scatter fraction; in one simulation, the scatter fraction was shown to increase from 45 to 60% as the energy threshold was decreased from 450 to 380 keV (15). Further, not only the magnitude but also the spatial distribution of scatter events changes as the energy threshold is changed. Narrowing the energy window in order to decrease acceptance of scattered photons decreases the certainty with which the scatter fraction can be estimated, based on statistical considerations. The scatter fraction increases by a factor of 2 to 5 when one moves from 2D to 3D imaging.

Count Rate

With its complications of singles, randoms, and scatters, the evaluation of count rate in PET is considerably more complex than in single-photon imaging. But in the absence of collimators, the count rate is a crucial determinant of system performance. The PET community has settled on the *noise-equivalent count rate* as the most appropriate quantitative expression of this performance measure:

$$\text{NECR} = \frac{N_{\text{true}}^2}{N_{\text{true}} + N_{\text{scaatter}} + kN_{\text{random}}} \quad (16\text{-}3)$$

where N_{true}, N_{scatter}, and N_{random} are the true, scatter, and random count rates, respectively, and k is a constant that has a value of 2 if the tomograph does online randoms correction or 1 if randoms are estimated from single-event rates and therefore are noise-free (16).

The derivation of the NECR formula starts with the assumption that the count rates for true, random, and scatter events obey the Poisson statistical model (17), and that each is high enough to be described by a Gaussian curve. The overall noise level in a PET acquisition is taken to be the square root of the sum of the three components: $\sqrt{N_{\text{true}} + N_{\text{scatter}} + N_{\text{random}}}$. The denominator in Equation 16-3 also includes the modifying factor to account for the differing noise levels in the two methods of randoms determination. The SNR is then the true coincidence count rate (the "signal") divided by the noise. The NECR is the square of the SNR (18). Thus we minimize the effect of noise by operating at the maximal attainable value of the NECR.

Figure 16-3 shows a representative graph of NECR vs activity concentration for a 3D system, along with the individual components contributing to it. The "ideal trues" line is extrapolated from the straight-line portion of the "measured trues" curve. As with all paralyzable radiation detectors, the measured trues rate reaches a maximum and declines at higher activity concentrations. But the added factors in the NECR cause its maximum to be reached at a lower activity concentration than that of the measured true coincidence rate, particularly due to the geometric increase of randoms with increasing activity concentration. The maximum of the NECR curve represents the best performance of the tomograph with the least amount of image noise, so the goal is to operate at or below the corresponding activity concentration (13, 19).

The NECR allows us to compare count rates from system to system and from situation to situation, taking

Sample Calculation 16-3   Noise-Equivalent Count Rate

The following data are obtained from an F-18-containing cylindrical phantom at two different activity concentrations:

Activity concentration:	25 kBq/ml	10 kBq/ml
Trues:	220 kcps/voxel	103 kcps/voxel
Randoms:	328 kcps/voxel	46 kcps/voxel
Scatters:	121 kcps/voxel	50 kcps/voxel

Calculate the NECR, using both k values of 1 and 2, for each activity concentration.

At 25 kBq/ml and using $k = 1$, the NECR is

$$\text{NECR} = \frac{N_{\text{trues}}^2}{N_{\text{trues}} + N_{\text{scatters}} + N_{\text{randoms}}}$$

$$= \frac{220^2}{220 + 121 + 328} = \frac{72.3 \text{ kcps}}{\text{voxel}}.$$

If $k = 2$, we get

$$\text{NECR} = \frac{N_{\text{trues}}^2}{N_{\text{trues}} + N_{\text{scatters}} + 2N_{\text{randoms}}}$$

$$= \frac{220^2}{220 + 121 + (2)(328)} = \frac{48.5 \text{ kcps}}{\text{voxel}}.$$

At 10 kBq/ml, the $k = 1$ calculation yields

$$\text{NECR} = \frac{103^2}{103 + 50 + 46} = \frac{53.3 \text{ kcps}}{\text{voxel}}$$

and the $k = 2$ calculation gives

$$\text{NECR} = \frac{103^2}{103 + 50 + (2)(46)} = \frac{41.9 \text{ kcps}}{\text{voxel}}.$$

The $k = 1$ value assumes that the method of estimation from singles includes less statistical variation, so that the signal-to-noise ratio is higher. Even though the activity concentration varies by 250%, the NECR varies only 36% ($k = 1$) or 16% ($k = 2$). The tomograph is unable to effectively use most of the extra counts of the higher activity concentration.

the combined effects of random coincidences and scatter events into account (**Figure 16-4**). Figure 16-4a compares 2D and 3D NECRs. The septa reduce the contributions of random and scatter coincidences to such an extent that the 2D NECR is close to the true coincidence rate and does not reach a maximum value at clinical imaging dosages (13). At low activity concentration, the 3D NECR

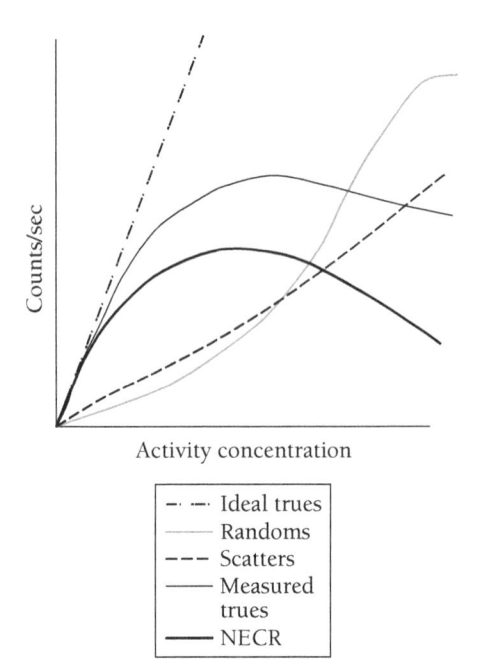

Figure 16-3 Components of the NECR. The NECR expresses the count rate in a PET acquisition in a way that takes into account the random and scatter event rates. It is recommended that the tomograph be operated at or below the activity concentration corresponding to the peak NECR.

curve is above the 2D NECR curve, because the random coincidence rate is not so high as to affect the SNR. But the 2D NECR reaches a higher peak NECR value, because its true coincidences are "purer" than the scatter- and random-contaminated 3D trues. The NECR in a 3D imaging situation can be significantly improved by shifting from a noisy ($k = 2$) to a noiseless ($k = 1$) randoms subtraction method (18).

Table 16-2 further illustrates the difference between 2D and 3D imaging as well as the value of the NECR as a performance measure. A direct-plane-only 2D-mode acquisition of a radioactive phantom was immediately followed by a strict 3D-mode acquisition. With septa in place, 79% of counts are true coincidences, whereas with septa retracted, only 24% are trues. The number of scatters is higher by a factor of almost 14, and the number of randoms by a factor of 67, in the 3D acquisition. But the two acquisitions have nearly identical NECR values, and thus similar SNRs, a fact that is not at all obvious from looking at the raw data.

The NECR graphs also demonstrate the advantage of switching to one of the newer scintillation materials (Fig. 16-4b). The use of LSO as the scintillator significantly increases

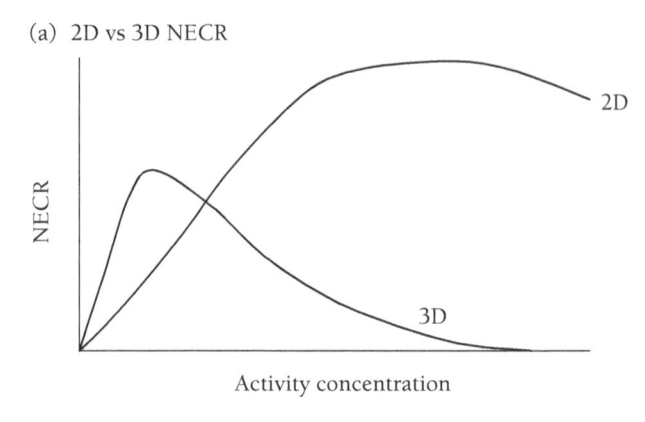

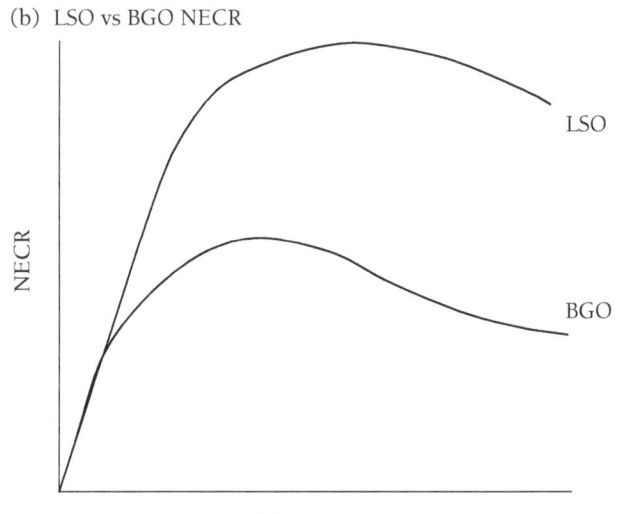

Figure 16-4 NECR vs activity concentration—two comparisons. Figure 16-4a shows NECR curves for 2D and 3D acquisitions. The NECR is initially higher for the 3D situation, but its peak is reached at a lower activity concentration and is a lower value than the peak 2D NECR. The 2D NECR rises only slowly, and its peak is generally not reached at clinically relevant activity concentrations. Figure 16-4b illustrates the benefits of the more recently developed scintillation material, LSO, compared to BGO. The timing characteristics of the type of scintillation crystal used have a significant effect on the NECR. Adapted from: Moses W. PET data acquisition and processing. *Basic Science of Nuclear Medicine* [CD-ROM]. Reston, VA: Society of Nuclear Medicine; 2001. Tarantola G, Zito F, Gerundini P. PET instrumentation and reconstruction algorithms in whole-body applications. *J Nucl Med.* 2003;44:756–769. With permission from the Society of Nuclear Medicine.

the activity concentration, producing the maximum NECR, as well as the value of the NECR itself. These improvements allow for shorter imaging times and/or better image quality. The NECR measurement is sensitive

Table 16-2

Sample Count Rates in Strict 2D and Complete 3D Modes

Mode	Trues	Randoms	Scatters	NECR	Trues % of Total
2D	39 kcps	4.7 kcps	6.0 kcps	30.9 kcps	79
3D	126 kcps	314 kcps	83 kcps	30.4 kcps	24

Data from: Phil Vernon, personal communication, 2004.

to a number of factors, including not only the tomograph and acquisition mode, but also the size and characteristics of the phantom used. It should be considered a global measure of the true counts available, not sensitive to regional variations.

Operator-Determined Parameters in PET

Nuclear medicine technologists will notice that a major difference between PET and single-photon imaging is that PET requires much less operator interaction. In single-photon imaging, the actions of the technologist have a significant impact on image quality. Choices such as collimator, matrix size, acquisition time/counts, and patient–collimator distance are all ultimately under the control of the technologist. In PET, by contrast, most of the choices are simply part of the acquisition protocol. The coincidence timing window and energy window are dependent on the choice of scintillation crystal. The method for determination of the randoms fraction is also fixed in most systems, and all corrections are automatically applied. Even the choice between 2D and 3D acquisition modes is either not available (in many newer tomographs) or programmed into the acquisition protocol. If the latter, all of the subchoices, such as the span or ring difference or the scatter estimation method, are also included in the preset protocol. Thus there is no table in this chapter to describe how to improve image quality.

This is not to say that the technologist's role is less important in PET than in SPECT. In fact, the technologist must be considerably more attentive in PET, particularly to details of patient preparation and data entry for quantitative results. The issue of patient preparation is beyond the scope of this text; suffice it to say that for some radiopharmaceuticals, the quality of the study is primarily dependent on the patient's compliance with the preparation instructions. Patient history may also be crucially important for the proper interpretation of PET studies, requiring an in-depth patient interview and/or review of records. The issue of quantitative results is addressed at the end of this chapter, but consider just one example of the importance of attention to detail in PET: Calculation of the SUV (see Eq. 16-4) requires an exact measurement of the dosage administered. The technologist must measure the syringe in the dose calibrator both before and after injection, and she or he must note the time of each measurement, in order to supply this crucial piece of information.

Technologist interaction in the imaging process is also crucial after the study is acquired. The emission and transmission data sets are acquired not simultaneously, but rather sequentially. If the patient moves such that the two do not match exactly, artifacts could result when the attenuation map is applied to the emission data set. The technologist may need to make the call that an unacceptable amount of movement has occurred, and to correct the situation by reacquiring both emission and transmission scans at that bed position. So while PET requires the careful attention of the technologist, it does so in ways that are somewhat different than what is required for single-photon imaging.

Factors Affecting Performance Measures

Many of the factors that affect PET performance measures are due to the design of the PET tomograph itself. Some are inherent to PET, others to the choice of multidetector ring geometry, and still others to the choice of acquisition mode or reconstruction methods. The following discussion tries to make clear which is which. In addition, design choices made by different manufacturers may make some of these factors more or less important in a particular tomograph. The discussion here is general and may not apply to all systems.

Inherent Limits on Resolution

The basis of PET is the imaging of annihilation photons that result from a positron-electron annihilation reaction. There are, within that sequence of events, two uncertainties that put lower limits on the attainable spatial resolution: positron range and noncolinearity of the annihilation photons. For commonly used PET radionuclides, the average positron range varies significantly (0.6 mm for F-18 vs 5.9 mm for Rb-82), such that resolution varies with the choice of radionuclide (Reference 13 has a nice illustration). The possibility that the two annihilation photons are not exactly 180° opposed adds uncertainty to the location of the annihilation event. This degrades resolution depending on the diameter of the detector ring, ranging from 0.9 mm for a 40-cm diameter ring to 1.8 mm for a 90-mm diameter ring (4). Both positron range and noncolinearity can be incorporated into the physics model used in iterative reconstruction (5).

Ring Geometry

The design decision to utilize many small detectors in a ring arrangement has several significant consequences (**Figure 16-5**). Figure 16-5a shows a single ring of 24 detectors and all the possible LORs. Note that the density of the LORs is greater in the middle of the ring compared to the perimeter. Where there are more LORs, we get better information about the location of the radiopharmaceutical and therefore better spatial resolution. Note also the periodicity of the LORs, with increased LOR densities in concentric circles. Spatial resolution therefore also varies to a small amount over the same concentric circles. Similarly, there are fewer LORs at the front and back rings of the tomograph, compared to the center, so axial spatial resolution varies depending on axial location.

Based on this analysis, it can be seen that as the detectors get smaller, and more LORs can be drawn, the resolution improves. The same conclusion is reached simply by recognizing that in most PET systems, the localization is only to the individual detector, not to an exact location within the detector, as in single-photon imaging. Decreases in detector size have driven much of the improvement in spatial resolution, from 17 mm in 1975 to about 4 mm

(a) Spatial distribution of LORs

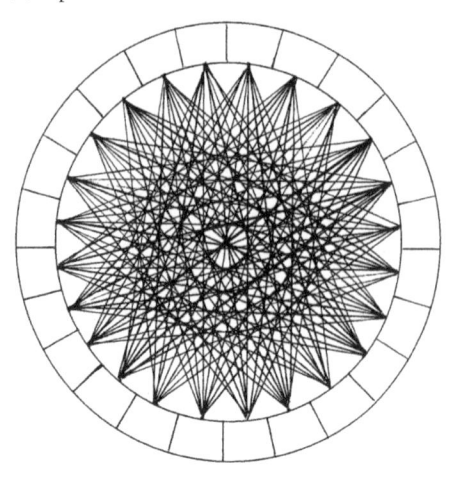

(b) Arc correction

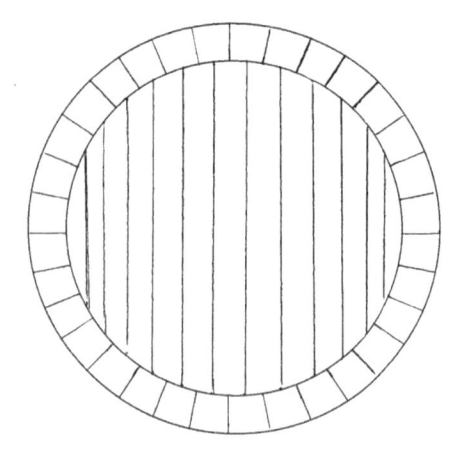

Figure 16-5 Issues of ring geometry. The choice of ring geometry brings several geometric factors into play. Figure 16-5a shows a single-ring system with 24 detectors; note how the LOR density varies within the patient port. Some areas have many LORs, while others have fewer, and the LOR density decreases drastically near the periphery of the ring. Using smaller detectors decreases this geometric effect.
Figure 16-5b illustrates that parallel LORs are not evenly spaced. As we move toward the periphery, they are closer together. This irregularity is accounted for in the reconstruction process.

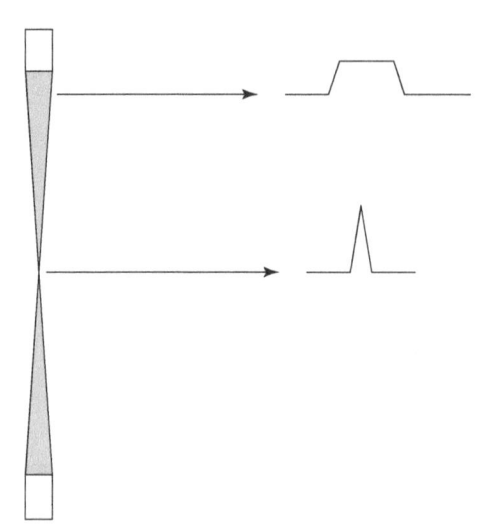

Figure 16-6 Geometric response functions. The shaded areas on the left show the locations in space of events that will interact with a single pair of detectors. At the center, the two detectors will detect only annihilation photons originating from the narrowest point, producing a triangular shape for the point-spread function, as shown on the right. Near the periphery, on the other hand, a much wider area of annihilation interactions produces coincidences detectable by these detectors. The point-spread function therefore becomes more trapezoidal near the ring periphery, implying a degradation of spatial resolution.

today. But as the detector size decreases, the detector's ability to stop annihilation photons also decreases, such that the trade-off between sensitivity and resolution must be considered. Current PET tomographs use crystals that are 4 to 6.5 mm square (the surface facing the gantry bore) by 20 to 30 mm long, giving extra length in the radial dimension for stopping the annihilation photons.

Another factor relating to the ring geometry is the *arc correction*. Figure 16-5b shows a set of parallel LORs. Near the edge of the gantry bore, the lines get closer together, an effect that is more significant for systems with larger bores. Arc correction occurs either in the reconstruction process or in the rebinning of the data prior to reconstruction.

The location of the annihilation interaction within the transaxial plane also affects the spatial resolution, irrespective of detector size. Consider the geometry of coincidence detection between a pair of detectors (**Figure 16-6**).

At the center point, only a small volume of the object produces annihilation photons that are detected by these two detectors, so the (idealized) point-spread function (PSF) at this location is triangular. If annihilation photons are being generated near the periphery of the ring, the PSF has a trapezoidal shape, indicating that the location of the annihilation reaction is known with less certainty.

A further loss of spatial resolution occurs when the source is located near the periphery and the line of coincidence does not intersect the face of the detector at a 90° angle (**Figure 16-7**). If an annihilation photon intersects the long, narrow detector at an oblique angle, there is some likelihood that it will pass through that detector and deposit its energy in the neighboring detector. In the reconstruction, however, such an event will be assigned to the detector where the energy is deposited, not in the detector the photon went through first. This cross-talk effect, called *parallax* or the *depth of interaction effect*, produces a skewed point-spread function. Again, the implication is that resolution is worse at the edge of the ring than at the center.

One way to deal with parallax is to determine the depth of the annihilation photon's interaction in the scintillation crystal. The two LORs shown in Figure 16-7a would both be assigned to the same pair of crystals in a standard PET tomograph. But in the LOR on the right, the two coincident photons interact deep in the two crystals, whereas the two coincident photons in the left LOR interact near the surfaces of the crystals. If we could detect this difference, we would be able to assign the LOR on the right to the neighboring set of crystals, through which the annihilation photons first passed. This can be accomplished by incorporating two scintillation materials (e.g., LSO and GSO)

(a) Coincidence detection in tangential direction

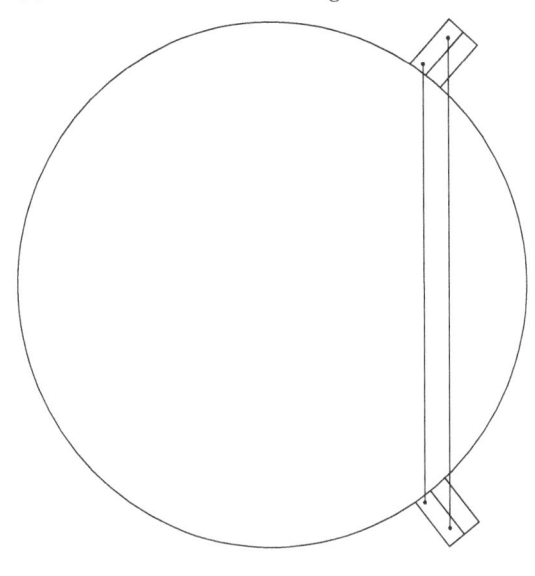

(b) Point-spread function in tangential direction

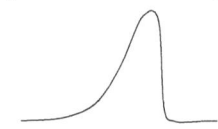

Figure 16-7 Parallax or depth of interaction effect. Annihilation photons are difficult to stop, and PET detectors are constructed to be most efficient at this task when the photon enters the detector at a 90° angle. When an annihilation photon does not enter the detector at an angle close to 90°, it may cross through the first detector it hits and deposit its energy in the neighboring detector (Fig. 16-7a). This leads to a skewed point-spread function (Fig. 16-7b). The end result is the same as in Figures 16-5a and 16-6: a degradation of spatial resolution near the periphery of the ring.

instead of one in each detector, an arrangement called a *phoswich*. The two scintillators must have different decay times, so that the location of an annihilation photon interaction can be identified based on the decay time of the scintillation light it produces. This has been shown to reduce the resolution loss from parallax error by a factor of two (13).

Thus, from multiple geometric arguments, resolution will degrade as a point source moves from the center to the edge of the ring. This is contrary to the situation in single-photon imaging, in which resolution is best at the collimator face and degrades as the source is moved away. The degradation in PET is in the range of 0.5 to 1 mm in the transaxial plane, according to published data (13).

The choice of a ring design also has a significant effect on sensitivity. Given a point source of radioactivity, the isotropic sphere of equal radiation intensity at a diameter of 80 cm (a common detector ring diameter) has an area of 20,000 cm^2. An 80-cm-diameter cylinder of height 15 cm (i.e., the circumferential area of the detector ring) has an area of 3,769 cm^2. Thus, less than 20% of the annihilation photons emitted from a point source have any possibility of intersecting with a detector. With the further requirement that both annihilation photons be detected, and the fact that detector efficiency for annihilation photon absorption is not 100%, PET systems register 0.2 to 0.5% of possible annihilations in 2D mode and 2 to 10% in 3D (13). Note that this is still 10- to 100-fold greater than gamma camera sensitivity.

The limitations of ring geometry result in two important consequences. First, the manufacturer's quoted resolution at the center of the tomograph is a best-case scenario, and some degradation should be expected in other parts of the gantry volume. Second, if resolution is critical for a particular organ, it should ideally be positioned as close to the center of the gantry bore as possible. The operator should also be aware that sensitivity drops off toward the gantry front and back (Fig. 15-11), and this should be taken into account when considering patient position.

Interplay among Administered Activity, Dead Time, and Noise-Equivalent Count Rate

The multiplicity of events in PET (trues, randoms, scatters, singles) leads to some confusion when discussing counting rates and activities. As the activity concentration in the FOV increases, the number of events (of all types) also increases (trues and scatters in an approximately linear fashion, while randoms and singles increase exponentially). But not all of these additional events provide useful information, and some of the new events are not registered due to dead time. So administered activity, the NECR, and the dead time are all interrelated.

The dead time in PET is primarily related to the singles rate, because each detected gamma ray incurs a pulse integration time. Because singles are distributed across the tomograph, a global correction factor is often applied. It makes sense that there should be some amount of local variation that corresponds to the distribution of the radiopharmaceutical, but not all systems correct dead time on an LOR-by-LOR basis. It is very clear, however, that dead time corrections need to be determined separately for 2D and 3D modes, and for emission vs transmission vs blank scans (when radionuclide sources are used for attenuation correction). When positron-emitting transmission sources are used, separate corrections must be available for preinjection vs postinjection transmission imaging. As discussed above, dead time causes both count loss and image degradation. Dead time count losses are "generally minimal" in clinical studies (13), but can reach as high as a factor of four (that is, 75% count loss due to dead time as calculated using Equation 17-3) (4).

Random and scatter coincidences cause image degradation and must be subtracted from the total number of prompt coincidences to produce a meaningful image. The subtraction has the effect of decreasing the SNR. The number of random and scatter events varies significantly depending on the tomograph design and the choice of 2D or 3D mode. As shown above, the NECR provides a way to compare the SNR in different situations. In 3D mode, the maximum NECR represents the optimum counting rate for a particular tomograph (20) and is thus an important consideration for determination of radiopharmaceutical dosage.

In 2D mode, the maximum NECR is not reached until clinically acceptable dosages have been exceeded, so the NECR is usually not a factor in deciding on an appropriate dosage.

2D vs 3D Acquisition

Clearly, the choice of septa vs no septa has a large impact on all performance characteristics. With septa in place, the scatter fraction and randoms are greatly reduced, the dead time is low, the NECR shows a slow increase with activity concentration, and spatial resolution is improved, especially in the axial direction. With septa removed, we must be concerned about the increased count rate, dead time, and scatter fraction, and with the variation in both sensitivity and spatial resolution in the axial direction. Studies acquired in 3D mode also take longer to process (by as much as a factor of 10 given the same computing power [13]) and require significantly different reconstruction methods.

But if we use the septa, we lose part of the advantage of PET, namely, the increased sensitivity achieved with electronic (as opposed to absorptive) collimation. Sensitivity is increased approximately five times in 3D PET vs 2D PET (11, 17). To take full advantage of the 3D mode, the new, faster scintillators are preferred (20). As computing power increases and reconstruction algorithms are refined, it appears that 3D PET is the wave of the future.

The bottom-line question is: Does 3D PET produce noticeably improved images compared to 2D? A recent article attempted to answer this question (21). Using a torso phantom, the study showed that for the equivalent of a 12-mCi (444-MBq) dose (a common clinical dosage), the 3D acquisition gives equal or better lesion detection compared to 2D. But 2D with a higher dosage (20-mCi [740-MBq] clinical equivalent) resulted in better lesion detectability than the 3D acquisition using 12 mCi. The maximum dosage for 3D imaging is determined by the maximum NECR, whereas in 2D the NECR doesn't reach a maximum in the clinical dosage range, allowing the physician to determine the dosage based on other factors, such as image quality.

Time-of-Flight Acquisition

Tomographs that utilize TOF techniques gain additional clarity by limiting the location of the annihilation to a small section of the LOR. Let us examine this a little more closely. According to Equation 14-1, the location of the annihilation relative to the middle of the LOR (Δx) is determined by the difference in arrival times of the two photons (Δt). The uncertainty in the location of the annihilation depends on the uncertainty in the determination of Δt. The accuracy of the localization in TOF-PET therefore depends on the precision with which the timing difference can be measured. Finer timing resolution more precisely identifies the location of the annihilation along the LOR. If the difference in photon arrival times can be measured to within 0.6 nsec, then the annihilation can be localized to a 9-cm portion of the LOR. A timing resolution capability of 0.1 nsec would limit the position uncertainty to about 1.5 cm (5). Timing resolution of 0.015 nsec would allow each event to be placed in a specific voxel, completely eliminating the need for reconstruction (14). But even imperfect localization can be helpful, as the smaller range of origin of the annihilation photons can be incorporated into either FBP or iterative reconstruction.

The chief benefit of TOF-PET is an improvement in the SNR in the reconstructed 3D image matrix. The reduction in noise is estimated to be roughly a factor of 2 to 10, using timing resolutions that are either currently available or within the reach of modern electronics (2). Moreover, improvement in the SNR increases as the object size increases. This means that contrast improves as the size of the object (i.e., the girth of the patient) increases, a result that has been demonstrated in both phantoms and patients (2). This would be extremely helpful in today's climate of increasing body weight.

Sample Calculation 16-4   Time-of-Flight PET

In a system with timing uncertainty of 0.4 nsec, two coincident photons are registered 1.2 nsec apart. Approximately how far from the middle of the tomograph did the annihilation occur?

According to Equation 14-1, the distance between the annihilation event and the center of the tomograph is equal to the difference between the two photons' detection times, multiplied by the speed of light and divided by 2:

$$\Delta x = \frac{\Delta t \times c}{2}$$

$$\Delta x = \frac{(1.2 \times 10^{-9} \text{ sec})(3 \times 10^{10} \text{ cm/sec})}{2}$$

$$\Delta x = 18 \text{ cm}$$

Thus the annihilation occured 18 cm from the center of the LOR. The uncertainty in this measurement is:

$$\Delta x = \frac{(0.4 \times 10^{-9} \text{ sec})(3 \times 10^{10} \text{ cm/sec})}{2} = 6 \text{ cm}.$$

This means we can limit the placement of this event to a section of the LOR 15–21 cm from its center, much smaller than its full length.

Standardized Uptake Value

The introduction to PET imaging highlighted the ability of PET to give quantitatively meaningful numbers. In the early days of PET, quantitation was performed by imaging a "jug" of known radioactivity concentration on the imaging table with the patient. Today, the ability to determine activity concentrations in various regions of interest is accomplished somewhat differently, but is still of major value.

The ability to obtain quantitatively correct activity concentration values in modern PET tomographs relies on a cross calibration between the tomograph and the dose calibrators and well counters used to measure activity values. This is commonly referred to as a *well counter* or *gamma counter calibration*, even though activity is more often measured in a dose calibrator than in a well counter. The calibration factor, usually given in units of (cps/voxel) ÷ (Bq/ml), in turn is dependent on several factors. Clearly, the choice of acquisition mode and reconstruction method will affect the calibration factor, but so will the dead time and the presence of noise in both the acquisition and the reconstructed 3D image matrix. For all these reasons, it is necessary to store well counter calibration factors for every combination of variables that is frequently encountered.

Clinical PET to date has primarily utilized a relative measure of radiopharmaceutical uptake in lesions of interest called the *standardized uptake value* (SUV), which is similar to a tumor-to-background ratio. The SUV is a unitless number calculated as follows:

$$\text{SUV} = \frac{\text{MBq}/\text{ml in area of interest}}{\text{injected dose (MBq)}/\text{pt. weight (g)}}. \quad (16\text{-}4)$$

The cps/voxel value in a region of interest is multiplied by the well counter calibration factor to get the numerator. The denominator is the injected dose divided by the patient's body weight. The calculation assumes that attenuation correction has been performed. (In fact, many systems display the attenuation-corrected images as "SUV images" in which the cursor held over a pixel displays an SUV value.) Given that each gram of tissue occupies a volume of approximately 1 ml, a completely uniform radiopharmaceutical distribution throughout the body would result in the numerator and denominator being equal. The resulting SUV of 1 provides a point of comparison for clinical measured SUVs. FDG uptake in tumors, for example, can generate SUVs of 3 to 50 or higher.

The determination of the best cps/voxel value for use in the SUV calculation needs further clarification (22). Several options can be considered. One way would be to draw a region of interest that encloses an area of increased activity and to determine the average count rate within it (referred to as the SUV_{avg}). But the value obtained would be variable depending on the size of the region of interest. Another possibility is to use the cps from the hottest voxel in the lesion (SUV_{max}). But while it is commonly used, SUV_{max} is subject to effects related to noise. And so the current preferred method is to create a small, fixed-size region of interest and to use it to find the highest average cps within the lesion. This SUV_{peak} method decreases the potential for a statistically high value. All three methods have been used, and some authors recommend reporting two or more (23).

The weight term in the denominator is a measure of the volume of distribution within the body, and a variety of metrics have been employed here as well. The patient's raw body weight is commonly used, but does not always work well. The radiopharmaceutical being used makes a

Sample Calculation 16-5   Standardized Uptake Value

In a tumor with elevated FDG uptake, the maximum count rate is 100,000 cps (all corrections having been applied). The system's well counter calibration is 50,000 cps/voxel per µCi/ml. The patient received 16.4 mCi F-18 FDG and weighs 175 lb. What is the SUV?

The activity concentration in the tumor is determined by multiplying the count rate in the tumor by the inverse of the well counter calibration factor:

Activity concentration =

$$100{,}000 \text{ cps in tumor} \times \frac{\mu\text{Ci/ml}}{50{,}000 \text{ cps}} = 2 \text{ µCi/ml}.$$

Convert from non-SI to SI units throughout:

$$\frac{2 \text{ µCi}}{\text{ml}} \times \frac{37 \text{ kBq}}{\mu\text{Ci}} = \frac{74 \text{ kBq}}{\text{ml}} = \frac{0.074 \text{ MBq}}{\text{ml}}.$$

$$16.4 \text{ mCi} \times \frac{37 \text{ MBq}}{\text{mCi}} = 607 \text{ MBq injected}.$$

$$175 \text{ lb} \times \frac{1 \text{ kg}}{2.2 \text{ lb}} = 79.5 \text{ kg} = 79{,}500 \text{ g}.$$

We can then calculate the SUV as

$$\text{SUV} = \frac{0.074 \text{ MBq/ml}}{607 \text{ MBq}/79{,}500 \text{ g}} = 9.69.$$

difference. For example, fat does not accumulate FDG, so the measured FDG SUV increases with increasing weight (which is mostly fat in adults). Body surface area or lean body mass is currently recommended (24).

The FDG SUV has much additional potential for error and uncertainty. Factors that can affect the measured value in FDG studies include the time between injection and measurement of lesion activity and the patient's blood glucose level at the time of injection. A high blood glucose level (i.e., a recent meal) causes the body to produce insulin, which forces FDG into the muscles, thus decreasing the measured SUV in a lesion of interest. Similarly, high uptake of FDG in particular tissues such as myocardium or brown adipose tissue can cause lesion uptake of FDG to be artifactually decreased.

It is not unusual to see SUVs reported in research studies on radiopharmaceuticals other than FDG. We do not know what factors impact the SUV for these radiopharmaceuticals, so it will be important not to assume that they will be the same as for FDG. For all these reasons, the SUV should be used with some degree of caution (25).

We also want to be careful in applying the SUV to clinical situations. In FDG oncologic imaging in the lungs, for example, an SUV of 2.5 or more in an area has been suggested as an indicator of malignant tissue. But such a cutoff value may be specific to the organ system involved. An appropriate cutoff value for a lung tumor, in an area of low background, would not be applicable to liver lesions, where the SUV of normal liver may be greater than 2. Add in 10 to 20% variability between sites and the diagnostic criteria of the physician involved, and the SUV as a demarcation point between benign and malignant becomes less meaningful. So from many points of view, it is important to interpret the SUV with a grain of salt.

Despite the potential for inconsistency, it is increasingly clear that the SUV will be a primary metric for quantitative evaluation in PET. The concept of evaluating uptake relative to a completely even distribution seems to work well for many radiopharmaceuticals, and SUV determination is built into the software and display of commercial tomographs. That being the case, standardization of image reconstruction parameters takes on greater importance. Scatter, random, and attenuation corrections must be applied. Correction for PVE should also be applied, according to some authors (23). Consistency in the numbers used in both the numerator and the denominator of Equation 16-4 will be essential.

PET studies, often using the SUV as the quantitative measure of radiopharmaceutical uptake, are being proposed as biomarkers for new drug trials. *Biomarkers* are biologic indicators of disease or of therapeutic effects that can be measured directly (26); an example of a biomarker is the blood level of prostate-specific antigen (PSA) as an indicator of recurrent prostate cancer. Many scientists believe that clinical trials for new therapeutic drugs can be completed more quickly if PET imaging is used to determine response, rather than waiting for anatomic or clinical evidence of drug effect; the formulation of the SUV makes it easy to utilize for this purpose. The Society of Nuclear Medicine has recently created the Clinical Trials Network, a consortium of institutions certified to provide data to FDA-approved trials. Certification means that the SUVs from the institution have been determined to be directly comparable to SUVs from other certified institutions. A prior experience of the American College of Radiology Imaging Network indicated interinstitutional variability in SUVs in the range of ±15% (27). So standardization of protocols and processing will be necessary, and institutions wishing to join the Clinical Trials Network will need to undergo testing with phantoms and test cases.

Summary

In many ways, a PET tomograph is more of a "black box" imaging device than a gamma camera, requiring less operator input and effort. While the image characteristics discussed in the beginning of this chapter are similar to those found in other types of nuclear medicine imaging, in PET less can be done to ameliorate their effects. However, given the ability to quantify radiopharmaceutical uptake, PET requires an accounting (and in most cases correction) for these characteristics. Performance measures provide the metrics for assessing the quality of the corrections. In addition, evaluation of tomograph performance is a crucial aspect of the effort to utilize PET study results as biomarkers of disease, metabolism, or drug effect. So while we need to recognize some inherent limitations on image quality, we are in no way excused from recognizing their effects on images, or from maintaining tomograph performance at the highest level possible.

References

1. Budinger T. Radionuclide enhancements above and beyond signal to noise: losing the background. Hal Anger Memorial Lecture, Society of Nuclear Medicine Annual Meeting, Salt Lake City, UT, June 8, 2010.
2. Karp JS, Surti S, Daube-Witherspoon ME, Muehllehner G. Benefit of time-of-flight in PET: experimental and clinical results. *J Nucl Med.* 2008;49: 462–470.
3. Muehllehner G, Karp JS. Positron emission tomography imaging—technical considerations. *Semin Nucl Med.* 1986;16:35–50.
4. Budinger TF. PET instrumentation: what are the limits? *Semin Nucl Med.* 1998;28:247–267.
5. Phelps ME, ed. *PET: Physics, Instrumentation, and Scanners*. New York, NY: Springer; 2006:9, 35, 63, 69.
6. Hoffman EJ, Huang S-C, Phelps ME, Kuhl DE. Quantitation in positron computed tomography: 4. Effect of accidental coincidences. *J Comput Assist Tomogr.* 1981;3:391–400.
7. Germano G, Hoffman EJ. A study of data loss and mispositioning due to pile-up in 2-D detectors in PET. *IEEE Trans Nucl Med.* 1990;37:671–675.
8. Huang SC, Hoffman EJ, Phelps ME, Kuhl DE. Quantitation in positron emission computed tomography: 2. Effects of inaccurate attenuation correction. *J Comp Asst Tomog.* 1979;3:804–814.
9. Henkin RE, Boles MA, Dillehay GL, et al. *Nuclear Medicine*. St. Louis, MO: Mosby; 1996:287.
10. Valk PE, Bailey DL, Townsend DW, Maisey MN. *Positron Emission Tomography: Basic Science and Clinical Practice*. London: Springer; 2003:142.
11. Soret M, Bacharach SL, Buvat I. Partial-volume effect in PET tumor imaging. *J Nucl Med.* 2007;48:932–945.
12. Rousset OG, Ma Y, Evans AC. Correction for partial volume effects in PET: principle and validation. *J Nucl Med.* 1998;39:904–911.
13. Zanzonico P. Positron-emission tomography: a review of basic principles, scanner design and performance, and current systems. *Semin Nucl Med.* 2004;34:87–111.
14. Pichler BL, Wehrl HF, Judenhofer MS. Latest advances in molecular imaging instrumentation. *J Nucl Med.* 2008;49:5S–23S.
15. Zaidi H, Koral KF. Scatter modeling and compensation in emission tomography. *Eur J Nucl Med Mol Imaging.* 2004;31:761–782.
16. Daube-Witherspoon ME, Karp JS, Casey ME, et al. PET performance measurements using the NEMA NU2-2001 standard. *J Nucl Med.* 2002;43: 1398–1409.
17. Moses W. PET data acquisition and processing. In Fahey F, Harkness B, eds. *Basic Science of Nuclear Medicine* [CD-ROM]. Reston, VA: Society of Nuclear Medicine; 2001.
18. Brasse D, Kinihan PE, Laritzien C, et al. Correction methods for random coincidences in fully 3D whole-body PET: impact on data and image quality. *J Nucl Med.* 2005;46:859–867.
19. Strother SC, Casey ME, Hoffman EJ. Measuring PET scanner sensitivity: relating count rates to image signal-to-noise ratios using noise equivalent counts. *IEEE Trans Nucl Sci.* 1990;37:783–788.
20. Tarantola G, Zito F, Gerundini P. PET instrumentation and reconstruction algorithms in whole-body applications. *J Nucl Med.* 2003;44:756–769.
21. Lartizien C, Kinahan PE, Comtat C. A lesion detection observer study comparing 2-dimensional versus fully 3-dimensional whole-body PET imaging protocols. *J Nucl Med.* 2004;45:714–723.
22. Wahl RL, Jacine J, Kasamon Y, Lodge M. From RECIST to PERCIST: evolving considerations for PET response criteria in solid tumors. *J Nucl Med.* 2009; 50:122S-150S.
23. Shankar L, Hoffman JM, Bacharach S, et al. Consensus recommendations for the use of 18F-FDG PET as an indicator of therapeutic response in patients in National Cancer Institute trials. *J Nucl Med.* 2006;47:1059–1066.
24. Sugawara Y, Zasadny KR, Neuhoff AW, Wahl RL. Reevaluation of the standardized uptake value for FDG: variations with body weight and methods for correction. *Radiol.* 1999;213:521–525.
25. Blodgett T. Best practices in PET/CT: consensus on performance of positron emission tomography-computed tomography. *Semin Ultrasound CT MRI.* 2008; 29:236–241.
26. Larson SM, Schwartz LH. 18F-FDG as a candidate for "qualified biomarker": functional assessment of treatment response in oncology. *J Nucl Med.* 2006;47: 901–903.
27. Scheuerman JS, Saffer JS, Karp JS, et al. Qualification of PET scanners for use in multicenter cancer clinical trials: the American College of Radiology Imaging Network experience. *J Nucl Med.* 2009:50:1187–1193.

Additional Resources

Budinger TF. PET instrumentation: what are the limits? *Semin Nucl Med.* 1998;28:247–267.

Cherry SR, Sorenson JA, Phelps ME. *Physics in Nuclear Medicine.* 3rd ed. Philadelphia, PA: Saunders; 2003:Chap. 19.

Muehllehner G, Karp JS. Positron emission tomography imaging—technical considerations. *Semin Nucl Med.* 1986;16:35–50.

Phelps ME, ed. *PET: Physics, Instrumentation, and Scanners.* New York, NY: Springer; 2006.

Tarantola G, Zito F, Gerundini P. PET instrumentation and reconstruction algorithms in whole-body applications. *J Nucl Med.* 2003;44:756–769.

Wagner HN, Szabo Z, Buchanan BS. *Principles of Nuclear Medicine.* 2nd ed. Philadelphia, PA: Saunders; 1995:Chapter 19, Sec. 2.

Zaidi H, Koral KF. Scatter modeling and compensation in emission tomography. *Eur J Nucl Med Mol Imaging.* 2004;31:761–782.

Zanzonico P. Positron-emission tomography: a review of basic principles, scanner design and performance, and current systems. *Semin Nucl Med.* 2004;34:87–111.

CHAPTER 17
Quality Control and Artifacts in PET

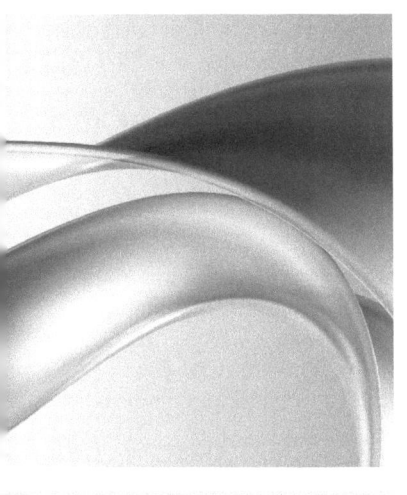

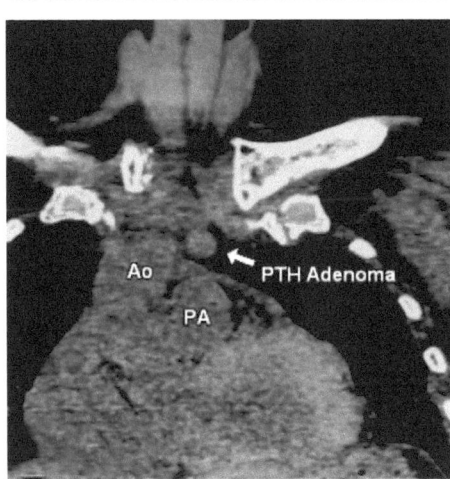

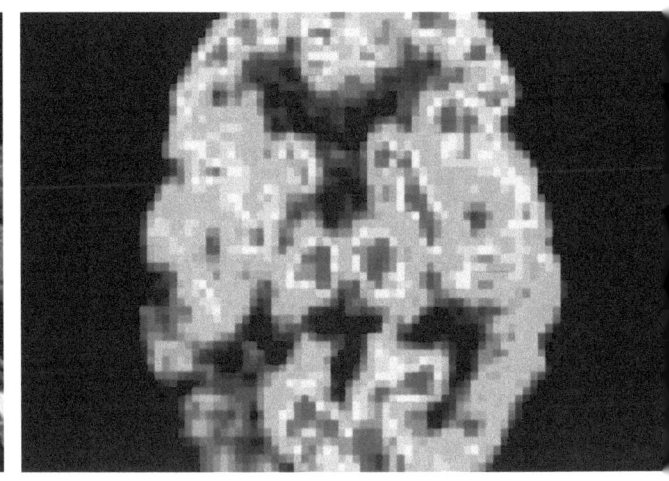

Learning Outcomes

1. Contrast quality control of PET tomographs with that for gamma cameras.
2. Describe acquisition and analysis and discuss the importance of routine quality control (QC) testing for PET tomographs, including:
   a. Normalization scan
   b. Well counter calibration
   c. Daily blank scan
   d. Uniformity assessment
3. Describe and explain the appearance of an electronics malfunction on a blank scan.
4. Briefly discuss infrequent quality control tests for PET tomographs, including measurement of NECR and dead time corrections, scatter fraction, and spatial resolution.
5. Discuss the appearance of artifacts on PET images.

Introduction

Modern PET tomographs require regular evaluation of their performance, as do all of the radiation-detecting instruments covered in this text. But the kinds of tests done are dissimilar from those used to evaluate gamma cameras. A PET tomograph is less susceptible to mechanical and electrical problems, and these are easily identified. So daily QC on a PET tomograph needs less effort than a flood on a gamma camera. The more important aspect of PET QC, namely, evaluation of the correction factors that are applied to each image, is done less frequently. In particular, the quantitative and semiquantitative aims of a PET study dictate that we verify their accuracy. So while PET QC may at first glance look easier than gamma camera QC, the former requires as much as or more attention than the latter. Table 17-1 shows a compilation of QC recommendations from PET physicists and from the PET Learning Center sponsored by the Society of Nuclear Medicine (SNM).

Acceptance Testing

As imaging systems become more complicated, the need for expert evaluation becomes more critical; PET tomographs are the most complex of all nuclear medicine instruments and hence require more extensive testing. Acceptance testing should be performed by a medical physicist with experience in PET system evaluation.

The PET community has collaborated on identification of standards for PET tomograph performance, the most recent publication of which is the NEMA Standard NU 2-2007, *Performance Measurements of Positron Emission Tomographs* (1). A similar set of standards, published by the International Electrotechnical Commission (IEC), is used in Europe. The methodology of the NEMA measurements for PET tomographs is in some cases relatively easy to reproduce, allowing the standards to serve as a reference

Table 17-1

Recommended Quality Control Tests for Dedicated PET Tomographs

Frequency	Quality Control Tests
Daily	• PMT baseline check and gain adjustment • Blank scan • Uniform cylinder or point-source scan
Weekly	• Uniformity check • Well counter calibration check • Coincidence timing check • Energy window calibration
Quarterly	• Preventive maintenance • Detector efficiency/normalization scan • Cross calibration

Annually	• NEMA NU 2-2007 testing
	  • Spatial resolution
	  • Sensitivity
	  • Intrinsic scatter fraction
	  • Scatter correction
	  • Count rate performance
	• Update of normalization factors and well counter calibration (may be required more frequently)

Daube-Witherspoon ME. Routine QA of dedicated PET systems. Paper presented at the 51st Annual Meeting of the Society of Nuclear Medicine, Philadelphia, PA, June 21, 2004.
Society of Nuclear Medicine. PET Learning Center Notebook for Technologist Attendees. Reston, VA: Author; 2004:Sec. 7.
Zanzonico P. Routine quality control of clinical nuclear medicine instrumentation: a brief review. *J Nucl Med*. 2008;49:1114–1131.

for more than just physicists. The NEMA document does not address quality control as such, but it does provide procedures for measuring tomograph performance that should be performed on at least an infrequent (e.g., annual) basis on all systems.

The need for acceptance testing and regular evaluation of system performance in PET cannot be overemphasized. A final PET image set is more removed from the raw data than a SPECT image set, with several layers of corrections in addition to the reconstruction needed to convert sinograms into a 3D image matrix. The operator must have good assurance that these corrections are accurate and are being applied properly. As a relatively new diagnostic imaging modality, PET is still in the process of proving its worth, and faulty diagnoses resulting from inadequate corrections or improper system operation will be detrimental to its cause.

Routine Quality Control

For the nuclear medicine technologist, routine QC in the PET suite seems like a vacation compared to the same job in a general nuclear medicine department. Much of the routine QC needed for a PET tomograph can be done in an automated fashion and requires only the verification that the system is functional. The kinds of problems that can be subtle in a gamma camera, such as a malfunctioning photomultiplier tube (PMT), are obvious in a PET sinogram. Conversely, the following section on nonroutine QC is more involved and more important, because it discusses how to verify that the corrections and the results of quantitative measurements are accurate.

Normalization Scan

The most important QC procedure is the acquisition and evaluation of the normalization correction factors that are applied to every study (Eq. 15-2). Because it is so crucial to image quality, the normalization scan must itself be of high quality, with as little noise as possible. Therefore it is generally obtained in a very long acquisition (many hours, usually over a weekend), using either the rod source(s) installed in the tomograph or a Ge-68 cylindrical phantom. A different approach to the acquisition of the normalization scan may be required for 3D PET systems, due to the high number of lines of response (LORs) and the extended acquisition time required to reach statistical significance in each LOR (2, 3). Scatter must also be corrected for in a 3D normalization acquisition before normalization correction factors are generated (4).

The normalization scan should be acquired under conditions of low dead time and no pulse pileup (5). Additional QC acquisitions that may be performed in conjunction with the normalization scan check for variations in the coincidence timing window alignment, block maps, and energy windows. Depending on the system, they may be done before or after the normalization scan is acquired. All are generally automated.

Once the normalization scan is acquired, it must be analyzed. One easy way to do so is to subtract the newly acquired normalization sinograms from the stored sinograms, and then apply a statistical analysis to the result. If there is no significant change, the results of the subtraction should demonstrate low statistical variability around a mean value of zero (6). If appropriate, the newly acquired sinograms may be stored along with the newly determined normalization correction factors. If the subtracted result shows no appreciable changes, the better choice may be to continue to use the stored normalization sinograms.

The normalization scan corrects for several of the issues that arise from the multicrystal, multi-ring geometry of the PET tomograph. Its first and most important job is to normalize the individual detectors so that they generate a uniform response to a uniform source. It accounts for sensitivity variations in the axial direction that occur with 3D imaging so that bed positions can be combined into a whole-body scan. It also corrects for the fact that the LOR density varies in the transaxial plane.

Given that a single normalization scan may require upward of 6 hr of acquisition time, it only makes sense that in a clinical environment, these acquisitions need to be done outside of working hours (e.g., over a weekend). This scenario in turn suggests that the acquisition could be started automatically and proceed without operator intervention. It is perfectly reasonable from a mechanical viewpoint for this to happen, but raises concerns from a radiation safety standpoint, because either the rod sources or a Ge-68 cylindrical phantom will be unshielded and unattended for a length of time. Arrangements should be discussed with department personnel and handled in ways that are acceptable to both the department and its radiation protection personnel.

Cross Calibration

If it is to provide quantitative information, PET requires a correlation with some external measure of radioactivity. In research settings where body-fluid sampling is done, the external measuring device may be a well counter, but in clinical PET it will more likely be a dose calibrator. In either case, the desire is to be able to express cps/voxel in terms of µCi/ml or kBq/ml. This calibration (generically called a *well counter calibration*, whether a well counter or a dose calibrator is used) is vital to the numeric results generated in clinical studies. It is in essence a measure of sensitivity that can be directly applied to images.

Performing a well counter calibration measurement is quite simple. A normal patient dosage is added to a 20-cm-diameter cylinder and is mixed very well. A 1-ml aliquot is removed for dose calibrator or well counter measurement. (If cross calibration with a well counter is required, it may be necessary to dilute the 1-ml aliquot to avoid the well counter's count rate limitations.) The phantom is then imaged in the tomograph. The count rate per voxel of the resulting reconstructed image matrix is determined, and the calibration factor is expressed as

$$\text{Well counter calibration factor} = \frac{\text{cps/voxel}}{\mu\text{Ci/ml or kBq/ml}} \text{ in phantom.} \quad (17\text{-}1)$$

A branching fraction (the fraction of radionuclide decays that occur via positron emission) can be included if the radionuclide used for the calibration factor determination is something different than the radionuclide being used for clinical imaging (5). The well counter calibration factor is then used to correct cps/voxel values in patient imaging studies:

$$\text{Activity concentration in voxel } (\mu\text{Ci/ml or kBq/ml}) = \frac{\text{cps in voxel in question}}{\text{well counter calibration factor}}. \quad (17\text{-}2)$$

As was true with the normalization scan, separate cross-calibration factors will be required for each acquisition mode and for different reconstruction algorithms. All corrections must be applied to the phantom study being used to determine a well counter calibration factor, and the accuracy of the well counter calibration value depends on the accuracy of the applied corrections. If the corrections are accurate and are similarly applied to clinical studies, then the resulting activity concentration should be accurate to about ±5% (5). A partial volume correction (see

Sample Calculation 17-1 Well Counter Calibration

Three mCi F-18 are added to a 6,000-ml cylindrical phantom and mixed well. A 1-ml aliquot is removed and assayed at 0.48 µCi. The phantom is then imaged, and all corrections are applied to the images during reconstruction. The average count density is measured at 102,700 cps/voxel. What is the well counter calibration factor?

$$\text{Well counter calibration factor} = \frac{102{,}700 \text{ cps/voxel}}{0.48 \text{ µCi/ml}}$$
$$= \frac{214{,}000 \text{ cps/voxel}}{\mu\text{Ci/ml}}.$$

In a patient study with this PET tomograph and dose calibrator, a voxel records a count rate of 55,000 cps. What is its activity concentration?

$$\text{Voxel activity concentration} = \frac{55{,}000 \text{ cps/voxel}}{214{,}000 \text{ (cps/voxel)/(µCi/ml)}} = 0.26 \text{ µCi/ml}.$$

Eq. 16-1 and Fig. 16-2) should be applied to small objects less than twice the system FWHM.

A simple method to verify operationally the accuracy of a tomograph's well counter calibration is to perform an SUV determination in an area with a known Standardized Uptake Value (SUV). For example, normal liver tissue has an F-18 fluorodeoxyglucose (FDG) SUV of about 2; if a calculated liver SUV over an area of normal liver is not around this value, one reason could be that the well counter calibration data are incorrect. Any discrepancy should prompt a recheck of the data and (potentially) acquisition and storage of a new well counter calibration factor.

Daily Blank Scan

Once the normalization scan and cross calibration are in place, it is only necessary to verify the functionality of the tomograph on a daily basis. This is done in a quick acquisition using the rod source(s) or a Ge-68 cylinder, called a *blank scan* (**Figure 17-1**); it is also called an *air scan* or *reference scan*. Some scanners automatically check and/or adjust PMT gains; such routines are generally run prior to acquiring the blank scan. Because the purpose of the blank scan is to elucidate equipment failures, which tend to be obvious in PET sinograms, a study with excellent statistics is not required. Instead, a short acquisition (in the neighborhood of 30–60 min) may be automatically started prior to the beginning of the work day (again, this practice should be discussed with radiation safety personnel). The study is visually inspected and quantitatively evaluated by the technologist (most often by normalization to and subtraction from the stored normalization sinograms). Any drift may prompt acquisition of a new normalization scan.

Figure 17-1 Blank scan. A blank scan is a short-time acquisition done at the beginning of the day to verify that the PET tomograph is operational for that day's work. If any detectors or blocks are not functioning, the sinogram will generally look abnormal, as seen in Figure 17-2. Image courtesy of Puget Sound Cancer Center.

Figure 17-2 Detector block failure. Failure of a PMT, a detector block or bucket, or other electronic component creates an obvious defect on the sinogram, such as the diagonal stripe seen in this figure. A single malfunctioning PMT produces alternating light and dark stripes on the sinogram, analogous to edge packing in a gamma camera. Image courtesy of Puget Sound Cancer Center.

The reason that equipment failure is more obvious in PET tomographs than in gamma cameras has to do with the detector block architecture. Because each block only has a small number of PMTs and uses only one set of electronic devices, a failure often affects the entire block. Further, the blocks are seen as diagonal lines on the sinogram, so a malfunction will be visualized along a diagonal. An example of detector block failure can be seen in **Figure 17-2**. Certainly the visual evaluation of a daily blank scan can be more cursory than evaluation of a gamma camera flood. Many laboratories record the count rate of the blank scan and look for any significant changes from previous blank scans as a way to track slow drifts in the system.

In non-CT PET systems, the daily blank scan is used to normalize the transmission LORs for attenuation correction, as shown in Equation 15-3. In this situation, it is imperative that the blank scan be analyzed every day, because an incorrectly acquired or outdated blank scan will produce errors in the attenuation correction process. In addition, the daily blank scan must be archived as it might be needed for reprocessing of patient data.

Uniformity

Uniformity of reconstructed 3D images should be measured and evaluated on a regular (daily or weekly) basis (4). This measure of system performance is not included in the NEMA standard. The procedure would be similar to that described for measurement of 3D uniformity in SPECT using a 20-cm-diameter cylindrical phantom (either a solid phantom containing Ge-68 or a liquid phantom filled with F-18 solution) reconstructed with a ramp filter. The slices generated are then evaluated visually and using 1-cm square regions of interest (ROIs) to determine positive and negative deviations from the average.

Infrequent Quality Control Tests

One prominent PET physicist (7) expressed the different levels of PET quality control as follows:

- Daily: Should we scan today?
- Weekly: How well is the scanner operating?
- Quarterly: Has the scanner changed over time?
- Annually: Is the scanner still performing at its best?

The more important but less frequently performed QC measures relate to the accuracy of calibrations and corrections. It is particularly important that these be performed properly, because they will be applied to imaging studies and the accuracy of quantitative results depends on them. The importance of these calibrations and corrections may justify the expense of contracting with a consulting medical physicist to verify their accuracy. As always, check the recommendations of the tomograph's manufacturer for specific procedures.

Energy Window Calibration and Detector Identification Maps

Even though all PET scans use 511-keV photons, it is still important to evaluate the energy of each event, in order to separate out scattered photons as much as possible via pulse height analyzer (PHA) exclusion. Energy window calibration is required only infrequently, but should be performed prior to acquisition of a new normalization scan and after repair (8).

Similarly, the flood histograms for each detector block and the resulting detector identification maps are not expected to change frequently, but should be checked occasionally, as they may degrade over time due to changes in the PMTs and the coupling compounds. PMT gains are closely linked to detector identification designs, so a gain adjustment may require a revalidation of the detector identification map. Some systems have methods to check PMT gain settings daily, to ensure the individual PMT gains are at the correct values for the detector identification maps. Keep in mind that a change in temperature may result in a change in system sensitivity, due to drifting of the PMT gains (8).

Coincidence Timing Calibration

All systems have procedures for generating corrections for coincidence timing between detector blocks so that all of the LORs can use the same timing window. Generally, such corrections are applied in the acquisition electronics prior to the coincidence circuitry. Some systems generate a histogram showing the timing distribution of accepted coincidences; checking the histogram for changes may be part of weekly or quarterly QC. Tomographs using time-of-flight techniques also need a measured set of timing differences between individual pairs of detectors (9).

Accuracy of Dead Time Corrections

Depending on the acquisition modes and types of clinical studies performed, dead time losses may range from insignificant to large (as high as 40–50%). If the latter, it is important to know that the dead time corrections are in fact accurate. To measure the dead time, a cylindrical phantom containing a high-activity concentration is scanned repeatedly, and the singles, trues, and randoms count rates are plotted vs remaining activity (determined by decay correction of the initial activity). The ideal (trues + scatters) rate is extrapolated from the low-activity measurement (**Figure 17-3**), and the percentage loss is given by

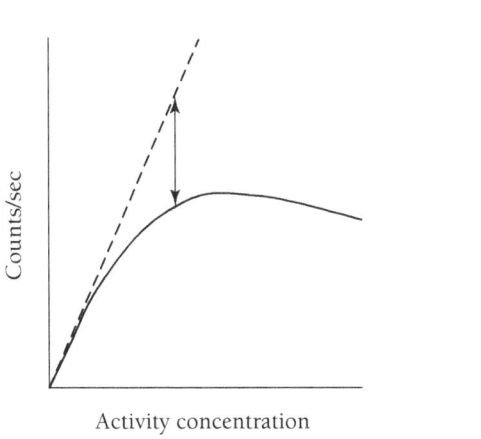

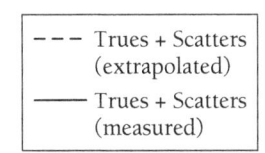

$$\% \text{ Dead time loss} = 100\% \times \frac{(N_{\text{trues}} + N_{\text{scatters}})_{\text{extrapolated}} - (N_{\text{trues}} + N_{\text{scatters}})_{\text{measured}}}{(N_{\text{trues}} + N_{\text{scatters}})_{\text{extrapolated}}}.$$

(17-3)

Figure 17-3 Measurement of count rate loss. The graph illustrates the determination of fractional count loss as a function of activity concentration. The ideal (trues + scatters) rate is extrapolated from the straight-line first part of the measured (trues + scatters) graph. The fractional count loss, shown by the double-headed arrow, is then calculated as in Equation 17-3.

where $(N_{\text{trues}} + N_{\text{scatters}})$ is the randoms-corrected prompt count rate (1, 10). The percentage of dead time loss is a function of activity concentration, as are N_{trues} and N_{scatters}. The activity concentration level at which the dead time loss is 50% should be noted and used as an approximate upper limit for detector operation (10). The random coincidence count rate in each measurement of the cylinder should also be noted; this provides an estimate for the proportion of events that are random coincidences at a specified activity concentration.

Accuracy of Scatter and Attenuation Corrections and Reconstruction Algorithms

Thanks to the quantitative abilities of PET, phantoms can be filled with known amounts of radioactivity, and the resulting images evaluated for the accuracy of the measured μCi/ml or kBq/ml values. We can therefore evaluate the corrections that are included in the reconstruction process as well as the reconstruction algorithms themselves. The NEMA document specifies the phantoms to be used for each test, and these phantoms should be used if comparison to NEMA specifications is desired. For general system evaluation without reference to NEMA tests, other phantoms may be substituted. Accreditation by the American College of Radiology (ACR) requires a quarterly or semiannual phantom study using a Jaszczak-type phantom with fillable cylinders and rods (similar to that shown in Figure 13-8). Cylinders containing air, nonradioactive water, and Teflon allow for measurements of residual scatter fraction, while the rods and fillable spheres provide a measure of spatial resolution for cold defects and hot spots, respectively.

Scatter Fraction

The scatter fraction in particular is an important indicator of the quality of the events being recorded. Scatter must be subtracted from PET images; approaches to this problem include modeling scatter and estimating its magnitude at the periphery of the field of view (FOV). But subtraction of scatter decreases the signal-to-noise characteristics of the data set, because subtraction decreases the count rate. Thus, knowing how much scatter is being subtracted is important information, and may guide further image manipulation. This is especially true in 3D PET, where scatter represents 20 to 50% or more of total counts (2).

The NEMA protocol for measuring the scatter fraction uses a solid polyethylene cylinder with a hole drilled off-center, through which a tube filled with radioactivity is threaded (1). The tube is to be 70 cm in length (even though most tomographs are less than 20 cm in axial dimension) in order to account for out-of-field activity, which is a major source of scatter events. At a low dead time, low randoms activity level, the scatter fraction is the ratio of scatter events (i.e., those in the area of the nonradioactive phantom) to total events in each slice of the reconstructed phantom. Note that this measurement does not say anything about the spatial distribution of the scatter events or the validity of the subtraction techniques employed; it is simply a global measure of the percentage of all counts that are scatter counts.

The NEMA torso phantom with hot and cold spheres and a lung insert provides a great deal of information. After reconstruction, the hot and cold spheres can be used to measure contrast, thereby providing a quantitative measure of image quality. The calculated activity concentration of the hot spheres is compared to their known activity concentrations. The lung insert (which is filled with a low-atomic-number, nonradioactive material) is used to measure residual error after scatter and attenuation corrections have been applied (1). Based on Equation 16-2, the residual scatter fraction (rSF) can be determined as (10)

$$rSF = 100\% \times \frac{cts/voxel\ in\ lung\ insert}{cts/voxel\ in\ surrounding\ phantom}.$$

(17-4)

The rSF can be measured similarly in any phantom that has a cold (nonradioactive) insert, using the cts/voxel in the center of the cold insert in the numerator of Equation 17-4. With perfect scatter correction, the cts/voxel in the center of the cold insert, and therefore the rSF, would be zero.

Spatial Resolution

To measure spatial resolution, a point source of F-18 is positioned at several locations within the tomograph's FOV, and resolution is measured in axial, radial, and tangential directions. The NEMA protocol specifies reconstruction by filtered backprojection (FBP) with a ramp filter, because iterative reconstruction is dependent on local activity distribution, of which there is little in this quality control situation. The measurements represent an ideal scenario: no scatter, low counting rate, and sharpest filter. The result of the NEMA test will therefore not be matched in clinical situations (11).

It is very important to use the same radionuclide for all spatial resolution measurements, as the measured value will change with the range of the positron. Fluorine-18 is the usual choice, and it is specified for this purpose in the NEMA standard (1). The NEMA protocol also requires a pixel size no greater than one-third of the expected FWHM. The spatial resolution measurement should be performed under low-activity conditions, so that random coincidence rates and dead time losses are not significant.

The spatial resolution provides an important gauge of the accuracy of quantitative measurements, such as the SUV. We know that the partial volume effect (PVE) causes inaccurate measurement of a lesion's activity concentration below a size that is about twice the spatial FWHM. Therefore, once the FWHM is known, lesions can be evaluated for PVE based on their size, and the SUV can be considered in light of the PVE.

Noise-Equivalent Count Rate (NECR)

The NECR provides a measure of the ratio of true counts to total events, at a given activity concentration. Using the same phantom setup as for the scatter fraction, the NECR is calculated from Equation 16-3 using the true, random, and scatter coincidence rates, at activity concentrations ranging from relatively high to quite low. The NECR should be plotted vs activity concentration, and its peak value should be noted (1).

The NECR is an important measure of image quality in the complex environment of a PET acquisition. It is described in one text as "that count rate which would have resulted in the same signal-to-noise ratio (SNR) in the data in the absence of scatter and random events" (2). Knowledge of the NECR in clinical situations allows the interpreter of the images to judge the relative statistical precision in each case, and by extension his or her confidence in the interpretation. Keep in mind, however, that like the scatter fraction, the NECR is only a global measure of the SNR and does not take into account regional variations (3). It should again be pointed out that all of the NEMA performance measurements will be better than those achievable in clinical situations (11).

System Sensitivity

The NEMA protocol for measuring sensitivity is an absolute measurement (cps per MBq) done in the absence of complicating factors. It uses a 70-cm length of plastic tubing, filled with a measured amount of radioactivity and suspended in the center of the transaxial FOV. A series of attenuating sleeves are used to attenuate the radioactivity, and emission acquisitions are obtained for each combination of sleeves. The count rates in a slice through the tube and attenuating sleeves are corrected for decay and for the attenuation of the sleeves, and compared to the known activity. The value for absolute sensitivity in many clinical situations is only about 10 to 100 counts (cts) per 1,000 radioactive disintegrations, demonstrating that even PET tomographs without collimators make scant use of the events available to them (3).

In real life, the *effective sensitivity*—the tomograph's ability to register true coincidences in the presence of random coincidences, scatter events, and dead time, and considering geometric efficiency—is far less than the absolute sensitivity measurement. A procedure for measuring effective sensitivity is given in Reference 12. A 20-cm-diameter cylinder is filled with F-18 solution at high activity, and trues, randoms, and scatters are measured repeatedly as the radioactivity decays. The ideal true coincidence rates (i.e., no dead time or random coincidences) and NECR are determined as a function of activity concentration, and effective sensitivity is calculated as

$$\text{Effective sensitivity}\ (A) = \frac{NECR\,(A)}{N_{\text{ideal trues}}(A)} \times \text{absolute sensitivity} \quad (17\text{-}5)$$

where NECR and $N_{\text{ideal trues}}$ are the noise-equivalent and ideal count rates, respectively. Both are functions of the activity concentration A in the cylinder. Absolute sensitivity is the value obtained in annual QC, according to the NEMA protocol just referenced.

Effective sensitivity allows for comparison between systems and between acquisition modes on one system. A couple of examples illustrate its value (12). The effective sensitivity of one PET tomograph was shown to be the same whether the energy window was set at 250 or 350 keV, indicating that the gain in total events counted with the lower threshold is offset by the increase in random and scatter events. Another PET tomograph exhibited a high effective sensitivity at low count rates, but a more significant decrease than other tomographs as the activity concentration increased. Effective sensitivity provides a meaningful way to make comparisons such as these.

Artifacts in PET

PET tomographs are complex pieces of machinery with multiple associated computers, which can experience difficulties in a wide variety of ways (Table 17-2). Some of these malfunctions produce artifacts. Additional artifacts arise from other causes in the context of clinical imaging. We concentrate here on those artifacts that can be attributed to the PET tomograph or its operator. It is important to recognize these and take steps to remove them, if possible. Some are similar to those seen in SPECT, while others are unique to PET.

Artifacts due to Electronics Malfunctions

The detector block design of most modern tomographs makes the identification of defects an easy task. Figure 17-2 shows an example. Because an electronic failure affects an entire detector block, a wide diagonal stripe is seen on the blank sinogram. Failure of a single PMT within a block produces a white stripe representing the failing PMT, and in some systems an adjacent black stripe where the mispositioned events are assigned. Failures may also occur in the coincidence-processing and event-sorting electronics.

Ray Artifacts

The source of ray artifacts is the same in PET as in SPECT: the use of FBP as the method of reconstruction. The essence of the problem is that backprojection puts the counts from a particular LOR into the entire column of the reconstruction image matrix corresponding to that LOR. A ramp filter is used to subtract out the excess counts around an area of increased activity. If this filtration is inadequate, some of the excess counts persist and are seen as a ray. The problem is most noticeable with a very intense focus of activity, which often happens with FDG oncologic imaging (Figure 17-4). It is diminished when iterative reconstruction techniques are employed.

Motion Artifacts

Nuclear medicine technologists are well versed in spotting motion on cines or sinograms of raw SPECT images. In PET, however, what is generally viewed is not the sinogram, but the reconstructed image. Figure 17-5 shows patient motion that is apparent at the base of the brain. The hot brain tissue is seen in two places with a photopenic area in between.

Misregistration Artifacts

Most whole-body PET protocols acquire emission and transmission data sets sequentially rather than simultaneously. If the patient moves during or between the two scans at a given bed position, or between the CT and PET scans, the data sets are no longer co-registered. This results in application of an erroneous attenuation correction to the emission data set. The applied correction may be either high or low, resulting in an artifactual hot or cold abnormality, respectively, on the reconstructed emission images. One way to identify such artifacts is to reconstruct non-attenuation-corrected images and to refer to these

Table 17-2

Sources of PET Tomograph Failure

Part of Tomograph	Possible Problems
Radiation detection system	• Detector/block/cassette malfunction • PMT malfunction • High-voltage gain drift • Temperature drift
Electrical system	• Power supply/cable/fuse failure • Coincidence timing malfunction • Memory location initialization failure • Circuit board component failure
Rod-source system	• Mechanical/robotic failure • Decrease in activity below usable level
Mechanical systems	• Failure of septa robotics • Imaging table or gantry misalignment/malfunction
Other	• Software failure

Data from: Christian PE, Waterstram-Rich KM. *Nuclear Medicine and PET/CT: Technology and Techniques.* 6th ed. St. Louis, MO: CV Mosby; 2007:336.

(a) Coronal slice from PET study reconstructed with FBP

(b) Same slice, reconstructed with iterative reconstruction

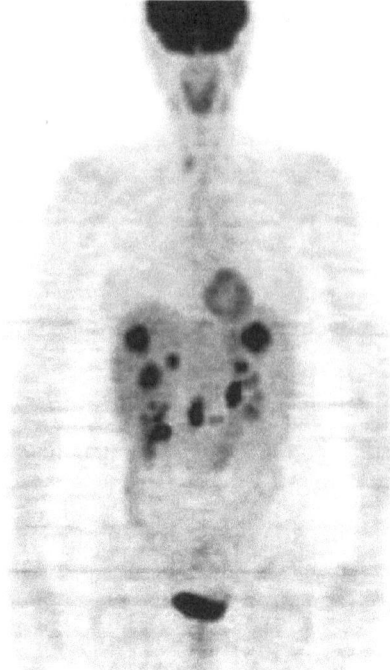

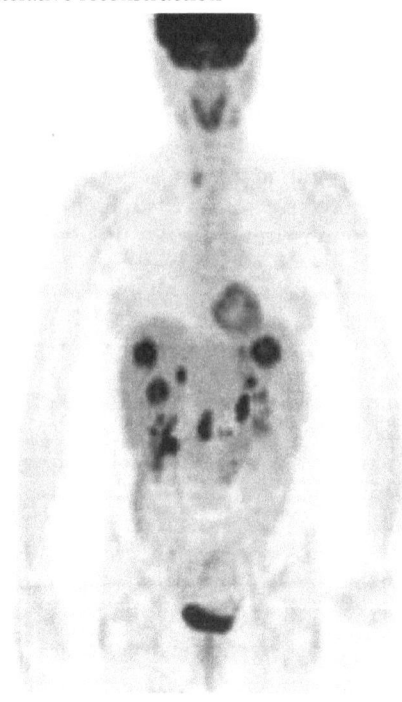

Figure 17-4 PET FDG study reconstructed with FBP and iterative methods. Figure 17-4a shows a coronal maximum intensity projection (MIP) image of an oncologic FDG study reconstructed using FBP, and Figure 17-4b shows the same image using iterative reconstruction. Note the ray artifacts in the FBP image that are not present in the iterative image. Images courtesy of City of Hope Medical Center.

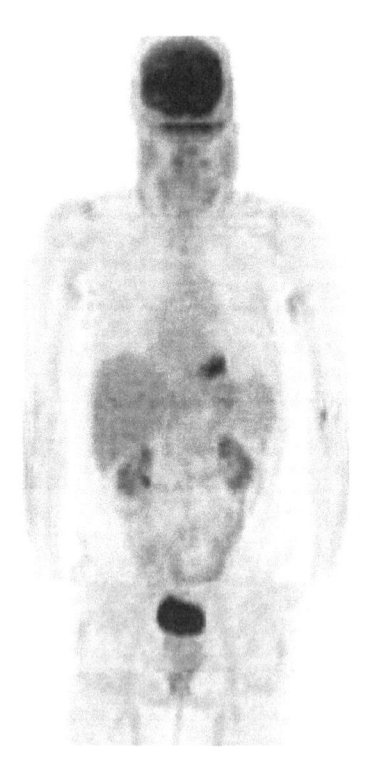

Figure 17-5 Motion artifact. Note the double exposure of the base of the brain on this FDG MIP image. The base of the brain appears as it should, an area of decreased FDG uptake appears just below it, and then intense brain uptake is seen again. The patient shifted between the two superior bed positions, so that some brain tissue was registered in the second bed position, below the base of the brain acquired in the most superior bed position. A second motion artifact can be seen just superior to the bladder. Image courtesy of City of Hope Medical Center.

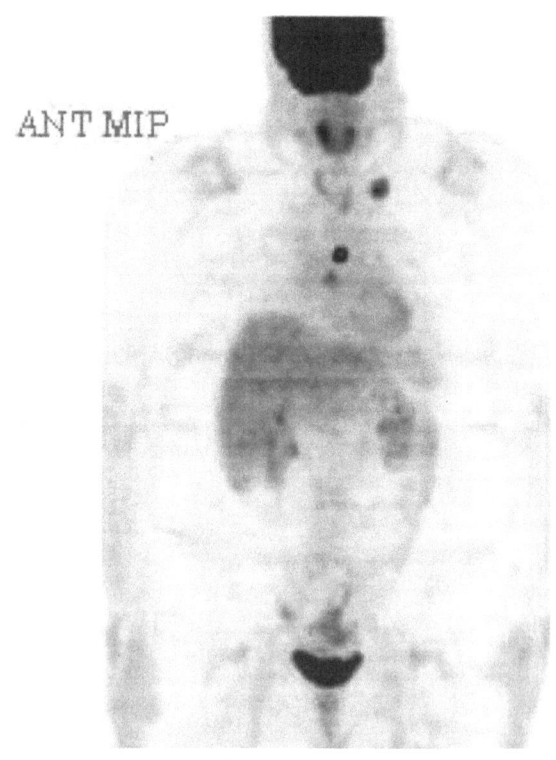

Figure 17-6 Bed overlap artifact. The degree of overlap that is needed between bed positions on a whole-body study is dependent on the choice of 2D vs 3D mode and the specific details of the acquisition (as discussed in Chapter 15). If the normalization study is not updated when needed, photopenic stripes will appear on the coronal images at the intersection of bed positions. The appearance of these stripes is a good indication that a new normalization study should be acquired. Image courtesy of City of Hope Medical Center.

images for any questionable area, and this is often routinely done in clinical practice. But clinical studies should always be checked for proper alignment before the patient leaves, so that reimaging can be done if needed.

Bed Overlap Artifacts

Recall that the normalization scan corrects for the decreased LOR sensitivity at the axial front and back of the tomograph. If this correction doesn't occur, horizontal photopenic stripes are seen at the junction of the bed positions (**Figure 17-6**). The appearance of such stripes indicates that a new normalization scan needs to be acquired. Every study should be analyzed from the standpoint of alignment of the bed positions; problems are most easily seen on coronal slices. Misregistration artifacts may also occur where bed positions overlap (13).

Hot-Spot Artifacts

A hot-spot artifact can occur when a positron-emitting source is used for attenuation correction (**Figure 17-7**). The underlying assumption of rod-source attenuation correction is that most of the counts in the rod window are coming from the transmission source. In an area of high activity, this assumption is not true, and the applied correction factors may not be as large as they need to be (5). In addition, the dead time is high in such areas, so that more of the true coincidences are coming from the hot spot than from surrounding areas, relative to the actual activity concentrations. This artifact may be seen in whole-body scans of FDG in the bladder area. A recent article noted a similar artifact resulting from a shifting pocket of gas in the rectum (14).

Partial Volume Artifacts

The PVE is an important image characteristic in tomographic imaging and especially in PET. We should thus be aware of the potential for partial volume artifacts. Small objects (less than twice the system FWHM) will appear larger and less intense than they truly are. "The smaller the tumor, the greater the underestimation of the uptake value" (15). This is especially problematic when tumor size is measured before and after therapeutic intervention. A tumor that shrinks will appear to have a lower SUV than when it was larger, just because of PVE (15). Additional effects can be expected if the lesion in question has increased surface area and if the background activity is changed. Corrections such as the recovery coefficient can be applied, but care should be used when evaluating small lesions.

Summary

The subject of quality control for clinical (as opposed to research) PET tomographs is not addressed completely in the literature at this time. While this gap will no doubt be filled as more PET tomographs are purchased, there is

(a) Non-attenuation corrected   (b) Attenuation corrected

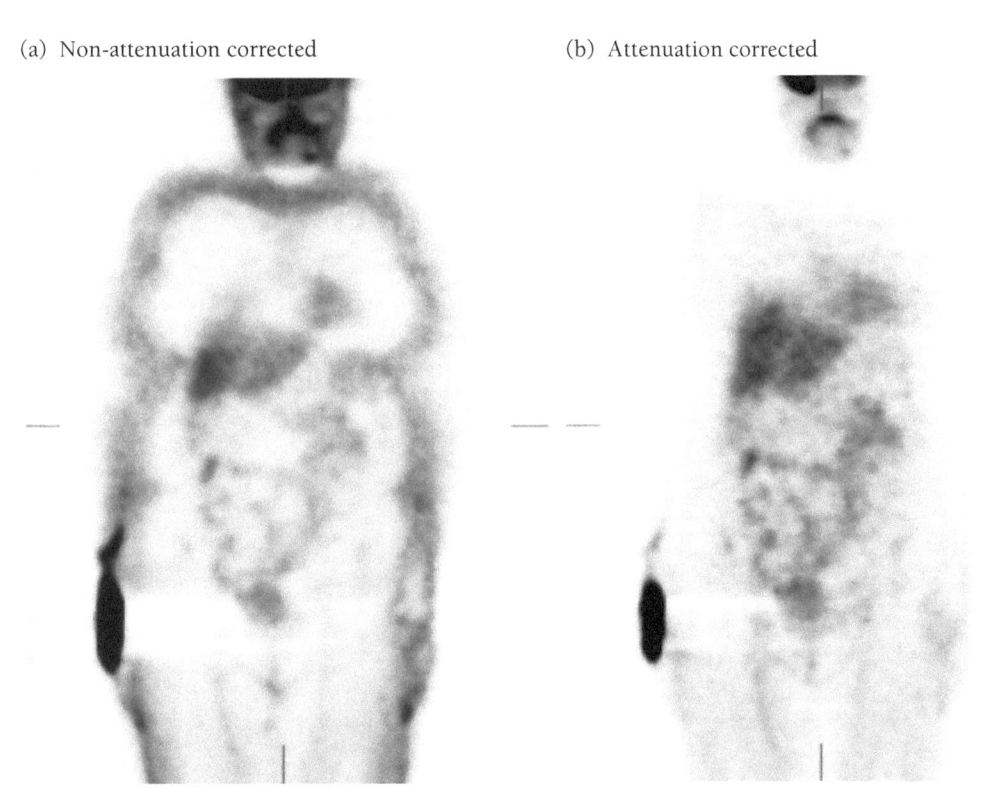

Figure 17-7 Hot-spot artifact. When a positron-emitting source is used as the transmission source, any annihilation photons detected in the transmission scan will be assigned to the attenuation map. This figure shows non-attenuation-corrected and attenuation-corrected coronal slices in a patient with retention of the radiopharmaceutical dose at the injection site. The non-attenuation-corrected slice shows a lack of counts in the body adjacent to the hot spot. This occurs because the high radioactivity swamps many of the true events originating in the nearby tissue. Attenuation correction (Fig. 17-7b) improves the situation somewhat but not completely. Images courtesy of Puget Sound Cancer Center.

certainly a lack of written materials at the moment. But clearly, the complexity of PET systems will require ongoing evaluation, especially of the correction factors needed to correct the raw data. As with all other aspects of nuclear medicine, PET will demand vigilance on the part of the physician, the technologist, and the service personnel.

References

1. National Electrical Manufacturers Association. *NEMA Standards Publication NU 2-2007: Performance Measurements of Positron Emission Tomographs*. Rosslyn, VA: Author; 2007:12, 27, 7, 17.
2. Valk PE, Bailey DL, Townsend DW, Maisey MN. *Positron Emission Tomography: Basic Science and Clinical Practice*. London: Springer; 2003:84, 85, 123.
3. Zanzonico P. Positron-emission tomography: a review of basic principles, scanner design and performance, and current systems. *Semin Nucl Med*. 2004; 34:87–111.
4. Zanzonico P. Routine quality control of clinical nuclear medicine instrumentation: a brief review. *J Nucl Med*. 2008;49:1114–1131.
5. Phelps ME, ed. *PET: Physics, Instrumentation, and Scanners*. New York, NY: Springer; 2006:4, 61–62, 93.
6. Buchert R, Bohuslavizki KH, Mester J, Clausen M. Quality assurance in PET: evaluation of the clinical relevance of detector defects. *J Nucl Med*. 1999; 40:1657–1665.
7. Daube-Witherspoon ME. Routine QA of dedicated PET systems. Paper presented at the 51st Annual Meeting of the Society of Nuclear Medicine, Philadelphia, PA, June 21, 2004.
8. Christian PE, Waterstram-Rich KM. *Nuclear Medicine and PET/CT: Technology and Techniques*. 6th ed. St. Louis, MO: Mosby-Year Book; 2007:334.
9. Surti S, Kuhn A, Werner ME, et al. Performance of Philips Gemini TF PET/CT scanner with special consideration for its time-of-flight imaging capabilities. *J Nucl Med*. 2007;48:471–480.
10. Wagner HN, Szabo Z, Buchanan JW. *Principles of Nuclear Medicine*. 2nd ed. Philadelphia, PA: WB Saunders; 1995:354, 356.
11. Daube-Witherspoon ME, Karp JS, Casey ME, et al. PET performance measurements using the NEMA NU 2-2001 standard. *J Nucl Med*. 2002;43:1398–1409.
12. Bailey DL, Meikle SR, Jones T. Effective sensitivity in 3D PET: the impact of detector dead time on 3D system performance. *IEEE Trans Nucl Sci*. 1997; NS-44:1180–1185.
13. Society of Nuclear Medicine. *PET Learning Center Notebook for Technologist Attendees*; Reston, VA: Author; 2004:Sec.7.
14. Lodge MA, Chaudhry MA, Udall DN, Wahl RL. Characterization of a perirectal artifact in 18F-FDG PET/CT. *J Nucl Med*. 2010;51:1501–1506.
15. Soret M, Bacharach SL, Buvat I. Partial-volume effect in PET tumor imaging. *J Nucl Med*. 2007;48:932–945.

Additional Resources

Christian PE, Bernier DR, Langan JK. *Nuclear Medicine and PET: Technology and Techniques*. 5th ed. St. Louis, MO: Mosby; 2004: Chapter 10.

Daube-Witherspoon ME. (June 21, 2004). *Routine QA of Dedicated PET Systems*. Paper presented at the 51st Annual Meeting of the Society of Nuclear Medicine, Philadelphia, PA.

Daube-Witherspoon ME, Karp JS, Casey ME et al. PET performance measurements using the NEMA NU 2-2001 standard. *J Nucl Med*. 2002;43:1398–1409.

National Electrical Manufacturers Association. *NEMA Standards Publication NU 2-2007: Performance Measurements of Positron Emission Tomographs*. Rosslyn, VA: Author; 2007.

Society of Nuclear Medicine. *PET Learning Center Notebook for Technologist Attendees*; 2004: Sec. 7.

Valk PE, Bailey DL, Townsend DW, Maisey MN. *Positron Emission Tomography: Basic Science and Clinical Practice*. London: Springer; 2003: Chapters 3, 5, 23.

Wagner HN, Szabo Z, Buchanan JW. *Principles of Nuclear Medicine*. 2nd ed. Philadelphia, PA: WB Saunders; 1995: Chapter 19.

Zanzonico P. Routine quality control of clinical nuclear medicine instrumentation: a brief review. *J Nucl Med*. 2008;49:1114–1131.

CHAPTER 18

Computed Tomography and Its Application to Nuclear Medicine

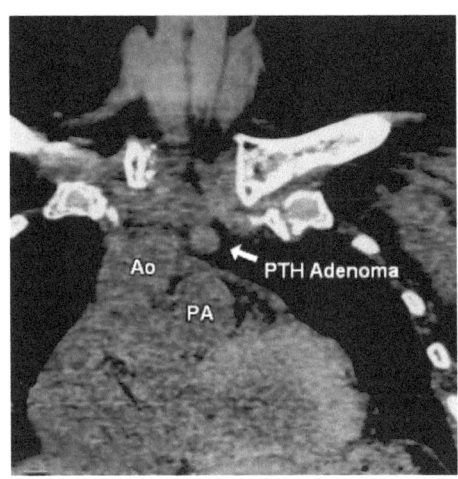

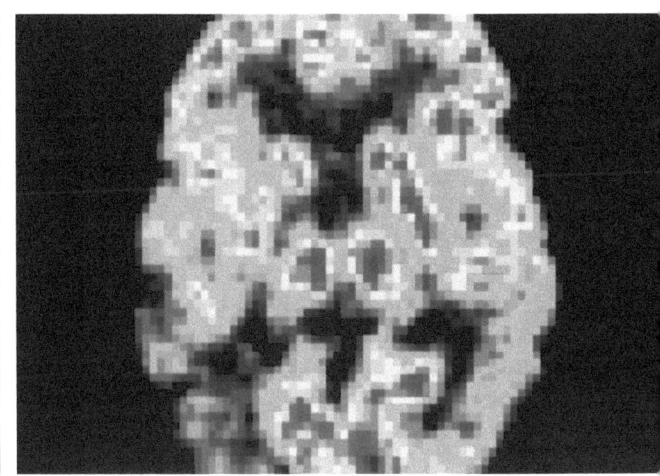

Learning Outcomes

1. Describe the production of x-rays in an x-ray tube and the resulting x-ray energy spectrum.
2. Diagram the essential parts of a computed tomography gantry, and state the purpose of the x-ray tube, filter, collimators, and detectors; discuss the operation of a multislice detector array.
3. Describe data acquisition in CT, including the concepts of helical scanning, pitch, and interpolation.
4. Explain how tissue attenuation coefficients and CT numbers are determined, and give approximate CT number ranges for air, soft tissue, and bone.
5. Outline the principles of image display in CT, particularly the need for different window-level combinations.
6. List the daily quality control (QC) procedures needed for a CT tomograph.
7. Discuss factors that affect image quality in CT.
8. Define the $CTDI_{100}$ and discuss ways that patient dose from a CT study can be decreased.
9. Discuss radiation protection methods used in CT.
10. List the steps in a PET/CT study in order of occurrence.
11. Discuss technical and regulatory issues involved in combining PET and CT.

Introduction

Nuclear medicine has flourished as a diagnostic imaging modality, because it does so well at demonstrating physiology. But its relative lack of anatomic information in many studies is an impediment. Identifying the location of a solitary area of increased activity on a nuclear medicine study, and correlating to separately acquired anatomic images such as computed tomography (CT) or magnetic resonance imaging (MRI), can be a distinct challenge. PET, with its ability to display metabolic information and quantitative capabilities, is especially in need of direct anatomic correlation.

Radiologists have performed "eyeball fusion" for years, hanging two sets of images side by side on a viewbox and moving back and forth between them. This method of co-registration works reasonably well except in the cases where it is most difficult but also most crucial. Computerized fusion of images acquired on two unconnected systems is complex and time-consuming, and it only works well in the brain (where it will continue to be important as standard databases are applied to various types of nuclear medicine brain imaging). But the best way to do image fusion would be to combine two modalities into one machine. So physical integration of nuclear medicine and x-ray computed tomographs was pursued, for both SPECT (1) and PET (2).

There are a number of significant benefits to the direct co-registration of nuclear medicine and CT images. First

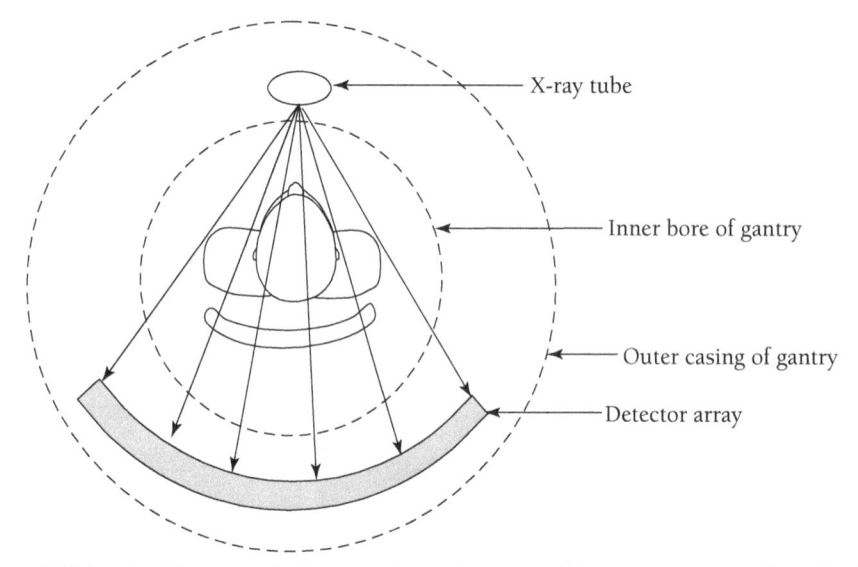

Figure 18-1 Basic geometry of CT imaging. The x-ray tube is on one side, and an array of detectors are on the other side of the patient and imaging table. These rotate together, such that the x-ray beam is always opposite the detector array, as the imaging table moves through the circular gantry. The combination of the two motions results in the tomograph making a spiral or helical path around the patient.

and foremost is anatomic localization; a hot spot on a SPECT or PET study can be directly correlated with an anatomic structure. This greatly enhances the diagnostic credibility of the nuclear medicine study and gives the clinician a more solid basis for considering treatment options. Second, the CT scan can be used for attenuation correction of nuclear medicine images, providing an attenuation map with greatly reduced noise (compared to the very noisy attenuation map generated by a radioactive source). Third, a co-registered PET/CT study is ideal for computer-assisted methodologies in radiation therapy such as *intensity-modulated radiation therapy* (IMRT). This technique uses radiation beams from multiple angles to provide a large dose of radiation to a malignancy while sparing neighboring normal tissues. The addition of physiologic imaging to anatomic information is extremely helpful for radiation therapy planning, especially in areas with tissue changes from prior radiation or surgery.

Computed tomography is considered a modality separate from x-ray, with its own training and certification requirements. CT imaging has many complexities beyond those discussed in this chapter, and this text in no way attempts to provide the nuclear medicine technologist with a complete course in CT. Rather, the goal is to provide an overview of x-ray and CT physics; image acquisition, reconstruction, and display; radiation dosimetry and protection; hybrid SPECT/CT and PET/CT tomographs; and technical and regulatory issues arising from the juxtaposition of the two modalities. The nuclear medicine technologist wishing to become certified in CT is directed toward courses and books designed for that purpose.

Basics of X-Ray and CT

Computed tomography uses x-rays produced in an x-ray tube as the source of photons. The x-ray tube rotates, and x-rays that pass through the patient or object being imaged are registered in solid-state detectors opposite the x-ray tube. The number of x-rays detected, when compared to the number produced, provides a measure of the attenuation that has occurred in the object. The basic concept is illustrated in **Figure 18-1**. By detecting x-rays from many angles around the object and combining them according to Radon's theory, we can create a 3D map of attenuation within the object. Before we discuss the specifics of the CT tomograph, let us look at the basics of x-ray production and detection, the attenuation of x-rays in tissue, and the mathematics of image reconstruction.

Production of X-Rays

X-rays are created in an x-ray tube, shown in **Figure 18-2**. Activation of the cathode filament circuit heats the filament wire due to its electrical resistance, causing it to release electrons by thermionic emission. The electrons are accelerated toward the anode by an electrical potential difference in the range of 50 to 150 kV. A high-frequency generator utilizes transformer technology to create this high potential difference. The accelerated electrons interact in the anode to produce x-rays.

The tungsten anode, due to its high atomic number of 74, is more efficient than most materials at inducing Bremsstrahlung interactions, which in turn produce x-rays. But the great majority of electrons will interact via collisional (ionization and excitation) interactions, which produce heat as a by-product. The target area on the anode (known as the *focal spot*) is very small, on the order of 1.2 mm in diameter, so this heat buildup is significant. Tungsten has an extremely high melting point and accommodates some of the heat internally. To further reduce heat buildup, the disc-shaped tungsten anode is attached to a rotor capable of revolving at a speed of several thousand revolutions per minute; hence a different part of the anode is being exposed each msec. Despite these mitigating factors, buildup of heat energy is the main limitation on

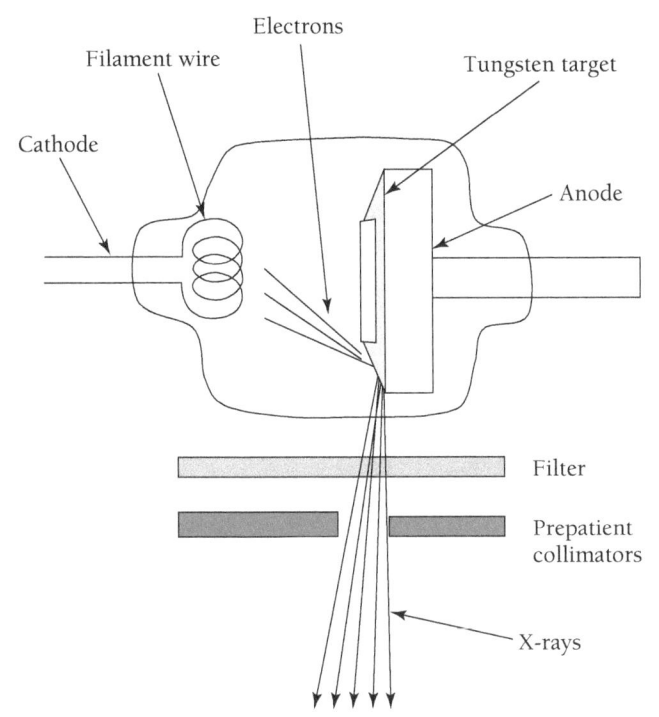

Figure 18-2 X-ray tube. The x-ray tube is an evacuated glass container, inside which a cathode (a heated tungsten filament) produces electrons that are accelerated toward the anode, which has a tungsten target. The electrons interact in the target via Bremsstrahlung and ionization interactions, both of which produce x-rays. Bremsstrahlung interactions produce many low-energy x-rays that do not contribute to the image; the purpose of the filter is to absorb most of these. The collimators absorb wide-angle x-rays so as to produce a compact x-ray beam.

x-ray production, and CT scanners have effective oil- or water-based cooling systems as well as operating protocols that take cooling times into account.

Figure 18-2 shows two additional components found outside the tube that modify the output of the x-ray tube. The *filter* is a low-atomic-number material such as aluminum. It serves to absorb lower-energy x-rays, which will contribute only to the radiation dose received by the patient and not to the image. A *collimator* assembly defines the beam shape (usually fan or cone shape) and protects the patient from excess radiation.

The operator controls the potential difference between the anode and cathode, the cathode filament current, and the time per 360° rotation. The potential difference (usually abbreviated kVp for kilovolt peak) determines the kinetic energy given to the emitted electrons (Eq. B-8), which in turn designates the maximum x-ray energy. The cathode filament current determines the number of electrons released at the cathode and therefore the number of x-rays created (Eq. B-6). It is measured in milliamperes, abbreviated mA. The operator thus controls both the number and the energy of the x-rays used for a radiograph. Typical settings for a CT scan are a kVp of 80 to 150 kV and 50 to 400 mA.

An x-ray tube produces many billions of x-rays per second. For example, a tube operating at 120 kVp and 200 mA produces a radiation exposure rate of about 500 mR/sec at a 50-cm distance, corresponding to approximately 1.2×10^9 x-ray photons/per mm^2/sec (3). A radioactive source producing the same photon flux at the same distance would have an activity of 112,000 Ci. This comparison should help the nuclear medicine technologist to appreciate the radiation levels involved in CT imaging.

The X-Ray Energy Spectrum

As noted, electrons can produce x-rays via ionization and Bremsstrahlung interactions (see Appendix A). *Bremsstrahlung x-rays* are formed when an electron passes close to the atomic nucleus. The electron is decelerated, and the energy lost in the deceleration appears in the form of a photon. Bremsstrahlung x-rays form the broad spread of x-rays seen in the energy spectra of **Figure 18-3**.

Ionization interactions involve an electron ionizing a tungsten atom by removing an atomic electron from an inner-shell orbital. A higher-shell electron in the tungsten atom must then fill the vacant spot in the lower orbital; this transition is accompanied by the release of a photon called a *characteristic x-ray*. In Figure 18-3a, the 69.5- and 57-keV characteristic x-rays of tungsten are seen as straight lines in the idealized energy spectrum.

Figure 18-3a shows that the x-rays produced in an x-ray tube are *polychromatic* (having many different energies), in contrast to the monoenergetic gamma rays used in nuclear medicine. The energy of the polychromatic x-ray beam can be specifically referenced in a couple of ways. The choice of kVp value determines the maximum energy that can be transferred to the x-ray in a Bremsstrahlung interaction, such that the kVp value equals the highest possible x-ray energy in the spectrum, in keV. We can also define the *effective energy* of the polychromatic spectrum as the monoenergetic energy that produces an equivalent half-value layer of aluminum (4). For example, a 120-kVp energy spectrum has a half-value layer of 7.89 mm of aluminum, equal to the half-value layer of a 49.9-keV monoenergetic x-ray. The effective energy of the 120-kVp spectrum is therefore 49.9 keV.

Figure 18-3a shows both filtered and unfiltered energy spectra. In the unfiltered spectrum, the low-energy x-rays are essentially useless, in that they do not have enough energy to pass all the way through the object being imaged. The filter shown in Figure 18-2 absorbs these x-rays and produces an energy spectrum that contains mostly higher-energy x-rays and is therefore suitable for imaging, with a lower limit of about 10 keV (5). Depending on the amount of filtration employed, the highest point in the x-ray energy spectrum occurs between one-third and one-half of the maximum x-ray energy.

Figures 18-3b and 18-3c show the effect of changing the kVp and mA, respectively. A higher kVp stretches the energy spectrum to the right by generating more higher-energy x-rays. A higher mA value increases the number of x-rays at each energy level, but does not affect their energy distribution. These figures also show a more realistic energy spectrum, as opposed to the idealized spectrum in Figure 18-3a.

While it is important to recognize the reason the x-ray spectrum is shaped the way it is, it is also important to

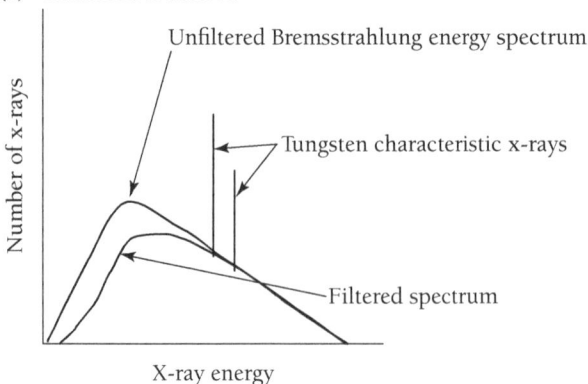

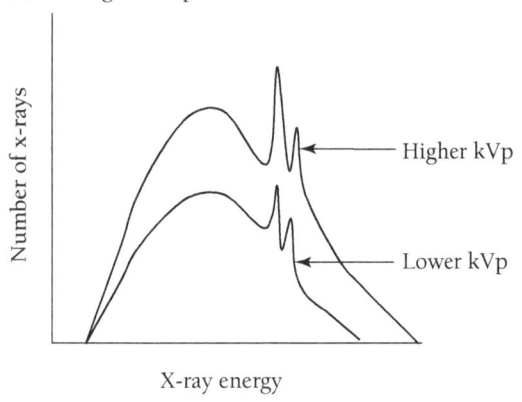

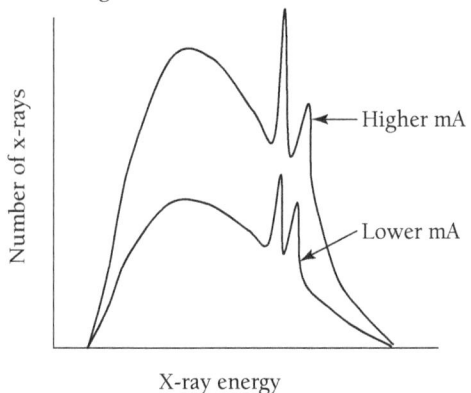

Figure 18-3 X-ray tube energy spectra. Bremsstrahlung interactions produce x-rays with a range of energies, from very low up to a maximum that is determined by the potential difference between the anode and cathode (the kVp value). Characteristic x-rays, the result of ionization interactions, are monoenergetic, producing sharp peaks (shown as idealized straight lines in Fig. 18-3a and as wider, more realistic peaks in Figs. 18-3b and 18-3c). Figure 18-3a shows the original Bremsstrahlung spectrum and the filtered spectrum. Some absorption of low-energy x-rays occurs in the glass envelope of the x-ray tube, but most occurs in the filter located just beyond the x-ray tube. Figure 18-3b demonstrates the effect of changing the kVp value; a higher kVp produces a Bremsstrahlung spectrum that ranges to a higher value. The tube current in mA determines the number of electrons released from the cathode and therefore the number of x-rays produced (Fig. 18-3c).

recognize that the spectrum represents only a small fraction of the electrons released from the filament. Only about 0.5% of the electron interactions produce Bremsstrahlung x-rays, and an even smaller number produce characteristic x-rays. More than 99% are simply absorbed in the anode in collision interactions, producing only heat and necessitating the need for cooling.

X-Ray Detection

The CT portion of a commercial PET/CT tomograph uses a scintillating material to detect radiation, usually either a ceramic material or cadmium tungstate ($CdWO_4$). The latter has very high density and a long decay time, which would seem to be a disadvantage. But CT is performed in current mode, so the long decay time is not consequential. The detectors are on the order of 0.5 to 1 mm on a side and are grouped together in large arrays. For example, a detector module might be a 16 × 16 square array of solid-state detectors, and 48 modules might be lined up circumferentially in the CT gantry, for a total of 12,288 detectors. The 16 rows of detectors in the axial direction would make this a "16-slice" CT tomograph. Different manufacturers have a variety of methods to produce different slice thicknesses, given a defined array of detectors; these details are beyond the scope of this text. Some tomographs have septa to absorb scattered x-rays. These are similar to those found in a 2D-mode PET tomograph, but oriented in the axial direction rather than circumferentially as in PET.

A photodiode takes the place of a photomultiplier tube (PMT) to convert scintillation light into an electronic signal. Photodiodes are smaller and less expensive than PMTs. They are more subject to electrical noise (5), do not amplify the signal created in response to the radiation as much as PMTs do, and are therefore not usable in most nuclear medicine applications. In CT, on the other hand, the large number of x-rays generated eliminates both of these concerns.

Tissue Attenuation

What happens between the production and the detection of the x-rays, namely, attenuation by the object, is what makes the CT image. The differential absorption of x-rays by bone, various types of soft tissue, and air results in varying numbers of x-rays passing through the object (**Figure 18-4**). The tissues in line with the x-ray beam determine the degree of attenuation of the beam. This is the basis for all x-ray imaging. The advantage of CT over plain-film x-rays is that reconstruction provides a means for 3D localization of linear attenuation coefficients, based on the measured attenuation from multiple angles. The resulting 3D image matrix therefore consists of the attenuation coefficients of each small volume of tissue.

Image Reconstruction

Three-dimensional reconstruction of an object imaged with a CT tomograph is based on the attenuation equation

$$I(x) = I(0)\, e^{-\mu_{tot} x} \tag{18-1}$$

(a) Linear attenuation coefficients vs energy

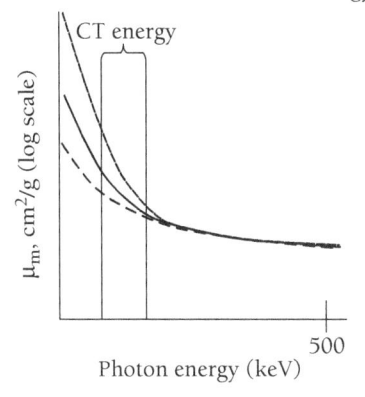

(b) Percentage of x-rays absorbed vs energy

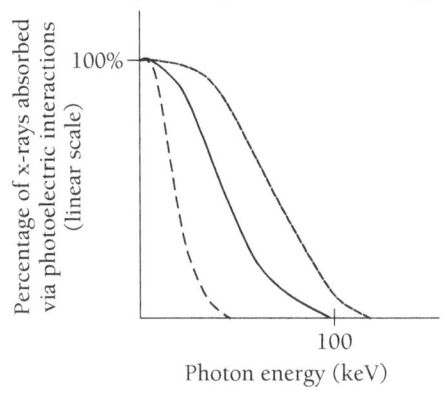

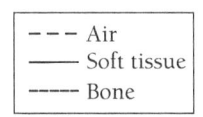

--- Air
— Soft tissue
----- Bone

Figure 18-4 Differential absorption of x-rays by tissue type, as a function of energy. The basis of all x-ray imaging is that different types of tissues absorb different fractions of an x-ray beam, and that this differential absorption is a function of x-ray energy. For biologic tissues, all of the attenuation coefficients converge at about 150 keV. Therefore, attenuation at CT x-ray energies is not linearly related to attenuation at 511 keV. Figure 18-4b shows the same relationship in a different way, specifically in terms of photoelectric interactions.

where $I(0)$ is the intensity of the unattenuated x-ray beam, $I(x)$ is the intensity of the attenuated x-ray beam (i.e., after going through the object), x is the thickness of the object, and μ_{tot} is the total attenuation occurring in the object. While the attenuation equation itself is familiar to us, in CT there are two important sources of complexity. The first is that the equation assumes a homogeneous photon beam, whereas the actual x-ray spectrum is polychromatic. This problem is solved by taking the $I(0)$ and $I(x)$ values to be equal to the numbers of x-rays detected.

The second complication is that if the object is a patient, then the different tissues attenuate different amounts of the x-ray beam. It is precisely this complexity that is the objective of CT imaging. We can envision the x-ray beam traveling through many small cubes of tissue within the object, each small cube with its own μ value. Thus the attenuation equation can be rewritten as

$$I(x) = I(0)e^{-(\mu_1 \Delta x)(\mu_2 \Delta x)(\mu_3 \Delta x)(\mu_4 \Delta x)...} \quad (18\text{-}2)$$

where Δx represents a short distance traveled by the x-ray beam. Thus x in Equation 18-1 is the sum of all the Δx's and μ_{tot} is the sum of all the μ values. In CT, the x-ray tube and detectors rotate around the patient, generating many $I(x)$ values. The goal of CT is to determine the individual μ values, by obtaining many measurements of μ_{tot} and reconstructing those values into a 3D image matrix.

Practical Aspects of CT Acquisition, Reconstruction, and Display

Instrumentation for CT has gone through a number of changes since its invention in 1972. These refinements have significantly improved image quality even as they have greatly decreased imaging time, from 4.5 min per slice with the original EMI Mark I tomograph to less than 1 sec per slice in new-generation helical-motion tomographs. There has been debate about the quality required in the CT portion of a hybrid machine, and some SPECT/CT hybrids employ CT tomographs with less than diagnostic quality (although the trend is toward incorporation of higher-end CT systems). The great majority of PET/CT sales have high-end, multislice CT tomographs that can perform diagnostic-quality CT studies. It would appear at this juncture that the future lies in the direction of hybrid tomographs that incorporate a high-quality, recent-generation CT tomograph.

CT Gantry

The CT gantry consists of an x-ray tube and an array of individual detectors aligned opposite the tube (**Figure 18-5a**). The whole assembly is able to rotate rapidly and continuously, thanks to slip-ring technology developed in the 1990s. A reference detector sits just beyond the pre-patient collimators and provides a measurement of $I(0)$; this measurement is called the *reference beam*. The *rotation time* is the time required for the whole assembly to rotate 360°. Modern systems have rotation times of less than 1 sec. The gantry surrounds an imaging table, which is allowed to slide through the gantry; its direction of movement defines the Z-axis. The other important directional term is the *circumferential direction*, which describes a circle around the Z-axis. The x-ray tube and detectors rotate in the circumferential direction.

A complete orbit of the x-ray tube/detector assembly is broken up into approximately 1,000 *views*, each view consisting of a parallel set of rays at a given angle. The number of rays (analogous to ray-sums in SPECT) is equal to the number of individual detectors in the circumferential direction of the detector array. To be parallel, the rays in a given view must each arise from a different position of the x-ray tube. These can be displayed in a sinogram form similar to that for PET (Fig. 18-5c); each complete rotation has a sinogram for each row of detectors.

The basic assumption of the filtered backprojection (FBP) reconstruction algorithm is that all of the image data being collected are from the same transaxial plane of tissue. A single-slice CT tomograph, with only a single row of detectors, meets this criterion by utilizing an x-ray

(a) Schematic of CT gantry

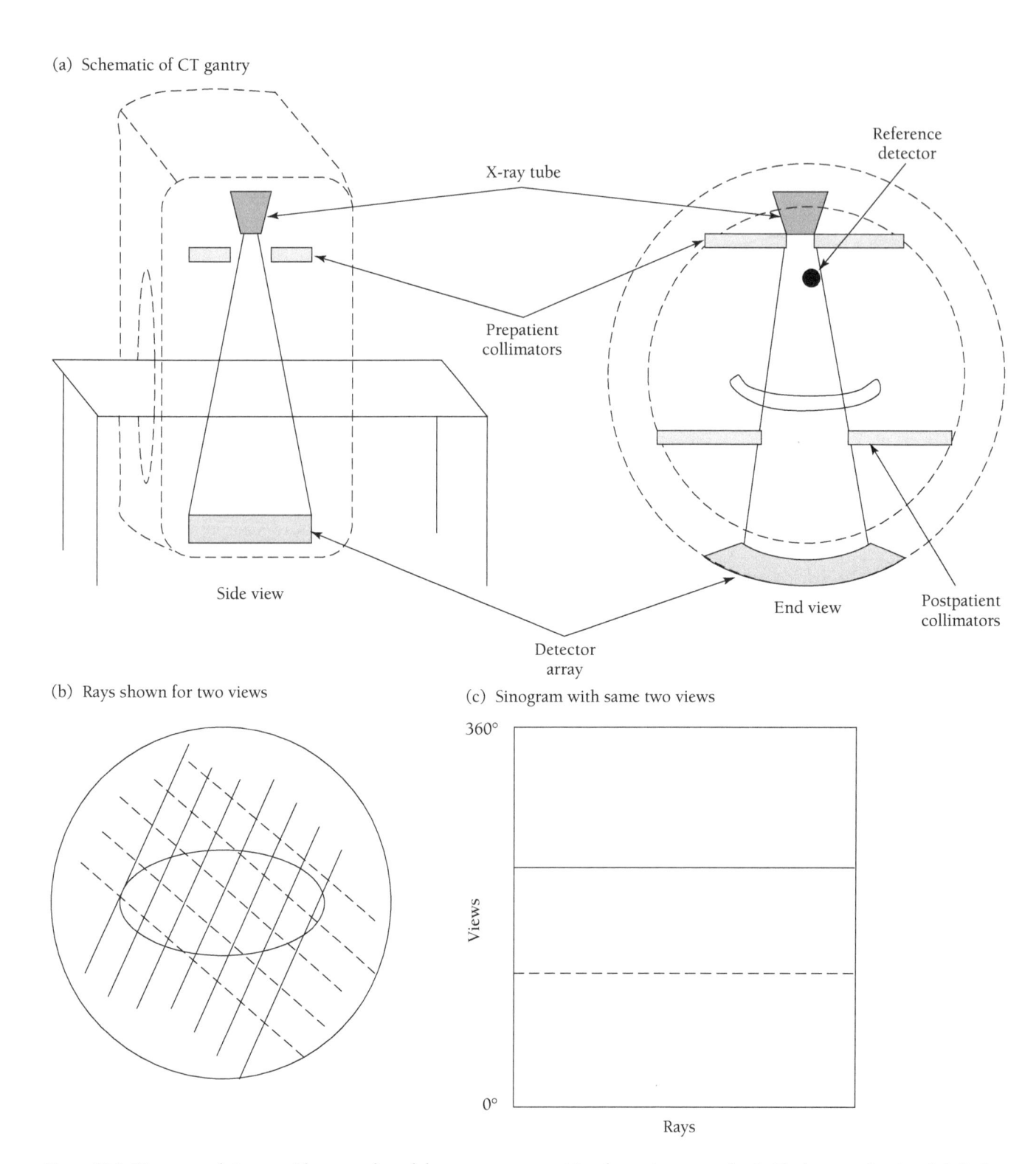

(b) Rays shown for two views

(c) Sinogram with same two views

Figure 18-5 CT gantry and sinogram. The x-ray tube and detector arrays are positioned opposite one another inside the gantry housing. In helical CT, the gantry rotates continuously as the imaging table moves. A single 360° rotation is separated into approximately 1,000 views, each of which is represented by a single horizontal line of the sinogram (Fig. 18-5c). A view consists of x-rays traveling at a particular angle relative to the gantry axis, analogous to a projection in SPECT (Fig. 18-5b). The X-axis of the sinogram represents the individual detectors in the circumferential direction. One sinogram represents one rotation of the gantry as viewed by a single row of detectors; for a 16-slice CT tomograph, 16 sinograms are needed to contain the raw data from one rotation.

beam in the shape of a fan that is as wide circumferentially as the row of detectors and is one slice thick. Once the detector array is widened to include multiple rows, the x-ray fan beam needs to widen in the Z direction, in order to irradiate the entire array. This is called *cone-beam geometry*. The increase in the beam divergence means that different parts of the beam are irradiating different planes of tissue, which in turn requires some modifications of the reconstruction algorithms. (The helical path of the x-ray tube around the patient requires that the acquired data be interpolated to generate information in transaxial slices, as discussed below.)

Between the x-ray tube and the detector array there are three entities designed to ensure that the x-rays are put to maximal effect. The filter absorbs low-energy x-rays that will not contribute to the image, but will only be absorbed in the patient. A bow-tie shaped filter that is thicker on the circumferential edges of the x-ray beam is used (**Figure 18-6**). It decreases the beam intensity where the x-rays will have a shorter path through the patient. *Prepatient collimators* shape the x-ray beam so that its intensity will be constant (except for absorption in the patient) at the detector array.

Postpatient collimators (Fig. 18-5a) sit between the patient and the detectors. These serve to absorb scattered gamma rays that would otherwise reduce the contrast in the image. They also determine the thickness of each slice in single-slice CT; in multidetector CT, the slice thickness also depends on the number of detector rows, the pitch (see definition in next section), and the reconstruction filter used (6). Slice thickness is an important determinant of image quality. Small objects can only be visualized with thin slices, but thin collimation limits the number of x-rays and therefore creates noisier images (7). Slice thickness thus involves a trade-off similar to that between resolution and sensitivity in gamma camera collimators.

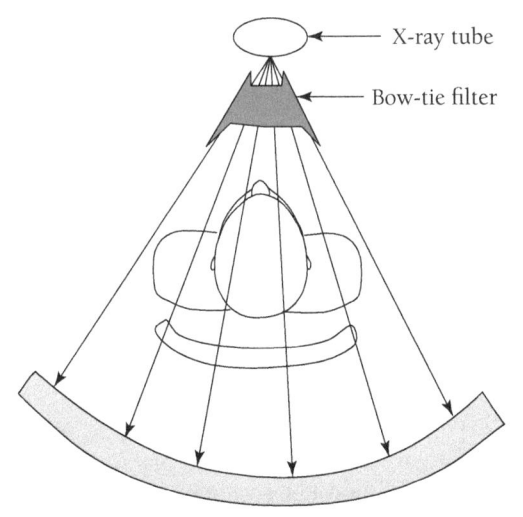

Figure 18-6 Bow-tie filter. This filter, made of aluminum or Teflon®, absorbs the low-energy x-rays that will not reach the detectors. It is thicker at the lateral edges of the x-ray beam, because this part of the beam will traverse much less thickness through the patient compared to other parts of the x-ray beam. The radiation dose to the lateral parts of the patient is therefore decreased to be approximately equal to that in the middle of the body.

The *data acquisition system* (DAS) transmits data from the detectors to the computer. Each slice needs its own DAS channel, and each individual detector has an input into the DAS. The radiation intensity measured at each detector is amplified, converted into logarithmic values, and sent to an analog-to-digital converter (ADC). The ADC has at least 12 bits, allowing for 4,096 digital values; modern CT tomographs often have 16-bit ADCs. The resulting ADC output values are transmitted to a computer using *optoelectronic data transmission*. This involves the use of lenses and light diodes, and it allows for data transmission at rates of 50 million bits per second.

Pitch

In modern CT tomographs, called spiral or helical CT systems, the imaging table and gantry move at the same time, resulting in the gantry tracing a *helical* path around the patient (**Figure 18-7**). In single-slice helical CT, the relationship between table speed and gantry rotation is referred to as the *collimator pitch*:

$$\text{Collimator pitch} = \frac{\text{table movement (mm) per 360° rotation}}{\text{collimator width (mm)}}. \quad (18\text{-}3)$$

A collimator pitch of 1.0 indicates that the table movement per rotation equals the slice width, producing contiguous slices. But we don't necessarily need contiguous slices; Figure 18-7b shows what happens when the pitch is changed. A collimator pitch of 2.0 implies that the table moves 2 mm for every 1 mm of detector width, such that only one-half of the object is directly imaged. The data for each desired transaxial slice are interpolated from the helical data, and this can be accomplished even if the pitch is greater than 1 (Fig. 18-7c). A collimator pitch of less than 1 indicates an overlap of rotations.

In multislice CT tomographs, the definition of pitch is complicated by the fact that each rotation produces multiple slices of information. The accepted terminology

---

Sample Calculation 18-1   Pitch in a Multidetector CT Tomograph

A CT tomograph is a 16-slice scanner, with 0.5-mm-wide detectors. The table is moving at a speed of 16 mm per rotation. What is the pitch?

According to Equation 18-4,

$$\text{Pitch} = \frac{16 \text{ mm}}{(16 \text{ slices})(0.5 \text{ mm/slice})} = 2.$$

The pitch of 2 indicates that only one-half of the tissue is actually being irradiated. We can also see this result when we realize that the sixteen 0.5-mm detectors measure a total width of 8 mm. When compared to the 16-mm table speed, it is clear that only one-half of the tissue is intercepted by x-rays in each rotation.

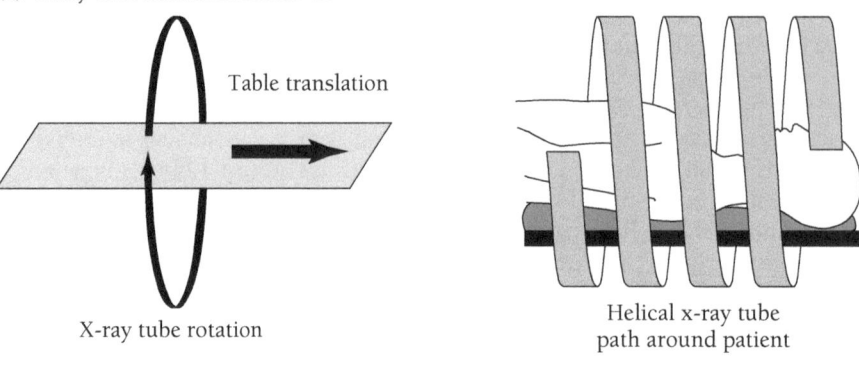

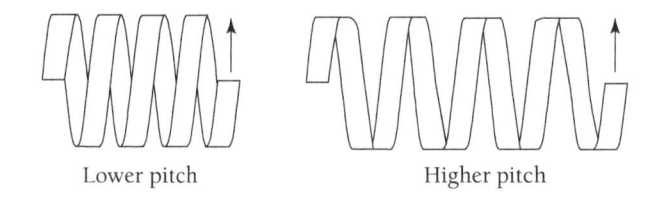

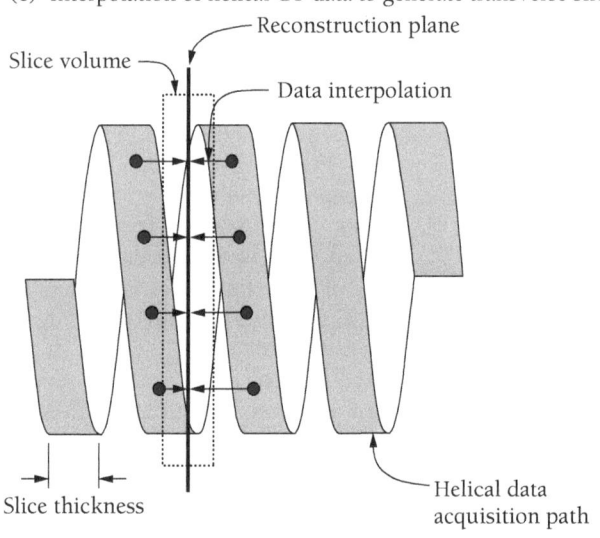

Figure 18-7 Pitch and slice interpolation. Helical motion allows CT scans to be completed in a very short time (Fig. 18-7a). The pitch describes the relative motion of the table and the rotating gantry; a higher pitch indicates greater table motion per rotation and therefore more widely spaced x-ray information (Fig. 18-7b). A transverse slice is created from interpolation of the helical passes on either side of the slice, such that each data point in the helical sinogram is added to the slice data weighted by its proximity to the slice location (Fig. 18-7c). Multiple slices can be interpolated between two helical rotations by using appropriate weighting factors. Reprinted from: Bushberg JT, Seibert JA, Leidholdt EM, Boone JM. *The Essential Physics of Medical Imaging*. 2nd ed. Philadelphia, PA: Lippincott Williams and Wilkins; 2002:338, 350. With permission from Lippincott Williams & Wilkins and Dr. Bushberg.

for pitch (sometimes called *beam pitch*) presents the equation as

$$\text{Pitch} = \frac{\text{table movement per rotation (mm)}}{(\text{number of slices})(\text{slice width [mm]})}. \quad (18\text{-}4)$$

Increasing the pitch decreases the number of views per linear scan distance, which in turn decreases radiation exposure. However, more noise is a consequence of increasing the pitch, so there is again a trade-off between exposure reduction and image quality.

Image Acquisition

A number of image acquisition protocols are used in CT, depending on the area of the body being imaged, the desired information, and several other factors. In non-PET diagnostic CT, each study of a specific part of the body has its own parameters. For example, a chest CT is started soon after the injection of intravenous (IV) contrast, employs a relatively low mA setting because of the low-density lung tissue, and needs a small slice thickness to resolve small lesions. An abdominal CT study needs thicker slices, higher mA, and/or higher kVp, and it is timed to coincide with the IV contrast reaching either the arterial or the venous system in the abdomen. A PET/CT study, in contrast, requires a continuous technique for the entire CT scan.

A CT acquisition commonly proceeds in the following order (this protocol assumes the administration of both oral and IV contrast, which are not used in all cases):

- The patient is interviewed, proper preparation is verified, and contraindications to IV contrast are checked (if appropriate for the study). An IV catheter is placed.
- Patient drinks 2 liters of dilute barium-based oral contrast over 1 hr. Water can also be used to provide contrast for the gastrointestinal tract.
- With the patient positioned on the imaging table, a 2D x-ray called a *topogram* or *scout scan* is acquired. In this scan, the gantry does not rotate; the x-ray tube is stationary above the patient, the detectors are below, and the table moves through the gantry with the x-ray beam on. The topogram provides an anatomical map from which the CT scan is planned.
- If IV contrast is to be administered, a test injection is given to measure the transit time of a contrast bolus from the IV site to the area of interest.
- The IV contrast is administered via a high-pressure injector (for example, 100–200 ml of contrast injected at 1.5–5 ml/min, per Reference 8).
- The CT acquisition is timed to start as the bolus reaches the aorta (or other vessel depending on the part of the body being imaged) and proceeds from superior to inferior. The entire acquisition takes only a few minutes at most. The patient may be asked to hold his or her breath during parts of the acquisition.

Many variations and alternative acquisition protocols are possible. But this outline will generally be followed for PET/CT scanning.

The choice of kVp, mA, time per rotation, table speed, and slice thickness is typically included in the acquisition protocol, and the effects of changing each are considered in **Table 18-1**. The kVp value is usually not changed, but may be modified in particular situations (e.g., for pediatric patients). More commonly, the mA value is adjusted for individual patients. For example, a very large patient might require an increase in mA to obtain a study of adequate quality. The number of x-rays is primarily determined by the mA and the rotation time; more x-rays mean better signal-to-noise characteristics, so a higher mA value is preferred when contrast resolution needs to be maximized. Some CT tomographs will recommend a current setting based on patient characteristics as measured in the topogram. Others allow the mA to be modulated automatically during an acquisition, so that more x-rays are only generated at the thicker parts of the body where they are needed (see radiation dosimetry section).

Image Preprocessing and Reconstruction

The data from the acquisition exist in raw form as a series of sinograms (Fig. 18-5c), but processing begins immediately. First, a calibration correction for the gains and geometric efficiencies of the different detectors is performed, based on an air scan quality control test (similar to the normalization scan in PET). Then the logarithm of each ray is determined from

$$\ln \frac{I(0)}{I(x)} = \mu_{tot} x \qquad (18\text{-}5)$$

where $I(0)$ is the beam strength (number of x-rays detected) in the reference x-ray beam, $I(x)$ is the beam strength through the object, x is the object thickness, and μ_{tot} is the total attenuation along the ray. The final preprocessing step is to interpolate the helical data into true transverse slices. Given that the transverse slices are based on interpolated data, they may be reconstructed to any desired thickness (7).

Next, an image matrix is created for reconstruction. Matrix dimensions in CT range from 340 × 340 to 1,024 × 1,024. A zoom factor can be included by choosing a smaller reconstruction diameter than the FOV. For PET/CT, it is important that the reconstruction diameter include the entire body, because otherwise the attenuation correction factors will not include all of the attenuating tissues. Table 18-1 considers reconstruction choices as well as acquisition parameters.

Image reconstruction in CT is based on the concept that the right side of Equation 18-5 is really the sum of tissue attenuations in each increment of tissue within the object:

$$\mu_{tot} x = \mu_1 \Delta x + \mu_2 \Delta x + \mu_3 \Delta x + \ldots + \mu_n \Delta x \qquad (18\text{-}6)$$

where $\mu_1, \mu_2, \ldots \mu_n$ represent the attenuation in each increment of tissue and Δx is the thickness of the increments. This statement of the reconstruction problem is then solvable using Radon's theory.

The most common reconstruction algorithm applied to CT is FBP using a ramp filter and either a Shepp–Logan or a Hamming filter (**Figure 18-8**). The Shepp–Logan filter cuts off sharply at the Nyquist frequency, which contradicts the requirement in SPECT that the filter roll off to zero amplitude. There are two reasons that the sharp cutoff can be used in CT. First, a CT scan uses many, many x-rays to create the 3D image matrix, and therefore it has virtually no noise. Consequently, a filter can apply a large amplitude to high-frequency components of the data, because these components represent true object data.

Second, a sharply cut-off filter should produce a ringing artifact. This artifact produces an overshoot that accentuates the boundary between bone and soft tissue, and the Shepp–Logan filter is specifically used to enhance the edges of bony structures. Soft tissue, because it has less contrast in density between different tissue types, needs a band-pass filter such as the Hamming. Filters may also

Table 18-1

Acquisition and Reconstruction Parameters in CT

	Range	Effect of Increasing	Benefits	Drawbacks
X-Ray Beam kVp	30–150 kV	Increases energy of x-rays, also produces more x-rays	• Greater penetration of object • Decrease in noise • Fewer beam-hardening artifacts	• Higher dose to patient • Reduction in tissue attenuation differences
mA	50–400 mA	Produces more x-rays	• Decrease in noise • Increase in contrast resolution	• Higher radiation dose to patient
Detectors Slice thickness	0.5–10 mm	More tissue is imaged in one rotation	• Decreased noise • Decreased imaging time	• More volume averaging • Degraded resolution
Gantry Rotation speed	0.3–1.0 sec	Faster rotation time	• Less possibility of patient motion • Lower patient radiation dose	• Reduced contrast resolution
Table motion	5–20 mm/sec	Greater table movement per rotation, larger pitch	• Decrease in scan time	• Not all parts of the area of interest are imaged directly
Reconstruction Reconstruction matrix	340 × 340–1,024 × 1,024	(e.g., 512 × 512 → 1,024 × 1,024) Smaller pixels in each transverse slice	• Improved spatial resolution	• Increased noise • Greater storage space required
Reconstruction FOV		Reconstruct a larger volume within the gantry	• Includes entire body in CT reconstruction (necessary for attenuation correction)	• Each pixel represents a larger area; less detail seen
Reconstruction kernel		(e.g., increasing the sharpness of the cutoff frequency) Reconstruction includes more high-frequency details	• Greater image detail, less smoothing	• Can accentuate statistical variabilities into appearing as real structures • Ringing artifacts

Christian PE, Waterstram-Rich KM. *Nuclear Medicine and PET/CT: Technology and Techniques.* 6th ed. St. Louis, MO: Mosby-Year Book; 2007:Chapter 11.
Seeram E. *Computed Tomography: Physical Principles, Clinical Applications, and Quality Control.* 3rd ed. Philadelphia, PA: WB Saunders; 2009:Chapter 9.

vary depending on the type of information needed, especially whether spatial resolution or contrast resolution (the ability to distinguish subtle differences in image contrast) is more important. For metastatic disease surveys, where contrast resolution needs to be high, a "softer" filter may be used.

CT Numbers

The tissue attenuation values of each voxel are expressed in *Hounsfield units* (HU)

$$HU_{ij} = 1{,}000 \times \frac{\mu_{ij} - \mu_{water}}{\mu_{water}} \tag{18-7}$$

where μ_{ij} is the linear attenuation coefficient of voxel ij and μ_{water} is the linear attenuation coefficient of water (which is about 0.195/cm, depending on the kVp setting) (8). In the 3D image matrix, each voxel is assigned a *CT number*, measured in Hounsfield units, based on that voxel's attenuation. The allowed range for CT numbers in most systems is –1,024 to +3,071, for a total of 4,096 (2^{12}) possibilities (9). **Table 18-2** gives approximate CT numbers for different tissue types. The quantitative nature of CT numbers has diagnostic significance; for example, in evaluating the potential for malignancy in calcified pulmonary nodules or in measuring bone density.

Image Display

The transaxial slices created by the reconstruction process can be stacked and then resliced in orthogonal projections to produce coronal and sagittal images. Orthogonal views have always been available in CT, but only recently have

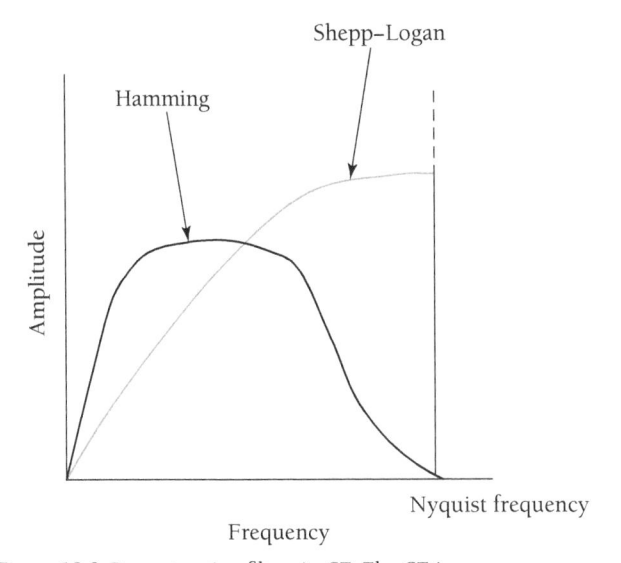

Figure 18-8 Reconstruction filters in CT. The CT images are reconstructed using FBP with a ramp filter combined with either a Hamming or a Shepp–Logan filter. For CT, the Nyquist frequency is determined by the size of the detectors used.

Table 18-2

Range of CT Numbers for Various Tissues and Contrast Agents

Tissue Type	Approximate CT Number (Hounsfield Units)
Air	−1,000
Lung tissue	−850 → −200
Fat	−250 → −30
Soft tissue	−200 → +200
Water	0
Oral contrast	+200 → +800[a]
Iodinated contrast	up to 300
Bone	+300 → +1,000

[a]The CT number of oral contrast increases as the contrast medium transits through the intestines and water is absorbed from it.
Christian PE, Waterstram-Rich KM. *Nuclear Medicine and PET/CT: Technology and Techniques.* 6th ed. St. Louis, MO: Mosby-Year Book; 2007:357.
Kinahan PE, Hasegawa BH, Beyer T. X-ray based attenuation correction for positron emission tomography/computed tomography scanners. *Semin Nucl Med.* 2003;33:166–179.

they been routinely utilized. The quality of the orthogonal views improves as the slice thickness and pitch decrease. Surface- and volume-rendering techniques may also be applied to CT, providing additional ways to visualize internal organs. Surface rendering of vascular contrast in vessels is especially dramatic. Thanks to its very small voxel size (about 1 mm^3), CT is also considered the best way to measure lesion volumes.

There are several differences in CT image display compared to nuclear medicine. One is that CT rarely uses nonlinear gray scales. Another distinction has to do with the range of pixel values employed. Nuclear medicine image display often uses the entire counts/pixel range

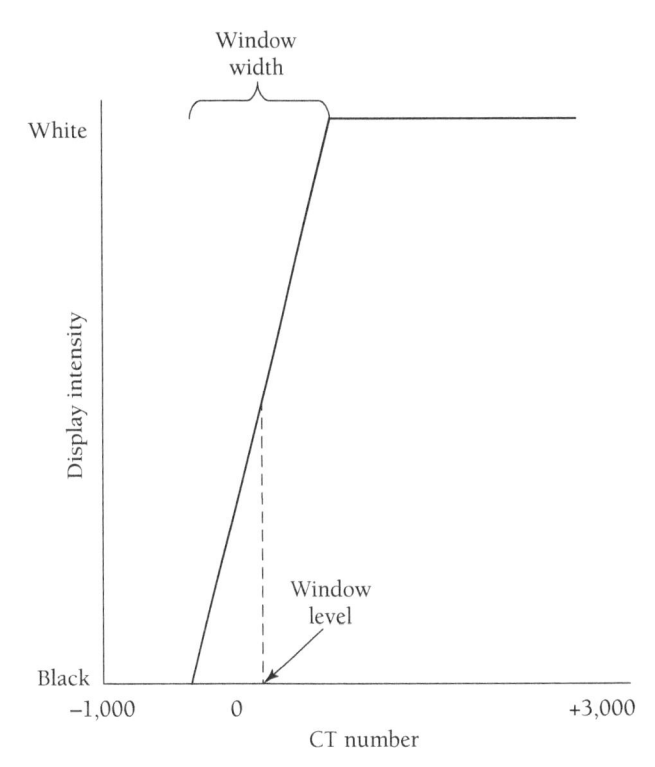

Figure 18-9 Windowing for CT image display. The range of CT numbers within the body far exceeds the ability of the eyes to register levels of a gray scale, so only small portions of the range of possible CT numbers are used. The window level and width are chosen to best demonstrate the anatomy of interest. Most systems have preset window level/width combinations to visualize lung vs soft tissue vs bone (see Table 18-3).

present in the image. This is reasonable because at most a few hundred different levels are required. In CT, on the other hand, the range of possible CT numbers is more than 4,000, as noted above, and if all were displayed, the contrast in clinically significant areas would be too small to be appreciable. So instead, a smaller range of CT numbers are singled out from the entire range of CT numbers and applied to a 256-level gray scale.

The appearance of CT images thus depends on the window and level set by the user. As shown in **Figure 18-9**, the *window width* is the range of CT numbers assigned to the display intensities, and the *level* is the CT number of the midpoint of the window. A narrower window increases contrast, because the diagonal line becomes steeper. Changing the level accentuates a different set of attenuation coefficients. CT images may be filmed at two or more window/level settings. A lung CT, for example, may be photographed first to show soft tissue, then to show vascular contrast in the lungs. Bones typically appear uniformly white at windows that are appropriate for soft tissues, but their internal anatomy can be demonstrated by setting a bone window. **Table 18-3** shows some sample window settings used in CT.

In the days before picture archiving and workstations, CT studies were filmed at appropriate combinations of window and level settings (usually only one or two for each study), and the reconstructed data were not saved. Now that many radiology departments have the

Table 18-3

Examples of Window/Level Combinations

Tissue Type	Window Level (HU)	Window Width (HU)
Lung	600	1,200
Soft tissue	45	250
Bone	700	600

Christian PE, Waterstram-Rich KM. *Nuclear Medicine and PET/CT: Technology and Techniques*. 6th ed. St. Louis, MO: Mosby-Year Book; 2007:358.

infrastructure to be "filmless," the transverse slices may be saved as digital files. This allows the radiologist to choose an appropriate window/level combination, not just for the study, but for an individual slice, and even for different structures within the slice. Reformatting into orthogonal planes, surface rendering, and so on are done at the workstation, and great savings in terms of film are realized. Filmless radiology is a boon to the CT department, as much as or more so than other modalities within radiology.

Quality Control

CT tomographs, like gamma cameras and PET tomographs, require performance assessment on a regular basis (10). Daily QC tests include warm-up of the x-ray tube; verification of the tube output and detector response at various kVp and mA settings; and evaluations of tomographic uniformity, CT number accuracy, and image noise at clinical scanning parameters. These tests are typically performed on a water-filled cylindrical phantom. Images of the QC phantom should be reconstructed and evaluated visually and quantitatively. Some of the QC requirements will vary depending on the type of CT tomograph being tested (e.g., low level vs high level); as always, manufacturer recommendations should be followed.

Other QC tests are required on a less frequent basis. Reference 10 recommends that the following be evaluated on a monthly or quarterly basis: image slice thickness, spatial resolution, linearity of CT numbers, and contrast resolution in both high-contrast and low-contrast situations. Annual QC should include assessment of the CT dose index (see "Radiation Dosimetry"). Alignment of the lasers between the PET or SPECT and CT tomographs should be verified regularly; this is generally accomplished with markers that are visible in both systems. And last but certainly not least, safety features such as the primary-door interlock (which turns off the x-ray tube if the primary barrier door is opened during an acquisition) should be inspected regularly.

Image Data Management

A single CT scan generates a very large data file. The raw projection data alone require a file size in the gigabyte range (11). The raw data are typically not saved to long-term storage, but are discarded after the study has been reviewed. The final set of reconstructed images for a PET/CT study has a file size of about 500 megabytes, still requiring frequent archiving to free up computer memory. With such large files, data transfer speeds are an important characteristic of the computer system. Throughput issues (simultaneous acquisition and processing, reconstruction speeds, system bandwidth, etc.) need to receive careful attention when installing a PET/CT system.

Image Quality in CT

As we have done with nuclear medicine imaging modalities, we will consider the components of image quality in CT. This text is not intended to be comprehensive, so our consideration will be brief. But even an overview of the factors contributing to image quality will point out the importance of various acquisition parameters (see Table 18-1). This discussion will also illuminate the trade-offs that are made when trying to decrease patient doses, which is discussed in the next section.

Image Contrast

The goal of x-ray imaging is to allow visualization of small differences in attenuation between normal and abnormal tissues. The ability to do this is the major strength of CT: whereas radiographs can only discriminate differences in tissue density of 10% or more, CT can discriminate differences of 0.5% (6). Contrast between two tissues is based primarily on their electron densities, which are in turn usually dependent on their mass densities. In terms of acquisition parameters, image contrast is affected most by the choice of mA, because small differences in density are easily overwhelmed by image noise when too few x-rays are used.

Spatial Resolution

A system's spatial resolution is its ability to resolve closely spaced objects. For CT imaging, spatial resolution is measured using small bar phantoms made of acrylic. Each bar plus its adjoining space is considered a line pair. A series of bar phantoms are imaged, and the system resolution is described as the smallest line pair that can be visualized. Factors affecting spatial resolution include the size and spacing of the detectors and the size of the focal spot (the target on the anode where the electrons interact). The reconstruction matrix and volume to be reconstructed also play a role, based on the sampling theorem. The reconstruction filter strongly influences spatial resolution.

Image Noise

Quantum mottle is the term used in radiography to describe the noise resulting from the finite number of x-rays used to make an exposure. In CT, quantum mottle is directly related to the number of x-rays detected by each detector: fewer x-rays result in greater noise. The variability in measured intensities from one detector to the next is described by Poisson counting statistics. This aspect of image quality is most affected by acquisition parameters.

Any change that results in more x-rays per detector will decrease image noise. Increasing the tube current (mA) or time per rotation will increase the beam intensity proportionally and thus diminish noise. Similarly, increasing the slice thickness decreases noise. So does increasing the kVp, although this may decrease contrast, as higher-energy x-rays are less likely to interact with tissues. A larger value for pitch increases noise, because fewer x-rays are generated per mm of table travel. The reconstruction filter can be chosen to blur out the noise or to accentuate it.

Because noise so profoundly affects image contrast and spatial resolution, the general aim in deciding on acquisition parameters is to reduce noise to the level that allows important pathology to be visualized. But whatever we do to reduce noise will simultaneously increase the radiation dose to the patient, because both are functions of the number of x-rays traversing the body. So there must be a point of compromise between excellent images and appropriate radiation dose. This point will be patient- and organ-system-specific. The goal is always to obtain adequate images at the lowest possible radiation dose.

Artifacts

Many artifacts can occur in CT, only one of which is described here. When a polychromatic x-ray beam passes through an attenuating material, more lower-energy x-rays are absorbed than higher-energy x-rays, an effect called *beam hardening*. The beam on the far side of the absorbing material thus has an energy spectrum that is skewed to the high-energy side. This effect is dependent not only on the composition of the tissue but also on the path of the x-ray beam (8). The bow-tie filter discussed previously provides some initial beam hardening, which removes the low-energy x-rays that would otherwise be absorbed in the patient. But in clinical CT images, bone and metallic objects may cause noticeable beam-hardening artifacts. Beam hardening produces variations in the final image that have to do with the path taken by the x-rays rather than the characteristics of the tissue itself. A beam-hardening correction algorithm is included in CT software, which helps to lessen the artifact, but many beam-hardening artifacts will nonetheless be observed. Beam-hardening artifacts can also generate attenuation correction artifacts in PET/CT scans. The operator of a hybrid tomograph should be aware of the potential for such errors.

Radiation Dosimetry

Sources of radiation exposure in diagnostic x-ray (including CT) include the primary radiation beam, scattered radiation, and leakage radiation from the x-ray tube. Radiation from scatter and leakage are most concerning to the technologist, and they are discussed at the end of this section. The radiation dose received by the patient comes from the primary radiation beam and is determined by the acquisition parameters, in particular the tube current (mA), the time of rotation, and the kVp. Radiation exposure from CT exams has recently been identified as the largest contributor to exposure of all diagnostic radiologic procedures. The dose from CT studies has increased in the last decade due to machines capable of very fast study times and multislice capabilities. Lately, much has been written about the health risk of the radiation dose from CT scans, and dose reduction has become a focus of industry, regulatory, and clinical efforts.

Radiation Dose Parameters

CT dose quantities are measured using two standard acrylic phantoms, a 16-cm-diameter cylinder to approximate the head and a 32-cm-diameter cylinder to approximate the torso. They are 15 cm in length and have a number of holes drilled in the longitudinal or axial direction to allow placement of various radiation detection devices. The holes are located around the outer edge and in the center of each phantom, thus providing for measurement of both peripheral and deep doses.

A pencil ionization chamber is inserted into one of the holes, and the phantom is imaged by a single rotation of the CT scanner. From this scan, a dose profile is generated (**Figure 18-10**). The full width at half-maximum (FWHM), the width of the dose profile at one-half the peak dose, is approximately the same as the slice thickness (12). The graph shows that tissue beyond the slice being imaged gets a significant amount of radiation.

It can be demonstrated that the amount of radiation dose given to other slices from a single rotation exposing a particular slice is reciprocated by the radiation dose received by that slice from other rotations around the phantom (12). Hence, from a single-rotation exposure, we can measure the total dose under the curve in Figure 18-10 and establish that it is equal to the total radiation dose received by that slice of tissue from a complete series of rotations. The total dose is measured using a 100-mm-long pencil ionization chamber inserted into one of the

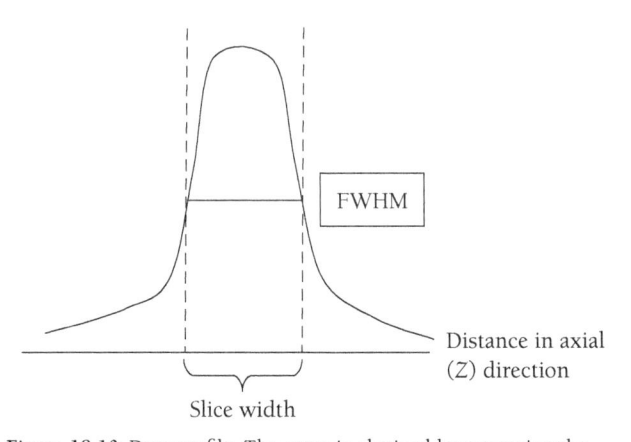

Figure 18-10 Dose profile. The curve is obtained by measuring the exposure from a single rotation around a phantom. The FWHM corresponds to the slice thickness, and the graph shows that there is a significant amount of radiation dose beyond the slice being imaged. The tails on either side of the FWHM, representing the dose given to other slices by this rotation, are matched in this slice by tails from other nearby rotations. Thus, the total area under the dose profile curve is equal to the radiation to this slice from a multirotation acquisition. The area under the curve is typically measured over a length of 100 mm, and it is called the $CTDI_{100}$.

holes of the phantom. The ionization chamber reading in milliroentgens (mR) (or air Kerma, a unit that is the starting point for human radiation exposure calculations) is converted to absorbed-dose units (rad or Gray) and converted from air to the tissue-equivalent value. This number is called the $CTDI_{100}$ (CT dose index over 100 mm), and it is the basic dose quantity used in CT.

The $CTDI_{100}$ represents the cumulative radiation dose to a single slice from a multirotation scan of the phantom (13). From the $CTDI_{100}$ two other measures of dose are derived. The weighted $CTDI_w$ takes into account the fact that in CT imaging, the surface of the body gets about twice as much radiation as the center of the body (13). It weights the measured surface and central values to account for this differential:

$$CTDI_w = \tfrac{1}{3} CTDI_{100, central} + \tfrac{2}{3} CTDI_{w, surface}. \quad (18\text{-}8)$$

The $CTDI_w$ thus represents the average absorbed dose within a central transaxial plane of the phantom, accounting for variation in the X and Y directions (i.e., within a transaxial slice).

The volume expression $CTDI_{vol}$ further accounts for the gaps or overlapping of the x-ray beam from consecutive rotations (i.e., the pitch):

$$CTDI_{vol} = \frac{CTDI_w}{pitch}. \quad (18\text{-}9)$$

It provides an estimate of the average absorbed dose over all three dimensions of space.

Finally the *dose-length product* (DLP) combines the $CTDI_{vol}$ with the scan length to provide an overall measure of total radiation dose from a complete acquisition:

$$DLP = CTDI_{vol} \ (mGy) \times scan\ length\ (cm). \quad (18\text{-}10)$$

It has been demonstrated that the DLP provides a good starting place for calculation of the effective dose, which equates to biological effect (13). The DLP is therefore the best value to use when comparing doses from CT scans to those of other radiologic exams. Most tomographs display the $CTDI_{vol}$ and the DLP for each study.

Sample Calculation 18-2 Dose Quantities in CT

A dose measurement for a CT tomograph produces values of 30 and 16 milligray (mGy) for $CTDI_{100, surface}$ and $CTDI_{100, central}$, respectively, using scan parameters typical for an oncologic PET/CT scan. Calculate $CTDI_w$, $CTDI_{vol}$, and DLP for a pitch of 1.5 and a scan length of 100 cm.

The surface and central dose values are combined in a 2:1 ratio, according to Equation 18-8:

$$CTDI_w = \tfrac{1}{3}(16\ mGy) + \tfrac{2}{3}(30\ mGy) = 25.3\ mGy.$$

The $CTDI_{vol}$ incorporates the pitch:

$$CTDI_{vol} = \frac{25.3\ mGy}{1.5} = 16.9\ mGy.$$

Finally, the DLP incorporates the scan length:

$$DLP = 16.9\ mGy \times 100\ cm = 1{,}690\ mGy.$$

Patient Radiation Doses

The $CTDI_{100}$ and its derived quantities should be measured for each set of imaging parameters used (for example, each combination of kVp, mA, and slice thickness). One might assume that these parameters must be maintained throughout an entire scan, but that is not the case. Since 2001, CT tomographs have employed automatic exposure control principles, which allow the tube current to be varied throughout the course of the scan, in both angular and longitudinal directions. Angular modulation (within the course of a single rotation around the patient) allows the tube current to increase as the x-rays travel through the body from one side to the other, and to decrease when they travel front to back. Longitudinal modulation takes into account the increased thickness of the body in the abdomen and pelvis as well as the decreased absorption of x-rays in the air-filled lungs. The tube current at a given time within the scan is determined by the number of x-rays registered in the corresponding part of the topogram and/or the last rotation. A level of desired image quality, chosen by the operator, determines the number of x-rays needed. Significant reduction in radiation doses can be achieved when tube-current modulation is applied (6).

Radiation dose is higher for CT than for most plain-film radiographic procedures. This is mainly because large mA values are needed to achieve the signal-to-noise ratio that allows this modality to realize such high image quality. CT doses are in the range of 1 to 15 millisieverts (mSv) (0.1–1.5 rem), approximately the same order of magnitude as patient doses from nuclear medicine studies (14). In one study, effective doses from four hospitals were calculated as 5.7 to 7.0 mSv (0.57–0.7 rem) from F-18 fluorodeoxyglucose (FDG) administration and 14.1 to 18.6 mSv (1.41–1.86 rem) from the CT study, with an average total dose (including topogram, CT, and nuclear medicine scans, and in some cases a low-dose CT scan) of about 25 mSv (2.5 rem) (15).

Public Health Concerns

The question of overexposure to individuals as a result of multiple radiologic imaging studies has recently been raised (16). In particular, the number of CT scans being performed annually in the United States has increased by a factor of 20 since 1980, with the largest increases in adult screening and pediatric studies (6–11% of all CT scans). The increase in pediatric scans is of particular concern, both because children are inherently more radiosensitive than adults and because they have many more years of life in which to develop malignancies as a result of radiation exposure. Several scientists have lifted up the value of 50 mSv (5 rem) per year (the value used by the Health Physics Society as an approximate lower threshold for radiation effects) and have pointed out that a patient receiving three or more CT scans in a year will most likely exceed that limit. Moreover, the overall increase in the number of CT scans and nuclear medicine studies performed means that radiation exposure from medical exams should be considered as a public health issue as well as a concern for individual patients.

Several steps have been taken to address this concern. Many radiologists have reconsidered their standard pediatric and/or adult acquisition protocols to ensure that unnecessary radiation exposure is not being incurred. Manufacturers of CT tomographs have reminded users about the dose modulation features mentioned above. While some would argue that the concern about increased public health effects is unwarranted, the controversy has clearly resulted in greater attention being paid to the radiation doses from CT, especially in the pediatric population.

Radiation Protection for the Technologist

The sources of radiation exposure to the operator of a CT tomograph are scattered radiation (due to interactions of x-rays in the patient) and leakage radiation (from the x-ray tube itself). The former is approximately 0.1% of the primary beam exposure at one m from the patient, but may be markedly different for head vs body CT. The leakage radiation is limited by federal regulation to no more than 100 mR/hr at 1-m distance (5). Information about radiation levels at various locations is supplied by the vendor in the form of isocenter lines (**Figure 18-11**). These diagrams and additional calculations are used to determine the appropriate location and shielding needed for the operator workstation (usually called a control room). Scatter and leakage radiation levels are measured annually using a large-volume ionization survey meter (6).

As noted above, the number of x-ray photons generated by a CT tomograph corresponds to radiation exposure levels much higher than those routinely encountered in nuclear medicine. Consequently, issues of radiation safety and radiation protection take on much greater importance. Technologists should be in the control room when the CT portion of a combined exam is being acquired. An "x-ray in use" sign should be lighted whenever the CT x-ray beam is turned on. All personnel need to be cognizant of this sign and avoid the area when it is lighted.

SPECT/CT Systems

Imaging systems consisting of a dual-head gamma camera and a CT tomograph have been commercially available for a longer time than PET/CT systems (1, 2). These systems are used to generate a patient-specific attenuation map, and can be used for anatomic localization as well. All of the major manufacturers of nuclear medicine equipment are producing SPECT/CT systems (**Figure 18-12**). Some

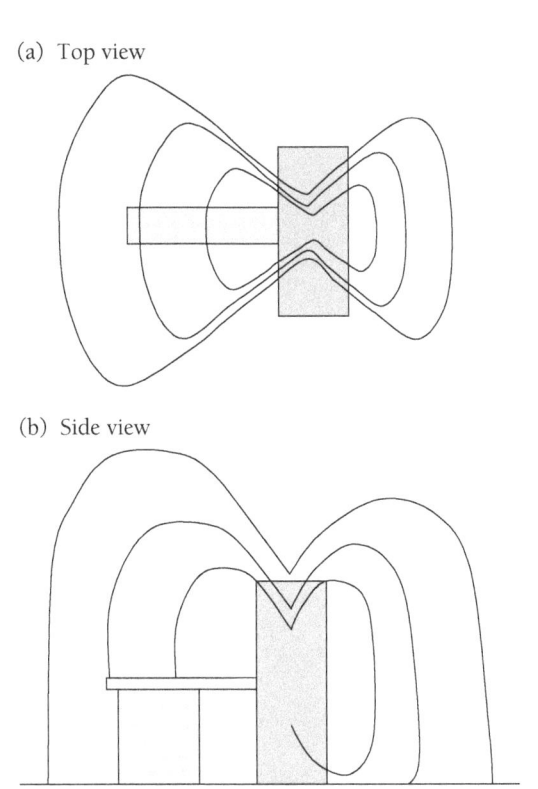

(a) Top view

(b) Side view

Figure 18-11 Isocenter lines showing scatter radiation from a CT tomograph. The manufacturer supplies a diagram that shows lines of equal radiation intensity around the CT gantry. The radiation level at each isocenter line is measured with an ionization survey meter, giving the mR from a single-slice exposure at a given mA. From this information and the expected number of slices to be done per week, one can estimate the total exposure at a given location. Each successive isocenter line (moving from the gantry outward) is a factor of 2 lower than the previous line.

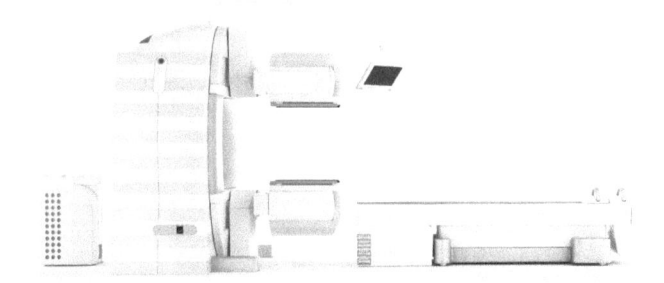

Figure 18-12 Commercial SPECT/CT system. The CT system is contained in the circular gantry at left, and the two gamma camera heads are attached to the front of it. The imaging table extends through the entire system. Photo courtesy of Siemens Healthcare.

of these systems are not capable of diagnostic CT imaging and hence have avoided some of the regulatory issues found in PET/CT. In particular, because of their limited capabilities, such "low-level" SPECT/CT systems may not require CT-certified personnel. The characteristics of one such low-level system will be used to illustrate their operation (17). The kVp and mA are fixed at 140 and 2.5, respectively, and slice collimation is 10 mm. The low value for tube current is what makes this system a low-level CT system. (**Figure 18-13** shows a quality control acquisition using low- and high-mA systems.) The absorbed dose to

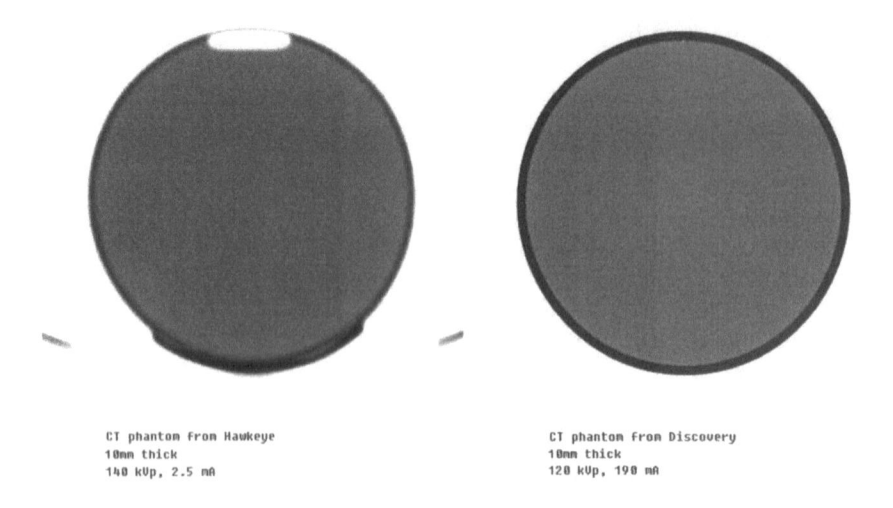

Figure 18-13 Low-mA vs high-mA CT scans. CT phantom images acquired on low-mA and diagnostic CT machines are shown on the left and right, respectively. Notice that the low-mA image shows a less distinct boundary between the edge and the central cavity of the phantom. It is this extra level of information density that a high-mA CT study supplies. On the other hand, if the CT image is to be used only for attenuation correction and anatomic localization, and not as a diagnostic study in its own right, the low-mA version is quite adequate in most cases. Courtesy of Virginia Mason Medical Center.

the patient from a low-level CT is considerably lower than a diagnostic CT (one-fourth or less according to one source [18]).

Even as PET/CT has taken off, SPECT/CT has also grown in popularity, and the CT systems incorporated into SPECT/CT are now commonly able to perform diagnostic-quality imaging. This has in turn led the major manufacturers to explore additional ways to improve SPECT resolution, to more fully take advantage of the anatomic localization capability of the combined-modality tomograph. They have done so primarily by improving attenuation correction, scatter compensation, and depth-dependent resolution recovery algorithms for iterative reconstruction. This effort has been very successful, improving the spatial resolution of a line source from about 10 to about 5 mm (19); two example studies are shown (**Figures 18-14** and **18-15**). We can look for more gamma cameras to be replaced by SPECT/CT systems.

PET/CT Tomographs

PET scans are routinely compared to anatomical imaging studies, usually CT scans. As PET moved into the clinical arena, it became apparent that "eyeball fusion" of PET and CT images was not going to be sufficient for many clinical cases. More exact co-registration was needed. In the late 1990s, efforts were made to incorporate PET and CT tomographs into a single machine, with the goal of providing diagnostic scans in both modalities as well as image fusion of the two studies.

Gantry

A schematic of the result of incorporating PET and CT tomographs is shown in **Figure 18-16a**, and a commercial example is shown in **Figure 18-16b**. Both tomographs are based on commercial models available separately, and only a few modifications are needed to combine them on a single gantry. From the standpoint of the CT capabilities, one of these modifications is significant. Stand-alone CT tomographs have the ability to tilt relative to the Z-axis. This allows the operator to define transverse planes according to anatomic definitions, with the tilt compensating for any irregularity in patient position and avoiding beam-hardening artifacts due to metallic structures such as dental implants. In the hybrid PET/CT tomograph, tilt is generally not allowed. Another issue with the hybrid gantry is its length, often 120 cm or longer. While the gantry bore is wide (60–70 cm in diameter), still many patients will experience claustrophobia. One manufacturer has physically separated the two tomographs with an open space of about 20 cm to alleviate this concern.

Image Acquisition and Display

The current use of hybrid PET/CT systems is almost entirely for oncologic studies with FDG, so we will use that as an example of how the two acquisitions are integrated. This discussion will also assume that both oral and vascular contrast media are administered for the CT scan, although there remains some controversy about the use of contrast for PET/CT (see the next section).

After the patient arrives and all information is verified (including diet prior to the study, patient history, current blood glucose level, and any allergies to contrast), she or he is given an IV catheter, oral contrast to drink, and the FDG injection. When the time for FDG uptake has passed, the patient is positioned on the imaging table and a neck/chest/abdomen/pelvis CT study is acquired. The CT study will be contaminated with 511-keV photons, but their number is overwhelmed by the many x-rays used in the CT scan. Once the CT acquisition is completed, the table

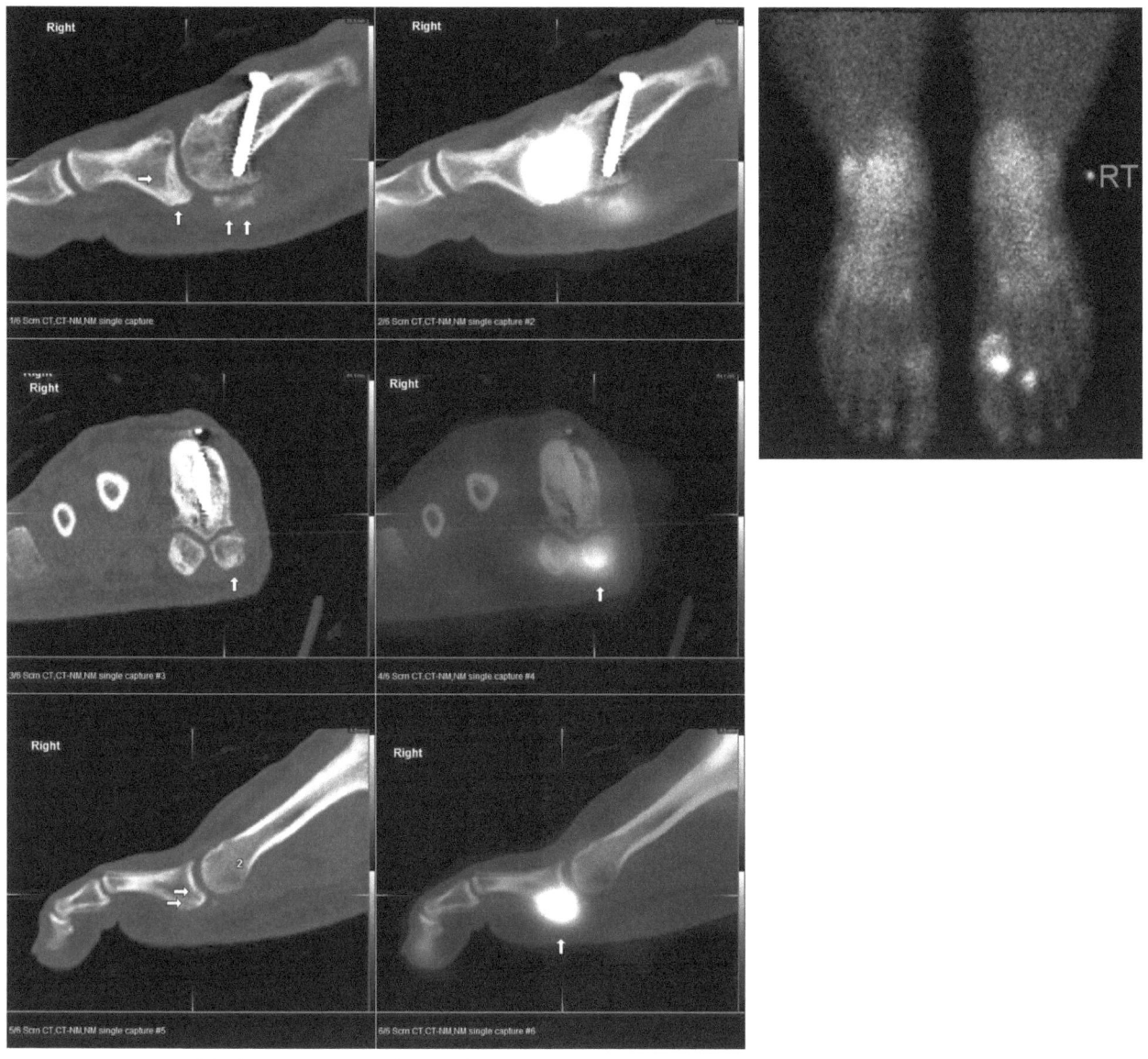

Figure 18-14 SPECT/CT of the foot in a patient with multiple abnormalities. The screw in the first metatarsal is not the cause of this patient's increased uptake on the bone scan (plantar image, upper right). There is increased activity in the first metatarsophalangeal joint and the medial sesamoid, seen in the top (sagittal) and middle (coronal) SPECT/CT images. In addition, an area of increased activity in the proximal phalanx of the second toe is seen on CT to be a nondisplaced fracture (bottom SPECT/CT images with arrows pointing to the fracture). The planar bone image, while showing two areas of increased activity, is not able to identify the exact location of each. (See color plate.) Images courtesy of Valley Medical Center and Valley Radiologists.

moves to the PET side of the system and the PET scan begins, moving in this example from the pelvis to the neck in 5 to 7 bed positions of 5 to 10 min each. The entire acquisition requires about 30 to 45 min (the newer PET scintillators allow for shorter scan times). Co-registration between the two acquisitions is based on bed position and the laser reference lines, and it is assumed that the patient has not moved between the two acquisitions.

The CT study is used to produce transverse slices, after which the CT 3D image matrix is downgraded to match the matrix characteristics of the PET study. The CT data must also be scaled to reflect attenuation at 511 keV (see the next section). The CT-generated attenuation map is used to create attenuation correction factors that are applied in iterative reconstruction. Finally, the PET and CT slices are displayed on either side of a workstation screen, with co-registered slices in the middle. Usually the CT is displayed in black and white, while the PET is displayed in color, allowing the viewer to visualize the information from both studies in a single image (**Figure 18-17**).

Technical Issues in PET/CT

The combination of PET and CT into one system raises a number of technical issues that are currently under discussion. As these controversies are still being sorted out, this text will attempt to give the current best answer; further

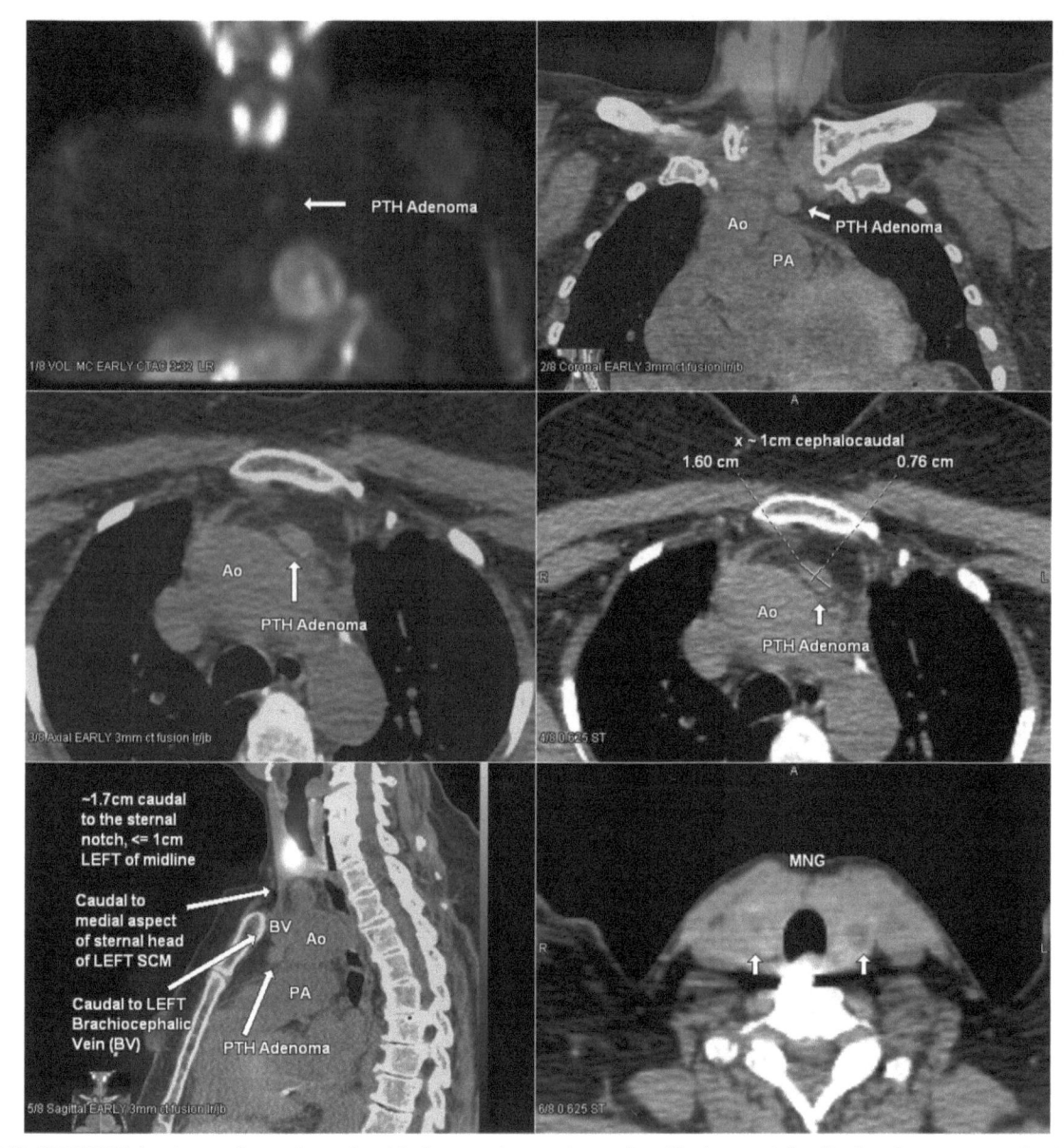

Figure 18-15 SPECT/CT showing a substernal parathyroid adenoma. An ectopic parathyroid adenoma is localized to the anterior mediastinum near the great vessels and behind the sternum. The annotation provides the surgeon with exact information about the adenoma's location and size. The CT scan incidentally identifies a multinodular goiter in the thyroid (lower-right image, arrows point at intrathyroidal nodules), but correctly locates the parathyroid adenoma elsewhere. (See color plate.) Images courtesy of Valley Medical Center and Valley Radiologists.

research and discussion may change opinions over time. Note also that these topics related to the combining of the two modalities are in addition to patient care and preparation issues specific to the particular studies being performed.

Low-Dose vs Diagnostic CT

If the patient has had a recent diagnostic-quality CT study in the context of his or her diagnostic workup, we should question whether another one needs to be performed. This is true not only from a reimbursement standpoint but especially from radiation dose considerations. A perfectly adequate attenuation map can be generated using many fewer x-rays (i.e., a low-current CT study, less than 20 mA), resulting in acceptable anatomic detail while decreasing the radiation dose by a factor of about 10 (15). (However, very low mA settings, combined with low kVp, may affect the attenuation correction process and alter SUV results by a small amount [19].) But good radiology practice requires that each study performed have a dictated report, and most radiologists would rather dictate based on a high-quality CT study. The trend at this time is toward a high-dose, high-quality CT; the ultimate solution is to incorporate the combined PET/CT study into diagnostic algorithms so that only one CT study is done.

Conversion of Hounsfield Units to 511-keV Attenuation

Prior to using the CT 3D image matrix as an attenuation map, it needs to be converted to attenuation at 511 keV.

(a) PET/CT schematic

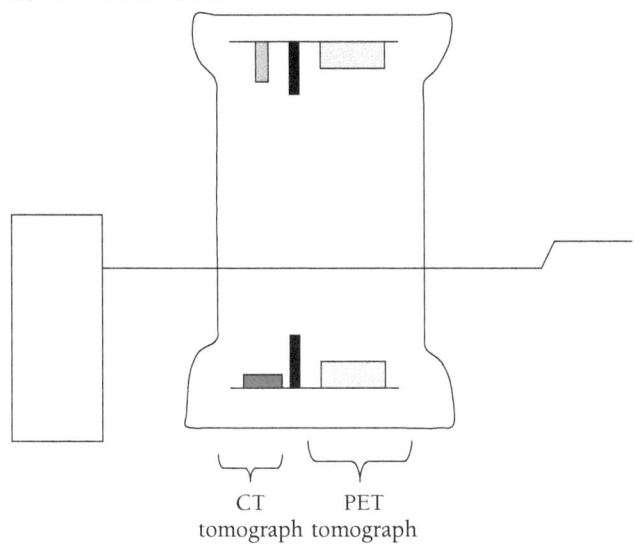

CT tomograph / PET tomograph

(b) Commercially available system

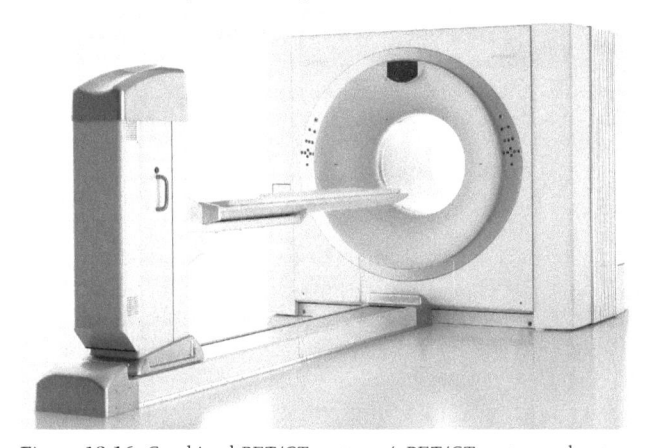

Figure 18-16 Combined PET/CT system. A PET/CT system colocates two tomographs within one housing, so that images can be co-registered based on the position of the imaging table. Figure 18-16a shows the schematic; a commercially available system is shown in Figure 18-16b. Adapted from: Beyer T, Townsend DW, Brun T, et al. A combined PET/CT scanner for clinical oncology. *J Nucl Med.* 2000;41:1370. With permission from the Society of Nuclear Medicine. Figure 18-16b courtesy of Siemens Healthcare.

This is not a straightforward linear conversion, because at CT x-ray energies, body tissues experience different degrees of photoelectric vs Compton interactions, whereas Compton interactions predominate in all tissues at 511 keV (Fig. 18-4a). This is particularly a problem for bone, such that different scaling factors need to be applied for bone vs soft tissue. **Figure 18-18** shows a bilinear conversion scheme, in which one linear conversion is employed for tissues with CT numbers less than 0 HU and a different linear conversion for tissues with CT numbers greater than 0 HU. More sophisticated schemes have been proposed, but this relatively simplistic model gives acceptable results (8).

Use of Contrast

Administration of contrast throws a wrench into the correlation between PET and CT attenuation factors. Both oral and vascular contrast agents have high CT numbers at x-ray energies, but they do not represent high-attenuation tissues in the body at annihilation photon energies. Attenuation correction artifacts are therefore possible when a contrast-containing CT study is used for attenuation correction. If an area containing contrast is interpreted as a high-attenuation tissue, the reconstruction algorithm will apply a higher attenuation correction factor to that area than the anatomy warrants. The resulting attenuation-corrected PET study may demonstrate an artifactual hot spot (**Figure 18-19**).

There are several ways around this dilemma. One is to view the non-attenuation-corrected images; if no hot spot is seen, then the attenuation-corrected hot spot is an artifact. Another method is to manually outline areas of contrast and reset their CT numbers to appropriate soft-tissue values. A third solution is to use the CT numbers themselves to distinguish between contrast and bone. Oral contrast is concentrated in the intestines as water is reabsorbed, and can reach CT numbers up to +800 HU. But, for the most part, IV and oral contrast have CT numbers between soft tissue and bone, in the +200–300 HU range. Algorithms have been written to assign soft-tissue rather than bone-tissue types based on CT numbers, but these have not been implemented in most PET/CT systems as of this writing.

As experience with PET/CT has accumulated, the emerging consensus is that venous phase IV contrast and dilute oral contrast result in minimal overcorrection, leaving only immediate postinjection and arterial phase IV contrast as the problematic issue (20, 21). The particular problem is IV contrast in the subclavian and brachiocephalic veins immediately after injection; a brief delay before starting the acquisition allows the contrast to exit these structures. A dual-port injector with a 30-ml saline flush also helps. The issue ultimately reverts to the type of CT study being done: if a diagnostic CT scan with arterial phase IV contrast is needed, then any accompanying artifacts need to be dealt with.

Misregistration

The assumption of the hybrid PET/CT acquisition is that the patient does not change position between the two acquisitions, so that the only change between the two is the table location. There are a number of reasons that this assumption may not be true. The most obvious, of course, is that the patient moved. The lasers used to determine positioning are based on the imaging table's position in all three dimensions, so if the imaging table bounces even slightly between the CT and PET acquisitions, they can become misaligned.

Arm location is one potential cause of patient movement. CT studies are typically acquired with the arms elevated over the head, mainly to eliminate the beam hardening that would occur if they were in the FOV. The scan time is so short in current-generation CT tomographs that this is tolerable for most patients. In a PET study acquired over 30 min, on the other hand, the arms-above-the-head position is very tiring. For radiation safety reasons, the technologist should not help to keep the arms in place

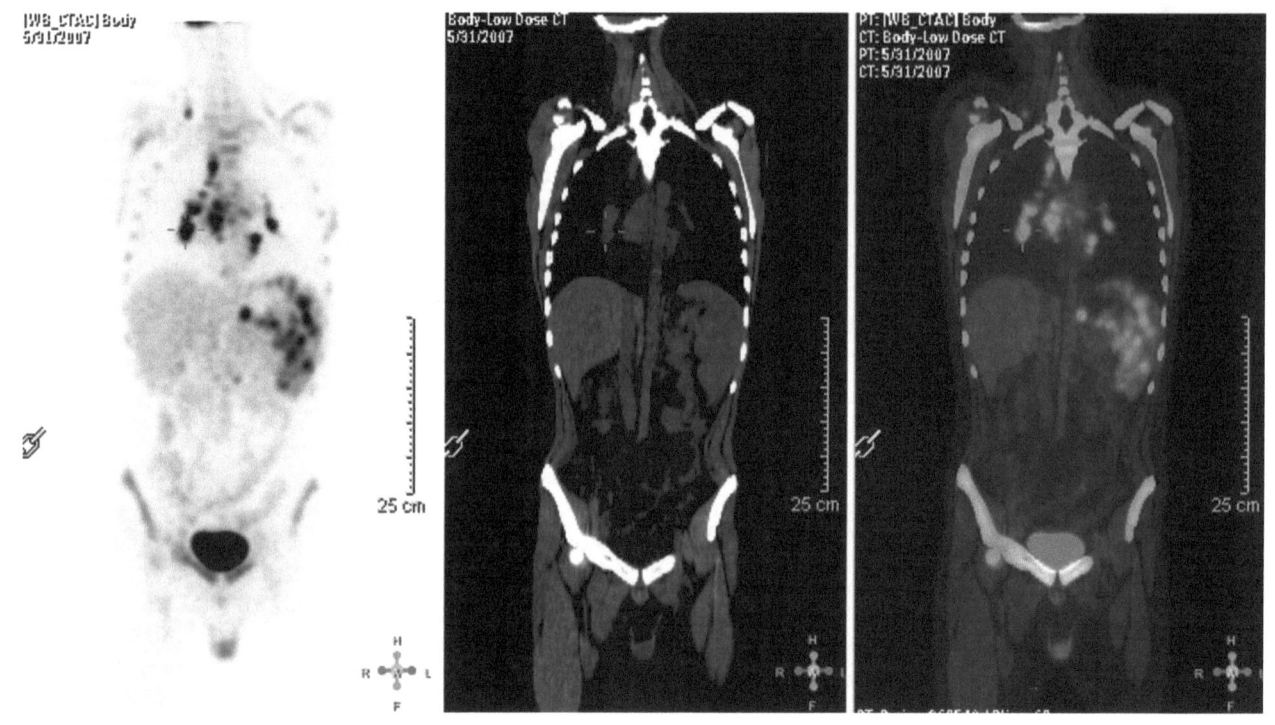

Figure 18-17 PET/CT scan. This standard display shows the PET coronal slice alone (left panel), the CT slice alone (middle panel), and the combined PET and CT slices (right panel). In the combined image, the CT information is shown in gray scale and the PET information in color, superimposed on the CT. (See color plate.) Courtesy of Philips Healthcare.

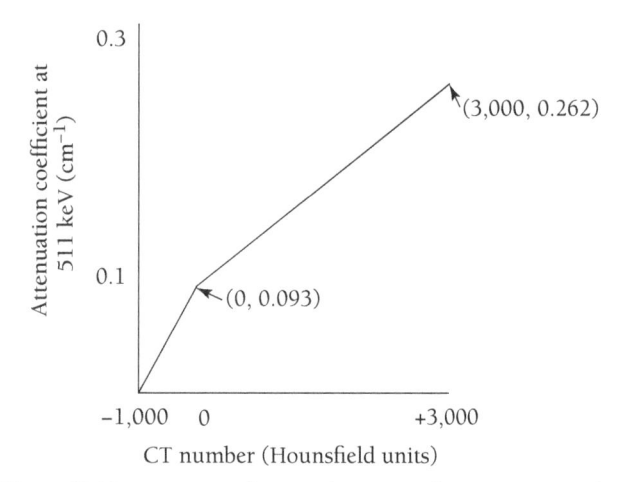

Figure 18-18 Conversion of CT numbers to 511-keV attenuation. The conversion from CT numbers to 511-keV attenuation coefficients is not linear. The line shows a proposed bilinear correlation between CT number and 511-keV attenuation coefficient in body tissues. Modified from: Nakamoto Y, Osman M, Cohade C, et al. PET/CT: comparison of quantitative tracer uptake between germanium and CT transmission attenuation-corrected images. *J Nucl Med.* 2002;43:1137–1143. Used with permission of the Society of Nuclear Medicine.

above the head. Investment in a comfortable arm support and frequent reminders to stay still may be the best solution to this problem.

Normal breathing is another source of misregistration artifacts. The location of the diaphragm is determined by the timing of imaging relative to the patient's respiratory cycle. For CT acquisitions, the patient is usually asked to hold at maximum expiration for the short acquisition times needed, but for a several-minute PET acquisition this would clearly be impossible. Some researchers are getting good results allowing patients to breathe shallowly during both the PET and the CT studies; others have found the best comparison to be a CT acquired while holding a normal expiration and PET with shallow breathing (22). **Figure 18-20** shows an example of misregistration at the diaphragm due to breathing. Respiratory gating can be added as an option in PET/CT tomographs so that artifacts due to organ motion can be reduced (23). This issue is especially important as PET/CT is applied to myocardial imaging (24).

CT Truncation Artifact

The gantry bore in a PET/CT system is 70 cm in diameter, but the CT FOV (as defined by the maximum angle between the x-ray tube and the outer-edge detectors) may be smaller (e.g., 50 cm). It is thus possible to put a large patient into the gantry but not to be able to produce CT scans that include the entire patient thickness. If this is the case, no attenuation correction will be applied to the parts of the patient not in the CT FOV, leading to artifactually incorrect PET results. Algorithms have been implemented on PET/CT scanners to interpolate the missing data and thus reduce artifacts in the truncated areas (25). This is an area of ongoing improvement, especially as the design factors involved in combining the two tomographs are worked out.

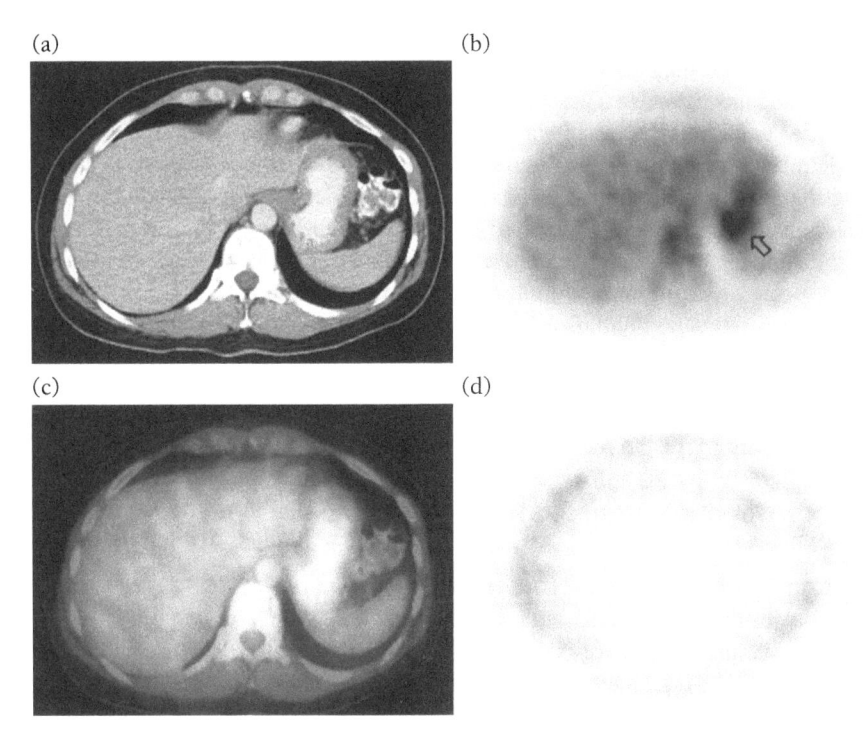

Figure 18-19 Contrast artifact in PET/CT. Contrast (both oral and intravenous) causes increased attenuation on CT, but not for 511-keV photons. Figure 18-19a is a CT transaxial slice following the administration of oral contrast, which can be seen as the white area in the stomach (on the right side of the image). In the attenuation-corrected PET FDG scan (Fig. 18-19b) and the co-registered PET and CT scans (Fig. 18-19c), that region is seen as an area of increased FDG activity. But the non-attenuation-corrected PET scan (Fig. 18-19d) shows no increase in the same area. Reprinted from: Antoch G, Freudenberg LS, Beyer T, et al. To enhance or not enhance? 18F-FDG and CT contrast agents in dual-modality 18F-FDG. *J Nucl Med.* 2004;45(Suppl 1):58S. Used with permission of the Society of Nuclear Medicine.

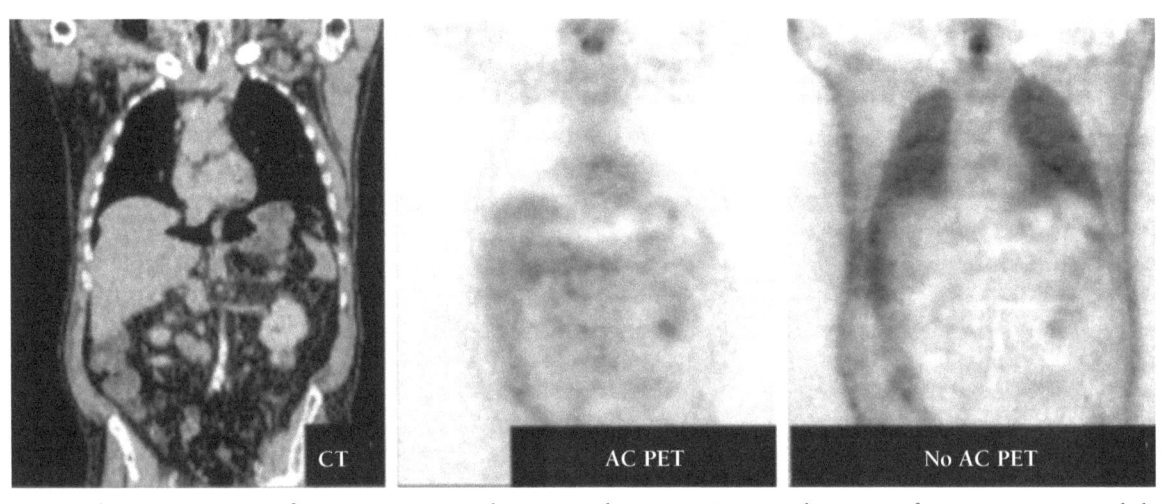

Figure 18-20 Diaphragmatic motion artifact. Because CT scans have a very short acquisition time, the amount of respiratory motion is slight. But PET scans require acquisition times of several minutes, such that respiratory motion is averaged out. The CT scan shows the dome of the liver in two different places, leading to a similar banana-shaped artifact on the PET attenuation-corrected scan. The artifact disappears on the non-attenuation-corrected image. Reprinted from: Beyer T, Antoch G, Muller S, et al. Acquisition protocol considerations for combined PET/CT imaging. *J Nucl Med.* 2004;45(Suppl 1):30S. Used with permission of the Society of Nuclear Medicine.

Regulatory Issues

The colocation of these two modalities into one machine raises several issues from a regulatory standpoint. One question is, "What type of technologist is allowed to operate this two-headed monster?" Scope-of-practice laws are defined and enforced at the state level, leading to different possibilities in different states. The industry recognized the need to find a more widely accepted solution and in 2002 convened a consensus conference to discuss the issue. The bottom-line concern of all involved was that both patient care and diagnostic results be maintained at a high level of quality.

The conclusion of the consensus conference was to allow persons already certified in nuclear medicine, radiography, or radiation therapy to become certified to operate a hybrid PET/CT tomograph (26). A nuclear medicine technologist may perform PET scans as a part of her or his scope of practice, but would need to pass the certification examination for CT in order to operate the CT portion of the hybrid tomograph. A radiographer certified in CT would likewise require education and training in PET and would take a PET certification examination. Both certification exams have been augmented to test not only the specific knowledge of PET and CT, but also the underlying principles of nuclear medicine and radiography, respectively. A similar consensus panel at the radiologist level identified appropriate training for interpretation of PET/CT studies (22).

But regulation of x-ray machines falls to the states rather than the federal government, and state statutes vary. In some states, licensure or certification is required for those who operate equipment that produces ionizing radiation; in others, no such laws exist. Regulations may be more or less specific in their definition of who might be covered. The Society of Nuclear Medicine Technologist Section (SNMTS) is working with the Council of Radiation Control Program Directors to try to reach some uniformity in regulation of dual-modality systems. The SNMTS is also pushing national legislation that would require states to regulate all persons using ionizing radiation for medical purposes for each modality an individual operates.

Some of the technical issues discussed come into play in this regulatory tangle. For example, in some states, a nuclear medicine technologist without x-ray or CT certification may be allowed to operate a low-dose CT tomograph, but a diagnostic CT unit requires personnel certified in diagnostic x-ray. Or the administration of intravenous contrast may be the key factor. The picture is further complicated by the fact that in some states, regulatory responsibility for nuclear medicine departments resides in a different part of state government than that for x-ray departments. There is still much work to be done in this area.

Summary

The strength of CT rests in its ability to measure accurately the attenuation of different types of tissues, and to display those differences over a wide range of attenuation values with excellent spatial and contrast resolution. This ability rests on the very large number of x-rays generated, the tomograph's small detectors and rotational capabilities, and the reconstruction of the resulting information by high-powered computers, using Radon's theory. The development of computed tomography represents one of the great medical advances in the 20th century.

The colocation of PET and CT tomographs into a single system is in many ways a similar revolution within the field of radiology. This is true in terms of not only the images that are obtained, but also the thought processes involved, from acquisition to interpretation to regulation. The swiftness of the revolution is astonishing, going from first publication of a prototype system in 2000 to encompassing the great majority of commercial sales in 2004. The benefits of the revolution are obvious, and the technical, regulatory, and reimbursement details are minor in comparison.

Nonetheless, the technical aspects of a combined-modality tomograph require the technologist to pay attention to new details and concerns. From the nuclear medicine standpoint, the use of radiographic contrast and the high radiation levels involved in CT imaging are significant additions to the requirements for good practice. Other aspects of combining modalities can be programmed into the reconstruction process. Quality control testing will be an important addition to the technologist's workload. In sum, it will be important for technologists operating combined-modality tomographs to have a good level of understanding of each modality.

References

1. Lang TF, Hasegawa BH, Soo Chin L, et al. Description of a prototype emission-transmission computed tomography imaging system. *J Nucl Med.* 1992;33:1881–1887.
2. Beyer T, Townsend DW, Brun T, et al. A combined PET/CT scanner for clinical oncology. *J Nucl Med.* 2000;41:1369–1379.
3. Seibert JA. X-ray imaging physics for nuclear medicine technologists. Part 1: Basic principles of x-ray production. *J Nucl Med Technol.* 2004;32:139–147.
4. Seibert JA, Boone JM. X-ray imaging physics for nuclear medicine technologists. Part 2: X-ray interactions and image formation. *J Nucl Med Technol.* 2005;33:3–18.
5. Bushberg JT, Seibert JA, Leidholdt EM, Boone JM. *The Essential Physics of Medical Imaging.* 2nd ed. Philadelphia, PA: Lippincott Williams and Wilkins; 2002:641, 760.
6. Seeram E. *Computed Tomography: Physical Principles, Clinical Applications, and Quality Control.* 3rd ed. Philadelphia, PA: WB Saunders; 2009:196, 236, 276, 499.
7. Christian PE, Waterstram-Rich KM. *Nuclear Medicine and PET/CT: Technology and Techniques.* 6th ed. St. Louis: Mosby-Year Book; 2007:353, 355.
8. Kinahan PE, Hasegawa BH, Beyer T. X-ray based attenuation correction for positron emission tomography/computed tomography scanners. *Semin Nucl Med.* 2003;33:166–179.
9. Kallender WA. *Computed Tomography: Fundamentals, System Technology, Image Quality, Applications.* 2nd ed. Erlangen, Germany: Publicis Corporate Publishing; 2005:30.
10. Zanzonico P. Routine quality control of clinical nuclear medicine instrumentation: a brief review. *J Nucl Med.* 2008;49:1114–1131.
11. Faasse T, Shreve P. Positron emission tomography-computed tomography patient management and workflow. *Semin Ultrasound CT MRI.* 2008;29:277–282.
12. Goldman LW. Principles of CT: radiation dose and image quality. *J Nucl Med Technol.* 2007;35:213–225.
13. American Association of Physicists in Medicine. AAPM Report No. 96: The measurement, reporting, and management of radiation dose in CT. College Park, MD: Task Group 23: CT Dosimetry members: McCollough C, Cody D, Edyvean S, Geise R, et al.; 2008.
14. McCullough CH. CT dose: how to measure, how to reduce. *Health Phys.* 2008;95:508–517.
15. Brix G, Lechel U, Glatting G, et al. Radiation exposure of patients undergoing whole-body dual-modality F-18 FDG PET/CT examinations. *J Nucl Med.* 2005;46:608–613.
16. Brenner DJ, Hall EJ. Computed tomography—an increasing source of radiation exposure. *New England J Med.* 2007;357:2277–2284.
17. GE Medical Systems. Infinia Users Guide, Direction 2411010-100. Rev. 1; 2005.
18. Keidar Z, Israel O, Krausz Y. SPECT/CT in tumor imaging: technical aspects and clinical applications. *Semin Nucl Med.* 2003;33:205–218.
19. Continuing Education Sessions titled *Clinical Implementation of Advanced Image Processing Techniques* and *SPECT/CT: Instrumentation and Clinical Applications.* Society of Nuclear Medicine 53rd Annual Meeting, San Diego, CA, June 5 and 6, 2006.
20. Shyn PB. Protocol considerations for thoracic positron emission tomography-computed tomography. *Semin Ultrasound CT MRI.* 2008;29:242–250.
21. Valk PE, Bailey DL, Townsend DW, Maisey MN. *Positron Emission Tomography: Basic Science and Clinical Practice.* London: Springer; 2003:205.
22. Goerres GW, Kamel EH, Heidelberg TNH, et al. PET-CT image coregistration in the thorax: influence of respiration. *Eur J Nucl Med.* 2002;29:351–360.
23. Pan T, Mawlawi O, Nehmeh SA, et al. Attenuation correction of PET images with respiration-averaged CT images with PET/CT. *J Nucl Med.* 2005;46:1481–1487.

24. Schwaiger M, Ziegler S, Nekolla SG. PET/CT: challenge for nuclear cardiology. *J Nucl Med.* 2005;46:1664–1678.
25. Beyer T, Bockish A, Kühl H, Martinez M-J. Whole-body 18F-FDG PET/CT in the presence of truncation artifacts. *J Nucl Med.* 2006;47:91–99.
26. SNM Technologist Section and American Society of Radiologic Technologists. Fusion imaging: a new type of technologist for a new type of technology. *J Nucl Med Technol.* 2002;30:201–204.

Additional Resources

American College of Radiology. ACR technical standard for medical nuclear physics performance monitoring of PET-CT imaging equipment. http://www.acr.org/~/media/5AL923DBCB254D8F9E29D082C1B28E79.pdf Accessed June 19, 2012.

Ballinger PW, Frank ED. *Merrill's Atlas of Radiographic Positions and Radiologic Procedures.* 10th ed. St. Louis, MO: Mosby; 2003:Chapter 33.

Bushberg JT, Seibert JA, Leidholdt EM, Boone JM. *The Essential Physics of Medical Imaging.* 2nd ed. Philadelphia, PA: Lippincott Williams and Wilkins; 2002: Chapters 3, 5, 13.

Kinahan PE, Hasegawa BH, Beyer T. X-ray based attenuation correction for positron emission tomography/computed tomography scanners. *Semin Nucl Med.* 2003;33:166–179.

Seeram E. *Computed Tomography: Physical Principles, Clinical Applications, and Quality Control.* 2nd ed. Philadelphia, PA: WB Saunders; 2001:Chapters 11, 12, 23.

Seibert JA. X-ray imaging physics for nuclear medicine technologists. Part 1: Basic principles of x-ray production. *J Nucl Med Technol.* 2004;32:139–147.

Seminars in Ultrasound, CT and MRI. Vol. 29, No. 4, August 2008.

Valk PE, Bailey DL, Townsend DW, Maisey MN. *Positron Emission Tomography: Basic Science and Clinical Practice.* London: Springer; 2003:Chapter 8.

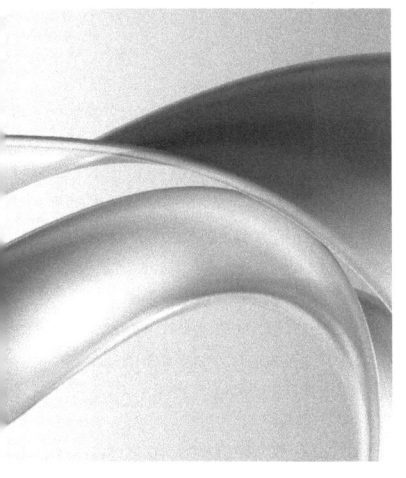

CHAPTER 19
Magnetic Resonance Imaging and Its Application to Nuclear Medicine

Authors: Fady Kassem and Jennifer Prekeges

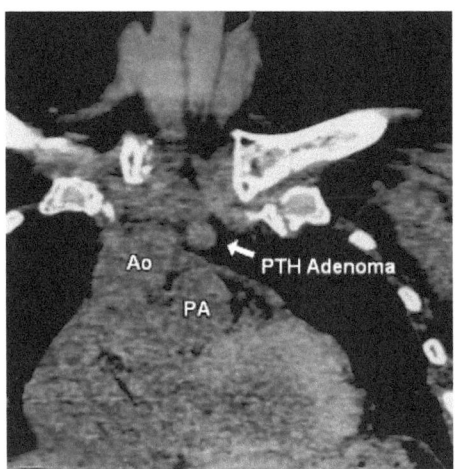

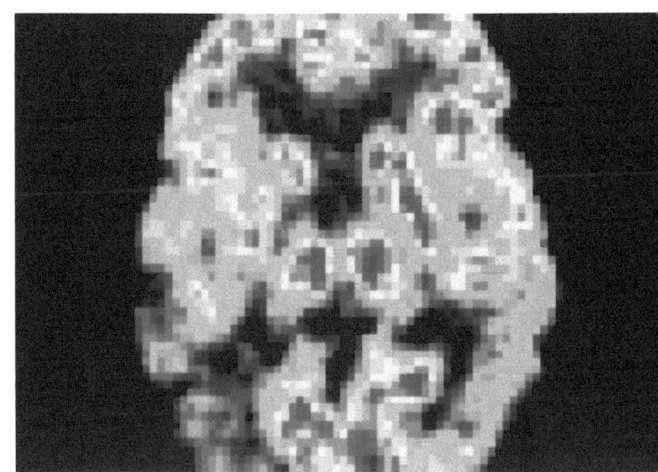

Learning Outcomes

1. Outline the relationship between electricity and magnetism, and discuss the magnetic properties of the hydrogen nucleus.
2. Illustrate the effect of a magnetic field and a radiofrequency pulse on hydrogen atoms in an object being imaged, including the effect of both 90° and 180° pulses.
3. Distinguish between T1 relaxation and T2 relaxation (or spin-lattice and spin-spin relaxation).
4. Describe the spin echo pulse sequence, and define the echo time and repetition time.
5. Identify the three magnetic gradients needed to accomplish spatial localization of magnetic resonance (MR) signal information.
6. Identify the components of an MR tomograph.
7. Discuss safety considerations in magnetic resonance imaging, including the screening of individuals prior to entry into the MR suite, shielding of the MR suite, effects on metallic implants, and acoustic noise.
8. Briefly discuss the use of contrast agents in MRI.
9. Briefly describe the benefits to be gained by combining MRI with PET and the challenges to colocating the two tomographs.

Introduction

Magnetic resonance imaging (MRI) is considered an advanced imaging modality, in terms of its physical complexity but even more so because of the superior quality of the resulting images. MRI utilizes electromagnetic radiation, a powerful electromagnet, and a computer to form images of the internal structures of the body. MRI is capable of diagnosing many disease processes much earlier than competing diagnostic imaging modalities. CT scanning employs x-rays to produce an image matrix of tissue attenuation values. MRI utilizes a similar computerized technique; however, MRI images reflect the chemistry of body tissues without using ionizing radiation.

The physical phenomenon of *resonance* dictates that under certain circumstances energy can be transferred efficiently from one entity to another, causing the receiving entity to vibrate at the same frequency as the sending entity. The property of magnetic resonance was discovered by Edward Purcell in 1946. In that same year, Felix Bloch proposed that protons inside the nucleus of the atom act like tiny magnets. According to Bloch's theory, the protons inside the nucleus of the atom behave as if they are spinning on an axis, and emit a miniscule magnetic field as they spin. These two important theories led to the development of the *nuclear magnetic resonance* (NMR) *spectrometer,* a chemistry lab instrument used to determine the atomic structure of unknown materials.

Raymond Damadian and Paul Lauterbur experimented with these spectrometers in the 1960s, focusing their attention on the production of anatomic images based on the molecular composition of different tissues. These two investigators produced the first MRI images in 1969. In 1971, Damadian found that different kinds of animal tissue emit response signals that vary in length, and that cancerous tissue emits response signals that last much longer than noncancerous tissue. In the early days of magnetic resonance imaging, the term *nuclear magnetic resonance* was carried forward from the laboratory instrument. But the word *nuclear* seemed to reference radioactivity, which is not used in this imaging technique, so the name was changed to *magnetic resonance imaging*. (In reality, the term *nuclear* as it is used in NMR refers to the nucleus of the atom.) By the late 1980s, the new name was widely accepted, and MRI had become a respected imaging modality. Lauterbur and Peter Mansfield shared the Nobel Prize for Physiology or Medicine in 2003, but Damadian is considered the inventor of the MR tomograph.

Creating a situation of magnetic resonance requires three components: hydrogen atoms (or another atom with an unpaired proton in its nucleus), a powerful magnet, and radio-frequency (RF) energy. Fortunately hydrogen protons are plentiful in the body. With the patient inside the powerful magnet, RF energy (similar to that used for commercial AM radio) is released in pulses. In response, the hydrogen nuclei emit characteristic signals that depend on their immediate environment. These signals are quantitative and easily measured. One of the greatest advantages of MRI is its ability to differentiate tissues based on their chemical composition.

MRI provides unique information that is quite unlike what is obtained in other imaging modalities. MRI is able to characterize tissue due to differing physical and biochemical properties (such as the content of water, iron, or fat in a tissue). Blood flow, joints, and even nerves can be imaged. Restricted diffusion of water, such as happens immediately following an ischemic stroke, can be measured. Calcium emits no signal with some MRI pulse sequences, so tissues surrounded by bone, such as the contents of the posterior fossa of the skull and the spine, can be imaged without the beam-hardening artifacts that are seen in CT scans of these areas.

Other advantages of MRI over other imaging modalities include the following:

- MRI produces cross-sectional images of equal resolution in multiple planes without moving the patient or the tomograph, yielding precise diagnostic value to the clinician.
- MRI produces excellent delineation of anatomic structures stemming from its superior contrast resolution.
- MRI acquisitions can be set up to look for radio frequencies of specific molecules (a technique called *MR spectroscopy*).
- MRI does not utilize ionizing radiation and has no documented biological effects to the patient, making multiple examinations on one patient a worry-free imaging option.

The mathematics and physics required to understand MRI in depth are quite daunting. We have chosen to take a less rigorous approach, "MRI lite" if you will, while at the same time attempting to reach a level of detail that explains not only the MRI signal but also the generation of 3D images and the composition of the MRI tomograph. The learning outcomes and sample calculations are accordingly less demanding than in other parts of this text. Many other texts are available for those who desire a more thorough understanding of the science behind this imaging modality. We believe that the level of presentation in this chapter approximates what nuclear medicine technologists need to know about this technology at this time.

In addition, we have made a strategic decision not to cover topics that would be quite pertinent to an MRI technologist, including the variety of different pulse sequences, artifacts, the effect of various image parameters, and quality control. Given the complexities of MRI, it makes more sense to emphasize the basics than to provide a comprehensive overview in a single chapter. Nuclear medicine technologists who aim to operate MRI tomographs will want to explore the field in much greater depth than we can present here.

Electromagnetism and Its Effect on Hydrogen Atoms

The term *electromagnetism* implies a connection between electricity and magnetism. In simple words, whenever a charged particle moves, a magnetic field is created. Similarly, a magnetic field can cause charged particles to move, creating a current in a conducting wire. Think of the description of electromagnetic radiation as consisting of alternating electrical and magnetic fields: the electrical field induces the magnetic field, and vice versa. MRI takes advantage of the fact that electromagnetic radiation can be used to alter magnetic fields, and it measures the subsequent changes in magnetic field via current changes in the electronic circuitry.

Certain nuclei have properties that cause them to display magnetic characteristics. Of all the nuclei with magnetic characteristics, hydrogen is the most abundant in the human body and is therefore used in clinical MRI (1). The following characteristics of the hydrogen atom make it magnetically active:

- It has a single, unpaired proton.
- It has mass.
- It has a positive charge.
- It spins on its axis, resulting in a magnetic field around the proton termed its *magnetic moment*.

In the human body, hydrogen exists primarily in two molecules, water and fat, which are two very strong physiological markers (1). We note here that what we more commonly think of as bulk magnetic properties of materials, such as ferromagnetism or diamagnetism, depend on electron pairing, whereas MRI is based on the much smaller magnetic effects of unpaired protons.

Net Magnetization

Because the hydrogen proton, often called a *spin*, has a magnetic moment, it exhibits certain behavior when placed in a large, externally applied magnetic field, which we shall indicate as B_0. Within seconds of the tissue being placed in a magnetic field, the hydrogen protons will assume one of two possible quantum spin states or energy levels: high energy or low energy (**Figure 19-1**). One way to explain the spin states is to speak of protons as aligning either with or against the external magnetic field (note that the hydrogen atoms themselves do not move to new locations in the same way as iron filings align with a magnetic field). Spins aligned parallel (i.e., with the direction of B_0) are in a low-energy state. Spins aligned antiparallel (i.e., against the direction of B_0) are in a high-energy state. At any given time, there will be slightly more spins in the low-energy state. The magnetic moment of spins in the high-energy state cancels the effects of an equal number of spins in the low-energy state, leaving a small net magnetic effect from those excess spins in the low-energy state (1).

The net magnetic moment is the sum of the magnetic moments of all the protons exposed to the main magnetic field. The behavior of protons can be far more easily visualized and understood if we consider the effects of the RF and magnetic fields on large populations of protons rather than individual protons. This is most easily expressed as a vector, a mathematical quantity that has direction as well as magnitude (**Figure 19-2a**). In the presence of the external magnetic field, the slight excess of parallel-aligned hydrogen nuclei results in a net magnetic vector in the direction of the magnetic field. We will define this direction as the Z direction, and we call this vector M_Z. The magnitude of M_Z is the result of the excess low-energy spins that are not canceled out by the high-energy spins.

Precession and the Larmor Equation

The magnetization of each proton does not line up perfectly with the main magnetic field without ever moving, but instead wobbles in response to the magnetic field with a motion called *precession* (Figs. 19-1c and 19-1d). This precession is brought about by the interaction of the main magnetic field with the proton's magnetic moment. The rate at which the magnetization precesses is described by a relationship called the *Larmor equation*,

$$f_0 = (\gamma/2\pi)B_0 \qquad (19\text{-}1)$$

where f_0 is the linear frequency of precession, B_0 is the applied magnetic field, and γ is a constant called the *gyromagnetic ratio*. This equation is of critical importance in MRI. The Larmor equation states that the rate at which the proton's net magnetization wobbles is directly related to the strength of the magnetic field in which the protons are placed. The f term in the Larmor equation represents the rate, or frequency, of the wobbling of the net

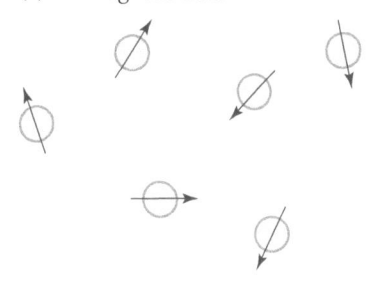

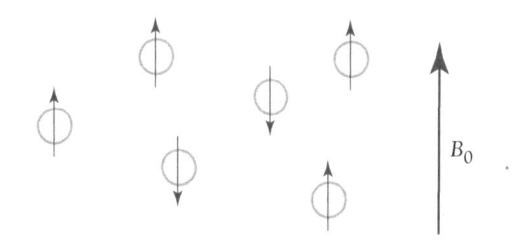

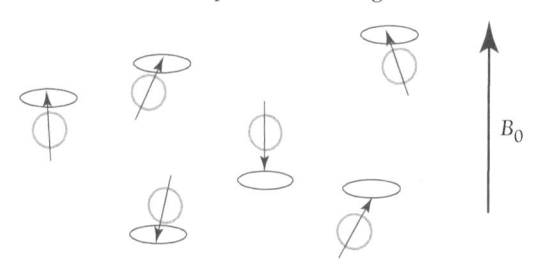

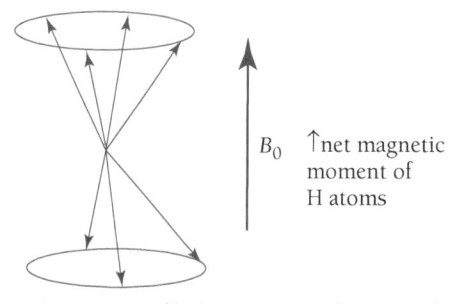

Figure 19-1 Magnetic properties of hydrogen atoms. The unpaired proton of a hydrogen atom behaves as a tiny magnet. In the absence of a magnetic field, the magnetic field of the protons may be oriented in any direction (Fig. 19-1a). In the presence of an external magnetic field (designated B_0), the magnetic fields of the hydrogen nuclei align themselves either with or against the field. The alignment with the field is the lower-energy state, so slightly more of the protons will align with the field, as shown in Figure 19-1b. Even under the influence of the external magnetic field, Figure 19-1c shows that the protons are precessing around their main directional axis in a random distribution. The consequence of the application of the external magnetic field is that there is a net magnetic force from the hydrogen atoms in the direction of the external field, but because their precessions are not in phase, there is no magnetic field in any other direction. Figure 19-1d shows the same situation in a different way.

(a) M_Z vector

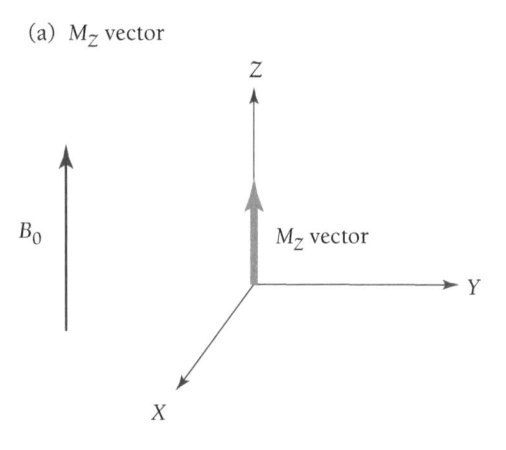

(b) M_{XY} vector

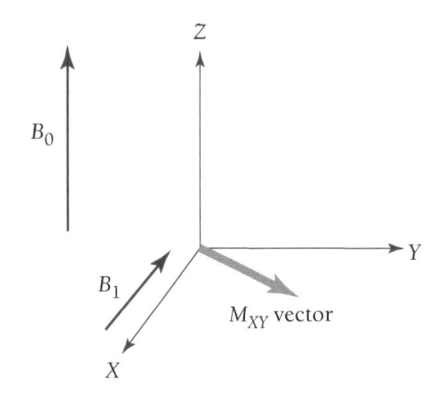

(c) Axis designations in a standard MR tomograph

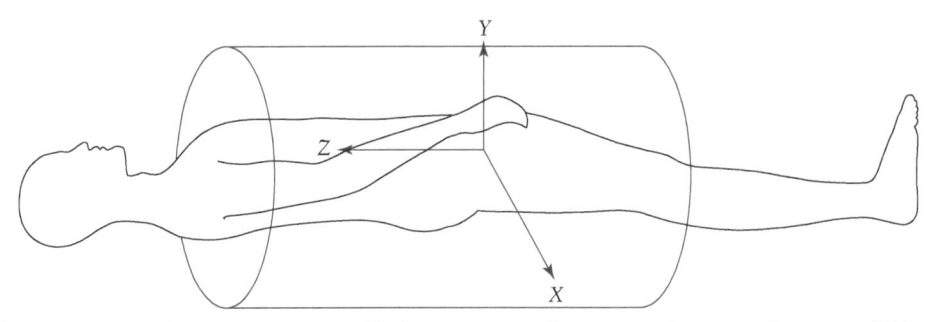

Figure 19-2 Axes and vectors in MRI. The net magnetization of hydrogen atoms in the presence of an external magnetic field is best expressed as a vector. The M_Z vector in Figure 19-2a represents longitudinal magnetization, while the M_{XY} vector in Figure 19-2b indicates a transverse magnetic vector. The vector moves into the transverse plane due to the application of a second magnetic field, denoted B_1. Note that the Z-axis is pointed up in order to make it easier to see M_{XY} in the transverse (X–Y) plane, but in actual MRI the Z-axis is the long axis of the patient and the gantry bore (Fig. 19-2c).

magnetization, called the *precessional frequency*. Frequency is measured in units called hertz (Hz), which are equivalent to revolutions or cycles per second. The B in the equation stands for the magnetic field strength, which is measured in units called *tesla* (abbreviated T; 1 T is about 15,000 to 40,000 times Earth's magnetic field). The constant γ, the gyromagnetic ratio, is different for each different atom with an unpaired proton. For hydrogen, it is equal to 42.6 MHz/T. The Larmor equation can also be written as $\omega_0 = \gamma B_0$, where ω_0 is the angular frequency of precession in radians per second (rad/sec) and the other numbers are as described above. The 2π factor in Equation 19-1 converts from radians per second to revolutions per second.

The subscript 0 in the Larmor equation indicates that this equation is true at a state of resonance. For nuclei other than hydrogen, their unique gyromagnetic ratios lead to values of γ other than 42.6 MHz/T, and therefore they resonate at different values of B_0. It is possible to perform MR imaging with nuclei other than hydrogen, simply by applying an RF pulse at a frequency that causes those nuclei to resonate. Examples of nuclei that are used for research MRI include C-13, F-19, and P-31. But all conventional MR imaging is done using the hydrogen nucleus. So for clinical imaging, the Larmor frequency is equal to 42.6 MHz times the magnetic field strength in which the protons are sitting.

Sample Calculation 19-1 Larmor Frequency

Calculate the Larmor frequency for hydrogen atoms exposed to magnetic fields of 1, 1.5, and 0.5 T.

We apply Equation 19-1 to the three magnetic field values given:

$$1 \text{ T} \times 42.6 \text{ MHz/T} = 42.6 \text{ MHz}.$$

$$1.5 \text{ T} \times 42.6 \text{ MHz/T} = 63.9 \text{ MHz}.$$

$$0.5 \text{ T} \times 42.6 \text{ MHz/T} = 21.3 \text{ MHz}.$$

Thus, if the protons are put in a stronger magnetic field, their net magnetization precesses faster. If the protons are put in a weaker magnetic field, their net magnetization precesses more slowly.

To learn about individual tissues in the body, the net magnetization needs to be disturbed and the response of protons to that disturbance measured. The Larmor equation provides the mathematical basis for this process. A complete understanding of precessional frequency and the Larmor equation is fundamental to many MRI concepts.

Tissue Disturbance and Differentiation

The goal of any diagnostic imaging modality is to differentiate various normal tissues as well as to identify those that have some sort of pathology. To accomplish this in MRI, a signal from the body must be generated by upsetting the alignment of the protons' net magnetization with the main magnetic field. When the net magnetization is aligned in the *longitudinal direction* (parallel to the main magnetic field B_0), there is no measurable signal, that is, no information about the tissue. To learn about the tissue, the proton's equilibrium must be moved into the *transverse plane* (perpendicular to the B_0 field). The applied disturbance comes in the form of a brief pulse of electromagnetic radiation, the RF pulse. The RF pulse has a magnetic field B_1 that is perpendicular to B_0, which causes the hydrogen spins in the object to precess *in phase* with one another, at the Larmor frequency. "Precessing in phase" means that all of the arrows in Figure 19-1d converge, such that all the hydrogen spins precess in exact synchrony, while maintaining their alignment with or against B_0. Thus, the net magnetization vector is moved out of alignment with the main magnetic field (the longitudinal direction) and into the transverse plane (Fig. 19-2b). The RF pulse used to tilt the magnetization from the longitudinal direction into the transverse plane is called an *excitation pulse*.

Further discussion of the resonance phenomenon and the RF pulse is in order. For excitation to occur, the frequency of the energy being sent must match the frequency at which the receiving object resonates. *Radio-frequency* energy is electromagnetic energy in the same band of frequencies used by commercial radio stations and cell phones. Resonance is very similar to how a radio station works (2). If a radio station is broadcasting with a 101-MHz radio signal and people want to receive it in their car radio, then the car radio must be tuned to the 101-MHz channel. The same is true with protons. Recall that in a 1-T field, the net magnetization vector precesses at 42.6 MHz. To transmit energy into those protons, a special radio transmitter and antenna called an RF coil must be used to send out and receive energy at 42.6 MHz. If we vary the field slightly, say, to 1.02 T, then the radio frequency needs to change proportionately, to 43.4 MHz, to cause the protons to resonate. The signal received back from the protons will likewise have a frequency of 43.4 MHz.

RF Flip Angle

When the object is within the confines of the B_0 field before the application of the RF pulse, the net magnetization vector M_Z does not precess. The individual protons are precessing, but they are out of phase with one another, so there is no net magnetization in the *X–Y* plane (Figs. 19-1c and 19-1d). The RF pulse causes the hydrogen protons to precess in phase with one another in the *X–Y* plane, a phenomenon called *phase coherence*. This causes the net magnetic moment to precess in the M_{XY} plane (**Figure 19-3**). As time passes after the removal of the RF pulse, the protons lose this phase coherence, a process known as *dephasing*.

The stronger the RF pulse and the longer it is applied, the farther the net magnetization vector of protons will be deflected. The strength and the duration of the RF pulse therefore dictate the degree of deflection of the net magnetization into the transverse plane. The angle that the net magnetization is rotated away from the longitudinal direction is known as the *RF flip angle*. Any amount of flip angle into the transverse plane will generate an MR signal (3), but 90° and 180° flip angles are most commonly used. A 90° RF pulse, which deflects the entire net magnetization into the transverse plane, is used to begin the conventional spin echo pulse sequence. A smaller flip angle would only move part of the net magnetization into the transverse plane. A 180° RF pulse, which is applied for a longer time, causes the protons to flip 180° relative to the longitudinal B_0 field. The length of time the RF pulse is applied is in the microsecond range.

The Free Induction Decay Signal

The loss of the M_{XY} signal due to transverse dephasing generates a signal known as *free induction decay* (FID). The FID represents the precessing signal in the transverse plane; this is what is measured as the MR signal. As dephasing continues, eventually the magnetization of the protons will decay to zero and there will be no signal left for sampling. Thus the FID decreases over time, and the decrease is measured by the exponential curve shown enveloping the FID in Figure 19-3d. The pace at which the FID decays varies by the type of tissue, so this signal

(a) Before 90° pulse

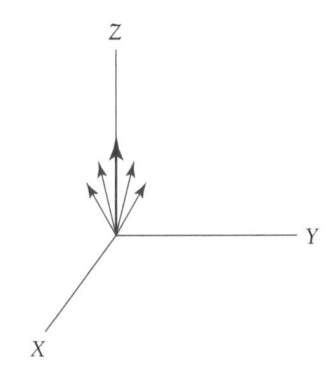

(b) Immediately after 90° pulse   (c) Dephasing after 90° pulse

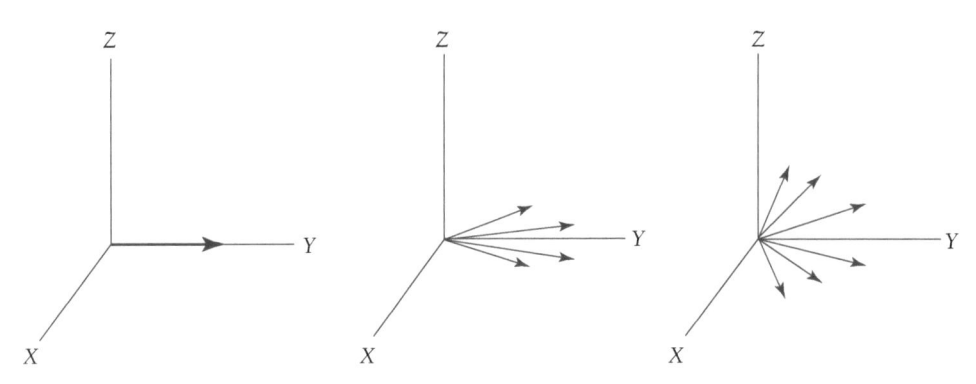

(d) FID pulse

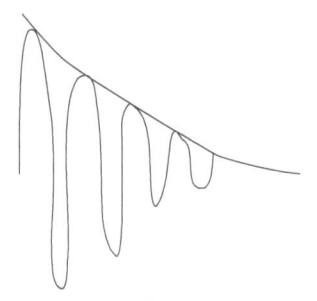

Figure 19-3 Effect of 90° RF pulse. After the protons are aligned with (or against) the external B_0 field, their precessions are out of phase (Fig. 19-3a). An RF pulse at the Larmor frequency is added. This causes the precessions to become aligned (phase coherence), which in turn generates net magnetization in the X–Y plane (Fig. 19-3b). As time goes on, however, the protons dephase (Fig. 19-3c), and this dephasing produces a measurable electronic current in the receiver called a free induction decay signal (Fig. 19-3d). The curve enveloping the FID in Figure 19-3d is reflective of T2* relaxation (see text for further explanation).

contains important image information. The FID is measured by an antenna within the MR tomograph called the receiver coil.

Relaxation

Let us look more closely at what happens as the spins dephase. As the nuclei stop precessing in phase with one another and return to equilibrium (that is, M_z aligned in the longitudinal direction), they lose energy by transferring it to the surrounding environment. The process by which energy is lost to the environment is called *relaxation*. Relaxation occurs via two mechanisms known as T1 relaxation and T2 relaxation (**Figure 19-4**). Both relaxation processes occur simultaneously but independently (3).

T1 Relaxation

When the RF pulse is switched off, the magnetization vector M_z, which was tilted away from the direction of B_0, will begin to regrow or recover due to the pull of the main magnetic field. T1 relaxation is the process of recovery of the net magnetization back into the longitudinal direction. Because different tissues in the human body experience T1 relaxation at different rates, this is one way that tissues in an MR image are differentiated. The primary mechanism

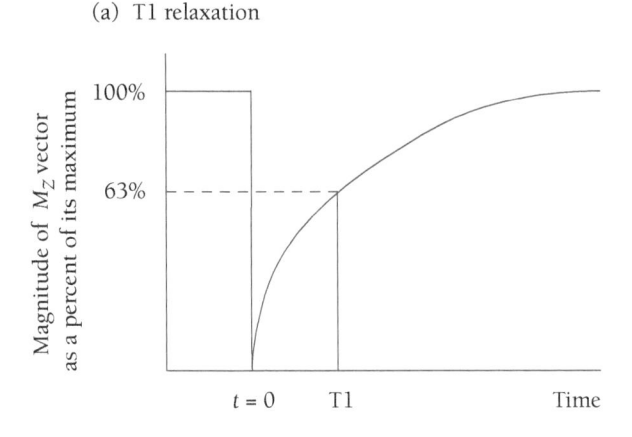

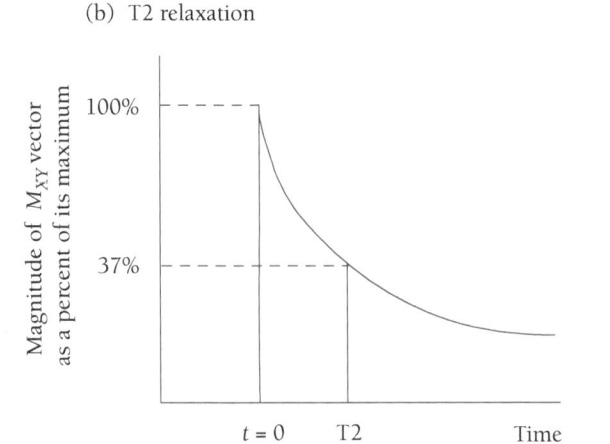

Figure 19-4 T1 and T2 relaxation. In each graph, $t = 0$ is the time of the 90° RF pulse. T1 relaxation is a measure of how long it takes for a tissue to return to its equilibrium position along the Z-axis (Fig. 19-4a). T2 relaxation measures the time needed for dephasing to occur (Fig. 19-4b). The time scales of the two graphs are not the same; T2 relaxation happens much more quickly than T1 relaxation.

of T1 recovery is the loss of the spins' energy to the surrounding molecular lattice. For this reason, T1 recovery is also known as *spin-lattice relaxation*. The *T1 relaxation time* is defined as the time required for the net magnetization in the Z direction to grow to 63% of its final amplitude. The T1 time for a given tissue is determined by measuring the increase in the maximum point on successive FID curves following a series of 90° RF pulses.

T2 Relaxation

T2 relaxation is the rate at which the net magnetization decays in the transverse plane. Dephasing of the spins results in a loss of transverse magnetization. Dephasing occurs as the spins interact with the magnetic fields of neighboring hydrogen molecules (known as *spin-spin interactions*) and with local magnetic field inhomogeneities. The *T2 relaxation time* is, by definition, the time required for transverse magnetization to decay to 37% of its maximum amplitude, due to spin-spin interactions. It is measured by determining the decrease in the peak FID after successive 180° RF pulses (each 180° pulse causes the magnetic field inhomogeneities to reverse, such that they cancel one another out). T2* relaxation includes not only spin-spin interactions but also the variations related to inhomogeneities of the magnetic field; in some imaging techniques, the latter effect must be taken into account specifically. T2* relaxation can be measured directly from a single FID (Fig. 19-3c).

The Pulse Sequence

A *pulse sequence* is a series of RF and gradient pulses that occur in a given order based on certain selected parameters, in order to disturb the orientation of the net

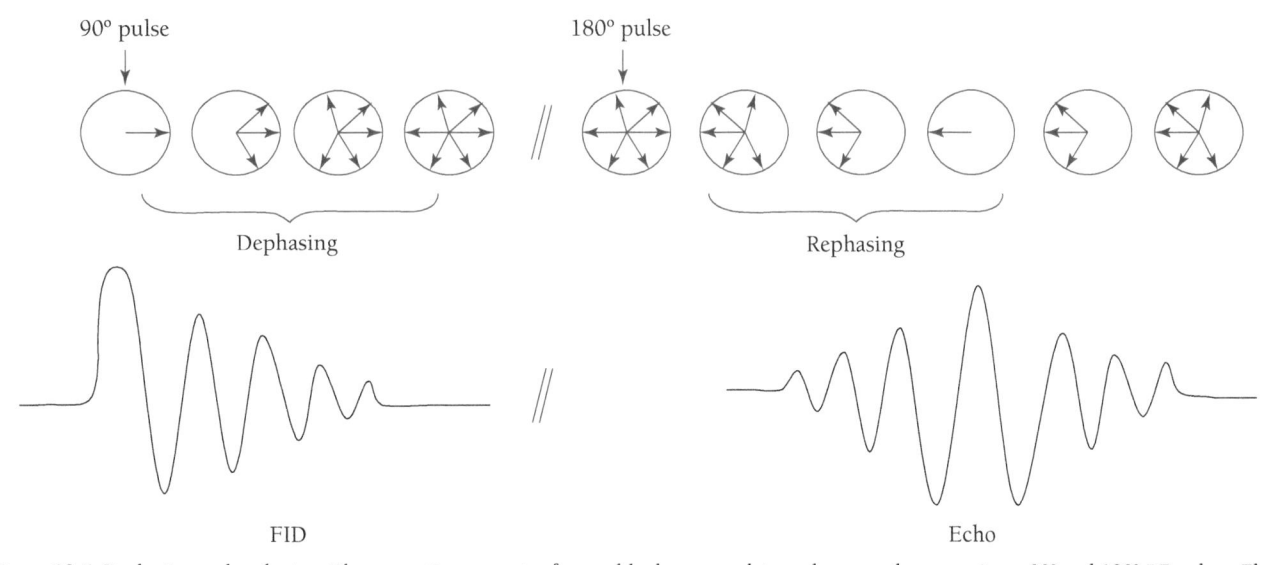

Figure 19-5 Dephasing and rephasing. The magnetic moments of several hydrogen nuclei are shown as they experience 90° and 180° RF pulses. The initial circle shows them all in phase in the X–Y plane. They dephase over time. The 180° pulse essentially reverses their dephasing, so that they come back into phase, generating the echo. The two slashes between the FID and the echo indicate that more time passes than the figure would indicate. The effect of the 180° pulse can be compared to causing runners on a track to turn around and go in the opposite direction. If the runners all started out together and continue at the same speed after the reversal, the 180° flip angle will cause them to come back together at the starting line.

magnetization of the protons and to spatially encode the information received as they return to equilibrium. Different pulse sequences generate a variety of images accenting various tissue qualities, each with unique benefits for diagnosis. New pulse sequences are generally developed either to be faster than an existing sequence or to better visualize specific anatomy or pathology.

The most elementary pulse sequence, and the only one to be discussed in this text, is called a *spin echo sequence*. This sequence consists of a 90° RF excitation pulse (which moves the protons into the transverse plane) followed by a 180° RF pulse (which aligns the protons in phase) and then the *echo*, the detected MR signal from which we measure the dephasing of the spins and regrowth of the M_Z vector (**Figure 19-5**). The time from the excitation pulse to the time at which the signal (the echo) is recorded is known as the *echo time* (TE), and the time from the excitation pulse until the cycle is ready to be repeated with the next excitation pulse is known as the *repetition time* (TR). (TE and TR are shown graphically in Figure 19-8.) The size of the echo is dependent on the T1 and T2 relaxation processes as well as the number of protons generating the echo, which is known as the *proton density*. This pulse sequence can be used to acquire any of the three most common types of images (T1-, T2-, or proton density–weighted), by varying TE and TR. The echo is the signal that is used to actually make the MR image. After the first echo is measured, a certain amount of time must be allowed to pass for some relaxation to occur, and then the process is repeated to obtain the next echo. This is repeated hundreds of times to achieve sufficient information density for the MR image.

Forming the Magnetic Resonance Image

As with other forms of tomographic imaging, our desire is to end up with slices of the body in the three orthogonal planes: transverse, coronal, and sagittal. These are defined relative to the patient and the three axes of the MRI tomograph: the Z-axis is the longitudinal (head-to-toe) axis, the X-axis crosses the body from left to right, and the Y-axis is the floor-to-ceiling or anterior-to-posterior direction (Fig. 19-2c). The most common MRI scenario is that the main magnetic field, B_0, is oriented with the Z-axis, causing a net magnetic moment M_Z in that direction. A 90° RF pulse causes the hydrogen protons to reorient into the X–Y or transverse plane. The signal to be measured is an estimate of how long it takes the protons to dephase and to realign with the B_0 magnetic field. The next question we need to ask is, "How do we get spatial information out of this scenario?"

Magnetic Gradients

In MR, several *magnetic field gradients* are used to spatially encode the information collected from echoes. A magnetic field gradient is simply a small, linear, incremental change in the magnetic field along a particular axis, expressed in milliteslas per meter (mT/m). This small change is achieved by sending an electric current through a loop of wire called a *gradient coil* located in the magnet. Each pulse sequence uses three different magnetic field gradients to spatially localize the information generated by each echo in three directions. Hence the MR tomograph has three gradient coils, which are designated the *slice selection* gradient, the *frequency encoding* gradient, and the *phase encoding* gradient. Each is described below.

By applying a magnetic field gradient along the Z-axis to a patient placed in the MR system with a 1-T magnetic field, we increase the magnetic field to be greater than 1 T in the head, decrease the magnetic field to be less than 1 T in the feet, and remain 1 T in the middle of the body. For the Y-axis gradient, the increase occurs in the anterior direction, the decrease occurs in the posterior direction, and the middle remains the same. For the X-axis gradient, the increase occurs to the left, the decrease occurs to the right, and the middle remains the same. In any axis, there is a point in the middle where the gradient is equal to the nominal value of the magnetic field. This point is called the *null*. **Figure 19-6** shows the B_0 field with its applied gradient. On one side of the null, the magnetic field is less than B_0; on the other it is greater than B_0. At the null, the field is equal to B_0.

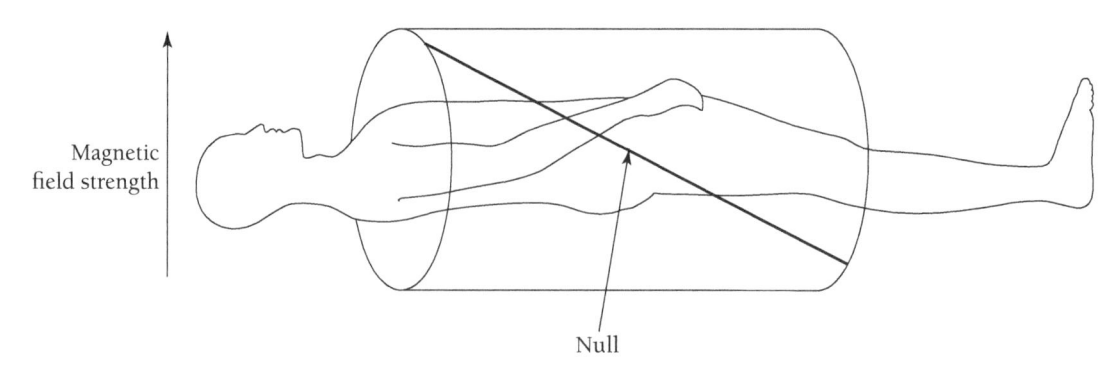

Figure 19-6 Slice selection gradient and null. The MR tomograph has a large magnet that creates the main magnetic field B_0. But to get information from different slices, a gradient or slope is applied to B_0, as illustrated by the heavy line in the diagram. The fact that the actual magnetic field varies in the longitudinal direction allows the tomograph to obtain information separately from each slice of the body, based on the proportional variation in the Larmor frequency. The null is the point at which the actual magnetic field is equal to the nominal value of B_0.

The gradient in the magnetic field causes the net magnetization's precessional frequency to vary depending on the position along the axis to which the gradient is applied. In other words, the magnetization vector at one end or side of the patient precesses more slowly, and moving along the gradient toward the other end or side of the patient, the magnetization vector precesses more and more quickly. To identify the received signal in three dimensions, three main functions are performed during data acquisition: *slice selection, phase encoding,* and *frequency encoding*. Generally, when one refers to the gradients by function rather than direction or orientation, the *logical notation* is used.

Logical Notation

It would be possible to use any of the gradients in any direction, but MR tomograph manufacturers generally apply them as follows (**Table 19-1**):

- The gradient used to perform slice selection is referred to as the Z gradient.
- The gradient used to perform phase encoding is referred to as the Y gradient.
- The gradient used to perform frequency encoding is referred to as the X gradient.

A good way to remember the logical notation is to place them in logical order or alphabetically (X, Y, Z). The functions are then in alphabetical order with the corresponding gradients (frequency, phase, and slice). In practice, when one refers to a physical gradient or gradient magnetic field direction, the physical notation is used. **Figure 19-7** summarizes the effects of the three gradients.

Data Storage

Let's take a moment to review the basic concepts of digital imaging. MRI can only be acquired digitally because the MR signal does not interact directly with a viewable medium as x-rays do with radiographic intensifying screens, or as gamma rays do with a scintillation crystal. Because MR is a digital imaging modality, the image information must be expressed in terms of discrete numbers. Digital images are numerical representations of an object that can be recognized and processed by a computer.

Prior to beginning the acquisition, the computer needs to allot space for data storage. The acquisition protocol specifies both the field of view (FOV) size and the matrix to be used. Common matrix sizes include 128, 192, 256, and 320, but there is not a requirement for the two matrix directions (the phase encoding and frequency encoding directions) to have equal numbers of pixels, as in gamma camera imaging. The FOV can be adjusted so as to apply the chosen matrix to a smaller area than the entire space within the MR bore. This allows for magnification of a small region, with a concomitant improvement in spatial resolution.

The actual data storage location is a mathematical map referred to as *k-space*. One direction in a *k*-space matrix represents phase information, and the other direction represents frequency information (physicists often use the letter *k* when referring to frequency). The number of data points in *k*-space is determined by the number of phase and frequency encodings specified in the acquisition protocol, which in turn is determined by the desired matrix. The more data points collected during the acquisition, the greater the detail on the image and (in some cases) the longer the scan time. Each transverse slice of the acquisition will have its own *k*-space matrix. When all the data points have been collected, the MR raw data (*k*-space data) are sent to the computer and the image is reconstructed by a mathematical process known as *Fourier transformation*.

Slice Selection

The first gradient to be applied is the slice selection or Z gradient. The slice selection gradient must be on during any application of RF pulses. In the spin echo sequence, the slice selection gradient is applied during both the 90° RF pulse and the 180° pulse. The slice selection gradient causes each transverse slice of the body to resonate at a different frequency. The RF pulses therefore must vary in frequency in order to excite the protons in each transverse slice, one slice at a time. The slice thickness is determined by the amplitude (slope) of the Z gradient. If a thinner slice is desired, higher amplitude is required; a thicker slice uses lower amplitude. The frequency bandwidth of the RF pulse may also be varied to control slice thickness. The slice location of the MR signal is determined by the center frequency of the RF pulse.

Frequency Encoding

The second gradient is called the frequency encoding gradient, and it is applied in the X-axis (patient's left–right) direction. Within the single slice of tissue that is being excited by the RF pulse, each column's hydrogen atoms precess with a slightly different signal frequency, due to this frequency encoding gradient. The receiving coil, which is registering the echoes, receives these signals, which are now a composite of both the Larmor frequency (the same for all the atoms in this slice) and the additional frequency from the gradient (which varies per column of tissue). These two components are decoded by the Fourier transform. The frequency encoding gradient is also called the *readout gradient,* because it is applied as the signals are being received.

Table 19-1

Directional Notations for Spatial Gradients

Physical Notation	Logical Notation	Gradient Direction
Head/foot	Slice selection	Z
Right/left	Frequency encoding	X
Anterior/posterior	Phase encoding	Y

(a) Slice selection

(b) Frequency encoding

(c) Phase encoding

Gradient 1

Gradient 64

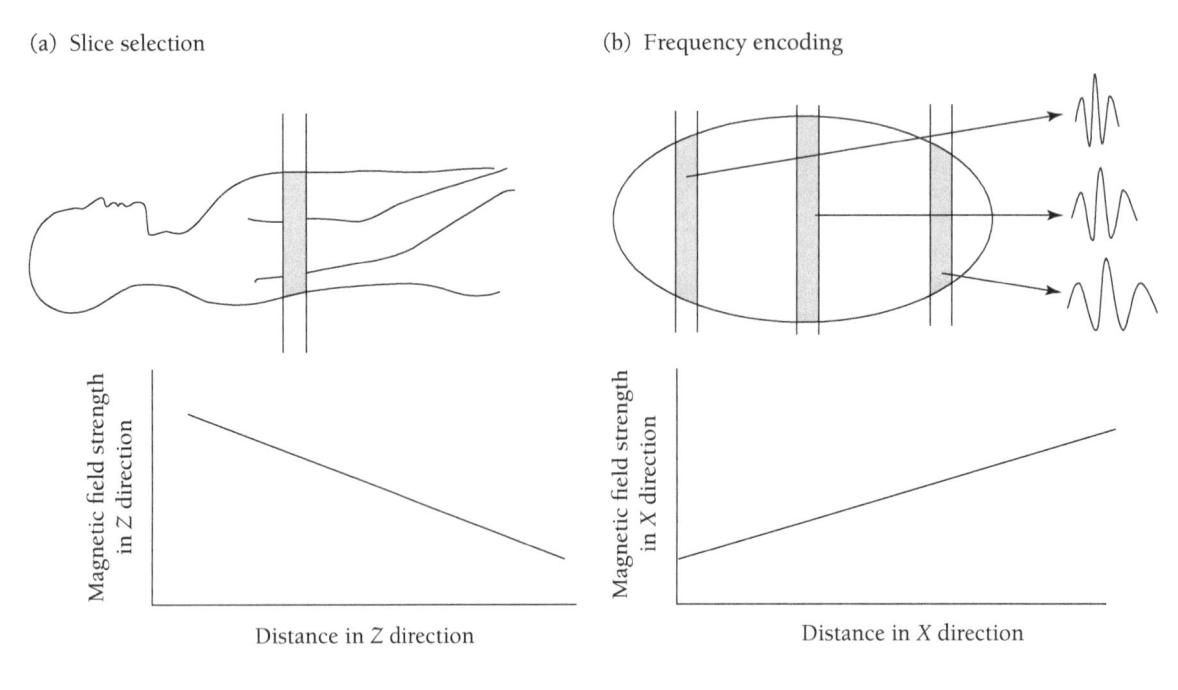

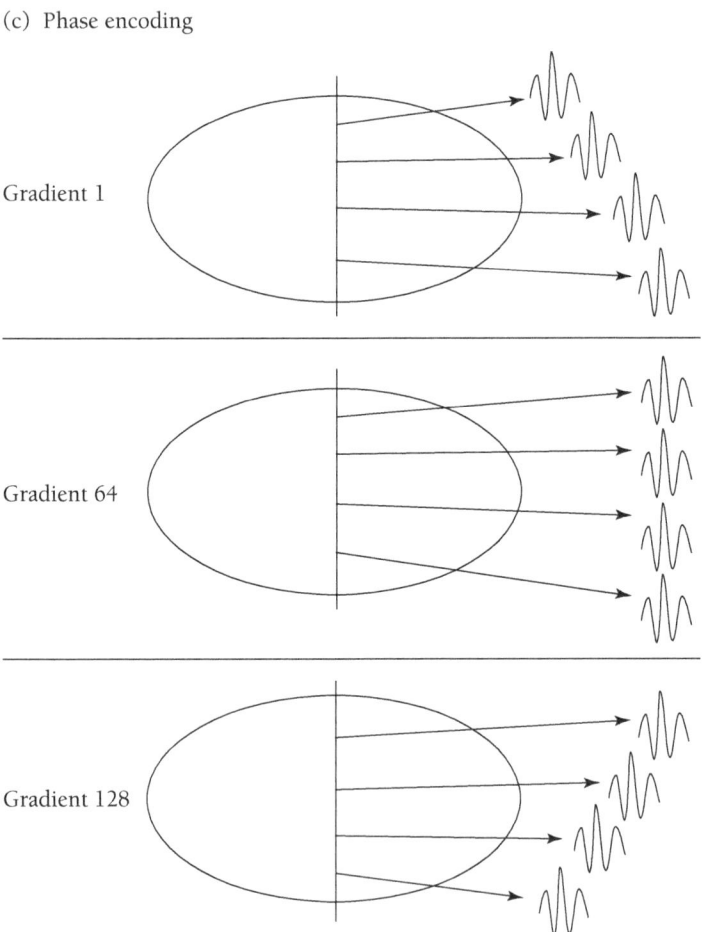

Gradient 128

Figure 19-7 Spatial encoding of the MR signal. To obtain information in three dimensions, the MR tomograph applies magnetic gradients (changing magnetic fields) at three times during the pulse sequence. The first gradient, the slice selection gradient, creates a variation in resonance frequency in the Z direction, which can then be matched by the RF frequency. Thus, only one slice of tissue is excited in a given moment (Fig. 19-7a). The frequency encoding gradient is turned on during the signal readout, causing echoes from different columns of the tissue (i.e., the X direction) to have slightly different frequencies around the slice's Larmor frequency (Fig. 19-7b). The phase encoding gradient shifts the phase of the echo from different vertical points. Figure 19-7c shows a single vertical column of tissue and three different phase encoding gradients. At the null point (gradient 64), the tissue experiences no phase shift (all of the wave forms are exactly aligned). But at other points, the echo phase shifts (the echo pulse moves left or right) depending on the vertical location of the protons generating the signal. The phase encoding gradient must be applied once for each matrix element in the Y direction.

Sample Calculation 19-2   Effect of the Slice Selection Gradient

For a particular acquisition, B_0 is 1T, the B_0 gradient is 0.01 T/m, and the RF pulse bandwidth is 0.005 MHz. Calculate the RF pulse frequency needed at the 1-T null point and at 10 cm on either side of this point. Also calculate the slice thickness, based on the bandwidth.

We have already calculated the RF pulse frequency for a 1-T field in Sample Calculation 19-1:

$$1\,\text{T} \times \frac{42.6\,\text{MHz}}{\text{T}} = 42.6\,\text{MHz}.$$

Given the gradient of 0.01 T/m, a slice 10 cm (0.1 m) to either side of the null point should have a magnetic field of

$$1\,\text{T} + (0.1\,\text{m})\left(\frac{0.01\,\text{T}}{\text{m}}\right) = 1.001\,\text{T}$$

$$1\,\text{T} - (0.1\,\text{m})\left(\frac{0.01\,\text{T}}{\text{m}}\right) = 0.999\,\text{T}.$$

These correspond to RF pulse frequencies of

$$1.001\,\text{T} \times \frac{42.6\,\text{MHz}}{\text{T}} = 42.64\,\text{MHz}$$

$$0.999\,\text{T} \times \frac{42.6\,\text{MHz}}{\text{T}} = 42.56\,\text{MHz}.$$

The RF bandwidth of 0.005 MHz corresponds to a magnetic gradient change of

$$0.005\,\text{MHz} \times \frac{1\,\text{T}}{42.6\,\text{MHz}} = 0.00012\,\text{T}.$$

This in turn can be related to the magnetic field gradient to determine the slice thickness:

$$0.00012\,\text{T} \times \frac{1\,\text{m}}{0.01\,\text{T}} = 0.012\,\text{m} = 12\,\text{mm}.$$

We can compare frequency encoding to notes from a piano (4). Piano keys have spatial locations, with the low-frequency keys on the left side of the keyboard and high-frequency keys on the right. If a low note is heard, we know it came from a key to the left of center; if we are well versed in the piano, we may be able to determine which key was struck to produce the note. Similarly, the frequency of a particular signal after frequency encoding indicates the part of the body where the signal originates. How many columns of tissue will we get? If 256-frequency encoding is selected, the system will sample the echo at 256 different frequencies. This process will produce 256 *columns* of data, which are plotted in the frequency or *X* direction of the *k*-space matrix.

Phase Encoding

The phase encoding (*Y* direction) gradient is applied during the free induction decay. The purpose of phase encoding is to encode spatial information into the MR signal representing the line in *k*-space on which the data will be plotted during the readout period. The phase encoding gradient is applied for a short duration, causing a linear variation in precessional frequency from anterior to posterior. After this gradient is turned off, the FID signals from the different rows of tissue revert to the Larmor frequency, but now have phase shifts incorporated in them that are relative to their position within the column of tissue. The protons remain in phase with one another within a row of tissue, but out of phase with other rows.

The phase encoding gradient must be applied a number of times to obtain phase encoding for each row of pixels. If a phase resolution of 256 is desired, then the pulse sequence must be repeated 256 times, with the phase encoding gradient having a different slope each time. Spatial resolution may be increased in the phase direction by acquiring a greater number of phase encoding steps, but this increases the scan time because the pulse must be repeated an equivalent number of times.

Data acquisition is accomplished as follows: The phase encoding gradient is held constant for one TR (generally 0.5 to several seconds). During the TR, each slice is excited and sampled in succession by applying the slice selection and frequency encoding gradients. The number of slices that can be sampled, therefore, depends on the length of the TR and the time required for sampling the signal for each slice (which is on the order of milliseconds). It is common to repeat the same sequence more than once to get an average signal, rather than just a single measurement for each data point in *k*-space. This is a parameter entered into the acquisition protocol, and it is called the *number of excitations* (NEX) or the *number of signal averages* (NSA). After the necessary data points at one phase encoding gradient have been stored in *k*-space, it is changed and the next set of data points is acquired. Each sample contains data from the entire slice, but different parts of the slice have different frequencies and phases. Again, the data are decoded by the Fourier transformation process.

Let us review the need for and the timing of application of the three gradients (**Figure 19-8**). If the 90° and 180° pulses were applied without the simultaneous application of the slice selection gradient, the RF energy would cause every proton in the vicinity of the transmitting RF coil to be disturbed. Therefore, to restrict the external energy's disturbance to a single slice, the slice select gradient must be turned on whenever the RF energy is being transmitted. Frequency encoding occurs during the time that the signal in the echo is being sampled. The range of the frequency or readout gradient determines the range of frequencies encoded in the echo, which in turn depends on the number of *X* elements in the image matrix. The phase encoding gradient is turned on between the 90° RF pulse and the

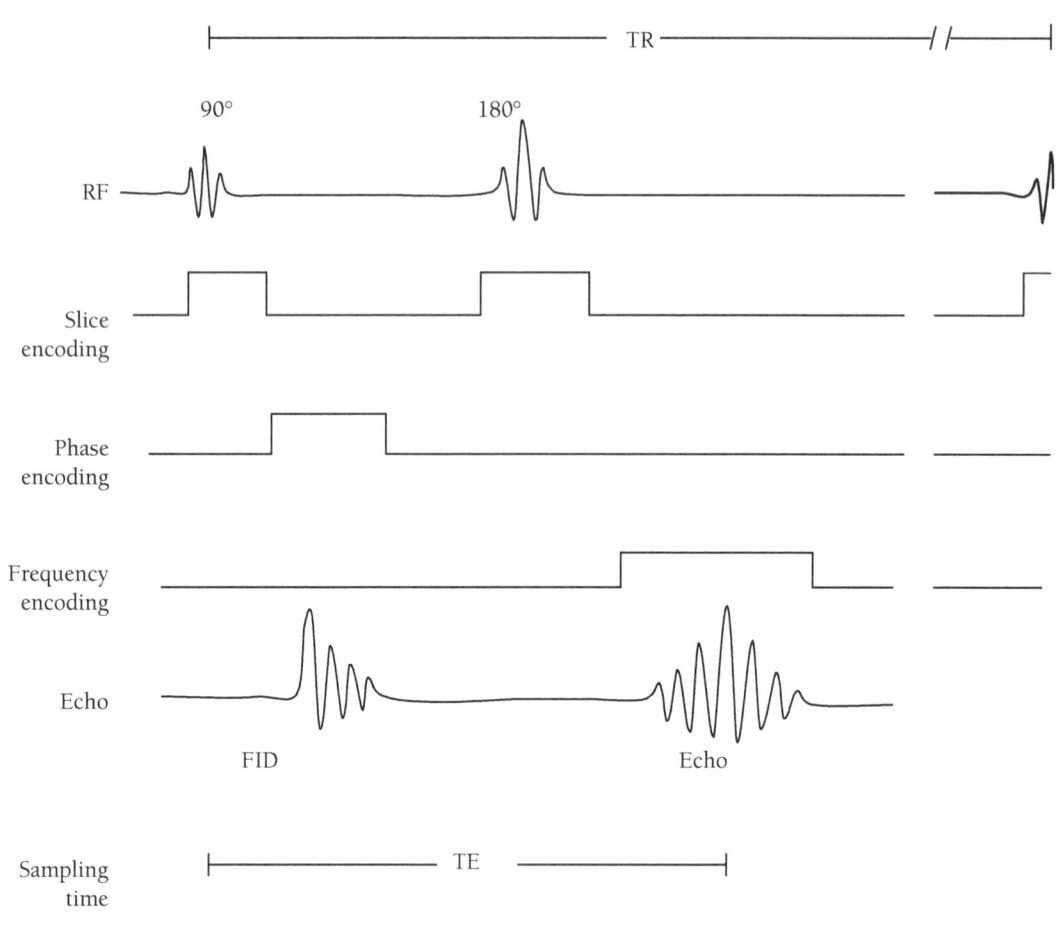

Figure 19-8 Pulse sequence and application of gradients. This figure shows when, within the spin echo sequence, each encoding gradient is applied. The slice selection gradient must be applied when the RF pulses are transmitted, because the slice selection involves setting a different Larmor frequency for each slice. The phase encoding gradient is applied between the 90° and 180° pulses, so that the resulting signals have the phase offsets necessary for spatial encoding. The frequency encoding gradient is applied during the readout, giving each column of tissue within the slice its own readout frequency. The sampling time occurs during the time that the echo is present. Each TR is aquired with a different phase encoding gradient, and each slice is sampled within the TR.

180° RF pulse. The number of phase encodings must equal the number of Y elements in the image matrix.

We can envision a k-space matrix as a chest of drawers (4). Each phase encoding gradient corresponds to one drawer. Within the drawer, items are placed according to their frequency, which depends on the frequency encoding gradient. When the next phase encoding gradient is applied, we have moved to the next drawer. But remember that we have many slices, so we really have many chests (each slice has its own k-space matrix). The acquisition sequence puts information into the same drawer of each chest during a single TR, and the contents of the chests (i.e., of k-space) are built up drawer by drawer.

Summary of Image Formation

Spatial encoding is accomplished by the application of magnetic gradients in all three orthogonal directions. All signals from the same slice are recorded in a single k-space data matrix, which is in turn processed to form an image of the slice plane. Within the k-space matrix, frequency is encoded along the X-axis and phase along the Y-axis. Frequency spatial encoding is applied only briefly, during signal reading. Phase encoding involves repeating the imaging sequence for data collection, with each repetition at a different point in the phase encoding gradient. In classic spin echo sequences, a single phase encoding gradient is applied during each TR. TR values can be up to 3 sec in length, so phase encoding always takes much longer than frequency encoding. The k-space matrix, when complete, contains the proton density, T1, T2, and flow information about each pixel within a single slice of tissue.

MRI Instrumentation

The essential components of an MR tomograph are: a magnet to provide the main external magnetic field, the gradient coils needed for spatial localization, a transmitter of the RF pulses, a receiver of the echo signals, and a computer to reconstruct the images. Each of these has its own complexities, and the incorporation of all of them into a working tomograph requires a considerable amount of engineering. The coverage given here is very brief, with the intent of describing the most common choices and briefly touching on the complexities.

Magnets

There are four main types of MR magnet: air-core resistive magnets, iron-core electromagnets, permanent magnets, and superconducting magnets. Nearly all clinical scanners are superconducting magnets and are typically a horizontal bore design (as shown in Fig. 19-2c). Superconductivity is a physical property of some materials in which there is essentially no resistance to electric current at very low temperatures. These magnets are made up of superconducting alloys of niobium and titanium. The state of zero electrical resistance needs to be maintained, and this is achieved by cooling the magnet to what is termed the *critical temperature* (a physical feature of the individual magnet). Critical temperature is maintained through the use of liquid helium, in which the magnet windings are immersed. Liquid helium levels must be monitored and replenished as needed. Systems needing less strong magnetic fields may employ resistive electromagnets, and some early machines even used permanent magnetic cores.

The homogeneity of the magnet is very important to the production of high-quality images. Open and short-bore design MR imaging setups have less homogeneous magnetic fields than their longer, closed-bore counterparts. Homogeneity is maintained through a service engineering procedure called *shimming*. Some passive shimming is done at the time of manufacture by fixing sheets of metal at certain points. Active shimming is achieved by manipulating the currents passing through the individual sets of magnet windings. It is usually checked at installation and after major repairs.

Magnetic fields from MR tomographs can extend 10 m or more (5). Shielding of the MR suite is obviously necessary so that the high magnetic fields do not impact individuals outside of the MR suite. Clinical scanners are both passively and actively shielded. Passive shielding consists of thick metal walls; active shielding utilizes opposite-direction current in external windings to counteract the main B_0 field. The magnet itself is housed in a specially constructed room with copper lining the walls and ceiling to create what is known as a *Faraday cage*. This ensures that extraneous RF signals cannot penetrate the room, as these would superimpose on the RF signals emanating from the MR tomograph and create artifacts in the clinical images. In addition to shielding, most departments designate zones of safety or danger in relation to the MR tomograph. Only trained personnel are allowed to be in the most dangerous zone when the tomograph is operating. The level of magnetic field considered to be safe is generally given as 0.0005 T. Safety concerns are addressed at greater length later in the chapter.

Gradients

Additional *coils* (loops of wire carrying current) are needed within the magnet to provide the gradients for each imaging plane. Typically a pair of coils is utilized to provide the Z-direction gradient, whereas two differently shaped coils are utilized for the X and Y directions. Oscillating eddy currents are induced by the varying magnetic field gradients, and these in turn induce magnetic fields in the conductors surrounding them. These contribute to noise and geometric distortions within the clinical image and therefore require additional shielding.

Gradient performance is specified in terms of the *slew rate* (how quickly the magnetic gradient reaches its final value), defined mathematically as the maximum amplitude divided by the rise time (time required to go from zero amplitude to maximum value). A typical modern scanner may have an amplitude of 40 mT/m and rise time of 200 msec, giving a slew rate of 0.2 mT/m per msec.

High-power audio frequency amplifiers are needed to supply the current required to produce the gradient fields. The higher the field size, the greater the requirement for high peak-gradient amplitudes. This in turn drives up the costs of the amplifier associated with the magnet, as the need for rapid electric current generation through the coils is critical for artifact-free imaging.

RF Coils

To provide the B_1 field necessary for transmission and to receive the signal, RF coils are required, either working separately or as a single coil (called a *transceiver*) in which both functions are combined. RF coils are located within the main magnet. They are designed for specific purposes, such as imaging different areas of anatomy, different study purposes, different FOV requirements, or different signal-to-noise (SNR) levels. Image quality is further influenced by the performance characteristics of the individual coil. The simplest coil design is a surface coil, consisting of a single loop of wire. It can function as a receiver only, and provides excellent signal from tissues closest to it. Transceiver coil designs are available for utilization on larger body parts, such as head and body coils. The performance characteristics of the latter usually translate into lower signal intensities, but often provide a more homogeneous magnetic field and produce a more uniform clinical image. Let us consider each aspect of the RF system separately.

RF Pulse Characteristics

The transmitter must generate RF pulses with unique and defined frequencies, bandwidths, amplitudes, and phases. This is a requirement in order for excited nuclei to be sampled and spatially located within the sampled slice or scan volume. The pulse's center frequency determines the strength and location of the slice selection gradient. Slice thickness is controlled by the bandwidth of the RF pulse. Bandwidth is in turn determined by the geometric shape and duration of the RF pulse profile. The RF pulse amplitude determines the amount of flip angle that can physically occur. RF pulse profiles are digitally produced in modern scanners.

Transmit Coils

The coil used to generate the RF pulse must produce a uniform field B_1 at right angles to the static magnetic field. Transmit coils are usually large in size in order to optimize their uniformity characteristics and increase the FOV size. Appropriate transmit coil selection protects the receiver circuitry from the very high voltages applied during pulse transmission and also prevents the small MR signal from being lost in the electronic noise generated by the transmitter in its "off" (nonreading) state. The body coil is the main transmitter and is usually wrapped around the inside of the MR gantry. Body coils are generally large and have nonuniform transmission fields. Body coils are not sensitive receivers. A head coil is a helmet-like piece that fits over the patient's head for imaging. It may serve as both transmitter and receiver.

Receiver Coils

The function of a receiver coil is to raise the efficiency of signal detection and keep the noise contribution to the clinical image at a minimum. Coil dimensions and scan volumes must be appropriately matched to the FOV size so that the SNR of the clinical images is maximized. At the same time, we need to keep the homogeneity of the magnetic field at a level that will give the clinician accurate images over the whole FOV. There are two types of receiver coils: volume and surface. Volume coils encompass the total anatomy of interest and are often dual-use transceiver coils. Surface coils are used for receiving only. Surface coils are excellent in detecting signals near the surface of the patient, but signal detection drops off exponentially for tissue that is farther away from the coil. Receiver coils may operate in various arrangements and orientations, and they can constructively fuse together in a phased array to enhance the reception of signals in an efficient manner. The signal response of a surface coil is nonlinear with depth, resulting in an intensity reduction for deeper tissues, making these desirable primarily for surface anatomy.

Computer

MR computer systems are composed of many subsystems, owing to the large number of tasks that are involved in generating and processing the MR signal. These are linked to the main host computer and derive their commands and language from the main host. Typically, the host computer will define scan parameters such as pulse sequence selection, TR and TE matrix size, and geometric orientation of data collection. These acquisition parameters are then converted into commands which in turn are transferred to another microprocessor system, termed the *pulse programmer* (PP). The PP ensures synchronization of data such as the RF, the gradient applications, and data acquisition. A separate computer system known as the array processor is the image reconstruction subsystem. The host computer controls the image display settings, processing tools, and image reconstruction methods applied by the operator.

Tissue Characteristics and Image Appearance

The basic types of images obtained in MRI are T1-weighted, T2-weighted, and proton density–weighted images. The different weightings are achieved by varying the acquisition parameters, particularly TE and TR. As we have seen, T1 and T2 refer to the relaxation times as the M_Z vector regrows and the M_{XY} vector decays, respectively. What makes these two quantities useful for imaging is that their values depend on the composition and neighborhood of the tissue in which the hydrogen atoms reside. Note that we do not have to measure T1 and T2 for each voxel in each scan. Rather, we set TE and TR such that either T1 characteristics or T2 characteristics are favored, or (if neither is favored) proton density weighting is illustrated. Each of these image types is discussed below. In addition, we discuss what happens when a fluid (such as blood) is moving during the acquisition of the MR signal.

Relaxation Characteristics

T1- and T2-weighted images can be produced using the spin echo or other pulse sequences. T1-weighted images usually have excellent contrast: the fluids are usually dark, water-based tissues are medium gray, and fat-based tissues are extremely bright. T2-weighted images are great for pathologies, as areas of inflammation or edema are represented as bright objects against the dark background belonging to normal tissue. A good example would be a tear of the meniscus in the knee, which is easily delineated by the observer because the synovial fluid in the tear is brighter than the cartilage. Let us consider how each of these images is generated, using the brain as an example organ (**Figure 19-9**, **Table 19-2**, and **Figure 19-10**).

T1 Relaxation Effects

A T1-weighted image is an image that emphasizes T1 relaxation characteristics by using a short echo time to minimize the T2 contrast and a short repetition time to maximize the T1 contrast in an image. *Spin lattice* is another name for T1 relaxation because the energy is dissipated from protons into the surrounding molecular lattice during the relaxation process. How quickly the protons can move the energy they absorbed into their surrounding molecular environment is unique for each tissue. T1 relaxation times can range from about 0.2 sec to several seconds. As the magnetic field strength of an MR system increases, the T1 relaxation time of tissue also increases. Tissues with short T1 relaxation times regrow along the longitudinal direction quickly, while tissues with long T1 relaxation times regrow along the longitudinal direction slowly. Tissues that have a short T1 time such as fat will appear bright on a T1-weighted image, and tissues that have a long T1 relaxation time such as cerebrospinal fluid (CSF) will appear darker.

T2 Relaxation Effects

A T2-weighted image is an image that emphasizes T2 relaxation characteristics by using a long TE to maximize the T2 contrast and a long TR to minimize the T1 contrast in an MR image. *Spin-spin* is another name for T2 relaxation, because energy is transferred from one spinning proton to another during the decay process. The rate at which the protons can exchange energy is unique for each type of tissue. T2 relaxation times range from 0.01 to 0.33 sec, much shorter than T1 relaxation. Unlike T1 times, T2 times do not depend on the magnetic field strength. Tissues with short T2 relaxation times lose transverse magnetization very quickly. Tissues with long T2 relaxation times lose transverse magnetization more slowly, resulting in higher signal intensity. Fat and white matter have similar T2 relaxation times. White matter is primarily made up of myelin (a lipid-based protein), so both transverse magnetizations behave similarly. Fat is an example of tissue with a short T2 relaxation time that will appear dark on a T2-weighted image; cerebrospinal fluid is an example of tissue with a long T2 relaxation time that will appear bright.

Proton Density Weighting

Proton or *spin density* refers to the density of magnetizable hydrogen atoms in a tissue. Tissues containing a large number of hydrogen atoms, such as fats and aqueous fluids, have a higher proton density than tissues consisting primarily of proteins. Proton density–weighted images are obtained by making TR long to minimize T1 differences and making TE short to minimize T2 differences. In the brain, fat and cerebrospinal fluid are relatively bright, and white matter has lower signal intensity than gray matter. Image contrast is generally less in proton density–weighted images than in either T1-weighted or T2-weighted images.

Appearance of Moving Fluids

Now consider what happens when a moving fluid such as blood is included in an MR acquisition. The initial RF pulse interacts with the hydrogen atoms in the slice of tissue that is excited. But by the time the echo makes its appearance, the blood that was initially excited has moved out of the slice. So our first guess would be that a moving fluid would show as an area of no signal, a *flow void*. However, moving fluid can be enhanced with certain pulse sequences and/or by injecting a paramagnetic contrast agent such as gadolinium. The appearance of a moving fluid also depends on the velocity and turbulence of its flow. So the identification of a particular structure as containing a moving fluid is not always obvious. Moving fluids can also create artifacts in the final image.

Safety Issues

The issue of safety in the context of MRI has many different aspects, requiring the technologist to keep a number of possibilities in mind at all times. As with any procedure that involves application of energy fields, we need to be aware of the potential negative effects these might have on the body. The potential for negative side effects increases significantly when a patient has a prosthesis, an aneurysm clip, or any other foreign object that can be affected by a magnetic field. Even for persons outside of the MR suite itself, the magnetic field can cause changes in pacemakers and other electronic devices. And last but not least, we should consider the

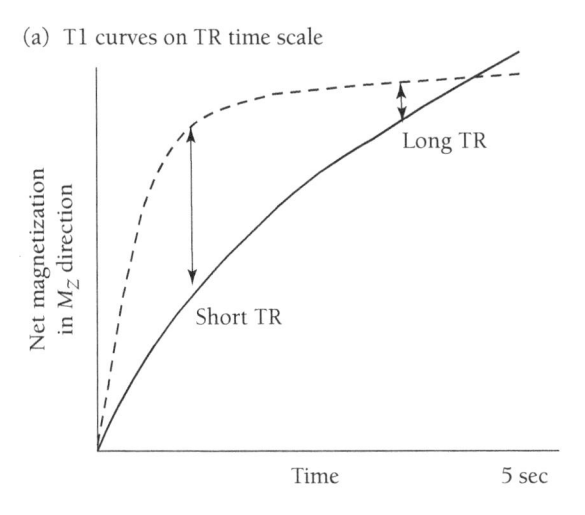

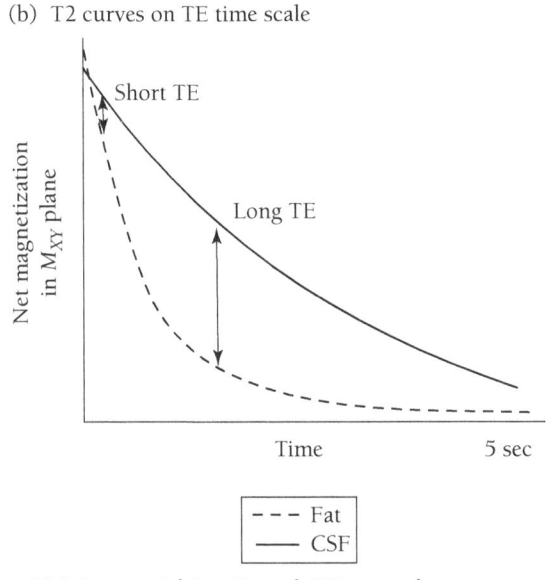

Figure 19-9 Image weighting. Fat and CSF are used as two components of images that have very different T1 and T2 relaxation curves. Because different tissues have different spin-spin and spin-lattice relaxation rates, we can manipulate the resulting images by judiciously choosing TR and TE. Figure 19-9a shows the relative regrowth of longitudinal magnetization for fat and CSF. Choosing a short TR emphasizes the difference between their T1 characteristics, while choosing a long TR deemphasizes those differences (notice the different lengths of the double-headed arrows). Figure 19-9b shows the relative loss of magnetization in the M_{XY} plane. A short TE deemphasizes the T2 characteristic differences of the two (the lines are closer together and the arrow shorter), whereas a long TE accentuates the difference. If we deemphasize both T1 and T2, the resulting image reflects the proton density.

Table 19-2

Parameters for Different Image Types

To Obtain:	TE	TR
T1-weighted images	Short	Short
T2-weighted images	Long	Long
Proton density–weighted images	Short	Long

(a) T1-weighted image   (b) T2-weighted image   (c) Proton density–weighted image

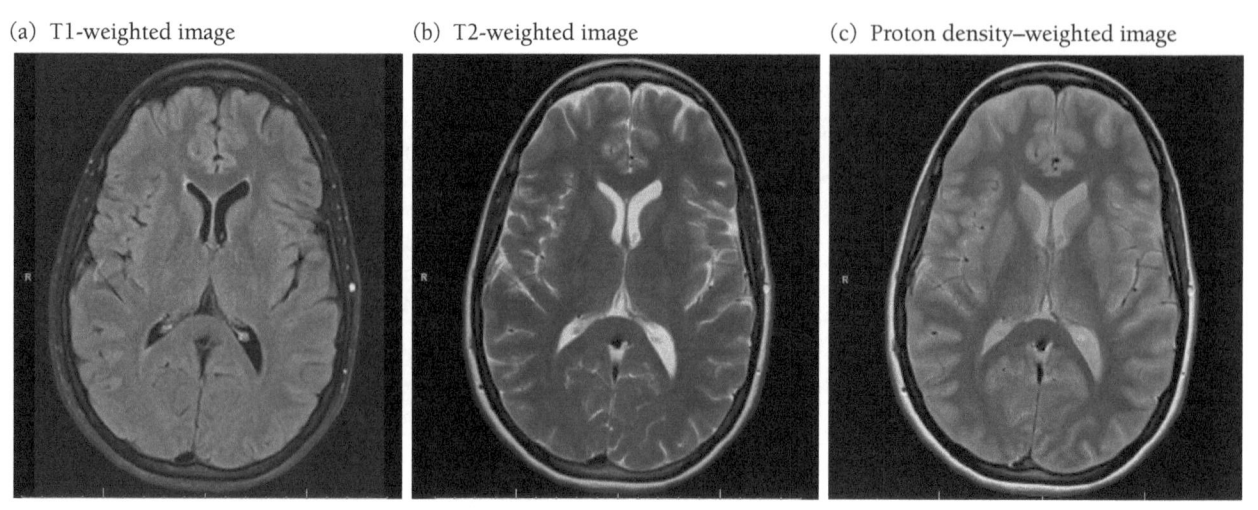

Figure 19-10 Examples of T1-, T2-, and proton density–weighted images. T1-weighted images have excellent contrast and effectively demonstrate anatomy. T2-weighted images show aqueous fluids at higher intensities than other tissues, and they are considered very good at showing many types of pathology. Proton density–weighted images reflect the total number of hydrogen atoms generating the signal in each pixel. Courtesy of Virginia Mason Medical Center.

potential for harm from MR-sensitive contrast agents such as gadolinium.

Bioeffects of Static Magnetic Fields

One of the ostensible benefits of MRI over other imaging techniques is that it does not involve ionizing radiation (RF electromagnetic radiation is much too low to cause ionization of electrons). Research is ongoing in regard to the effects of strong magnetic fields on living tissues. Temporary and reversible conditions that arise when individuals are exposed to large magnetic fields include these:

- Localized tissue and core body temperature heating
- Tingling sensations
- Peripheral nerve stimulation (involuntary muscle contractions)

At this time, none of these appear to be significant in the long term. The long-term safety of exposure to MR-strength magnets remains to be fully understood. Clinical MRI has been available for only about 30 years, but no carcinogenic or other chronic effects have yet been identified (4).

One area of concern is the ability of an MRI scan to cause temperature increases in tissues. Evidence can be found in the literature supporting both the theory of no temperature change and the potential for elevated temperature within the patient. RF energy does heat tissues (not by a significant amount with current system configurations and hardware), but the static magnetic field does not. The testes and the eyes are the organs of interest that would experience the largest temperature increase. Even tattoos can heat up in the MR tomograph; tattooed eyeliner is considered a contraindication to an MRI scan due to the potential effect on the eyes. The temperature issue is highly significant in patients with implanted metallic objects, as we shall see.

Another obvious issue is the pregnant patient. To date, fetal effects from magnetic fields have not been conclusively identified (4). While MRI (particularly in the first trimester) is not generally recommended for pregnant women, it can be an alternative to a more invasive or harmful test if the situation warrants. Pregnant employees may continue to work in the MR suite, but it is recommended that they not be in the tomograph room when it is in operation (5).

Magnet Safety

All patients and visitors must be thoroughly screened by qualified personnel before being exposed to an MRI environment. Most MR-related injuries have been a direct result of deficiencies in screening methods. It is essential that the topic of magnetic safety be thoroughly understood by all staff involved in the daily operation of the MRI scanner. The magnetic field can seriously damage or impair the following personal items:

- Cameras, cell phones, music players, watches, etc.
- Credit and bank cards
- Hearing aids, pacemakers, and implants (especially those made from materials with magnetic susceptibility)

It is vital that persons entering the MR suite identify to the staff any implants or other metal in their bodies. All removable items of clothing need to be removed, and patients should be clothed only in a hospital gown and robe.

Persons with metallic implants of any kind can suffer serious injuries in an MRI scan. Implants with magnetic properties will experience torque and heating, in addition to creating significant artifacts on the images. The magnetic field interaction with the implant in some instances has been strong enough to dislodge an implant (4). Even nonferrous metal implants can be heated by the magnetic field, because they are unable to dissipate the heat generated by absorption of the RF pulse (4). This eliminates a good portion of the population from eligibility for MRI scans. Dental amalgams and heart valves seem to be acceptable, but most other implanted materials should be allowed only with great care.

Every person entering the MR suite, including staff and visitors, must be screened to the same extent as those who will actually be scanned. Physical screening is intended to identify objects or materials that would be dangerous if brought into the MRI room, including both ferromagnetic objects that may become projectiles and electrically conductive materials that may experience focal heating during the MR exam. Even a paper clip can cause harm when traveling at high velocity toward the magnet. Many MRI providers now use screening systems such as metal-detecting wands to help ensure that patients, staff, and visitors do not accidentally bring ferromagnetic objects into the MRI room. There are anecdotal stories of various objects (guns, oxygen tanks, etc.) being pulled into MR tomographs.

Claustrophobia and Acoustic Noise

The most memorable aspects of an MRI scan for most patients are the amount of noise that is involved and the relatively small size of the gantry bore. The banging noise (sometimes described as a jackhammer or a machine gun, among other characterizations) results from the rapidly changing electric currents in the gradient coils. Noise levels can be as high as 90 decibels (6). Patients are offered earplugs or headphones to block out the noise, but for many they are only partially effective. Persons working in the vicinity of an MR tomograph can experience significant hearing loss over time.

Claustrophobia is another unavoidable point of patient discomfort. Some departments use relaxing medications for patients who are particularly bothered by the closeness of the gantry or the head coil, which must fit fairly closely over the face. There are reports of individuals who developed claustrophobia as a result of MRI scans (4).

MR Contrast Agents

Enhancement agents are routinely used in MRI to improve the contrast between normal and abnormal tissues, or between blood vessels and other tissues. The most common element used as a contrast agent is gadolinium (Gd), which has seven unpaired electrons. This makes it a paramagnetic metal, in that a Gd atom's magnetic moment will align with an external magnetic field. Gd is most often used in a chelated form, such as Gd-DTPA. When injected, a Gd contrast agent causes the T1 relaxation times of nearby water molecules to be shortened (4), thus enhancing the signal intensity of water-containing regions.

The safety of Gd contrast agents has come under some scrutiny in recent years. The chelation with DTPA leaves a negative charge that must be balanced in the injectate, usually by a molecule called meglumine. This makes Gd-DTPA an ionic contrast agent, similar to those used in CT, and in fact the safety profile for Gd-DTPA is similar to that of iodinated contrast (4). There is a small risk that patients on dialysis who receive Gd contrast agents can develop nephrogenic systemic fibrosis, a disease similar to scleroderma. This recently led to a "black box warning" placed on all Gd-based MRI contrast agents by the FDA (6).

PET/MRI

Work on combining PET with MRI started about the same time as the efforts to combine PET and CT. Now that PET/CT has become a reality, scientists have been making a concerted effort to fully develop PET/MRI. Using MRI as the anatomic imaging modality in conjunction with PET has several important advantages. One is that the tissue contrast is often better in MRI than in CT. Another is the ability to obtain images accenting different aspects of structure and function, as we have seen with T1, T2, and proton density weighting. A very intriguing possibility is that the PET tomograph can be made to be "invisible" to the MRI imaging process, allowing the PET tomograph to be located *inside* the MRI tomograph. And last but certainly not least, in this time of concern about medical radiation, MRI does not involve exposure to ionizing radiation.

Combined PET/MRI tomographs have recently come into the commercial market, and the three main manufacturers have each taken a different initial approach (7). GE Healthcare developed a table/track mechanism that allows a patient to have both PET/CT and MRI studies without moving. This provides a way to evaluate the clinical efficacy of PET/MRI relative to PET/CT, without a large research expenditure. Philips Healthcare took its already developed time-of-flight PET tomograph and aligned it in tandem with a separate MRI system (**Figure 19-11**). Siemens Healthcare took on the challenge of simultaneous PET/MRI, putting its redesigned PET tomograph inside the bore of a 70-cm-diameter MRI tomograph (**Figure 19-12**).

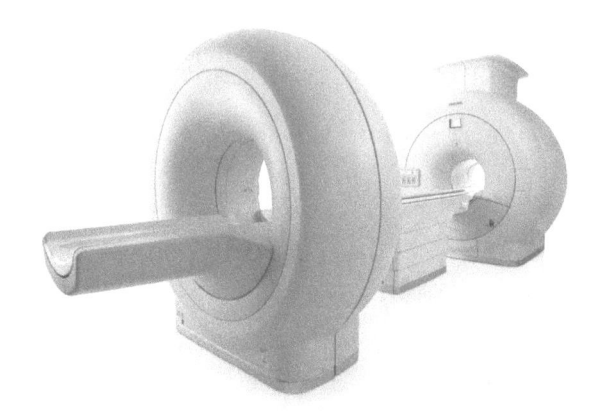

Figure 19-11 Philips Ingenuity time-of-flight PET/MR. This system combines PET (on the left) and MRI (on the right) tomographs. It accomplishes patient transfer between the two by means of a patient table (between the 2 units) that can be turned end for end. Courtesy of Philips Healthcare.

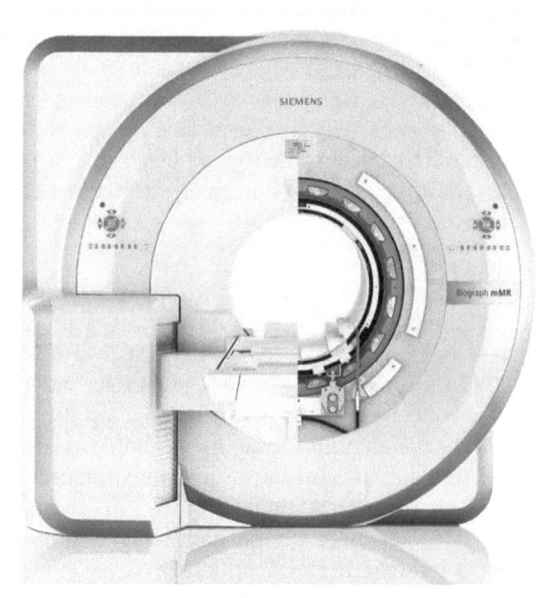

Figure 19-12 Siemens Biograph® mMR system. One of the possibilities that exists for PET/MRI and not for PET/CT is that the PET tomograph can be located inside the MRI gantry, allowing for truly simultaneous imaging with both modalities. The system shown here has made this concept a reality. Courtesy of Siemens Healthcare.

The company claims both a time savings and the elimination of misregistration artifacts with this system.

Technical Challenges

Let us consider the major technical obstacles involved in combining PET and MRI in a single gantry (8). The PET imaging process includes the creation of free electrons, most notably in the photomultiplier tubes (PMTs). These electrons would be redirected by the strong magnets used in MRI. One solution to this issue is to put the PMTs outside of the MRI bore, connecting them to the scintillation crystals via optical fibers. A second possibility is to replace the PMTs with avalanche photodiodes (described in Appendix B); this requires preamplifiers with greater gains, which can be distorted by the MR electronics (9). A thin layer of copper shielding between the MR and PET tomographs is necessary to remove this layer of interference.

Second, the PET tomograph must be "transparent" in terms of the magnetic resonance imaging process. Its presence must not affect the magnetic fields of the gradients, or the RF pulse, in any way. Some scintillators, notably gadolinium oxyorthosilicate (GSO) and lutetium gadolinium orthosilicate, have magnetic susceptibilities and produce significant artifacts in MR images (9). Lutetium oxyorthosilicate (LSO) is currently the scintillator of choice for a PET tomograph located within an MR gantry bore.

Another problem is that the voxel intensities in an MR image do not correlate with tissue density in the same way that CT voxel intensities do. This makes attenuation correction a very different challenge. For example, bone and air both show essentially no signal in MRI, but their 511-keV attenuation characteristics are very different (9). Several researchers have published MRI-based attenuation correction schemes, most based on segmentation of the tissues into bone, soft tissue, lung, fat, and/or air. These techniques use a variety of MRI pulse sequences as well as anatomic atlases to identify the different types of tissues, to which known 511-keV attenuation coefficients are applied.

A different kind of technical question mirrors that posed by PET/CT: What kind of training and education is required to operate a PET/MRI tomograph? Certification in MR is a postprimary path offered by the American Registry of Radiologic Technologists. Eligibility requirements include completion of an accredited MRI educational program as well as documentation of specific competencies. Candidates for MR certification must have a primary certification in radiography, nuclear medicine, radiation therapy, or sonography.

From the regulatory standpoint, PET/MRI presents issues distinct from those raised about PET/CT. Many state regulations limit the operation of equipment that produces ionizing radiation to persons who have completed a training program in radiography or radiation therapy. An MRI tomograph does not produce ionizing radiation, so it does not fall under this constraint. In fact, many states do not regulate MRI in any way, for the simple reason that radiation protection concerns do not apply. On the other hand, laboratory accreditation (see Appendix F) generally requires certification in any specialty in which a technologist is employed.

Clinical Benefits

The use of MRI as the anatomic localization modality for PET has some important advantages. The superb soft-tissue contrast of an MR image makes it ideal for pairing with molecular imaging probes that have very small amounts of uptake. The ability to obtain truly simultaneous image sets will make issues of registration and attenuation correction more exact and therefore more correct. Motion can be corrected for on a msec-by-msec basis in MR, then applied to PET data, opening up the possibility of gated PET/MRI studies (10).

But MRI has more to offer, because it can generate many different types of images. It can be used to detect oxygen utilization and perfusion (the blood oxygen level dependent [BOLD] technique, more generically known as functional or fMRI). MR spectroscopy allows quantification of specific chemicals on an organ-by-organ basis (9). MRI is also able to image hypoxia and growth of new blood vessels (angiogenesis), two conditions that allow cancers to grow and/or circumvent therapeutic efforts.

These different MR imaging techniques can be coupled with PET imaging to provide simultaneous, co-registered, temporally varying pictures of multiple physiologic processes. They allow for dynamic imaging following a pharmacologic intervention, using two different modalities. PET/MRI has particular applicability in areas that are not well imaged with CT, such as the base of the brain and the pelvis. It is thought that PET/MRI will be an ideal way to monitor therapeutic effects of oncologic treatment regimens (8). An added benefit in this setting is that the added radiation dose of a CT scan is avoided. Neuroscientists are especially interested in using PET/MRI to study white matter tracts, which may be the pathologic entities in a number of mental illnesses and brain injuries (10). In addition to these clinical applications, PET/MRI will be an excellent preclinical tool for evaluation of metabolism pathways of new drugs, with PET identifying tissues with drug uptake and MRI adding high-resolution imaging of the same areas (11). One major researcher hopes to achieve PET resolution of 0.5 mm, to be used in mouse studies (12).

Summary

PET/MRI is 10 or so years behind PET/CT, and we are just starting to understand its potential. The speed of adoption of this new multimodality system will likely be slower than that of PET/CT, due to both economic considerations and the simple fact that PET/CT was first. But in many ways, the possibilities with PET/MRI outstrip those we have already experienced with PET/CT. So it will be the forward-thinking nuclear medicine technologist who starts the effort to understand MRI, and who considers certification in MR as a near-term career goal.

References

1. Faulkner W, Seeram E. *MRI: Basic Physics, Instrumentation, and Quality Control.* Oxford, UK: Blackwell Publishing; 2001:13, 14.
2. Nielson C, Kaiser DA, Femano PA. *The MR Crosstrainer.* Clifton, NJ: Medical Imaging Consultants, Inc.; 2002:30.
3. Nielson C, Kaiser DA, Femano PA. *The MRI Registry Review Program.* Clifton, NJ: Medical Imaging Consultants, Inc.; 2002:8, 9.
4. Westbrook C, Roth CK, Talbot J. *MRI in Practice,* 3rd ed. Oxford, UK: Blackwell Publishing; 2005:69, 82–85, 331, 334, 335, 337, 346, 357, 361.
5. Bushberg JT, Seibert JA, Leidholdt Jr EM, Boone JM. *The Essential Physics of Medical Imaging.* 2nd ed. Philadelphia, PA: Lippincott Williams & Wilkins; 2002: 462, 465.
6. Burghart G, Finn C. *Handbook of MRI Scanning.* St. Louis, MO: Mosby; 2011:xvii, 352.
7. Fornell D. PET/MRI enters the U.S. market. *Imaging Technology News*, 28 Nov 2011.
8. Pichler BJ, Kolb A, Nagele T, Schlemmer H-P. PET/MRI: paving the way for the next generation of clinical multimodality imaging applications. *J Nucl Med.* 2010;51:333–336.
9. Pichler BJ, Wehrl HF, Kolb A, Judenhofer MS. Positron emission tomography/magnetic resonance imaging: the next generation of multimodality imaging? *Semin Nucl Med.* 2008;38:199–208.
10. Rosen B. PET and MRI: a match made in heaven, or the odd couple? Henry N. Wagner, Jr. Lectureship, SNM Annual Meeting, June 5, 2011.
11. Cherry SR. Multimodality imaging: beyond PET/CT and SPECT/CT. *Semin Nucl Med.* 2009;39:348–353.
12. Harvey D. PET/MRI: new fusion. *Radiology Today* 2008;9(11):20.

Additional Resources

Bushberg JT, Seibert JA, Leidholdt Jr EM, and Boone JM. *The Essential Physics of Medical Imaging.* 2nd ed. Philadelphia, PA: Lippincott Williams & Wilkins; 2002:Chapters 14 and 15.

Bushong SC. *Magnetic Resonance Imaging: Physical and Biological Principles.* 3rd ed. St. Louis, MO: Mosby; 2003.

Faulkner W, Seeram E. *MRI: Basic Physics, Instrumentation, and Quality Control.* Oxford, UK: Blackwell Publishing, 2002:13, 14.

Nielson C, Kaiser DA, Femano PA. *The MR Crosstrainer.* Clifton, NJ: Medical Imaging Consultants, Inc.; 2002.

Westbrook C, Roth CK, Talbot J. *MRI in Practice.* 3rd ed. Oxford, UK: Blackwell Publishing; 2005.

(a)

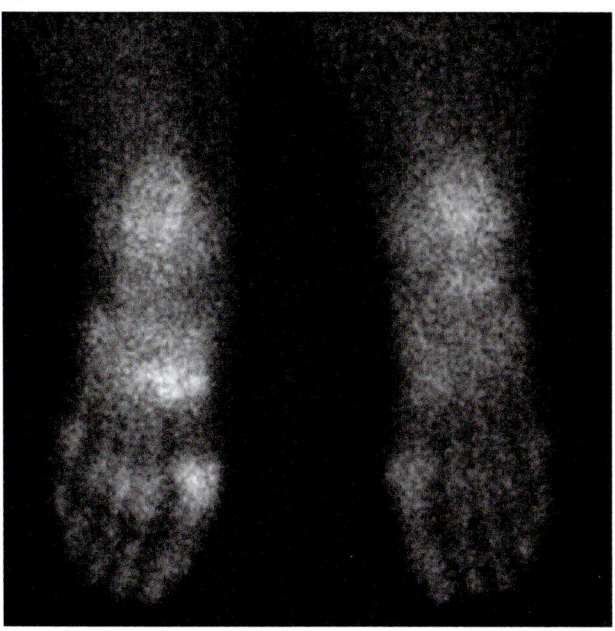

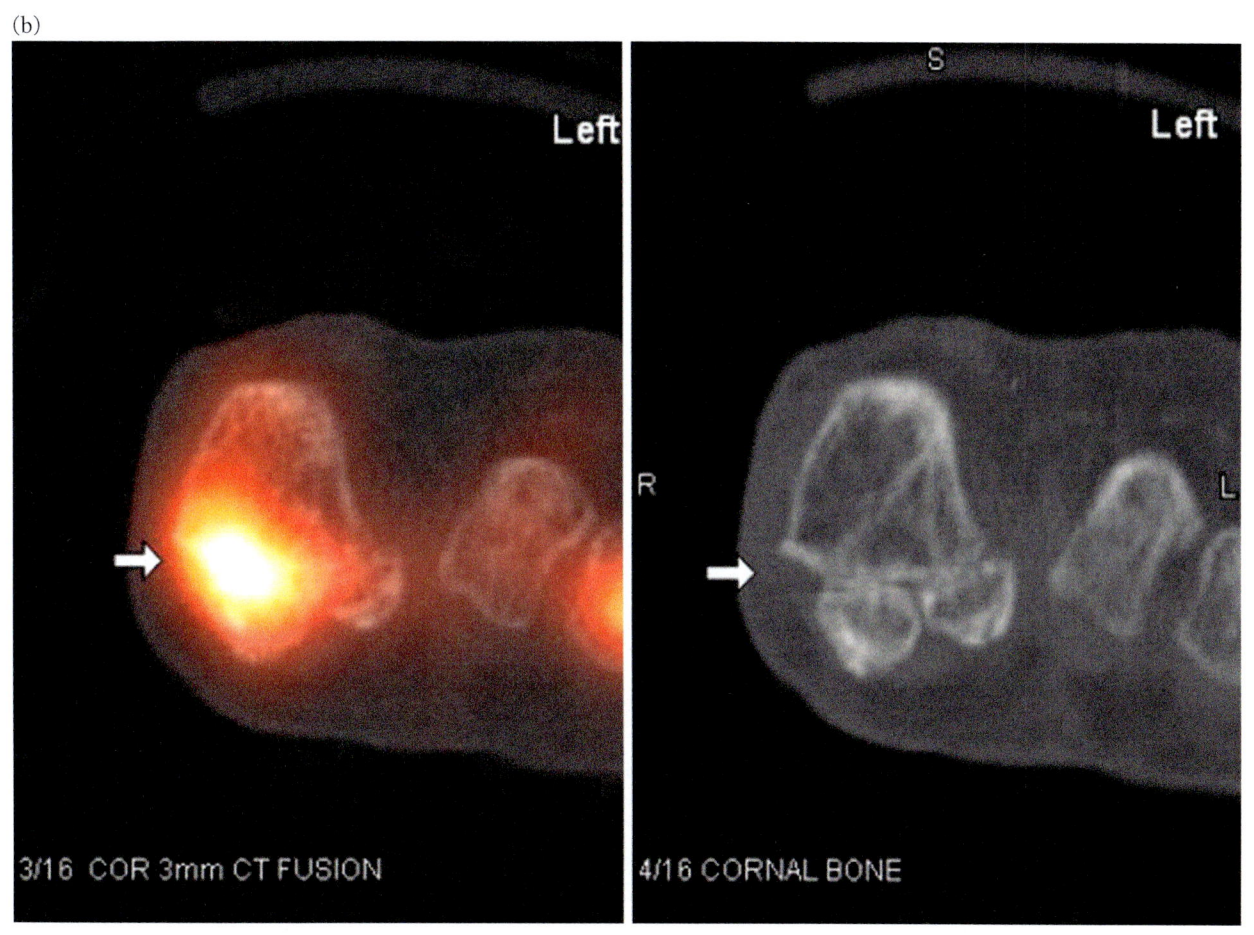

(b)

Figure 12-11 Planar bone scan image vs SPECT using Philips Astonish software. The upper image shows a plantar view of the feet in a patient being imaged for evaluation of arthritic changes. Increased activity is seen in the area of the first metatarsophalangeal joint of the left foot, but cannot be localized any more precisely. The lower-right image is a transverse CT slice through the metatarsophalangeal joint space, showing the head of the first metatarsal and tibial and fibular sesamoid bones. The lower-left image, in which the SPECT study processed with SC/RR/NR is overlaid on the CT slice, shows that the increased activity is localized to the joint space between the first metatarsal and the tibial sesamoid. The fibular sesamoid is not involved. Images courtesy of Valley Medical Center and Valley Radiologists.

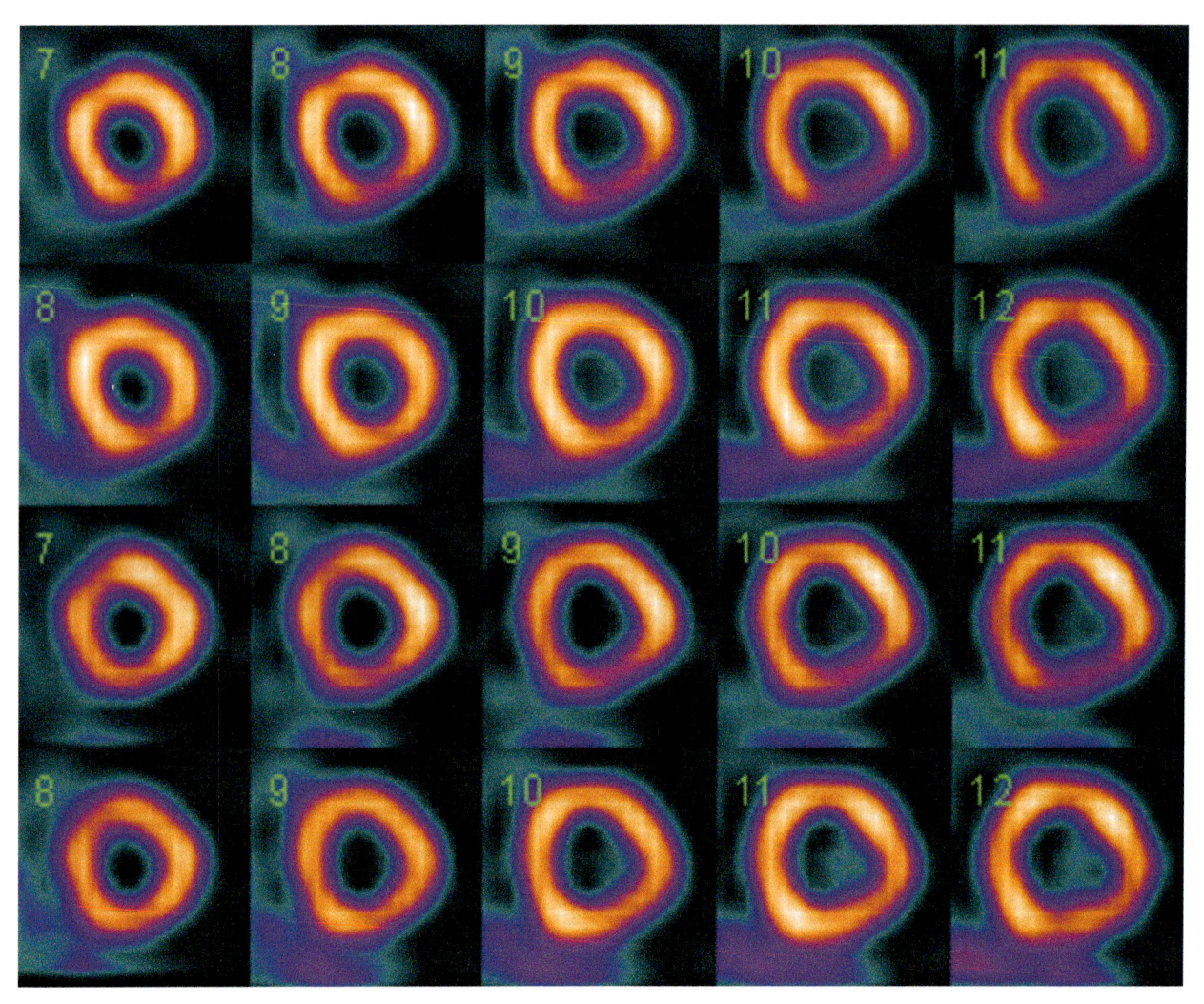

Figure 12-15 Myocardial perfusion SPECT without and with attenuation correction. The top two rows of this image show stress and rest short-axis views of a patient's myocardium. A significant inferolateral defect is seen, which is larger at stress but also apparent at rest. This could be interpreted as evidence of a prior infarction. Application of attenuation correction using Gd-153 rod sources (bottom two rows) causes the inferolateral wall to appear more normally perfused at rest, increasing the likelihood that the stress defect represents ischemia. Courtesy of Philips Healthcare.

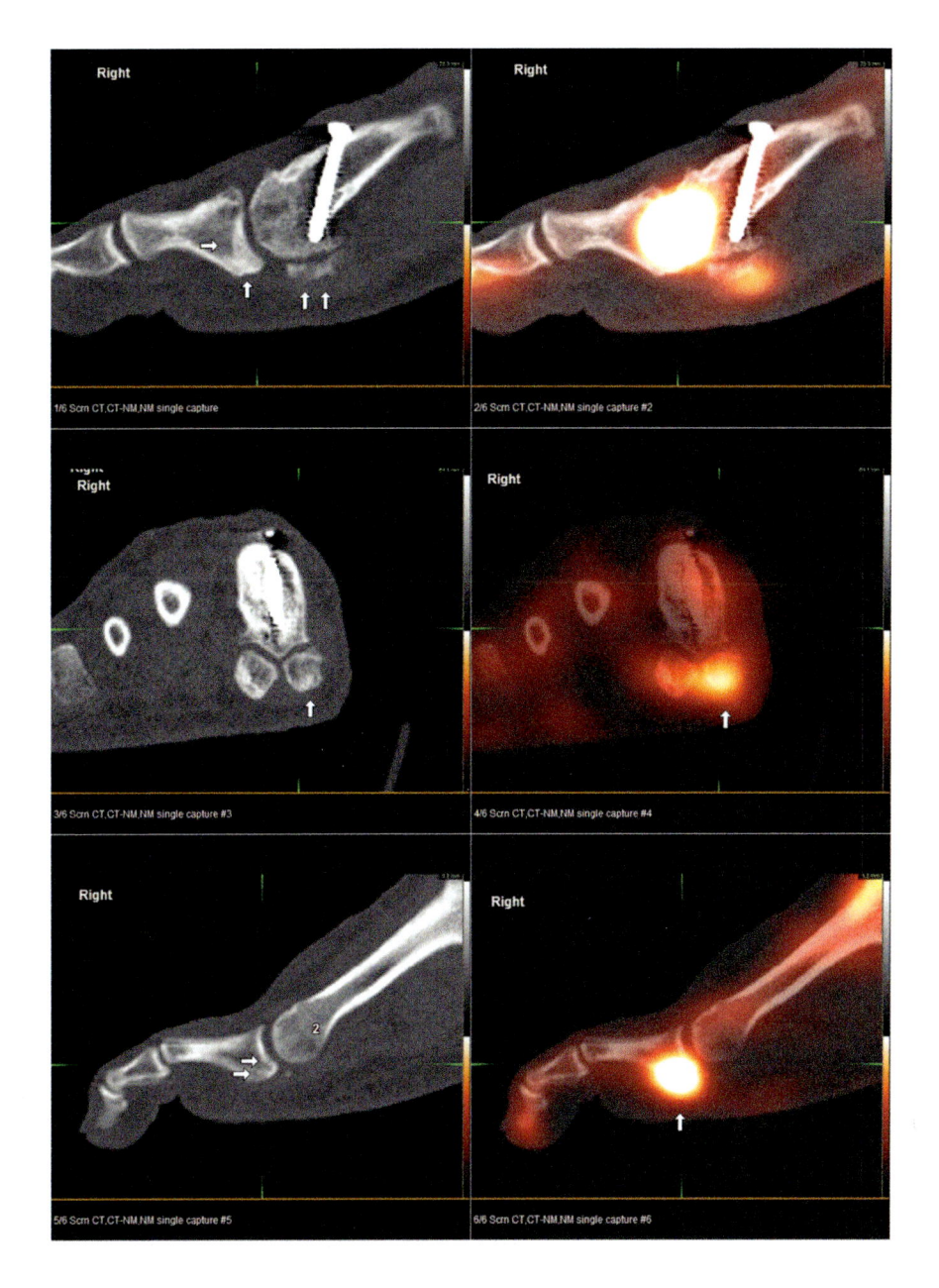

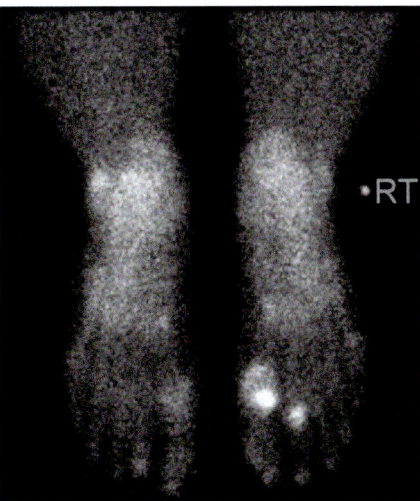

Figure 18-14 SPECT/CT of the foot in a patient with multiple abnormalities. The screw in the first metatarsal is not the cause of this patient's increased uptake on the bone scan (plantar image, left). There is increased activity in the first metatarsophalangeal joint and the medial sesamoid, seen in the top (sagittal) and middle (coronal) SPECT/CT images above. In addition, an area of increased activity in the proximal phalanx of the second toe is seen on CT to be a nondisplaced fracture (bottom SPECT/CT images with arrows pointing to the fracture). The planar bone image, while showing two areas of increased activity, is not able to identify the exact location of each. Images courtesy of Valley Medical Center and Valley Radiologists.

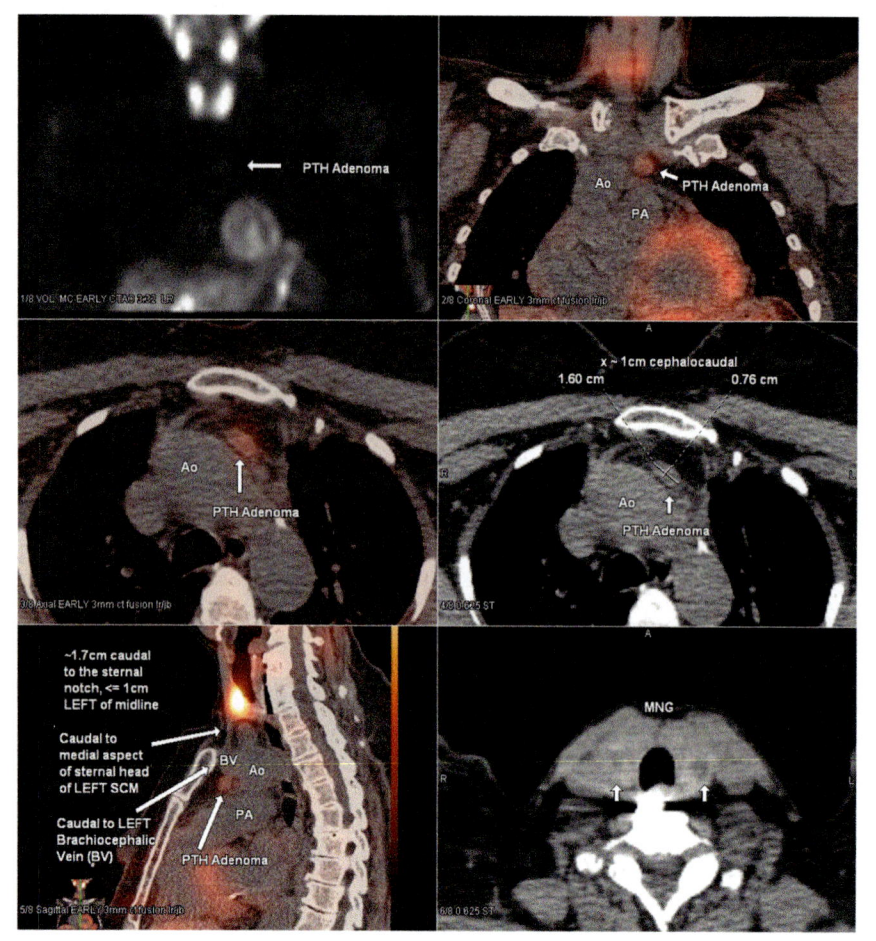

Figure 18-15 SPECT/CT showing a substernal parathyroid adenoma. An ectopic parathyroid adenoma is localized to the anterior mediastinum near the great vessels and behind the sternum. The annotation provides the surgeon with exact information about the adenoma's location and size. The CT scan incidentally identifies a multinodular goiter in the thyroid (lower-right image, arrows point at intrathyroidal nodules), but correctly locates the parathyroid adenoma elsewhere. Images courtesy of Valley Medical Center and Valley Radiologists.

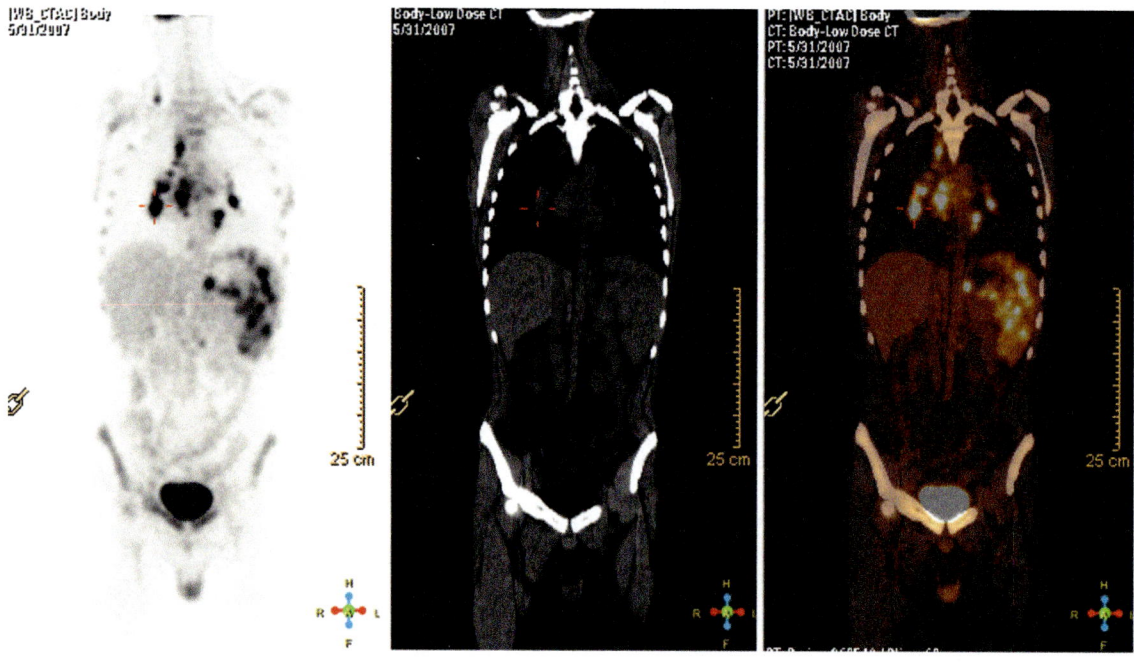

Figure 18-17 PET/CT scan. This standard display shows the PET coronal slice alone (left panel), the CT slice alone (middle panel), and the combined PET and CT slices (right panel). In the combined image, the CT information is shown in gray scale and the PET information in color, superimposed on the CT. Courtesy of Philips Healthcare.

APPENDIX A

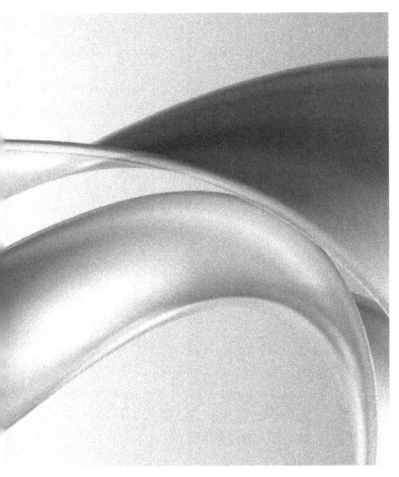

Atomic Structure and Interactions of High-Energy Radiation

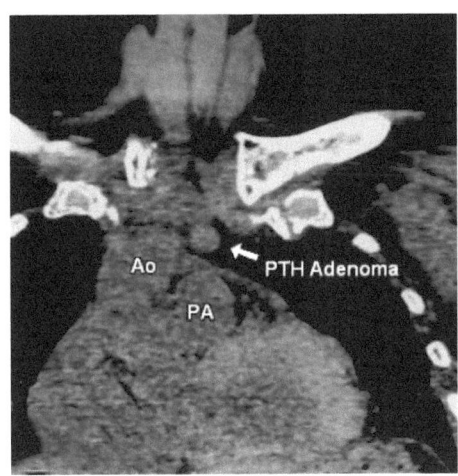

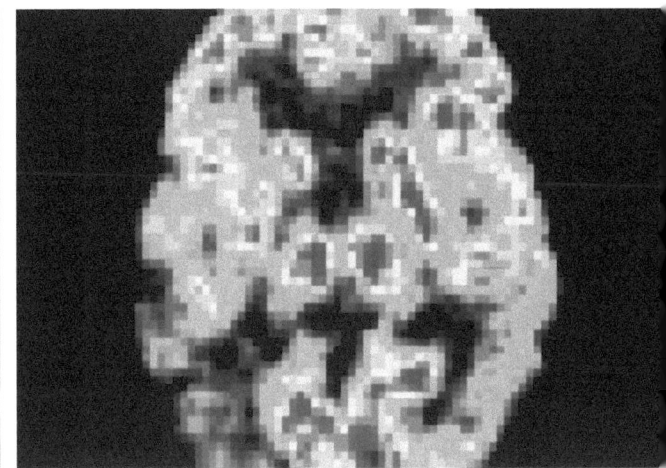

Learning Outcomes

1. Describe the structure of an atom, and in particular the relative binding energies of electrons in atomic orbitals.
2. Describe the interactions of photons and charged particles, and state the most important difference between the two.
3. Given the initial photon energy and the electron's binding energy, calculate the energy of a photoelectron; given the initial photon energy and scattering angle, calculate the energy of the scattered photon and the Compton electron.
4. Describe the possible events and ions produced following the interaction of radiation in a gas or a scintillation crystal.
5. Distinguish between the use of *range* for charged particles and *mean free path* for photons, and give estimates of the distance traveled for each in solids and in air.
6. Define the linear attenuation coefficient, and discuss how it changes with photon energy and with atomic number of the attenuating material.
7. Use the linear attenuation coefficient to determine the number of photons absorbed in a given attenuator or the thickness of an absorber needed to attenuate a given amount of photon radiation.

Introduction

This appendix reviews the concepts of atomic structure and interactions of charged particles and photons with matter. These subjects are covered well in most general nuclear medicine textbooks; most readers of this book have studied them already. The appendix therefore provides an at-hand review and concentrates on topics pertinent to this text.

Radiation detection instruments work by detecting the products of radiation interaction. The gamma rays that provide the basic information for a nuclear medicine image or measurement are not detected as gamma rays. Instead, we detect the product(s) of their interaction as well as (in many cases) the subsequent interactions of these products. We will also be dealing with radiation that is in the form of charged particles, such as beta-minus particles and positrons. So we will discuss charged-particle interactions as well.

The primary event in this process is an *ionization*, which in its general sense refers to the removal of an electron from its atom (a more specific meaning is discussed below). The result of ionization is the creation of an *ion pair*, which consists of the now-free electron and the positively charged atom that it came from. To be capable of causing an ionization, the radiation entity (particulate or photon) must have a minimum energy of 10 eV. Below the 10-eV threshold, radiation is not "ionizing" and is not detectable by the instruments discussed in this text.

A thorough understanding of radiation interactions requires that we have a good grasp of the basic composition of the atom. This appendix begins with a review of atomic structure. After consideration of the individual interactions of charged particles and photons, we will look at the consequences of these interactions, including the big-picture outcomes, the likelihood of different interaction types, and the attenuation equation and linear attenuation coefficient.

Atomic Structure

For the purposes of this discussion, we will utilize the shell model of the atom first proposed by Niels Bohr in 1913. Bohr was working at that time with Ernest Rutherford, who had proved that the nucleus of an atom is orders-of-magnitude smaller and more dense than previously thought. In Bohr's model, the nucleus of an atom (containing both protons and neutrons) is very small (about 10^{-14} m), and the electrons orbit around it in shells or orbitals, out to a diameter of about 10^{-10} m. Electron orbitals can be conceived (somewhat simplistically) as a series of discrete concentric spheres. Each orbital is defined by its principal quantum number, and the orbitals are distinctly separate in terms of the potential energy of the electrons in them (**Figure A-1**). Each orbital includes a number of subshells with more closely spaced energy levels. Electrons fill the orbitals starting with the K shell, which is closest to the nucleus, and hence has the most negative potential energy of all the orbitals.

Electrons are held in the orbitals by their electrical attraction to the nucleus. This form of potential energy is known as the electron's *binding energy*. Electrons in farther out orbitals have smaller binding energies than those in orbitals closer to the nucleus, because the electrons feel less of the attractive force of the protons. The more protons in the nucleus (i.e., the higher the atom's atomic number Z), the greater the binding energy. For example, the K-shell binding energy of carbon (Z = 6) is 0.284 keV, whereas for tungsten (Z = 74), it is 69.5 keV. The ejection of an electron from an atom requires an input of energy to overcome the electron's binding energy; this is often exactly what happens in an interaction with some form of radiation.

When an electron from an inner-shell orbital is ejected from its atom, a vacancy is left in that inner-shell orbital. Logically, it follows that the vacancy will be filled by an electron in a farther out orbital, which can reach a more favorable potential-energy state by making the transition. As the electron moves from the higher-energy orbital to the lower-energy orbital, there is a net energy change equal to the difference between the two orbitals' energy levels. This energy is seen in one of two ways. It may appear as a *characteristic x-ray*, a photon with kinetic energy equal to the energy difference. The x-ray is characteristic of the element involved because the orbital energy separations are specific to each element. The other possible outcome of the electron orbital transition is that the energy is used to eject another electron from the atom. This second electron is called an *Auger electron*. As we account for the energy produced by radiation interactions, we will need to keep both of these possibilities in mind.

Interactions of Charged Particles

Charged particles include alpha and beta particles, free electrons, positrons, protons, and ions of any kind. (We will call alpha and beta particles *primary charged particles* to distinguish them from electrons ejected in the interactions described below.) Because they carry an electric charge, charge particles interact with other entities that have an electric charge, via a force of nature called the *Coulomb force*. The Coulomb force is further described in Appendix B. The most important aspect of the Coulomb force from the standpoint of radiation interactions is that it occurs over a distance. Thus, charged particles are always interacting with the atoms of the medium through which they are traveling. The distance between a particular charged particle and a particular atom of the medium determines which type of interaction occurs and the amount of the charged particle's kinetic energy that is transferred.

Ionization

The more specific meaning of the word *ionization* refers to a particular type of interaction experienced by charged particles. A charged particle passing an atom can either pull or push an electron out of its atomic orbital (the distinction between "pulling" and "pushing" depends on whether the charged particle is positively or negatively charged, and beyond that it is immaterial to this discussion). In this *ionization interaction*, some of the charged particle's kinetic energy is transferred to the orbital electron. As a result, the electron is ejected from its orbital, and it becomes a free electron, at which point it behaves as any other free electron.

The energy transfer can be described by

$$E_0 = E_{0'} + E_K + E_B \tag{A-1}$$

where E_K and E_B are the kinetic energy and binding energy of the ejected electron, respectively, E_0 is the energy of the incident charged particle, and $E_{0'}$ is the energy of the charged particle after the interaction. The binding energy E_B will eventually be returned in the form of a characteristic x-ray or Auger electron.

The distance between the charged particle and the atom, as well as the binding energy of the orbital electron, determine how much kinetic energy is given to the orbital electron. In a particularly close encounter with a primary charged particle, an electron may get a significant amount of energy, enough that it is able to cause its own ionization interactions. These are called *secondary electrons* or *delta rays*. Most ejected electrons, on the other hand, leave the interaction with kinetic energy less than 10 eV; these are not able to cause ionization interactions, but because they are free from their atoms, they can be measured in an electrical system. These we will call *tertiary electrons*.

(a) Bohr's model of the atom

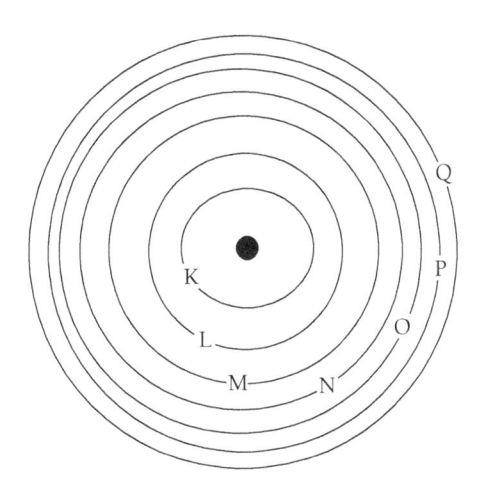

Shell	Maximum number of electrons
K	2
L	8
M	18
N	32
O	50
P	72
Q	98

(b) Energy diagram

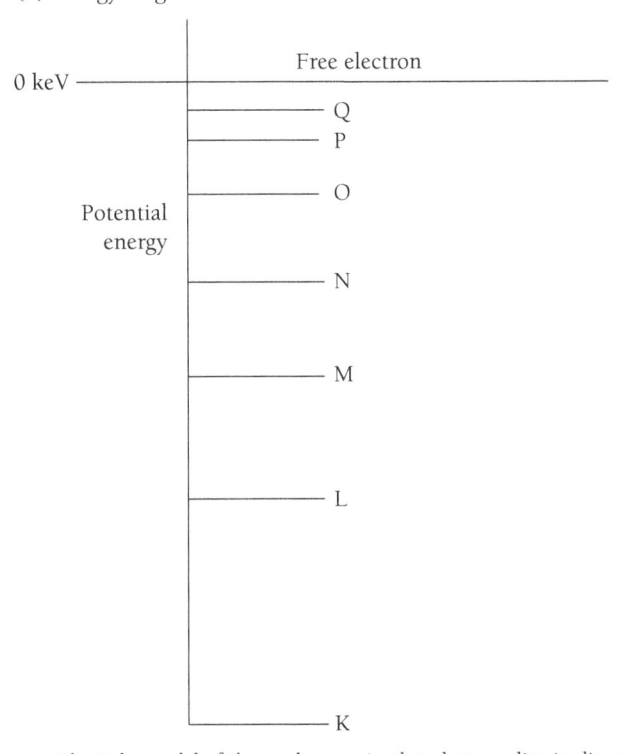

Figure A-1 Structure of the atom. The Bohr model of the nucleus posits that electrons live in discrete spheres around the nucleus (more sophisticated models have since been developed, but this is sufficient for our purposes). We use the nuclear physics convention of designating the orbitals with capital letters, beginning with the K shell closest to the nucleus. In the energy diagram in Figure A-1b, the potential energy of an electron that is not part of an atom by convention is assigned 0 eV. Bound electrons, by virtue of their position in an atom, have negative potential energy (they are "happier" than a free electron because of their association with a positively charged nucleus). The binding energy of electrons in a given orbital is the amount of energy required to jump an electron up the energy scale to the level of a free electron.

After an ionization interaction, the incident charged particle may still have considerable kinetic energy, and it will continue to interact with other atoms. A light charged particle, such as an electron or positron, will be deflected at each interaction, so that the actual path is quite convoluted. A heavy charged particle, such as an alpha particle, will have a much straighter track, as its inertia will keep it traveling in the same direction after the interaction. Eventually, having lost all (or almost all) of its kinetic energy, the charged particle will combine with an appropriate entity (such as an atom missing an electron) and become neutral, at which point it is no longer detectable.

Excitation

Let us return for a moment to the atomic orbital diagram in Figure A-1a. In their lowest energy state, the great majority of atoms do not need the P and Q shells. But those shells are inherent to the structure of the atom. An electron that is given a small amount of energy (not enough to overcome its binding energy) can jump up into any higher orbital not already fully occupied by electrons, including the P and Q orbitals. These higher-energy unoccupied orbitals are called *excited-state orbitals* (sometimes referred to as "higher levels").

Most of the time, a primary charged particle does not come close enough to an atom to cause an ionization interaction. Instead, it transfers a very small amount of energy, just enough to cause an electron to move into a higher-level orbital. This is an *excitation interaction*. At some point, the atom will return to its ground state, and the excess energy gained by the excited electron will be released. The energy may be released as a characteristic x-ray, an Auger electron, an ultraviolet photon, or a mechanical vibration. But if several excitation interactions occur in one atom or molecule, it is possible that the kinetic energies can come together in one spot to cause an ionization. Both ionization and excitation are referred to as *collisional interactions*, even though a physical collision is not necessary and in fact rarely occurs.

Bremsstrahlung Interaction

For light charged particles, specifically electrons and positrons, a third type of interaction can occur. In this interaction, a fast-moving primary charged particle does not interact with an electron in an atomic orbital. Instead, it interacts with the nucleus of an atom in such a way that the electrical field of the nucleus deflects it. In being deflected, the charged particle is decelerated, and the lost kinetic energy appears as a photon. The word *Bremsstrahlung* is German for "braking radiation," and this type of interaction is a *Bremsstrahlung interaction*. It is also referred to as a *radiative interaction*.

The energy of the Bremsstrahlung photon depends on how close the charged particle comes to the nucleus. It can thus range from very low energy all the way to the charged particle's preinteraction kinetic energy (**Figure A-2**). Bremsstrahlung radiation is the primary constituent of an x-ray beam. The energy given to the Bremsstrahlung photon is not lost, because it is subject to Compton and photoelectric interactions, which in turn will produce detectable charged particles.

Interactions of Photons

Photons in this context refers to various forms of electromagnetic radiation, including gamma rays (which result from nuclear transitions), x-rays (which result from electron orbital transitions), and ultraviolet photons. Photons have no electric charge and therefore do not interact at a distance as do charged particles. Instead, they must physically collide in order to lose kinetic energy. Again, the major criterion for the interactions to be discussed here is that the photons have kinetic energy greater than 10 eV. Photon interactions look different than charged-particle interactions, although the end result is much the same. A comprehensive overview would include additional interactions, but we can limit ourselves to the two interactions most pertinent to nuclear medicine.

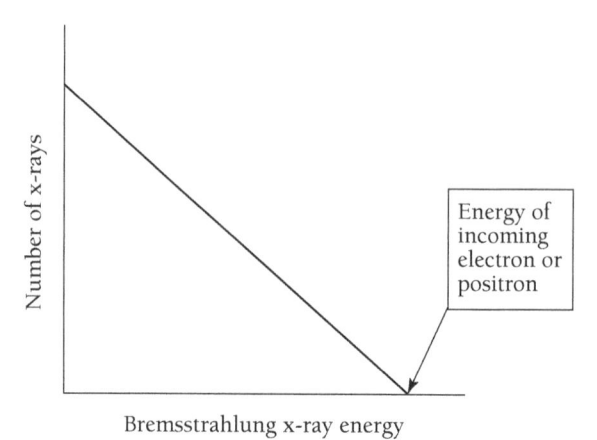

Figure A-2 Bremsstrahlung energy spectrum. When an electron or positron passes close to an atomic nucleus, it decelerates and loses energy. This results in the emission of a Bremsstrahlung x-ray, the energy of which depends on the amount of deceleration. Thus the energy spectrum from a Bremsstrahlung interaction in a particular material includes many lower-energy x-rays and fewer x-rays at higher energies. The number of x-rays at each energy decreases linearly, up to a maximum equal to the energy of the incoming electron or positron.

Photoelectric Effect

In a *photoelectric interaction*, a photon interacts with an inner-shell orbital electron, which is ejected from the atom. For this to happen, some of the photon's kinetic energy must be used to overcome the binding energy of the orbital electron. The remainder is given to the now-free electron as kinetic energy, as described by the *photoelectric equation*:

$$E_\gamma = E_k + E_B \qquad (A\text{-}2)$$

where E_γ is the incident photon's energy and E_K and E_B are the kinetic energy and binding energy, respectively, of the ejected electron. The photon thus disappears (we say it is *absorbed*), and the ejected electron (now called a *photoelectron*) behaves as a charged particle, moving about and having charged-particle interactions (if it has sufficient energy, which is usually the case). The vacancy left by a photoelectric interaction will be filled by another electron in the atom, following which a characteristic x-ray or Auger electron will be released. The photoelectron is considered a secondary electron, and a characteristic x-ray is considered a secondary photon.

Compton Effect

If a photon interacts with an outer-shell electron, it does not lose all of its energy. Instead, it transfers some kinetic energy to the electron and retains some for itself, in a *Compton interaction*. Because the interaction is with a loosely bound outer-shell electron, the binding energy of the orbital electron is very small in relation to the photon's energy and is explicitly taken to be zero. Again, the electron (in this case called a *Compton* or *recoil* electron) is released and acts as any other secondary electron. The photon's direction of travel is changed (we say it is *scattered*), and it moves on to have further photon interactions.

The energy retained by the photon is related to its incident energy and the scattering angle according to the *Compton equation*:

$$E_{\gamma'} = \frac{E_\gamma}{1 + (E_\gamma/511\,\text{keV})(1 - \cos\theta)} \quad \text{(A-3)}$$

in which E_γ is the energy of the photon prior to the interaction, θ is the scattering angle, and $E_{\gamma'}$ is the photon's energy after the interaction. The E_γ term in the denominator must be in units of keV to cancel with 511 keV, after which $E_{\gamma'}$ has the same units as E_γ in the numerator. Once $E_{\gamma'}$ is determined, the kinetic energy of the Compton electron is equal to the difference between it and the photon's preinteraction energy.

Sample Calculation A-1   Photon Interactions

A radionuclide emits 200-keV gamma rays. Calculate the energy of a photoelectron if one of these gamma rays interacts with a lead K-shell electron (binding energy = 88 keV) and the energy of the Compton-scattered photon and Compton electron for a 45° scattering angle.

For the photoelectric interaction,

$$E_K = E_\gamma - E_B = 200 - 88 = 112\,\text{keV}.$$

For the Compton interaction,

$$\cos 45° = 0.707$$

$$E_{\gamma'} = \frac{200\,\text{keV}}{1 + (200\,\text{keV}/511\,\text{keV})(1 - 0.707)} = 179\,\text{keV}$$

$$E_{\text{compton electron}} = E_\gamma - E_{\gamma'} = 200 - 179 = 21\,\text{keV}.$$

Note that any scattering angle is possible in a Compton interaction, from 0° (no deflection of the photon) to 180° (a reversal of the photon's direction). The probability of a given scattering angle depends on the photon's preinteraction energy, according to the Klein–Nishina equation (1). The main finding of the Klein–Nishina equation is that in the energy range encountered in nuclear medicine, scattering in a forward direction (<90°) is more likely than scattering at an angle greater than 90°, and this tendency becomes more pronounced as the photon energy increases (1).

It will be quite clear in reading the text that our detection methods are all based on electronic systems. It is therefore important to recognize that all photons will sooner or later undergo interactions that produce free electrons, which can be detected electronically. If a photon has a Compton interaction, the scattered photon will continue to experience Compton interactions and ultimately a photoelectric interaction. All of the energy released in an interaction will be eventually transferred to electrons, which are the basis for all detection processes.

Consequences of Radiation Interactions

Let us look next at the consequences of these interactions. The first goal of this section is to paint a picture of the series of interactions that can follow the passage of a photon or charged particle through some kind of absorbing material. The second part of this section addresses how far photons and charged particles travel. Finally, we will consider the attenuation equation and linear attenuation coefficient as mathematical mechanisms to describe the likelihood of photon interactions in different absorbing materials.

Big-Picture Outcomes of a Radiation Interaction

Let us start with a simple situation, a gamma ray from a Tc-99m decay passing through the gas chamber of a dose calibrator. The low density of the argon gas in the chamber makes it unlikely that the gamma ray will interact with very many gas molecules, so we will assume that it has only a single Compton interaction and then exits the gas chamber without having any other interactions. This interaction leaves in its wake a single secondary electron and a positively charged argon atom. The secondary electron is attracted to the anode of the dose calibrator, and as it moves toward the anode, it interacts with other argon atoms, by virtue of its electrical field. Many tertiary electrons, and maybe another secondary electron or two, are produced by the excitations and ionizations that the Compton electron experiences. A few of the interactions may result in the release of a characteristic x-ray or UV photon; these will quickly be absorbed in photoelectric interactions of their own, producing more tertiary electrons. All of the tertiary electrons produced in these interactions contribute to the electric current measured by the dose calibrator.

Take the same gamma ray, but now let's imagine it traveling through a sodium iodide crystal. A photoelectric interaction occurs, releasing a photoelectron with significant energy (107 keV for interaction with an iodine K-shell electron, 135 keV for an L-shell interaction). The photoelectron undergoes many ionization and excitation interactions. Again, the result of these interactions is a large number of tertiary electrons, as well as a smaller number of energetic secondary electrons and some characteristic x-rays and UV photons that will produce even more tertiary electrons. Some of the tertiary electrons are those that jump from the valence band to the conduction band of the sodium iodide crystal. As with the dose calibrator, it is these low-energy tertiary electrons that create the signal that is measured by our radiation-detecting instruments.

Any interaction that results in the ejection of an electron from an atom or molecule leaves in its wake an ion pair. The electron will move under the influence of an electrical field. The positive ion also moves because of the electrical field, but it moves more slowly because it is much heavier. In some detectors, such as Geiger counters, the positive ions become a factor in the detection process. In other situations, it does not contribute to the detection process in any significant way. Eventually the positive ion will combine with a free electron and return to a neutral state.

Distance of Travel

One of the questions we might ask at this point is, "How far do various radiations travel?" The answer depends on the type and the energy of the radiation as well as the composition of the material it is traveling through (the latter is discussed in the next subsection). Charged particles are always interacting with the electrons of whatever substance they are traveling through. Thus, they lose energy quickly and travel only a short distance before coming to rest (μm to mm in solids and cm to m in air). Charged particles are considered *nonpenetrating radiation* for this reason.

Photons, on the other hand, travel cm to m in solids and m to km in air and hence are called *penetrating radiation* (this category includes neutrons as well). The reason that photons travel so much farther than charged particles is because they must actually collide with an electron or atomic nucleus in order to have an interaction. The likelihood of such a collision depends on the energy of the photon and on the electron density of the material through which the photon is traveling. Further, the probabilities are different for a photoelectric interaction vs a Compton interaction.

The likelihood of a Compton interaction decreases as photon energy increases, but does so relatively slowly (**Figure A-3**). The likelihood of a photoelectric interaction also decreases with increasing photon energy, but more rapidly with increasing photon energy, such that at some point it becomes less likely than a Compton interaction. The exact shape of the graph in Figure A-3a, and the energy at which the Compton effect becomes dominant, is a function of the type of absorbing material being considered. Figure A-3b shows a probability-vs-energy graph that includes an *edge*. The edge energy corresponds to an orbital-shell binding energy in the absorber. When the photon's energy is above the electron orbital binding energy, a photoelectric interaction becomes more likely.

Let us return for a moment to the issue of "distance traveled." A group of charged particles (e.g., β− particles) with the same initial energy will travel about the same distance, because they all experience similar Coulomb-type interactions with neighboring atoms. If we aim a beam of β− particles at sheets or slabs of some kind of absorbing material, we find that at some reproducible thickness of the absorber, no more β− particles are measured on the far side. The absorber thickness is sufficient to stop all of the β− particles. We call this thickness the *range* of the β− particles in that material. The main point is that charged particles slow down and stop, and given enough of an absorbing material (even a low-density material such as air), all of the charged particles will lose their kinetic energy and become undetectable.

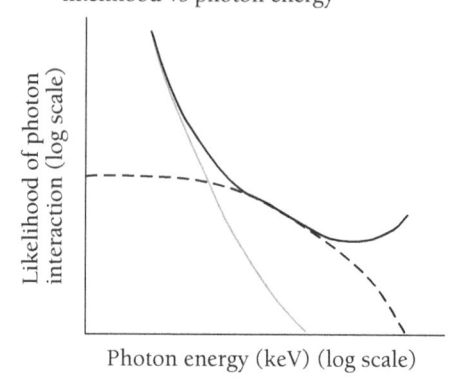

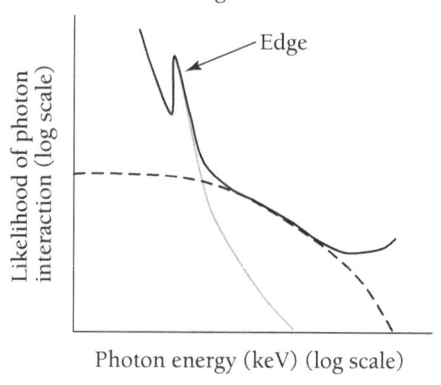

Figure A-3 Energy dependence of photon interaction types and probabilities. In a given material, photoelectric interactions dominate at low energies, with Compton interactions becoming significant when photoelectric interactions become unlikely. (The graph increases again at very high photon energies due to the pair production interaction, which is not discussed in this text.) The point at which this transition occurs depends on the characteristics of the absorbing material, but the general shape applies in most cases. Discontinuities in the graph will be seen at photon energy levels corresponding to electron binding energy levels in the absorbing material, as shown in Figure A-3b. The likelihood of a photoelectric interaction becomes much greater when the photon energy is at or just greater than the binding energy of a particular orbital shell.

Photons behave quite differently. The likelihood of a photon interaction in a given material is a matter of probability, and it shows an exponential decrease with increasing absorber thickness. There is no thickness at which we can be absolutely certain that all of a beam of photons has been absorbed. So instead of the range, we use the concept of the *mean free path*, which is the average distance a photon travels in the absorber before it has an interaction. The mean free path for a particular absorbing material depends on the energy of the photons being absorbed. For a specific photon energy, the mean free path in general decreases as the electron density of the absorber increases. Another way of saying this is that higher-density materials have greater *efficiency* for interactions with photons.

Attenuation Mathematics

This leads us to a brief discussion of the mathematics of attenuation. First, a definition: *attenuation* is the removal of a photon from the incoming beam by either absorption (a photoelectric interaction) or scattering (a Compton interaction). The likelihood of attenuation is therefore related mathematically to the likelihood of the two interaction types. We can express the likelihood of an interaction of any kind as being equal to the sum of the likelihoods of the two separate interactions, per cm of travel through the absorbing material of interest. We call this number the *linear attenuation coefficient* (μ_ℓ), and it is equal to the probability of an interaction in a cm of the absorbing material. The value of μ_ℓ depends on characteristics of the absorbing material and the energy of the photons, generally decreasing with increasing photon energy and increasing with increasing density of the absorbing material. The *mean free path* is equal to the inverse of μ_ℓ.

Given a particular absorber and photon energy, we can use the *attenuation equation* to calculate the decrease in beam strength for a given thickness of absorber:

$$I(x) = I(0)e^{-\mu_\ell x} \tag{A-4}$$

where $I(0)$ is the intensity of the photon beam before the absorbing material, $I(x)$ is its intensity after the absorbing material, and x is the thickness of the absorbing material in cm (**Figure A-4**). The equation is strictly accurate only if the radiation source is a well-collimated point source, but it is often used to estimate the amount of radiation that will be transmitted through different absorbing materials. Equation A-4 is commonly used for shielding calculations, but we can also apply it to the materials used to detect radiation, such as scintillators.

Sample Calculation A-2 Interaction Likelihood vs Gamma Ray Energy

Sodium iodide has μ_ℓ values of 2.09/cm at 140 keV and 0.33/cm at 511 keV. Calculate the number of photons interacting in a 30-mm-thick sodium iodide crystal, if the number of gamma rays reaching the crystal is 1,000/sec, for both Tc-99m photons and annihilation photons.

The attenuation equation (Eq. A-4) can be used with $I(0) = 1,000$ gamma rays/sec, and with the 30-mm thickness of the crystal converted to 3 cm, in order to cancel units in the exponential portion of the equation. At 140 keV:

$$I(3\,\text{cm}) = \left(1{,}000\,\frac{\text{photons}}{\text{second}}\right)e^{-(2.09/\text{cm})(3\,\text{cm})} = 1.89 \text{ photons.}$$

At 511 keV:

$$I(3\,\text{cm}) = \left(1{,}000\,\frac{\text{photons}}{\text{second}}\right)e^{-(0.33/\text{cm})(3\,\text{cm})} = 371 \text{ photons.}$$

The left side of the equation ($I(x)$) is the number of photons transmitted through the material of thickness x. Hence, a 3-cm-thick sodium iodide crystal stops virtually all of the Tc-99m gamma rays but less than one-third of the 511-keV photons.

Summary

The most important consequence of radiation interactions, from the standpoint of detection of radiation, is to

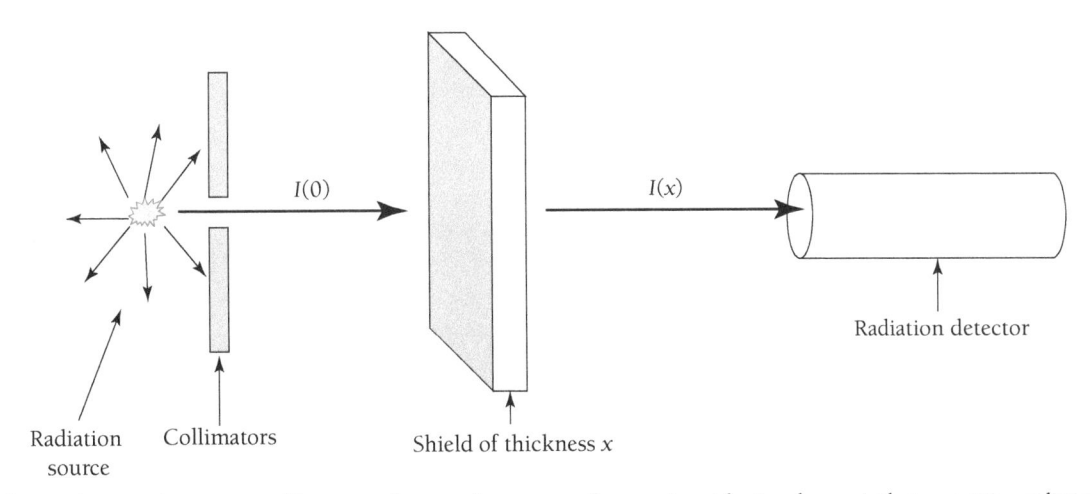

Figure A-4 Attenuation equation geometry. The attenuation equation assumes the experimental setup shown. A photon-emitting radiation source (that is emitting photons isotropically) is shielded with collimators to eliminate off-angle photons. The solid arrow on the left represents the unattenuated photon beam, with an intensity of $I(0)$. After the beam has gone through the shield, its intensity is represented by $I(x)$. The intensity values can be measured in radiation units such as mR/hr, or in terms of photon flux/sec, or even $I(x)$ as a percentage of $I(0)$. An important assumption of the equation is that the beam after the shield (and therefore $I(x)$) only includes photons that did not undergo any kind of interaction in the shield. Chapter 12 discusses the more realistic situation, which is that the radiation detector measures not only the unattenuated photons but also photons that have been scattered.

realize that the number of ionizations bears some relationship to the amount of radiation present. If we can count ion pairs or other products of radiation interaction such as tertiary electrons, which we are able to do using electric circuits and devices, then we can correlate their number to the quantity of radiation present. The proportionality is different for different instruments and different situations, but there is a proportionality that is the essence of nuclear medicine instrumentation. We can utilize the mathematics of attenuation to compare how well different radiation detection instruments will detect photons. These mathematical tools, by providing the means to perform calculations such as those in this appendix, allow us to see what happens under a variety of circumstances.

Sample Calculation A-3 Calculation of Absorber Thickness

We can use the attenuation equation to calculate the thickness of a given absorber required to stop a given amount of photon radiation. For example, after completing Sample Calculation A-2, we might ask, "How thick would the sodium iodide crystal need to be to stop 90% of 511-keV photons?" In other words, we need to identify x such that

$$0.1I(0) = I(0)e^{-\mu_\ell x}.$$

First, collect the $I(0)$ terms on the left side of the equation, and leave the exponential term by itself on the right:

$$\frac{0.1I(0)}{I(0)} = e^{-\mu_\ell x}.$$

Then take the natural logarithm of both sides:

$$\ln 0.1 = \ln e^{-\mu_\ell x}.$$

But the natural logarithm of Euler's number raised to some power is the power itself (i.e., $\ln e^x = x$). So the equation reduces to

$$\ln 0.1 = -\mu_\ell x$$

$$-2.30 = -\left(\frac{0.33}{\text{cm}}\right)x.$$

Solve for x:

$$x = (-2.30) \div \left(\frac{-0.33}{\text{cm}}\right) = 6.96 \text{ cm}.$$

The sodium iodide crystal must be 7 cm thick to stop 90% of the 511-keV photons.

Reference

1. Knoll GF. *Radiation Detection and Measurement*. 3rd ed. New York, NY: John Wiley & Sons; 2000:51–52.

Additional Resources

Cherry SR, Sorenson JA, Phelps ME. *Physics in Nuclear Medicine*. 3rd ed. Philadelphia, PA: Saunders; 2003: Chapter 6.

Knoll GF. *Radiation Detection and Measurement*. 3rd ed. New York, NY: John Wiley & Sons; 2000: Chapter 2.

APPENDIX B

Basic Electronics and Devices

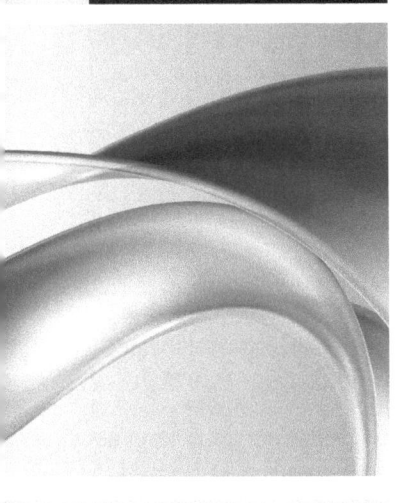

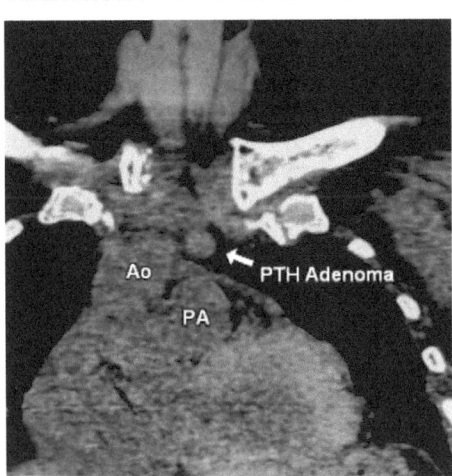

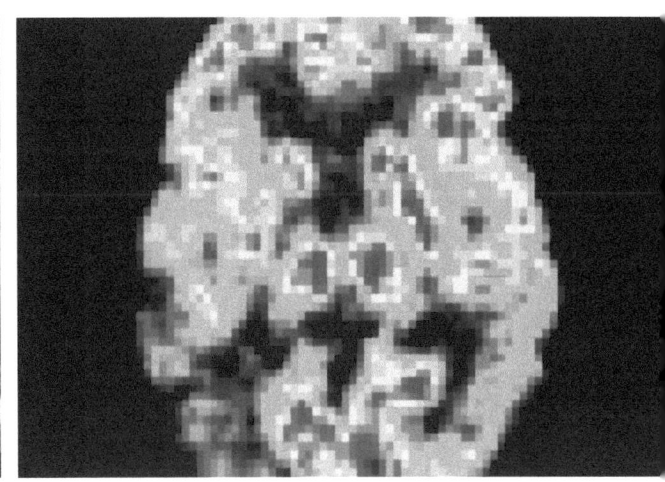

Learning Outcomes

1. Describe the behavior of electrons in an electric field, and identify the basic components of an electric circuit.
2. Distinguish between covalent and delocalized molecular bonding, and briefly describe the delocalized bonding diagrams for insulators, conductors, and semiconductors.
3. Define and utilize basic terms and units of electricity, including the coulomb, current, voltage, resistance, and capacitance.
4. Diagram a resistor-capacitor circuit and discuss its uses in radiation detectors and in pulse shaping.
5. Diagram a transistor and discuss its use as an amplifier and as a logic circuit.
6. Identify important characteristics of the following electronic modules used in radiation detectors:
   a. Amplifier
   b. Photodiode
   c. Power supply
7. Briefly describe the operation of the following image display devices:
   a. Cathode ray tube
   b. Video display monitor
   c. Liquid crystal display monitor

Introduction

All types of radiation detectors rely on electric circuits. Therefore, a complete understanding of these instruments includes basic knowledge about electronics. The main body of this text covers the concepts of the instruments themselves, and will be a sufficient level of understanding for many readers. This appendix is designed for those who desire a more in-depth look at the electronics involved in radiation detection instruments. Our starting point is the nature of electric charge and its manifestation in atomic structure and molecular bonding. The appendix also discusses some of the electronic components of radiation detectors as well as the electronic operation of image display devices.

Behavior of Electric Charges

Coulomb's Law

The most basic fact about electric charges is that like charges repel and opposite charges attract one another. This attraction/repulsion is mediated by a force of nature called the *Coulomb force*, which is inherent to any object having electric charge and which affects any other object with electric charge. The Coulomb force f

for spherical charge distributions is described by *Coulomb's law*

$$f = \frac{kq_1q_2}{r^2} \tag{B-1}$$

where q_1 and q_2 are the charges on the two objects, r is the distance between their centers, and k is a proportionality constant. The force is attractive if q_1 and q_2 are oppositely charged and repulsive if q_1 and q_2 are either both positive or both negative. Coulomb's law applies exactly only when the physical size of the charged objects is small compared to the distance between them, but the concept holds for electrically charged objects of any size and distance. The attraction/repulsion force gets stronger as the distance between the two objects decreases.

Electric Field

The Coulomb force creates a force field around an electrically charged object called an *electric field* (**Figure B-1**). According to convention established by Benjamin Franklin, the electric field of a positively charged object shows arrows pointing away from the object, whereas the electric field of a negatively charged object is represented by arrows pointing toward the object. These arrows represent a static property of space that points in the direction that a positive charge would move if released at that location in the field. A negative charge released from the same point will move in the opposite direction of the field. (Similarly, arrows in circuit diagrams show the direction of movement of a positive charge, even though it is actually negative charges [electrons] that move in almost all cases.) The implication of electric field lines is that energy is released when a positive charge is moved in the direction the arrows are pointing, and energy is required to move a positive charge against the arrows.

Figure B-1b shows a positive and a negative charge in the vicinity of each other, separated by a small enough distance that their electric fields interact to a significant degree. This is called a *dipole*. A negatively charged object (such as an electron) released into the middle of the electric field lines would spontaneously move toward the positively charged object, being both attracted to it and repelled by the negatively charged object. Energy would be released as the electron reached a more stable state. On the other hand, energy would be required to move the electron toward the negative side of the dipole. Coulomb's law provides a way to measure the forces involved but is complex to apply. A simpler approach is to consider the work done when moving a charge from one location to another in the field between the two sides of the dipole. The work done corresponds to a change in energy per unit charge. This difference is called the *electric potential* and is given the symbol ΔV.

(a) Electric fields for separated positive (left) and negative (right) charges

(b) Electric dipole

Positively charged object

Negatively charged object

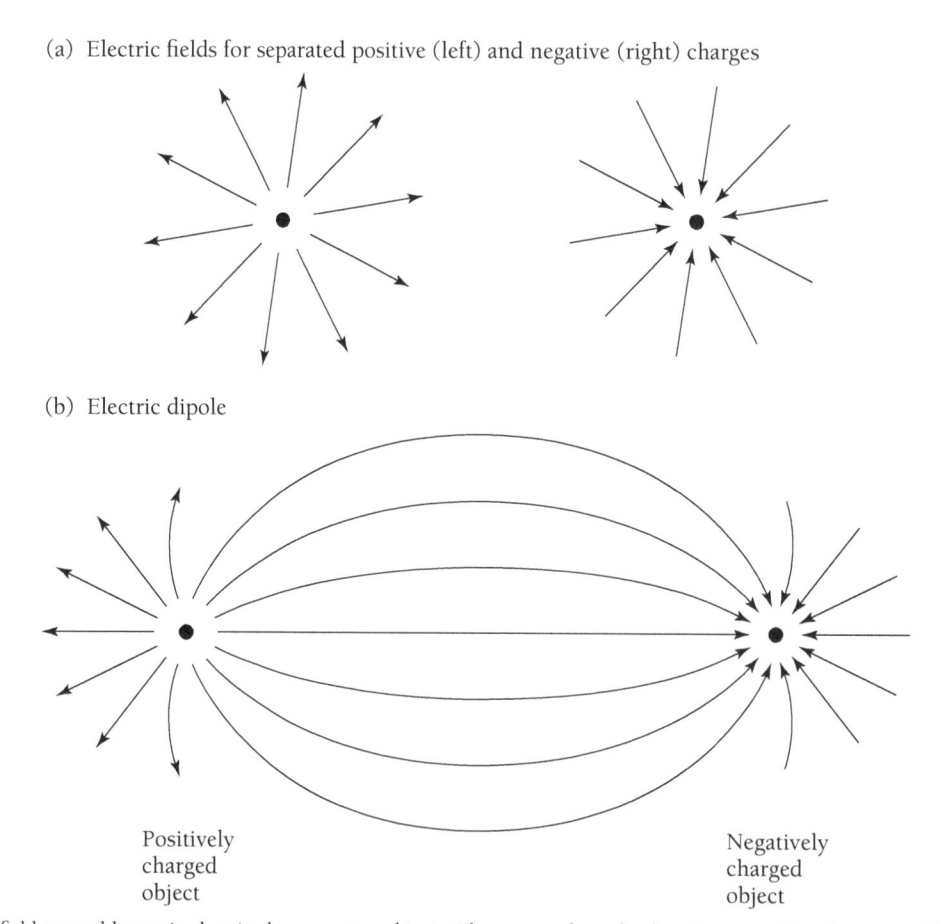

Figure B-1 Electric field created by static electric charge on two objects. The arrows show the direction a positive charge would travel if placed in the electric field. This is the standard convention for all electrical diagrams, even though it is the electrons that do the actual moving. Figure B-1b illustrates an electric dipole, in which the electric fields of oppositely charged entities interact.

We can illustrate the concept of electric potential using the familiar situation of a sock in a clothes dryer. The sock starts out in a neutral state (i.e., no excess of either positive or negative charge). As it tumbles in the dryer, it loses electrons to the dryer barrel and becomes positively charged. As the positive charge accumulates, the sock's remaining electrons are held more tightly to it, and greater effort is required to remove an electron. Meanwhile, the barrel is becoming more negative and the electrons are repelling one another, so more work is required to transfer additional electrons onto it. One can think of the electric potential as a kind of "pressure" that opposes attempts to push the electrons or positive charges closer together as they accumulate and repel one another.

Molecular Bonding

Electronics at its most basic level involves the movement of electrons within the bounds of a circuit. The ability of electrons to move depends on the characteristics of the materials that compose the circuit, the most important of which is the nature of the molecular bonding in those materials. As discussed in Appendix A, electrons are found in electron orbitals around the nucleus of an atom. Electrons in inner-shell orbitals (the spherical shells closer to the nucleus) are tightly bound to the atom and generally do not participate in interactions with other atoms. In most cases, only the *valence* electrons (those in the outermost orbital[s]) are available to bind to other atoms. It is these electrons that can create molecular bonds of the two types described below.

Covalent Bonds

In a covalent bond, the outermost electron orbitals of two atoms interact with one another to form two molecular orbitals, a *bonding orbital* and an *antibonding orbital*. As the names imply, a bonding orbital holds two atoms together in a molecule, whereas an antibonding orbital pushes them apart. The bonding and antibonding orbitals are shown both pictorially and in an energy diagram in **Figure B-2**. Because the antibonding orbital is a higher-energy state than the bonding orbital, both electrons are normally found in the bonding orbital. Electrons in a covalent (bonding) orbital are more or less tied to the

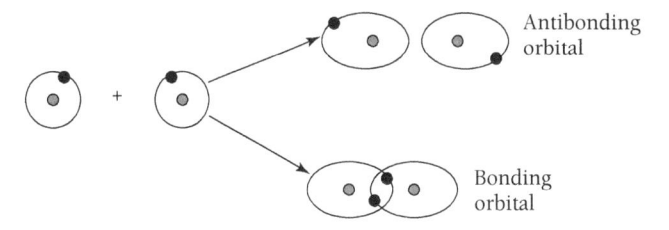

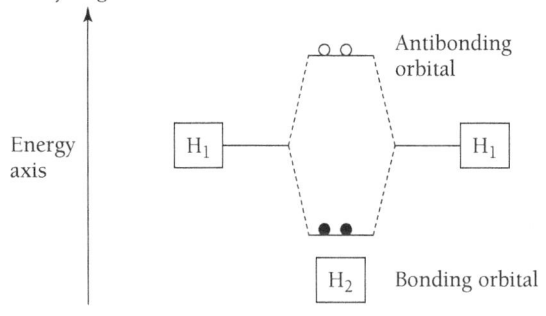

Figure B-2 Covalent bonding and antibonding orbitals. An H_2 molecule is shown pictorially (Fig. B-2a) and as an energy diagram (Fig. B-2b). Each atom contributes one electron to the molecular bond. The bonding orbital is at a lower energy level than the antibonding orbital, so electrons are typically found there.

space between the two atoms and are not free to move; materials with covalent bonds are often poor conductors of electricity. Covalent bonds are found in most organic compounds and in many common inorganic molecules.

Delocalized Bonds

Other types of materials essentially share all of their electrons in a band of electron orbitals. Instead of bonding occurring between two individual atoms, this delocalized bonding binds many atoms together. As with covalent bonds, it is possible to combine the electron orbitals in such a way as to get a delocalized band of antibonding orbitals at a higher energy (**Figure B-3**). The group of bonding orbitals is called the *valence band*, and the group of antibonding orbitals is the *conduction band*. Each band contains a large number of electron orbitals at very closely spaced energy levels. Within a band, if there are vacancies

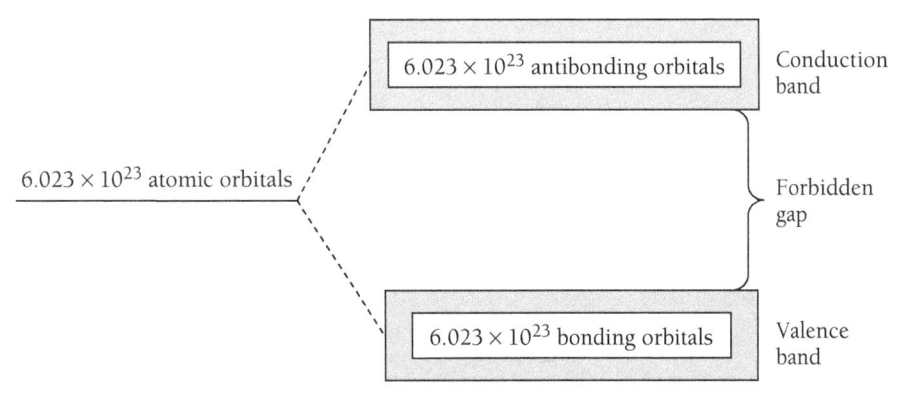

Figure B-3 Energy diagram showing bonding and antibonding orbitals in a delocalized molecular bonding situation. In this example, a mole's worth of metal atoms combine their valence electrons and become a "molecule."

in that band, electrons are relatively free to move about, but they cannot jump from the valence band to the conduction band unless they get additional energy. The height of the forbidden gap determines how much energy is required for this to happen, and ultimately it defines whether a material is an insulator, a conductor, or a semiconductor (see below).

Metals represent one example of delocalized bonding. In a metal, the "molecule" created by delocalized bonding is the whole piece of metal. In regard to the valence and conduction bands, the chief characteristic of a metal is that the valence band and conduction bands overlap. Therefore, electrons can move easily about the metal, because only a tiny amount of energy is needed to put an electron into an unoccupied orbital. Hence, metals demonstrate high electrical conductivity.

Crystals also exhibit delocalized bonding, but do so in a slightly different manner. Bonds in crystalline structures are most commonly ionic or covalent. The electrons in the valence band are bound to specific locations within the crystal lattice. They can move into the conduction band only by getting enough energy to "jump over" the forbidden gap and enter the conduction band. In crystals, the valence band is completely filled, and the conduction band is empty. These materials are insulators unless an input of energy allows valence electrons to enter the conduction band.

Conduction Properties of Materials

With this understanding of molecular bonds, we can divide different materials into three categories based on their electrical conduction properties (**Figure B-4**).

- Conductors: In metals, the valence and conduction bands overlap, and the valence electrons are held rather loosely. They are easily induced to move about by the application of an electric field. Materials with this band structure are able to conduct electricity.
- Insulators: The valence band is filled, so the electrons are not free to move. The forbidden gap is 5 eV or larger, which prevents electrons from jumping into the conduction band without an input of energy. These materials will not conduct electricity. Many molecules with covalent bonds and atoms that exist singly in nature, such as argon and helium gases, are also insulators.
- Semiconductors: The valence band is again full, but the forbidden gap is small (about 1 eV). Only a small amount of energy is required for electrons to move into the conduction band, where they can move and therefore conduct electricity. At very low temperatures, a semiconductor acts as an insulator, but at somewhat higher temperatures (in some cases at room temperature) it conducts electricity.

Conduction of electricity in different materials depends on a physical property called *resistivity*. When we look at a list of resistivity values, we find that the difference between conductors and insulators is one of magnitude, not kind. Even conductors have some very small amount of resistivity, and even insulators will conduct electricity in the presence of a large enough electric field.

Electric Circuits

If we have a source of electrical potential, we can make an *anode* (a positively charged pole) and a *cathode* (a negatively charged pole). Electrons will spontaneously want to leave the cathode and move toward the anode. However, no significant amount of electric current will flow until we connect the anode and cathode with a conducting material. An *electric circuit* consists of a set of devices connected by conducting wires, such that if the right electric field is present and the right connections are made, electrons will flow through the circuit.

Closed-Loop Circuit

An electric circuit generally must have the form of a closed loop if the movement of electrons (known as *current*) is to be continuous. Often, the closed loop is created by way of a switch. Think, for example, of a flashlight. Its components are a battery (the source of electric potential), a lightbulb, and a switch. Flipping the switch to "on" connects the battery to the lightbulb via a conducting wire, allowing electrons to move through the lightbulb and heat up the filament, which as a result generates light photons. For continuous operation, the electrons start at the negative terminal (low potential), move through the circuit,

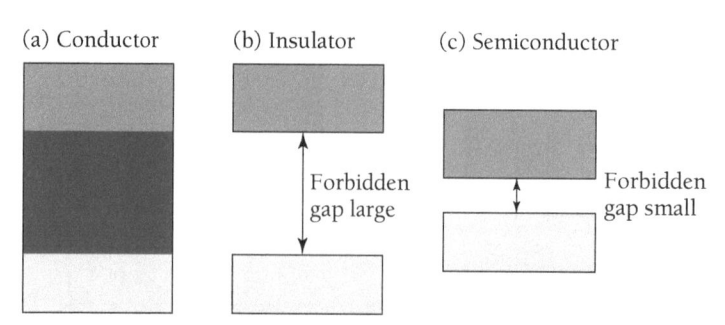

Figure B-4 Delocalized bonds in conductors, insulators, and semiconductors. In materials with delocalized bonds, the difference between materials that can conduct electricity and materials that cannot is the size of the forbidden gap. Conductors have overlapping valence and conduction bands, so electrons are able to move within the empty conduction band without requiring energy input. Insulators have a large forbidden gap, and so electrons in the valence band are unable to access the conduction band under normal circumstances. Semiconductors have a small forbidden gap, so electrons receiving only a small input of energy can jump into the conduction band.

and end up at the positive terminal of the battery. If the switch is flipped to "off," the connection is broken, electrons stop heating up the filament, and the light goes off.

The filament of the bulb in the flashlight has some resistance to the flow of electrons, and the battery is needed to overcome that resistance and get the electrons to move. This situation is described by *Ohm's law*

$$\Delta V = I \times R \tag{B-2}$$

where ΔV is the potential supplied by the battery, I is the current, and R is the resistance in the wire and lightbulb. (Ohm's law is not an absolute law of nature, but rather a rule of thumb for the behavior of circuits. Not all materials behave in the way that the law predicts; these materials are called *non-ohmic*.) For materials that obey Ohm's law, if the resistance is held constant, more electron movement (larger I) will only happen if the potential (ΔV) is increased. If ΔV is held constant, then I and R have an inversely proportional relationship.

We can use the analogy of water in a garden hose to understand the relationship among potential, current, and resistance. Imagine the garden hose has a spray nozzle on the free end, and the nozzle is closed. We can turn on the faucet to create pressure in the hose, but no water flows. Potential in an electric circuit is like the pressure in the hose: ΔV corresponds to the pressure difference between the hose side of the nozzle and the air side of the nozzle. Water flow (analogous to current) does not occur until the nozzle (analogous to resistance) is opened. When closed, the nozzle represents infinite resistance. The more open the nozzle (the lower the resistance), the more water will flow (the greater the current). Alternatively, we could leave the nozzle partially open (moderate resistance) and change the water flow rate (current) by adjusting the faucet to increase the pressure drop (ΔV) across the nozzle.

Capacitor

A different situation arises when the electric circuit is not a closed loop. A *capacitor* consists of two plates made of conducting material, separated by an insulator (**Figure B-5**). A potential source removes negative charge from one plate and places it on the other, causing a charge differential to be built up between the two plates. The electrons can't jump across the insulating gap under normal circumstances, so an electric field is created in the space between the two plates. The charge on the plates builds up to a maximum that depends on the size of the plates and the magnitude of the potential. At some point, no current flows through the circuit, because the electrons are crowded together and the potential source is not large enough to overcome their repulsion. So all movement of electrons stops, and the system is static.

The situation is similar to that of the sock newly removed from the dryer: because it has an excess of positive charge, its potential is high relative to its environment. The charged capacitor likewise has a high potential difference between the two plates, expressed by a simple algebraic relationship

$$C \times \Delta V = Q \tag{B-3}$$

where Q is the electric charge in coulombs on one plate, ΔV is the voltage across the capacitor, and C is the capacitance in farads (we'll get to units shortly).

This behavior makes capacitors quite useful. One common use is as a portable source of electric energy (i.e., an electronic battery). Once charged, the capacitor can be removed from its power supply without disturbing the charge buildup. It can then be connected to a second circuit, where it acts as the supplier of potential difference. Capacitors can also act as charge collectors, as they do in gas-filled detectors. A radiation interaction produces an electron and a positive ion (see Appendix A). If the interaction happens in the space between the two plates of a charged capacitor, the electron will move toward the positive plate and the positive ion toward the negative plate. From there each can be counted, to provide a measure of the radiation present.

Resistor

Resistors are another common component of electric circuits. They are made of materials with large resistivity (compared to other circuit components), and their primary function is to modulate current or voltage according to Ohm's law. For example, a resistor can be used to dissipate the power from the voltage source, when that much power is not needed. Or a resistor may be used to decrease voltage so as to keep the current at an acceptable level for a delicate circuit component. Like friction, resistance does its work by wasting energy as heat. We later explore the workings of a circuit containing both a resistor and a capacitor.

Electrical Units and Mathematical Relationships

Our comprehension of electric circuits is improved when we can apply some basic mathematical relationships to them. This will also provide a common understanding and terminology for the main body of the text. In nature, charge is most often found in a single-sized packet, namely, the amount of charge on an electron or proton:

$$1 \text{ unit of charge} = 1.602 \times 10^{-19} \text{ coulomb.} \tag{B-4}$$

Every object with electric charge has some integral multiple of this number, because electrons and protons are the physical bearers of negative and positive charge,

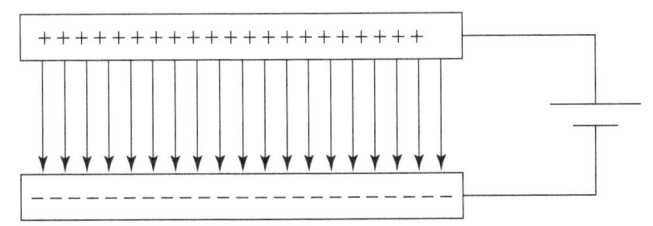

Figure B-5 Capacitor. A capacitor consists of two conductors connected to a voltage source and separated by an insulator. The voltage source moves electrons off one plate and onto the other. This creates a uniform electric field (shown by the arrows) between the two plates, with little or no electric field effects outside of this space.

respectively. The *coulomb* is therefore the basic unit of electric charge:

$$1 \text{ coulomb (C)} = \text{charge on } 6.24 \times 10^{18} \text{ electrons.} \quad \text{(B-5)}$$

The symbols Q and q are used to represent electric charge in equations.

Current is a measurement of the amount of charge moving past a reference point in a conductor per unit time. In electrical equations, current is denoted by either I or i and is measured in amperes:

$$1 \text{ ampere (A)} = \frac{1 \text{ coulomb (C)}}{\sec}. \quad \text{(B-6)}$$

Its magnitude in any given situation depends on both the characteristics of the conducting material through which it is traveling and the electric potential that is driving it.

Electric potential is, as the name implies, a source of potential energy. Electrons in an electric field feel the force of the field, and given the opportunity, they will move in the direction the force is pushing them. We can think of potential as electric pressure (back to the hose analogy). Positive charge moves from an area of higher potential (pressure) to an area of lower potential (pressure), while negative charges move from low potential to high potential. The only time electrical potential has a physical consequence is when there is a potential difference between two points and an object with electric charge is placed in the vicinity of that potential difference.

The joule is the unit of energy, so we can quantify the magnitude of potential in energy terms:

$$1 \text{ volt (V)} = \frac{1 \text{ joule (J)}}{\text{coulomb (C)}}. \quad \text{(B-7)}$$

Thus a potential difference of 1 V represents 1 J of energy given to each coulomb of charge, as the electric field does its work on the charge. We can bring this all the way down to the level of a single electron, where an electron volt (eV) is the potential energy given to a single electron as it moves across a potential difference of 1 V:

$$1 \text{ eV} = \left(1.6 \times 10^{-19} \text{ C}\right)\left(1 \text{ V}\right) = 1.6 \times 10^{-19} \text{ J}. \quad \text{(B-8)}$$

The eV and its multiples are used to describe the energy of gamma rays, beta particles, and other entities encountered in nuclear physics.

Because all physically significant instances of the electrical potential involve a potential change, it has become common to drop the use of the delta notation. Thus a 1.5-V battery really describes the difference in potential between the ends, but it is common to write $V = 1.5$ V rather than the more correct $\Delta V = 1.5$ V. This produces the unfortunate situation in which the quantity, electric potential, has the same symbol as its unit, the volt. Also, the student must learn from context and experience to distinguish those less common occasions where the term describes a single value rather than a difference. Here is an example: "This battery is a 9-volt battery because the positive terminal is at 9 volts." Unstated is the remaining phrase "... compared to the negative terminal at 0 volts." We will use V for potential difference through the remainder of this work unless there is a special reason to emphasize the absolute potential.

Resistance is opposition to electron movement, analogous to friction in the mechanical world. An electric potential difference is required to create a specified current in a circuit with resistance. The *ohm* is the unit of resistance:

$$1 \text{ ohm} = \frac{1 \text{ volt}}{\text{ampere}}. \quad \text{(B-9)}$$

The definition indicates that a circuit with resistance of 1 ohm requires 1 V of electrical potential difference for each ampere of current desired. In electrical equations and circuit diagrams, resistance is given the symbol R.

The *capacitance* of a capacitor is numerically equal to the charge on either plate divided by the potential difference between the plates; it is measured in *farads*:

$$1 \text{ farad (F)} = \frac{1 \text{ coulomb}}{\text{volt}} \quad \text{(B-10)}$$

A capacitor with 1-F capacitance holds 1 coulomb of electric charge for each volt of potential difference applied to it. If the voltage source is removed and the circuit remains connected, the capacitor charge will leak off. The letter C is used both to designate a capacitor in circuit diagrams and to indicate the value of capacitance in equations (e.g., $Q = C \Delta V$). It is always positive. (But be aware of a possible point of confusion: C is also used as the abbreviation for the Coulomb.)

Sample Calculation B-1 Conversion of Charge to Voltage

A radiation detector has a capacitance of 14 microfarads (μF). A radiation field creates 1 billion electrons in the radiation detector. What voltage will this number of electrons create?

$$1 \times 10^9 \text{ electrons} \times \frac{1 \text{ coulomb}}{6.24 \times 10^{18} \text{ electrons}}$$

$$= 1.6 \times 10^{-10} \text{ coulomb}.$$

$$\frac{1.6 \times 10^{-10} \text{ coulomb}}{14 \times 10^{-6} \text{ farads}} \times \frac{1 \text{ farad}}{1 \text{ coulomb/volt}}$$

$$= 1.14 \times 10^{-5} \text{ V} = 11.4 \text{ μV}.$$

RC Circuits

The most common electric circuit component used in radiation-detecting instruments is the resistor-capacitor circuit, or *RC circuit*. RC circuits have two features that make them quite useful in radiation detection. The first is that a size relationship is maintained between the input pulse and the output pulse. This is a requirement for energy-sensitive detectors such as scintillation detectors and semiconductor detectors. The second important feature is their ability to selectively filter electrical noise. In electrical systems, noise is any undesired fluctuation superimposed on a signal; it can have either low or high frequency.

Behavior

If we create a circuit containing a battery and a resistor, the current through the circuit reaches its final value (according to Eq. B-2) almost instantaneously. Similarly, in a circuit containing just a power source and a capacitor, the capacitor is fully charged soon after the circuit is connected. But when we include both a resistor and a capacitor in an RC circuit, its behavior changes markedly (**Figure B-6**). A battery is shown as the voltage source, but any type of power supply will do.

When the switch in Figure B-6a is put in contact with terminal A, the system is said to be *charging*, as electrons move onto one plate of the capacitor and are withdrawn from the other plate. When the switch is put in contact with terminal B, it no longer has an input voltage, but the stored charge on the capacitor supplies potential that causes the circuit to *discharge*. The effect of adding the resistor to the circuit is to slow the charging or discharging of the capacitor, so that both processes happen more slowly than if the resistor were not present. The circuit demonstrates a characteristic, finite time for charging or discharging, before constant values of capacitor charge (either the maximum charge on the capacitor in charging mode, or zero charge in discharge mode) are reached. The time behavior of the circuit is characterized by the circuit's *time constant* τ, which is the product of the resistance and capacitance. In Figure B-6c, for example, it takes about five times the τ value for the circuit's current to reach the plateau part of the curve.

We can describe the curves in Figures B-6b and B-6c according to characteristic exponential equations. During the charging phase, charge builds up on the capacitor according to the equation

$$Q(t) = V(0)C\left(1 - e^{-t/\tau}\right). \tag{B-11}$$

The current decreases as a function of time according to the equation

$$I(t) = \frac{V(0)}{R} e^{-t/\tau} \tag{B-12}$$

where $V(0)$ is the input voltage (the ΔV supplied by the battery). At the same time, the potential difference across the resistor decreases as the current diminishes, because the electric power originally supplied by the battery is now stored in the capacitor. Current stops flowing when the charge on the capacitor has reached its maximal value, and the charging phase ends.

(a) RC circuit

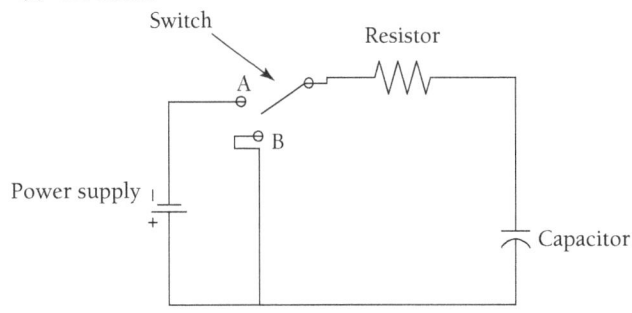

(b) Current

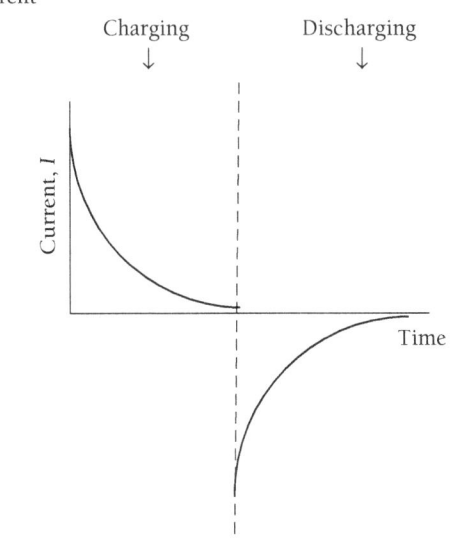

(c) Capacitor charge (and therefore potential)

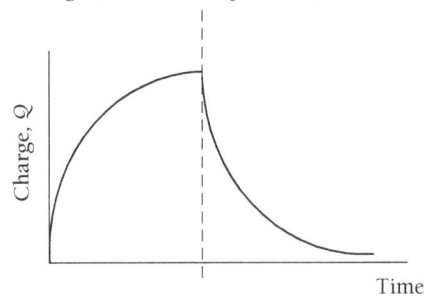

Figure B-6 Operation of an RC circuit. Figure B-6a shows a block diagram of the RC circuit. For Figures B-6b and B-6c, the circuit first is switched to connect at point A to charge the capacitor and then is discharged by connecting at point B. Figure B-6b shows that the current direction is reversed for discharge compared to its direction in the charging mode. The capacitor voltage is proportional to the charge (Eq. B-3) and therefore follows the shape of Figure B-6c.

In discharge mode, the stored charge on the capacitor drives the current. The current starts out high (but in the opposite direction of the changing phase), and decreases as the charge on the capacitor decreases according to the equation

$$q(t) = Q(0)e^{-t/\tau} \tag{B-13}$$

where $Q(0)$ is the charge on a capacitor plate at the beginning of the discharge phase. In the limit of $t \gg \tau$, the exponential terms in the above equations reach their limits, and Equations B-11 and B-12 reduce to Equations B-3 and B-2, respectively.

RC Circuits in Radiation Detectors

One common use of RC circuits is to convert charge to voltage. The initial result of radiation interactions in a gas-filled detector is the production of electrons, which are attracted to the positive and negative plates of the capacitor. As the electrons neutralize charge on the capacitor, the resulting signal is measured as a voltage signal, according to the equation

$$V(t) = \frac{q(t)}{C} \quad \text{(B-14)}$$

where $q(t)$ is the charge on either plate at any moment, according to Equation B-13. Voltage is generally easier to measure than current and is more useful in many situations.

Further, manipulation of the values of R and C can provide us with the exact output information we desire. **Figure B-7** shows two extreme possibilities for the time behavior of an RC circuit as electrons from radiation-induced ionizations are collected. If the resistor has a small value, then τ can be manipulated to be short relative to the charge collection time. In this situation, the output voltage signal $V(t)$ exactly duplicates the input signal in both time and amplitude (Fig. B-7b). The more common choice is to use a large resistor, making τ much larger than the charge collection time (Fig. B-7c). In this situation, charge from radiation interactions builds up on the capacitor and then discharges relatively slowly. This produces a signal whose amplitude accurately reflects the original charge signal, but with a very long tail. The detector must either wait until the tail has run its course or reshape the pulse to remove it. In either case, the RC circuit has acted as a transducer, converting charge into voltage, such that the relationship between the charge and the output voltage is linear.

RC Circuits in Pulse Shaping

Pulse shaping is an especially important aspect of producing a usable signal from a scintillation detector. **Figure B-8** shows three examples: an RC integrating circuit, a CR differentiating circuit, and a combined CR/RC circuit (1). The integrating circuit acts as a low-pass filter, passing low-frequency signals and blocking high-frequency signals. The differentiating circuit acts as a high-pass filter, registering high-frequency signals and suppressing low-frequency signals. Neither works optimally for radiation detection by itself, but when combined, they produce a pulse that is easy to deal with electronically. **Figure B-9** shows one example of how differentiating and integrating RC circuits change the shape of the signal as they amplify, ultimately producing the bipolar pulse shape that is optimum for signal evaluation. The important point about pulse shaping is that it maximizes the information content of the signal while minimizing the contribution of electrical noise.

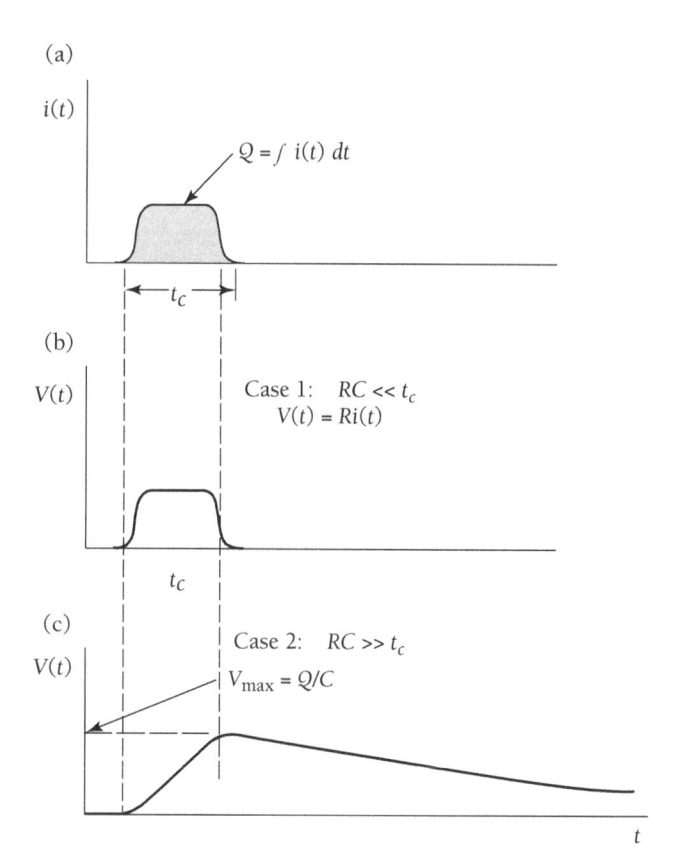

Figure B-7 Conversion of charge to voltage in a pulse-mode detector. Figure B-7a shows the original input signal, consisting of electrons arriving in the circuit due to the radiation interactions in the detector. If the time constant τ (= $R \times C$) is much smaller than the time required to collect the original electrons (t_c), then the voltage pulse is shaped identically to the charge pulse (Fig. B-7b). If τ is much larger than t_c (Fig. B-7c), then the output pulse is shaped by the circuit into a pulse with a very long tail. The amplitude of the pulse is directly proportional to the charge generated in the detector. Note that the value of V_{max} in Figure B-7c is much, much larger than the voltage signal in Figure B-7b. Reprinted from: Knoll GF. *Radiation Detection and Measurement*. 3rd ed. New York, NY: John Wiley & Sons; 2000:109, Fig. 4-1. Used with permission from John Wiley & Sons.

Transistors and Logic Circuits

The transistor was introduced in 1947 and was a critical technological advance that led to the development of computers. In fact, it is considered by some to be the greatest invention of the 20th century. The essence of a transistor is that a small signal controls a much larger signal. We consider first the operation of a transistor and then how it can function as an amplifier and as a switch. Transistors behave as they do because they are manufactured from semiconductor materials. They can be made in extremely small sizes, such that a million or more can be put onto a 1-inch-square integrated circuit.

Semiconductors and the Depletion Layer

Earlier in this appendix, a semiconductor was described as a material with a delocalized molecular bonding structure and a small forbidden gap. We can enhance the semiconductor properties of an intrinsic semiconducting material by adding impurities (a process called *doping*).

(a) RC (integrating) circuit and CR (differentiating) circuit

(b) Response of RC and CR circuits to input signal with high- and low-frequency noise

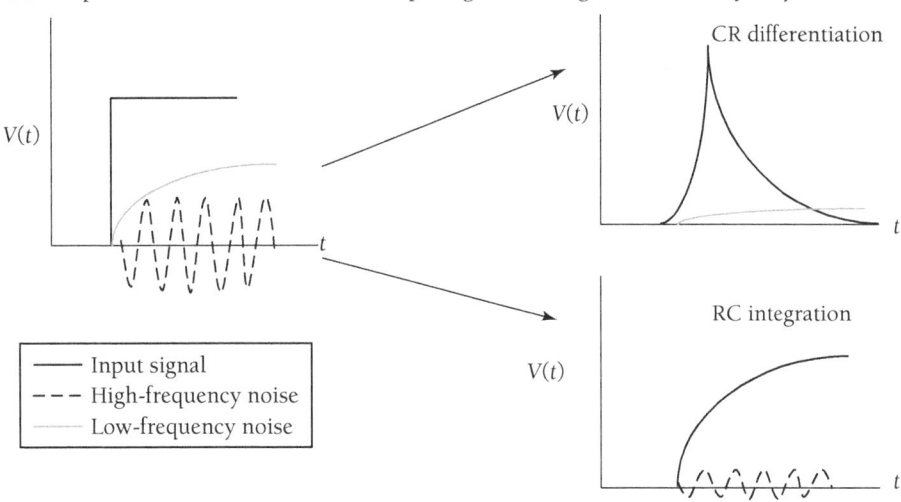

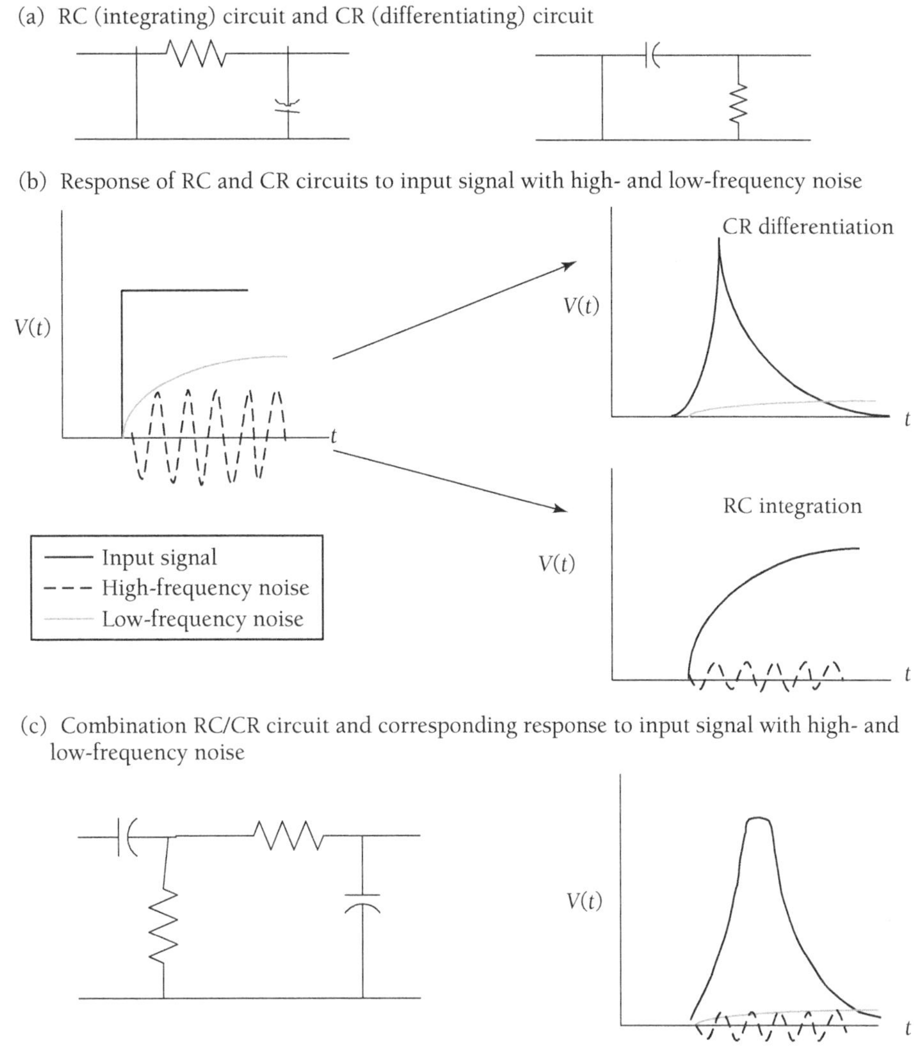

— Input signal
--- High-frequency noise
— Low-frequency noise

CR differentiation

RC integration

(c) Combination RC/CR circuit and corresponding response to input signal with high- and low-frequency noise

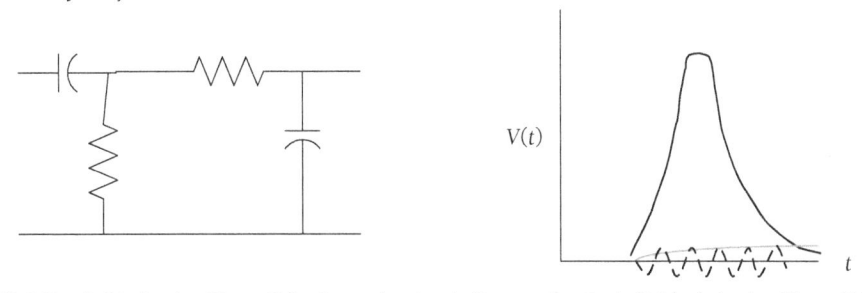

Figure B-8 Pulse shaping with RC and CR circuits. Figure B-8a shows the circuit diagrams for the individual circuits. Figure B-8b shows the effect of these circuits on an idealized input pulse, on which is superimposed high- and low-frequency noise. The X-axis in all the graphs is time. The CR (differentiating) circuit discriminates against low-frequency noise because its output is based on the rate of change of the signal. The RC (integrating) circuit discriminates against high-frequency noise because its output is based on the area under the input signal. Figure B-8c shows a combined RC/CR circuit and the final signal output of the combined circuit. Note that both the high-frequency and low-frequency noise signals are reduced in amplitude relative to their starting amplitudes. Adapted from: Cherry SR, Sorenson JA, Phelps ME. *Physics in Nuclear Medicine*. 3rd ed. Philadelphia, PA: Saunders; 2003:113, Fig. 8-4. With permission from Elsevier Science.

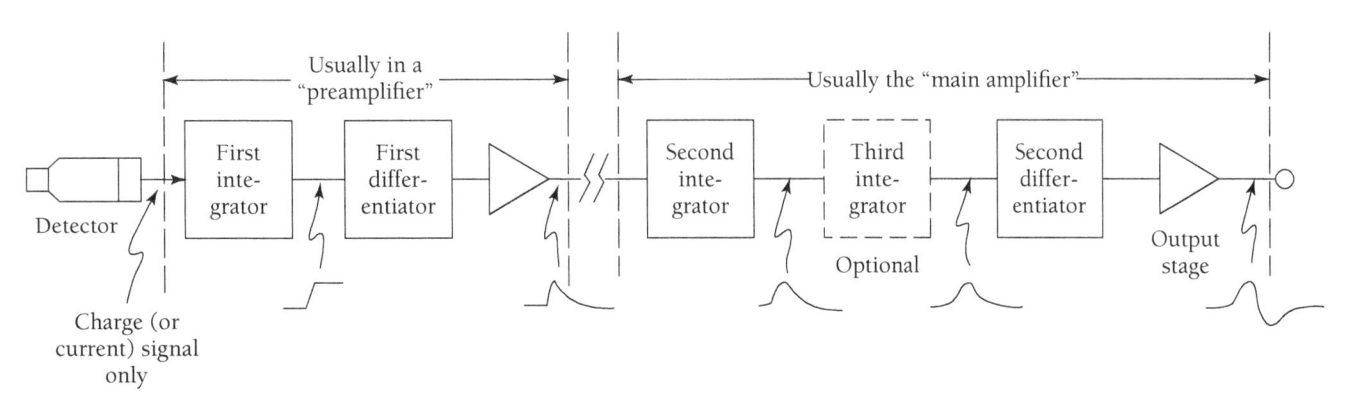

Figure B-9 Application of pulse shaping in a scintillation detector. The pulse shapes are shown after going through each RC or CR circuit, under the arrows below the chain of differentiating and integrating circuits. The triangular shape at the end of each section represents the amplification that is also occurring, but that is not reflected in the pulse shapes. The final output is a bipolar pulse (extending both above and below the electronic baseline); this is preferred from the standpoint of pulse separation. Reprinted from: Rollo FD, ed. *Nuclear Medicine Physics, Instrumentation, and Agents*. St. Louis, MO: Mosby; 1977:167. With permission from Dr. F. D. Rollo.

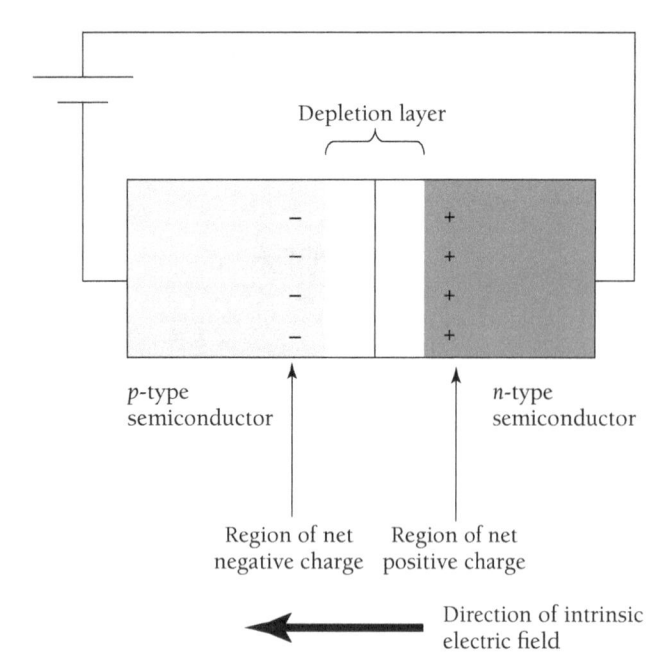

Figure B-10 A *p-n* junction. The *p*-type semiconductor contains an impurity with one less electron than is needed for the molecular structure, creating "holes" that can migrate through the semiconductor molecule. The *n*-type semiconductor has an impurity with an extra electron that is also mobile. When the two are brought together, the holes and electrons diffuse toward one another and combine, creating a depletion layer between the two sides with no mobile charge carriers. But the atoms "left behind" by the combining holes and electrons now have either a net negative charge (on the *p* side) or a net positive charge (on the *n* side). This creates an electric field gradient that opposes any further diffusion of electrons or holes. The power supply is shown providing a reverse bias.

An impurity that includes an extra electron beyond what is needed for the molecular structure is called an *n-type impurity*; one that is missing an electron is a *p-type impurity*. An orbital shell where the missing electron would live is called a *hole*. Figure 3-1 shows molecular and energy diagrams for pure, *n*-type, and *p*-type semiconductors.

A *p-n junction* (**Figure B-10**) brings the two types of semiconductors together, with some interesting and useful results. While both a *p*-type semiconductor and an *n*-type semiconductor are relatively conductive, when the two are brought together, a nonconducting region called the *depletion layer* is created. The electrons from the *n* side and the holes from the *p* side diffuse toward one another and combine, creating an area where there are no charge carriers. But that in turn means that the *p* side of the depletion layer has a net negative charge, and the *n* side has a net positive charge. Thus, even in the absence of any externally applied voltage, an intrinsic electric field exists across the *p-n* junction. This intrinsic field opposes the diffusion of electrons and holes, stopping their recombination.

The behavior gets even more interesting when we put the *p-n* junction into a circuit with a voltage source. If the *p* side is attached to the positive terminal and the *n* side to the negative terminal, a situation of *forward bias* is created. The excess holes remaining in the *p*-type semiconductor, and the excess electrons in the *n*-type semiconductor are driven toward the junction, reducing the width of the depletion layer. At some point as the voltage is increased, the intrinsic electric field is overcome, resistance to current flow is reduced, and current flows in the direction dictated by the applied potential.

If, on the other hand, the positive terminal of the external potential source is attached to the *n*-side and the negative terminal to the *p*-side, a *reverse bias* is created. The holes in the *p*-type semiconductor are pulled toward the negative terminal, and the electrons of the *n*-type semiconductor toward the positive terminal. The depletion layer (where there are no holes or electrons) thus gets wider, and the intrinsic electric field is supported and strengthened. Hence, no current is conducted across the *p-n* junction. The *p-n* junction acts as a *diode*—a one-way valve for current flow. The semiconductor radiation detector consists of a *p-n* junction with a reverse bias.

Transistor Operation

A transistor consists of a source and a drain made of *n*-type silicon, a gate and a base made of *p*-type silicon, and a coating of nonconductive material (**Figure B-11**). It therefore consists of two *p-n* junctions of the type described above, oriented back to back. The usual situation is that electrons are arriving at the drain (remember that the arrows point in the direction of movement for positive charges). Under normal circumstances they would move through the base easily, but they cannot cross through the depletion layer between the base and the drain. A positive charge applied to the gate draws the negative charge of the base toward the gate, reducing the depletion layer and allowing current to flow through the base (Fig. B-11b).

The behavior of the source-drain current is shown in Figure B-11c. If the gate voltage is less than A, not enough positive charge has been applied to create the electron channel between the source and drain; the depletion layer acts as a resistor to current flow. Once A has been exceeded, the current is proportional to the size of the gate voltage. At B, a maximal current is flowing, and the transistor is said to be saturated. Between A and B, the transistor is acting as an amplifier, and at B, it is acting as an on/off switch.

Logic Circuit Function

Logic circuits allow an electric device to perform sophisticated functions, because they provide a mechanism for the circuit's activity to change depending on its inputs. Logic circuits use a type of logic called *Boolean algebra*, based on set algebra and Venn diagrams, which is applicable to the binary numbering system used in computers. The transistor is the essential electrical component of most logic circuits. Whenever the transistor's base voltage is below A in Figure B-11c, it produces no output; when the base voltage rises above B, it produces maximum output. It thus acts as a yes/no output device for computer logic operations.

We use the anticoincidence logic circuit of a pulse height analyzer (PHA) as a simple example of a logic circuit. An electric signal generated by a gamma ray is evaluated by two voltage comparators called *discriminators*. If the signal is above the discriminator's preset level

(a) Transistor components

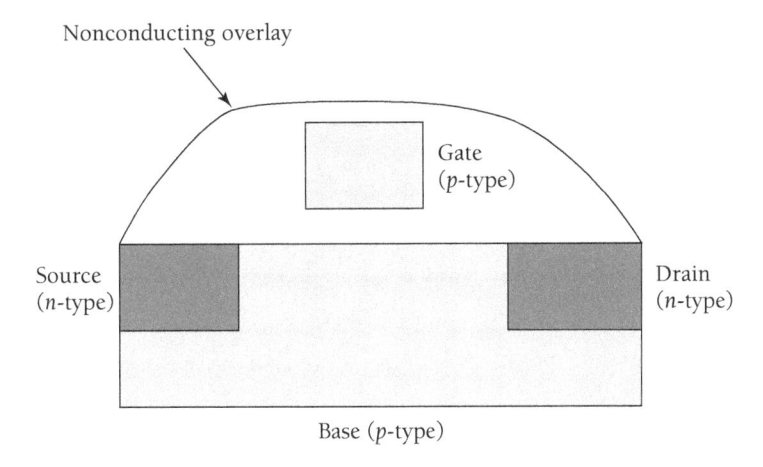

- Nonconducting overlay
- Gate (p-type)
- Source (n-type)
- Drain (n-type)
- Base (p-type)

(b) Transistor operation

- Controlling signal, V_s
- I_{in}
- I_{out}
- Bold arrow indicates direction of electron flow

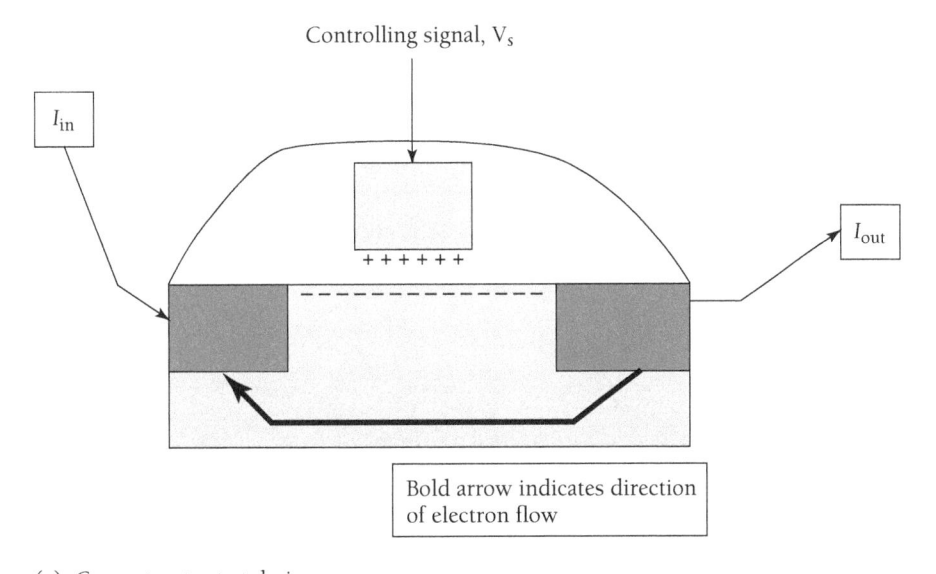

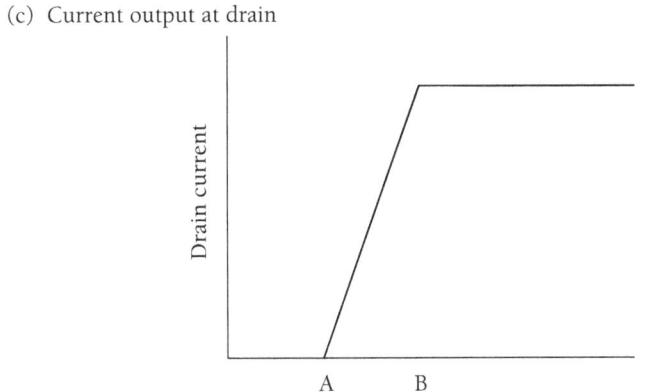

(c) Current output at drain

Drain current vs. Controlling signal, V_s, with thresholds A and B marked on horizontal axis.

Figure B-11 Transistor. The transistor allows control of electric currents using small input signals. It consists of a source and drain made of an n-type semiconductor material and a base and gate made of a p-type semiconductor material (Fig. B-11a). The gate is insulated from the other parts by a nonconductive material. Prior to application of an input voltage at the gate, the depletion layers between source and base and between drain and base prevent the flow of electrons from drain to source. Figure B-11b shows that a positive charge in the gate draws electrons to the edge of the base, shrinking the depletion layers and creating a channel through which current can pass from source to drain. For current to flow, the voltage at the gate must exceed a threshold, shown as A in Figure B-11c. Below A, the depletion layer has not been affected. Between A and B, the depletion layer is smaller but not completely gone. The size of the current in this region is related to the value of the gate voltage. Above B, the depletion layer no longer impedes current to any degree.

Table B-1
Operation of a Pulse Height Analyzer

Signal from Detector	LLD Output	ULD Output	Inverted ULD Output	Logic Circuit Output
Below level of LLD	0	0	1	0 (no source input)
Between levels of LLD and ULD	1	0	1	1 (input to both source and gate)
Above level of ULD	1	1	0	0 (no gate input)

(i.e., above B in Fig. B-11c), the discriminator produces a digital 1 as its output; if the signal is below, its output is a digital 0. We are looking for a signal that is between the lower-level discriminator (LLD) and the upper-level discriminator (ULD), such that the LLD output is a 1 and the ULD output is a 0.

Return to the description of the transistor given above. The LLD provides the source input and the ULD the gate input to the anticoincidence logic circuit. But the ULD's output signal is inverted before going to the gate, so that if the gamma ray signal is above the ULD, the gate input is a 0, and if below the ULD, it is a 1. The source receives input only if the gamma ray energy exceeds the LLD. Thus, when the LLD is exceeded and the ULD is not exceeded, signals are received at both the source and the gate. Only then does the electron channel open, causing the logic circuit to generate a 1 output signal. The possibilities are illustrated in **Table B-1**.

Amplifier Function

To demonstrate how a transistor can amplify a signal, we will use a three-terminal transistor called an emitter–collector amplifier as an example (**Figure B-12**). The emitter is held at a negative potential and the collector at a positive potential; the input signal is received at the base. When the base voltage is positive relative to the emitter potential, electrons are drawn from the emitter (which as an *n*-type semiconductor has many excess electrons) toward the base. But the amplifier has only a small region of *p*-type semiconductor, and therefore a low capacity to hold the many electrons that the emitter is sending. So the excess electrons get shunted toward the collector and from there to the next circuit component. The number of excess electrons at the collector is proportional to the signal at the base. Hence a small signal applied to the base can result in a large signal output, by as much as a factor of 1,000.

Electrical Components of Radiation Detectors

Radiation detectors require a number of electrical components. The previous sections on RC circuits and transistors introduce the operational details of these components, which in turn are employed in the various constituent devices that make up a given radiation detector. This section considers the constituent devices or *modules* that come together to form various types of radiation detectors,

(a) Construction of the emitter–collector amplifier

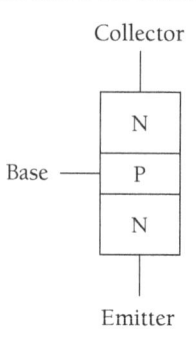

(b) Electrical diagram of an emitter–collector amplifier

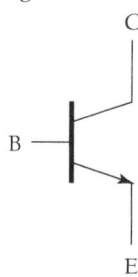

Figure B-12 Emitter–collector amplifier. This is one example of how an amplifier causes signal amplification. Figure B-12a shows the actual construction of the device from *n*-type (N) and *p*-type (P) semiconductors; Figure B-12b shows the electrical diagram representation. For the amplifier to transmit a signal, the input at the base (B on the diagram) must be positive with respect to the emitter (E) and negative with respect to the collector (C). When this is true, the extra electrons in E are attracted to B. But because B is small, there isn't enough room for them, so they are shunted off to C. Thus, the small input signal at B becomes a proportionately larger signal at C.

from the standpoint of what each module must do well if the detector is to work properly.

Amplifier

The signal resulting from a radiation detector is often quite small, and it may not be strong enough to allow its passage through subsequent modules. An *amplifier* enhances the small signal so that it can be passed through other electronic modules and analyzed for its size and other characteristics. The amount of amplification is commonly called the *gain*, expressed as the ratio of the output signal size to the input signal size. A wide variety of amplifier designs have been developed, too many to describe here; the above description of how a transistor can function as an amplifier is a sufficient level of understanding.

In a scintillation detector, the initial signal is so small that the first amplifier must be attached directly to the photomultiplier tube (PMT) anode; it is called a *preamplifier*. The amplified signal is then sent via a cable to another amplifier, whose gain can be controlled by the operator. The second amplifier not only increases the size of the signal, but also modifies its shape and removes some of the noise inherent in the electronics (Fig. B-9). Both the preamplifier and the amplifier need to be highly linear in order to produce uniform amplification over a wide range of input signal sizes. They also need to be quite stable, so as to not introduce any additional noise or other variation.

Photodiode

A *diode* is an electrical device that passes current in one direction much more easily than in the other direction. The vacuum tube found in the earliest computers is an old example of a diode. Today, most diodes are semiconductors, operating much as the p-n junction described above does.

A *photodiode* is capable of converting light into an electric signal, either current or voltage. It can thus substitute for a PMT in a scintillation detector, converting scintillation photons into a measurable electric signal. A conventional photodiode is diagrammed in **Figure B-13**. A semiconductor with n and p regions is aligned so that its p region abuts the scintillation crystal. Scintillation photons created by radiation interactions can pass through the thin p region and interact in the depletion layer. The energy of the scintillation photons (3–4 eV) is sufficient to bump an electron across the forbidden gap, allowing it to move into the conduction band. An applied voltage pulls the electrons toward the n region, where they can be collected and sent to the preamplifier.

Once the electric signal is created, the conventional photodiode does not further multiply it—it goes directly to the amplifier. This is a problem because photodiodes can generate a significant amount of electrical noise, which is then amplified along with the signal. This limits the ability of the conventional photodiode to operate in pulse mode, and in fact, most of its uses are in current-mode situations. Photodiodes coupled to scintillation crystals have worse energy resolution by a factor of about 2 compared to PMTs, because of noise (2). Another issue is that the photodiode itself can act as a semiconductor radiation detector, registering gamma rays and x-rays as well as scintillation photons. These interactions with high-energy photons produce much larger signals than those generated by scintillation photons. The problems of noise and detection of high-energy radiation are best addressed by keeping the photodiode small in all three dimensions. These factors have limited the applications of photodiodes in nuclear medicine, although they are commonly found in computed tomography scanners.

One way to get a bigger signal from a photodiode is to create additional ionizations as the electrons are drawn toward the n region. This is analogous to gas amplification in a gas-filled detector. The *avalanche photodiode* has an additional region of high voltage immediately in front of the n region (the dashed line in Fig. B-13). Additional ionizations, and hence signal amplification, occur only in this region, but this can nonetheless increase the signal size by a factor of several hundred. The signal is then easier to distinguish from noise, but is also subject to statistical fluctuation, resulting in degraded energy resolution. An avalanche photodiode is quite sensitive to changes in both high voltage and temperature, so the stability of these factors must be maintained. Avalanche photodiodes are starting to find applications in nuclear medicine, so we can expect to see more of them over time.

The main advantage of a photodiode or avalanche photodiode over a PMT is that there is no need for electrons to escape from the photocathode. The quantum efficiency (the number of electrons produced per incident scintillation photon) is in the range of 60 to 80% in a semiconductor

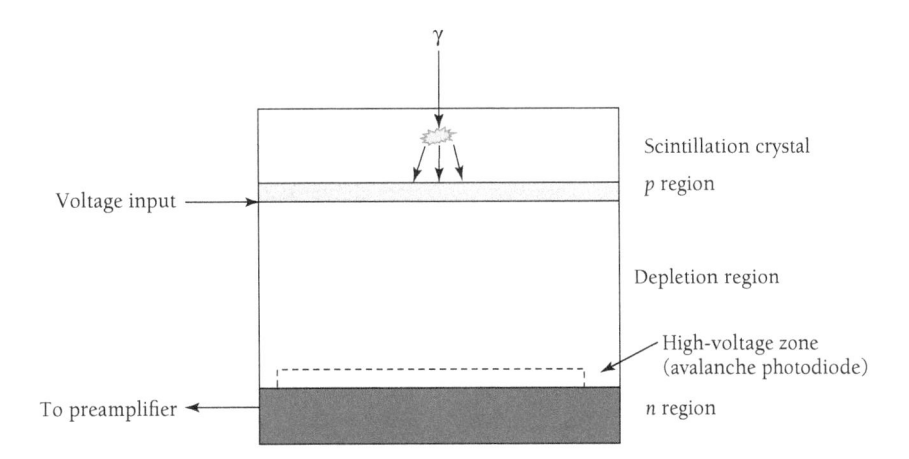

Figure B-13 Photodiode. A photodiode is a semiconductor device that creates an electronic signal in response to interactions of scintillation photons. The diagram shows the gamma ray interacting in the scintillation crystal, creating scintillation photons (small arrows). The scintillation photons are energetic enough to pass through the p region, which is kept as thin as possible. The scintillation photons then interact in the depletion region, creating electron-hole pairs. The applied voltage causes electrons to migrate to the n region, where they are collected and sent to the preamplifier. In an avalanche photodiode, an additional region of high voltage just prior to the n region causes the electrons to produce additional ionizations as they migrate, thus amplifying the electronic signal produced.

photodiode, compared to 30% or less for PMTs (2), so a larger initial pulse is produced. In addition, the photodiode responds to a larger frequency range of scintillation light than a PMT, further improving the quantum efficiency. Photodiodes offer significant advantages over PMTs, including lower power consumption, more compact size, improved ruggedness, and insensitivity to magnetic fields. Their main disadvantage is that the large multiplication factor supplied by the dynodes in a PMT is not replicated in a photodiode, so the final signal is several orders of magnitude smaller as a result.

Power Supply

An external power supply is a critical component of all radiation detection instruments discussed in this text. It produces the potential difference (often called *bias voltage*) that drives ion collection in gas-filled detectors and semiconductor detectors, and the electron multiplication that occurs in PMTs. The voltage source can be as simple as a dry-cell battery or as complex as alternating current from a wall outlet, converted into direct current within the detector. A rectification circuit (often called a *bridge*) is used to convert alternating current to the direct current needed by most instruments.

Power supplies can create three problems of note to nuclear medicine instruments. The first problem is electronic noise, which can result from mechanical vibration of circuit components, random thermal agitation of electrons, and unwanted discharges of circuit components. The goal is to have a high signal-to-noise ratio, so that noise from the power supply is not a significant contributor to the output. This is accomplished by adding a filter (e.g., a CR/RC circuit as in Fig. B-8c) to the circuit, in parallel with the bias voltage. The second problem is a *short circuit*, when the terminals of the power supply are connected directly, without any intervening resistance. This causes an unsafe current to flow. In a battery, a short circuit allows the chemical ions in the battery to recombine, thus potentially destroying the battery as well as making the detector inoperable. The third problem is that instruments can suffer a loss of bias voltage, as in a power outage or battery failure. Gamma cameras and positron emission tomographs are quite sensitive to power fluctuations and should always be protected by a surge protector.

Scaler/Timer

Scintillation and semiconductor detectors and gamma cameras display the total number of counts received and the time of the measurement using a device called a *scaler/timer*. The scaler consists of an electronic gate and a set of six or more decimal-counting assemblies (DCAs), each tied to a seven-segment light-emitting diode (LED). The gate is connected to external controls for stopping conditions (e.g., time or preset counts or the "stop" button) that can be set by the operator. Each pulse received from the PHA passes through the gate to the rightmost DCA, which is incremented by 1. When this DCA is at 9 and a new pulse is received, it is reset to 0 and a pulse is sent to the next DCA. The value of each DCA is displayed by its LED.

Meanwhile, the timer keeps track of the time and stops the counting measurement when time is selected as the stopping condition. Timers generally count the cycles of the 60 cycles/sec alternating current of the commercial power supply, so that they can easily produce an LED display down to tenths of a second, in a manner similar to that described for the scaler.

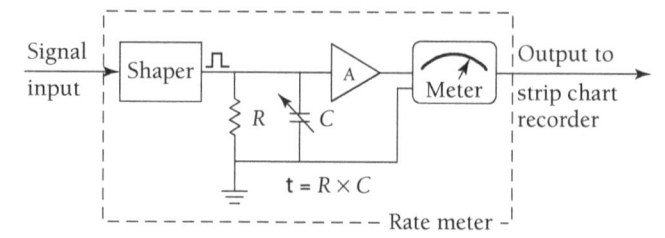

Figure B-14 Diode pump circuit used in rate meters. The box identified as "shaper" has produced output pulses of the type in Figure B-8, and the triangle labeled A is an amplifier. This is a typical CR differentiating circuit. The capacitor is overlaid by an arrow, indicating that it is variable, allowing the operator to control the rate at which the meter responds to changes in count rate. Reprinted from: Cherry SR, Sorenson JA, Phelps ME. *Physics in Nuclear Medicine*. 3rd ed. Philadelphia, PA: Saunders; 2006:123, Fig. 8-13. Used with permission from Elsevier Science.

Rate Meter

The rate meter provides a rough visual indicator of the counting rate. A common form of rate meter is the diode pump circuit shown in **Figure B-14**. The input into this system is a series of logic pulses (e.g., from a PHA). Each logic pulse deposits a small amount of charge on the storage capacitor. This charge is also continuously being discharged through the resistor. An equilibrium is established between the two, such that the output voltage reaches a steady value that is proportional to the rate at which logic pulses are arriving. This voltage in turn drives a needle in front of a scale, a digital readout, or some other type of display. As the rate of incoming logic pulses changes, the readout changes; the speed with which it registers a new count rate depends on the time constant τ of the diode pump circuit. The capacitor in the circuit shown is variable, allowing the operator to control the time constant and therefore the meter's response rate. A rate meter using a short time constant responds quickly to changes in count rate, but produces an erratic reading. A long time constant produces a steady reading, but responds more slowly as the count rate changes (this is illustrated in Fig. 1-8). The amount of amplification provides a multiplication factor (often logarithmic) that allows for measurement of a range of counting rates.

Image Display Devices

Nuclear medicine is primarily a business of images, so it is necessary to have a means of displaying those images. This aspect of the field has changed considerably since the development of the gamma camera. While the digital revolution has decreased the importance of hard-copy films for

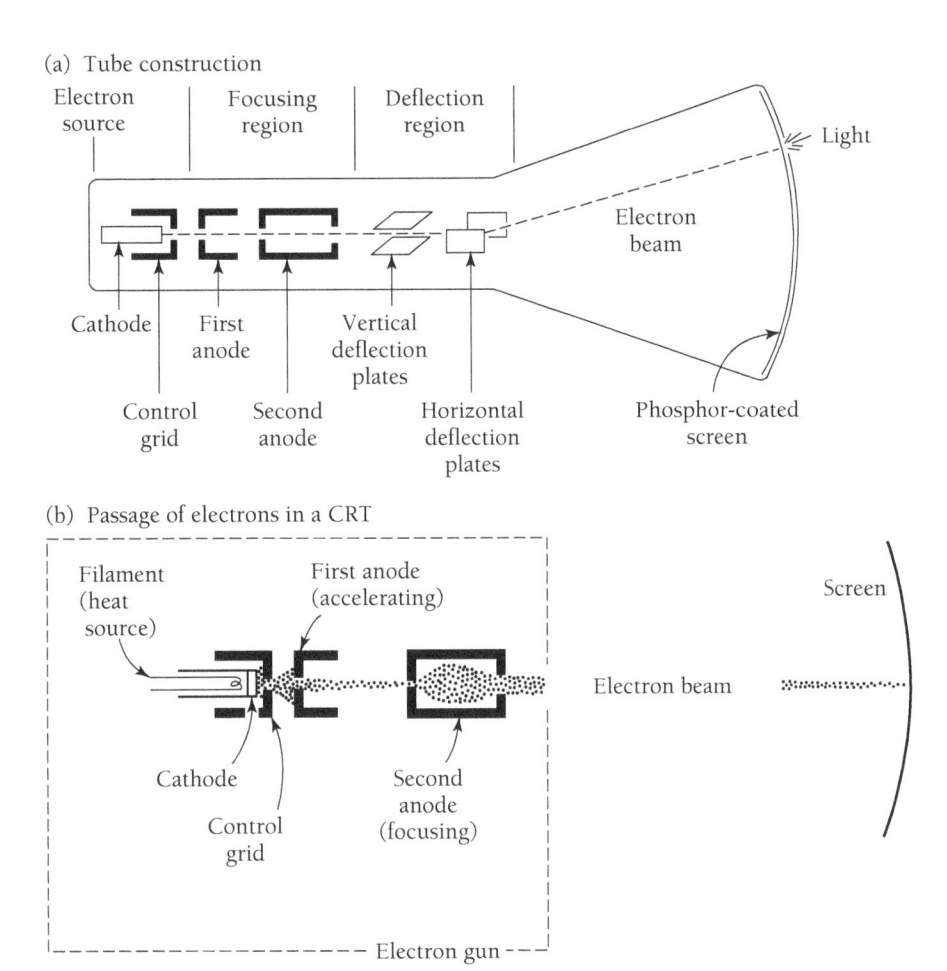

Figure B-15 Cathode ray tube. Figure B-15a shows the overall operation. The filament produces a beam of electrons; three anodes create a beam that is a small, finely focused point. The vertical and horizontal deflection plates, controlled by the Y and X signals, respectively, from the gamma camera, direct the electrons to the correct location on the screen. When the electrons hit the phosphor-coated screen, they cause the release of light that can then expose a film. Figure B-15b shows the action of each electrode on a burst of electrons at the filament. The control grid regulates the number of electrons in each dot. The accelerating anode accelerates them to high energy, and the focusing grid controls the spread of the electrons and therefore the sharpness of the dot. Reprinted from: Cherry SR, Sorenson JA, Phelps ME. *Physics in Nuclear Medicine*. 3rd ed. Philadelphia, PA: Saunders; 2006:126, 127, Figs. 8-16, 8-17. With permission from Elsevier Science.

long-term storage of nuclear medicine studies, image display is still vital. This section reviews the basic operation of several display devices.

Cathode Ray Tube

A *cathode ray tube* (CRT) aims short bursts of electrons at a phosphor-coated screen to make an image (**Figure B-15**). A filament is heated to release a batch of electrons. These electrons are given energy by an electrical potential and are formed into a pinpoint beam as they pass through a series of anodes. Vertical and horizontal deflection plates direct the electron beam to a particular location on the phosphor-coated glass screen. When they interact with the phosphor molecules, light is emitted.

Cathode ray tubes have been put to many uses over the years. Anger incorporated them into the gamma camera, a practice that continued until the 1980s. The television in its original form combined the CRT with the raster pattern of electron beam sweeps (**Figure B-16**). CRTs have been standard equipment for radiology viewing terminals for many years. Their major drawback is that they are power hogs, requiring a high-voltage power supply on the order of 1,000 V. They are therefore being displaced by liquid crystal displays and other more sophisticated and less expensive display devices.

Multiformatter

This device is commonly used to create a hard-copy image on x-ray film. The name stems from its ability to print multiple images on a single film, using a variety of image sizes and formats. Many types of multiformatters have been used in nuclear medicine. The images that are photographed in a multiformatter may be generated by a CRT or video display terminal (VDT) (described below). The image is multiplied by a gain-reduction factor corresponding to the desired image size, and a position offset puts the image in the correct location on the film. Or the image may be reduced to the desired size using one or more optical lenses, which are then offset to expose the desired portion of the film. Multiformatters are made in tower and tabletop models, indicating either straight-line or mirror optics, respectively. Laser light rather than visible light may be used to expose the film. Laser-exposed multiformatters require film that is sensitive to the laser's red light;

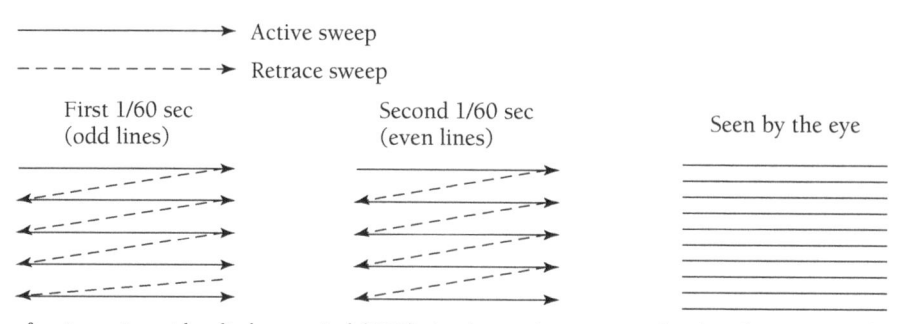

Figure B-16 Production of an image in a video display terminal (VDT). An electron beam sweeps the phosphorescent inside of the viewing screen in a raster fashion. The intensity of the light produced at each location on the screen is proportional to the intensity of the electron beam, which is in turn proportional to the brightness of the image at that location. Because the human eye responds somewhat slowly to changes in light intensity, the interlacing of odd and even lines is not noticeable to people. It will be noticeable if a standard camera with shutter speed less than $\frac{1}{30}$ sec is used to take a picture of a VDT screen.

this film cannot be exposed to the safelights used in dark rooms. While many multiformatters are designed for x-ray film, the same principles can be extended to laser printers and other hard-copy devices.

Video Display Terminal

A commonly utilized display device in modern nuclear medicine camera-computer systems is the *video display terminal* (VDT). A VDT consists of a screen in which are embedded tiny colored phosphors in groups of three (red, green, and blue) and CRTs to create three electron beams. When used in combination, they can form a wide array of colors, such that virtually any color scale can be replicated. (This is essentially the same system used by the human eye: cone cells contain pigments that are sensitive to red, green, and blue light.) When an image is sent to the VDT, each pixel is translated into appropriate intensities of red, green, and blue light to match the desired color scale. As the CRT moves from point to point, the three electron beams are modulated in intensity to create different colors according to the image data. The CRT sweeps the screen at a fixed rate according to a raster pattern (Fig. B-16), and the phosphors glow for a short time, until the next sweep of the electron beam. Additional circuits in the display interface allow the viewer to adjust the CRT contrast and brightness.

The information regarding the intensity of each picture element (or pixel) is stored in the computer as a digital value. The VDT holds this information in its own device memory and translates it into electron beam intensities as it scans. The number of bits used by a particular image format is an important factor in the final image appearance. A common configuration is to devote 24 bits to each pixel, 8 bits for each of the three colors. This allows for the creation of millions of different colors. In many VDTs, the digital signal indicating the pixel color is translated back into an analog signal, via a digital-to-analog converter, for use by the video monitor. This ensures optimal use of the VDT's capabilities, while still retaining the benefits of the digital image.

Spatial resolution of a VDT is determined by the number of phosphors struck by the electron beams per second, called *bandwidth*, and the number of scan lines displayed. For many years, most VDTs were made to match the U.S. television broadcast standard of 525 scan lines. The odd lines of data are displayed in $\frac{1}{60}$ sec, followed by an interlacing display of the even lines in the next $\frac{1}{60}$ sec. The resulting image as perceived by the human eye is complete, although a photographic picture of the screen taken with a quick shutter time shows only every other line. As radiology departments have increased their utilization of VDTs, the quality of VDTs has advanced. Current VDTs used to view x-rays have resolution of 1,600 × 1,200 resolution elements (or more) and refresh completely 75 times per second. Because they can display many more shades of gray or color than our eyes can distinguish, they do not impose any limits on the human eye, and for this reason they have become a preferred display device in most imaging applications.

Liquid Crystal Display Monitor

More recently, liquid crystal display (LCD) monitors have come to the fore. The phrase *liquid crystal* sounds like an oxymoron, but it actually describes a group of substances that exist in an intermediate state between a solid and a liquid. The particular class of liquid crystal used in electronic displays is called the twisted nematic liquid crystal. These molecules are naturally twisted, but the application of electric current causes them to untwist to varying degrees. In their twisted form, they allow polarized light to pass through. But the untwisted molecules block the polarized light, thus decreasing the intensity in that area and creating a black pixel. An LCD does not produce any light of its own; the monitor has fluorescent tubes built into it to illuminate the liquid crystals.

In an LCD monitor, each pixel has a nematic crystal and its own capacitor. A coating on the outer surface of the monitor face acts as a polarizer, allowing light from the monitor to pass through in one direction only. Pixel intensity is controlled by a grid of circuits that connect to each row and column. To turn on a particular pixel, that pixel's row is turned on and a charge is sent down the column containing the pixel. The capacitor at the location where the two cross is the only one to store the charge. The amount of charge given to the capacitor determines the degree to which the crystal untwists, thus controlling the amount of light blocked. The capacitor then keeps the pixel in that condition until the next refresh cycle.

Color LCDs work via three subpixels with red, green, and blue filters. A transistor controls each subpixel independently. In contrast to the VDT monitor, the LCD itself does not generate color. Instead, a tiny filter over the subpixel absorbs unwanted colors from white light, leaving only the color of interest to show through. The voltage at the subpixel is varied to precisely control the light intensity of each subpixel. The number of bits used by the LCD determines the total number of shades that can be created; a 24-bit color LCD system can generate 16.8 million colors.

LCD monitors are thinner and lighter than VDTs and require considerably less power than the CRTs that drive image display in VDTs. Because the capacitor holds the pixel or subpixel "on" until the next refresh cycle, flicker is much less of a problem than with VDTs. However, they have not completely supplanted CRTs as image display monitors, for several reasons. The first is the quality of the thin-film transistor matrix that can be created. As manufacturers strive for better resolution, they increase the chance of getting a bad transistor, which appears as a tiny black hole on the image. Thus the cost of high-resolution LCD monitors has been prohibitive. Also, a CRT image may be viewed from a wide range of angles, whereas an LCD monitor is best viewed from directly in front of the screen. But as LCD monitors have improved in quality and become less expensive, they are supplanting VDTs in many situations.

Hard-Copy Options

Traditionally, nuclear medicine relied on clear- or blue-based x-ray film and a standard x-ray processor to create a tangible, storable copy of its images (see Appendix C for more details). Many other options are now available. A "dry-process" system uses film that is heat sensitive rather than light sensitive. It employs a thermal print head that heats the film to produce levels of gray. The process is dry because no wet chemicals are required to develop the film. These devices are set up to accommodate several different types of film and can also print on paper, via a dye sublimation process. Dry-process systems are quite flexible and can receive input from multiple sources, but are often quite expensive.

A color printer may use a ribbon, ink, or toner coming out of a print head, or layers of ink overlay to create a colored image. In all cases, the actual colors of ink used are limited to three, as in the VDT; the printer driver (the computer program that runs the printer) translates the VDT colors into appropriate combinations of the three inks so that the image colors are reproduced exactly. A color printer may be a low-cost alternative to an expensive multiformatter or dry-processing film device; most models have comparable resolution and the ability to produce a wide range of colors.

A laser printer consists of a laser light, a cylindrical drum called a photoreceptor, and the input information from a display screen, stored digitally as a bitmap. (A bitmap gives the color and brightness of each bit [or pixel] of the image. This method of image storage can be contrasted to text formats, in which the document information is stored as letters rather than as a picture of the document.) To begin the reproduction process, the photoreceptor is given a negative electric charge. This negative charge is retained as long as the photoreceptor is in the dark, but is neutralized by light from the laser. The information about each pixel of the image to be printed is sent to the laser, which shines on the photoreceptor in relation to the bitmap's information. The laser light thus forms a latent image on the photoreceptor, consisting of negative and positive pixels on the photoreceptor's surface. The photoreceptor is then exposed to toner, which is composed of fine particles of plastic mixed with coloring agents. The toner particles are negative and hence stick only to the positive portions of the photoreceptor. Finally, paper is pressed over the photoreceptor to print the image and then heated to fuse the toner to the paper.

A color laser printer works in much the same way, but requires multiple passes with different colored toners. It is very important that the alignment of the system be perfect, lest a misregistration occur between the different passes (this effect can occasionally be seen in color photographs in a newspaper). Like a color VDT, a color printer takes advantage of the excellent color perception abilities of the human visual system.

Summary

Electronic circuits form the essential foundation for all of the equipment used in nuclear medicine. While we can operate these devices without an in-depth understanding of their inner workings, it is this author's belief that a basic level of knowledge makes for better, more careful technologists. The level presented is designed to be adequate for most nuclear medicine technologists, without delving into details that are beyond the needs of the field.

References

1. Cherry SR, Sorenson JA, Phelps ME. *Physics in Nuclear Medicine*. 3rd ed. Philadelphia, PA: Saunders; 2003:113, 125–128.
2. Knoll GF. *Radiation Detection and Measurement*. 3rd ed. New York, NY: John Wiley & Sons; 2000:287, 288.

Additional Resources

Bushberg JT, Seibert FA, Leidholdt EM, Boone JM. *The Essential Physics of Medical Imaging*. 2nd ed. Philadelphia, PA: Lippincott Williams and Wilkins; 2002: Appendix A.

Cherry SR, Sorenson JA, Phelps ME. *Physics in Nuclear Medicine*. 3rd ed. Philadelphia, PA: Saunders; 2003:Chapter 8.

Halliday D, Resnick R. *Physics: Parts I and II, Combined*. 3rd ed. New York, NY: John Wiley & Sons; 1978:Chapters 26, 27, 29–32.

Knoll GF. *Radiation Detection and Measurement*. 3rd ed. New York, NY: John Wiley & Sons; 2000:Chapters 4, 9, 16, 17.

Lee KH. *Computers in Nuclear Medicine: A Practical Approach*. 2nd ed. Reston, VA: Society of Nuclear Medicine; 2005:Chapter 4.

Patrick DR, Fardo SW. *Understanding DC Circuits*. Boston, MA: Newnes Press; 2000.

Rollo FD. *Nuclear Medicine Physics, Instrumentation, and Agents*. St. Louis, MO: Mosby-Year Book; 1977:Chapters 3, 4, 10.

Wang CH, Willis DL, Loveland WD. *Radiotracer Methodology in the Biological, Environmental, and Physical Sciences*. Englewood Cliffs, NJ: Prentice-Hall; 1975:Chapters 4, 5.

APPENDIX C: Film and Film Processing

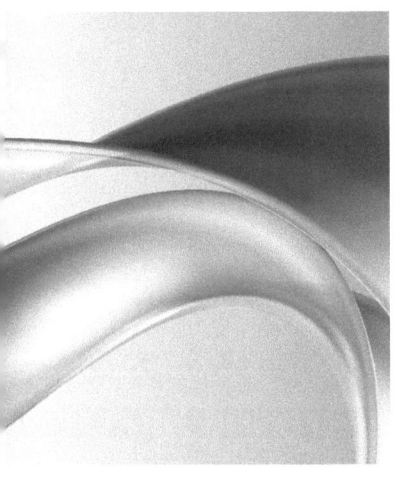

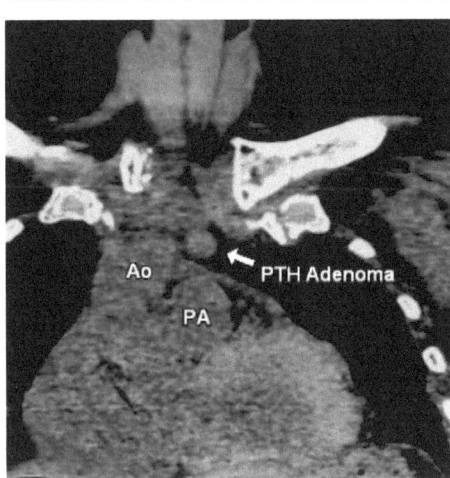

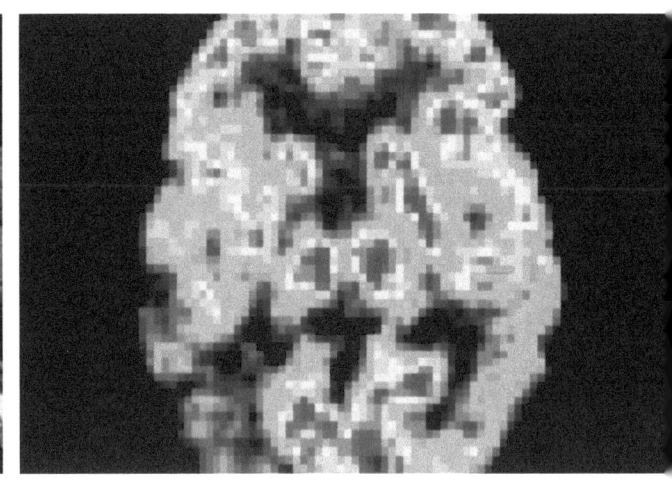

Learning Outcomes

1. Describe the composition of film and the chemistry of creating a latent image.
2. Identify the steps involved in film processing.
3. List important aspects of processor care.
4. Describe optical density, diagram a characteristic curve, and define speed and latitude.

Introduction

In contrast to radiology, where until recently an understanding of film has been essential, nuclear medicine textbooks have concentrated on the details of image formation in gamma cameras and have often ignored the physics of causing that image to appear on a sheet of film. This attitude misrepresents the importance of film; for many years, nuclear medicine images had a long-term existence only if they were on film. More recently, as nuclear medicine systems have become digital, it is more common to store images digitally and to view them on video display terminals (VDTs). Many departments are entirely filmless. Notwithstanding this advance, an understanding of the physics of creating and making visible an image on film, the developing process, and film characteristics may still be of value to nuclear medicine technologists.

Film Composition

A film sheet consists of a base of polyester or acetate, on which is laid down a thin layer (0.0005 in thick) of *photoactive emulsion*, which is a suspension of silver halide crystals in gelatin. The silver halide crystals will create the image; the gelatin keeps the silver halide crystals dispersed. The base may be clear or blue-tinted (to make viewing easier on the eyes). On the other side of the base, an *antihalation coating* absorbs any light that passes through the emulsion and the film itself. X-ray films are often of the double-emulsion type, with both sides of the base coated with emulsion, but nuclear medicine images appear sharper on single-emulsion film.

The silver halide crystals are usually silver bromide, with 1 to 10% of the bromine atoms replaced with iodine atoms. They exist as grains about 1 to 1.5 μm in diameter, each grain containing 1 million to 10 million silver atoms. The emulsion also contains a sulfur compound, such as allylthiourea, which reacts with silver atoms on the surface of the grain to form silver sulfide, called a *sensitivity speck*.

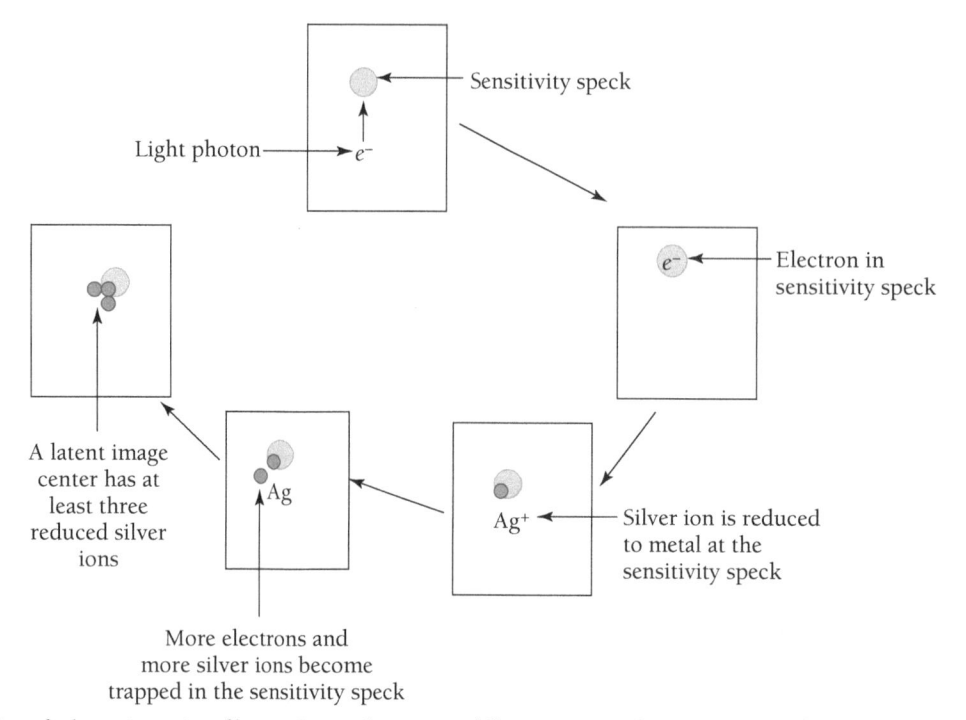

Figure C-1 Formation of a latent image in a film emulsion. The essence of film exposure is the accumulation of several silver atoms within a grain of silver halide in the emulsion. The process begins when a light photon causes an ionization of a bromine atom, and the resulting free electron is attracted to a sensitivity speck. This in turn attracts silver ions, which are reduced to metallic silver. The image is latent (not visible) until it goes through the developing process.

Film Exposure

When light photons interact with the silver bromide grains, they cause ionizations in the bromine atoms, producing free electrons that collect at iodine impurities and at sensitivity specks. Silver ions in turn attract the free electrons and combine with them to become metallic silver, which is black. The bromine atoms (now neutral in charge) leave the crystal and are taken up in the gelatin and are no longer pertinent to the exposure process. More silver ions and more electrons are attracted to the metallic silver, producing a "clump" of silver atoms called a *latent image center*. A minimum of 3 to 5 metallic silver atoms can produce a latent image center (1). Thus, after exposure to light photons, there is a *latent image* that is physicochemically present, but is not visible until the film is developed. The sequence of events occurring in the exposure process is diagrammed in **Figure C-1**.

Film Developing

Development is the chemical process by which the latent image is amplified by a factor of 10^9 or so to form a visible image. Its four steps of developing, fixing, washing, and drying usually take place in a self-contained film processor (**Figure C-2**). The processor has three baths that contain developing, fixing, and washing solutions and an air blower for drying. The developing and fixing solutions are automatically replenished from nearby tanks. A steady supply of water is required, both for washing the films and for cooling the processor.

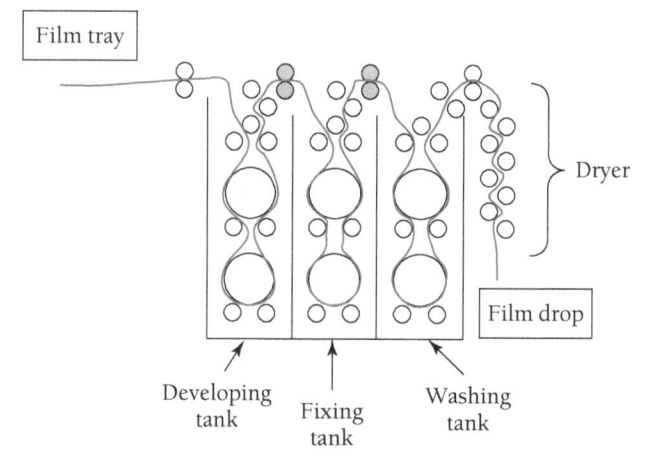

Figure C-2 Schematic of a film processor. The film tray is inside a darkroom, which has a red light (x-ray film is made to be insensitive to the wavelength of red light). The film, guided by the rollers (not all rollers are shown), transits through the developing, fixing, and washing tanks, and then it is dried by the dryer. The crossover rollers are shown in gray; they tend to accumulate chemicals from the developing and fixing tanks and need to be rinsed daily.

Processor Chemistry

The developer consists of reducing agents (commonly hydroquinone and phenidone) that reduce (give electrons to) silver ions to make them metallic silver. Development works on a grain-by-grain basis, with the latent image center catalyzing the reduction reaction. If the film is left in contact with the developer for a long period, eventually all of the crystal grains will be reduced, subsuming the image. The timing of the developing process is therefore critical—it must be long enough to maximize the development of exposed grains, but short enough to minimize the development of unexposed grains. Temperature also plays a role in minimizing the development of unexposed grains, so the developer tank should stay within a narrow range (90–95°F or 32–35°C). Even with the proper time and temperature, however, there is always some development of unexposed grains, leading to *fog* (a background tint) on the film.

The developing solution is key to the operation of a film processor, and it contains several additives to ensure that the image quality is maintained. The developing solution is kept at an alkaline pH (10–11.5), which increases the developing power of the developing chemicals and also acts as a buffer, neutralizing the hydrogen ions created in the development process. Sodium sulfite is also added as a preservative, to reduce the rate at which hydroquinone oxidizes in alkaline solution. Finally, dilute potassium bromide is added to decrease the amount of fog.

Fixing removes the undeveloped crystal grains. The fixing agent is thiosulfate, which forms water-soluble complexes with silver ions. It also contains a substance that hardens the gelatin. Washing removes the fixing-bath chemicals. Because the wash water also cools the processor, it is critical that it not be turned off. Finally, drying evaporates the wash water.

The Darkroom Environment

The radiology department darkroom is considered a scientific laboratory by the Occupational Health and Safety Administration (2). This in turn requires that darkroom operators maintain the environment properly and give consideration to their own health and safety. Attention must be paid to the darkroom temperature, humidity, and ventilation. Static electricity can cause artifacts to appear on x-ray films, so work surfaces and floors must be grounded. There are occupational exposure limits for the various processing chemicals. Activities such as eating, drinking, and smoking are prohibited.

Film Processor Quality Control

Like any other instrument, the film processor requires verification that it is working properly. This is typically split into two parts, one done by the technologist staff and the other by the company servicing the processor. Every morning, before using the processor for clinical film processing, the developer temperature should be checked and a densitometer test strip (**Figure C-3**) should be run. At the end of the day, the crossover rollers are rinsed; if possible, the processor is turned off and left open to cool. The personnel using the processor generally perform these tasks.

At least once a week, the developing tank pH and water temperature should be checked and the replenishment rates for developer and fixer adjusted. The time required

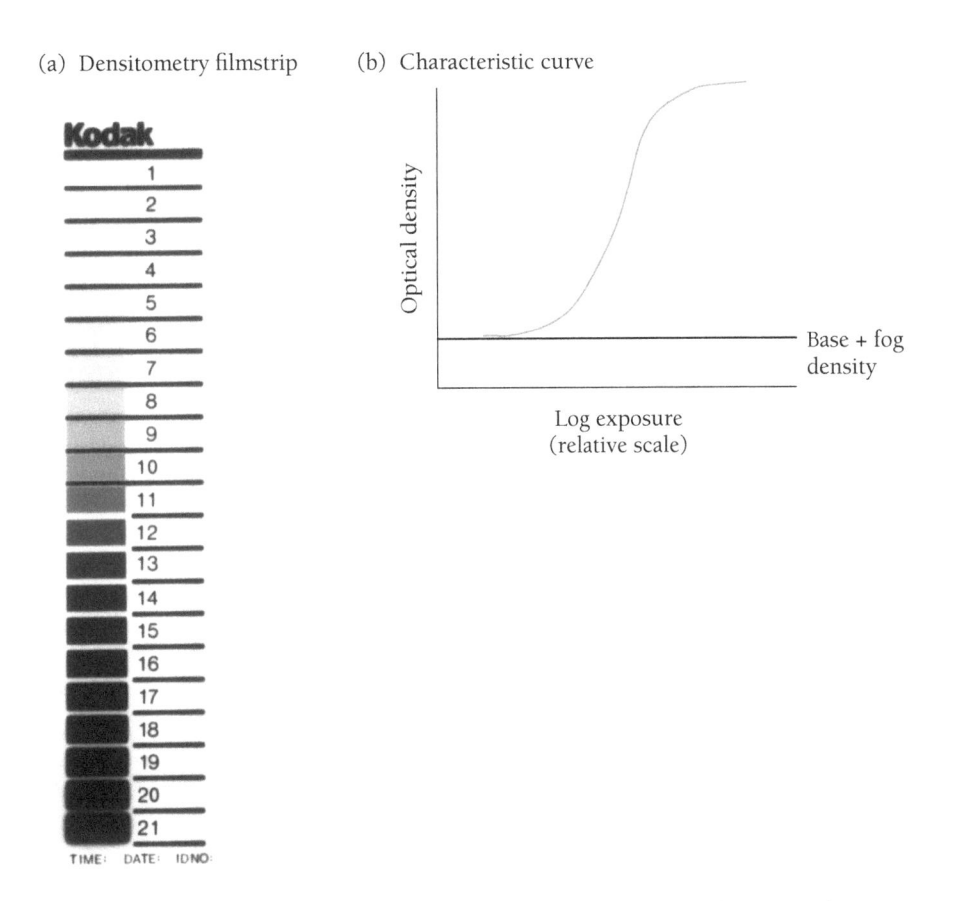

Figure C-3 Film processor quality control. Figure C-3a shows a densitometry strip; Figure C-3b illustrates a characteristic curve. Optical density (as measured from the test filmstrip) is plotted vs relative exposure (on a logarithmic scale). Image courtesy of Virginia Mason Medical Center.

for film transit should be checked. Monthly tasks include a thorough cleaning of tanks and rollers and replacement of the fixer and developer with fresh solutions. Personnel of the company servicing the processor more commonly perform the weekly and less frequent tasks.

Film Densitometry

The essence of a film processing system is to produce shades of darkness on a sheet of film. Its ability to do so is evaluated on a regular (usually daily) basis. A *sensitometer* is used to expose a filmstrip to precisely controlled steps of increasing light intensity. A *densitometer* reads the blackness of each step by measuring the amount of light that is transmitted through the film. A test filmstrip is shown in Figure C-3a.

Optical Density

The films used in nuclear medicine produce a negative image, meaning that exposure to light causes blackness on the film (the opposite of most photographic film). The degree of blackness can be quantified by its *optical density*:

$$\text{optical density} = \log\left(\frac{I_0}{I}\right) \quad \text{(C-1)}$$

where I_0 is the light intensity incident on the film and I is the light intensity transmitted through a given step on the test filmstrip. If a step is perfectly clear, the optical density is zero ($I = I_0$, so $I_0/I = 1$). An optical density of 1 corresponds to $I_0/I = 10$, or transmitted light intensity equal to 10% of incident light, corresponding to a gray film. At an optical density of 2, $I_0/I = 100$, or $I = 1\%$ of I_0, which is a dark film. The range of optical densities visible to the human eye is about 0.25 to 2.25, or approximately 2 orders of magnitude (because the formula for optical density puts it on a logarithmic [base-10] scale).

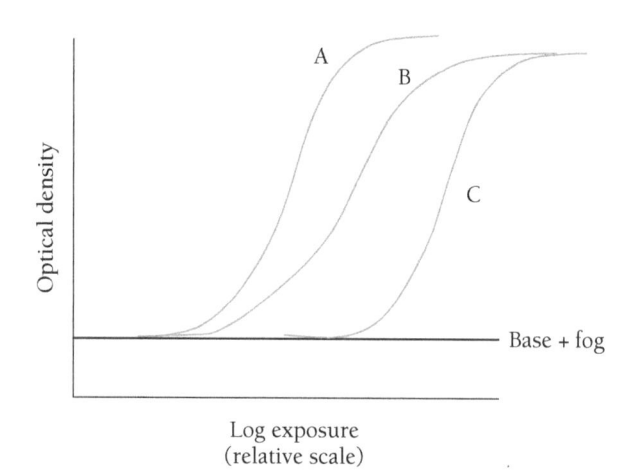

Figure C-4 Characteristic curves illustrating the concepts of speed, latitude, and contrast or gamma. Curve A has a faster speed than curve C, because it achieves a given level of optical density at a lower exposure. Curve B has a wider latitude than curves A and C, producing distinguishable optical densities over a wider range of exposures. Curves A and C have the same gamma, because the slope in the linear portion of both is the same.

Characteristic Curve

The optical density of the filmstrip is plotted vs sensitometer exposure on a curve known as a characteristic curve. It may also be called an H&D curve (after Hurter and Driffield, two amateur photographers who developed the curve [2]), or a D–log–E (density–log–exposure) curve. An example is shown in Figure C-3b. These curves can be used to track the performance of the processor and to compare different film types. Working from the

(a) Characteristic curve for a single densitometer strip

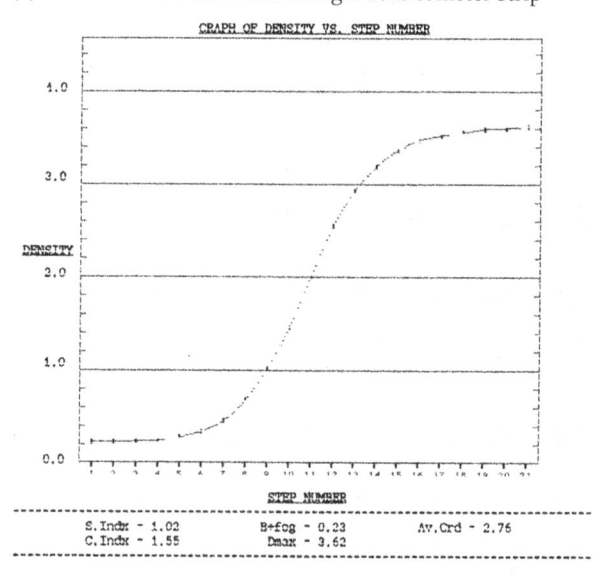

(b) Levy–Jennings plots of processor parameters

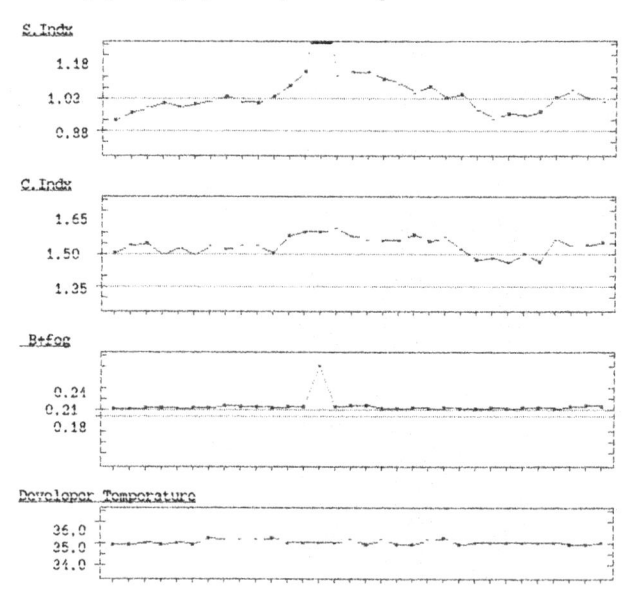

Figure C-5 Characteristic curve and Levy–Jennings plots for a particular processor. The characteristic curve is based on one day's filmstrip reading on a densitometer (Fig. C-5a). The densitometer printout lists the speed index, contrast index, base + fog, maximum density, and average gradient for this densitometry strip. In Figure C-5b, the values determined for the processor, including speed index, contrast index, base + fog, and developer temperature, are plotted to show changes over time (X-axis is days). Images courtesy of Virginia Mason Medical Center.

characteristic curve, we can define several terms that relate to film quality. The underlying cast or film darkness in unexposed areas is called *base+fog*. A film's *gamma* is defined as the maximum slope of the characteristic curve. It is a measure of contrast, which as a general term refers to the difference in optical density between two areas of the film. *Latitude* is the range of exposures that produce optical densities between 0.25 and 2.00. The *speed* of a film is defined as the exposure required to obtain an optical density of 1.0 above base+fog. When a single film processor is used, the gamma, latitude, and speed are qualities that can be used to distinguish different types of films (**Figure C-4**). Different applications require films of different film qualities; the characteristic curve provides a useful tool for comparison.

Densitometry Strip Evaluation

On a daily basis, the characteristic curve is used to test the functionality of the film processor. A sensitometer-exposed filmstrip is run through the processor after it is allowed to warm up, but before clinical films are run. Several quantities are measured, including base+fog density, the speed index (the density of a predetermined step), and the contrast index (the density difference between two predetermined steps). These are plotted over time in Levy–Jennings plots. Examples of a characteristic curve and Levy–Jennings plots for a film processor are shown in **Figure C-5**. The temperature should also be recorded daily. As mentioned previously, the developer temperature has a large effect on film quality. A film run through a processor with a too-low developer temperature will look pink-tinged, while a too-high developer temperature has a higher base+fog and a darker cast compared to films run at the correct temperature. If the developer concentration or pH is too low, the film will similarly show excessive optical density, and underreplenishment of the developing solution leads to a decrease in the optical density (2).

Summary

The creation of an image on a film is thus a matter of chemistry, and evaluation of film processor function one of some simple physics. We can put these concepts to work in analyzing problems with film quality. As with other aspects of nuclear medicine practice, attention to detail and quality control pay big dividends.

Of all the chapters in this text, this appendix is the most likely to become obsolete. But as long as film is used, even occasionally, this information needs to be available to nuclear medicine technologists. And as the overall use of film decreases, the ability to troubleshoot problems when it is used becomes even more important.

References

1. Bushberg JT, Seibert JA, Leidholdt EM, Boone JM. *The Essential Physics of Medical Imaging*. 2nd ed. Philadelphia, PA: Lippincott Williams & Wilkins; 2002: 177.
2. Papp J. *Quality Management in the Imaging Sciences*. 3rd ed. St. Louis, MO: Mosby Elsevier; 2006: 33–35, 65, 71.

Additional Resources

Bushberg JT, Seibert JA, Leidholdt EM, Boone JM. *The Essential Physics of Medical Imaging*. 2nd ed. Philadelphia, PA: Lippincott Williams & Wilkins; 2002: Chapter 7.
Kodak. *Operator's Manual, Process Control Densitometry System*, 1995.
Papp J. *Quality Management in the Imaging Sciences*. 3rd ed. St. Louis, MO: Mosby Elsevier, 2006: Chapters 3–5.

APPENDIX D: Computer Fundamentals and Systems

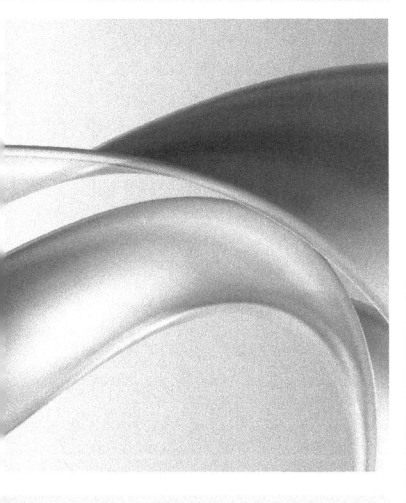

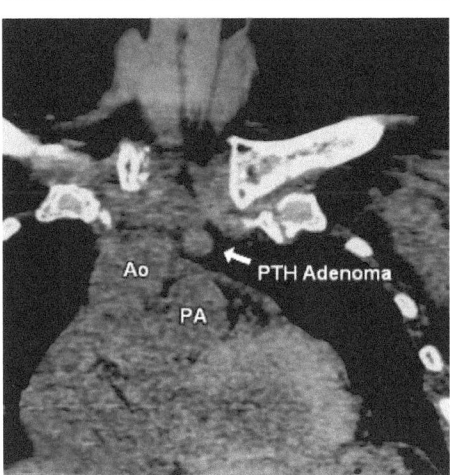

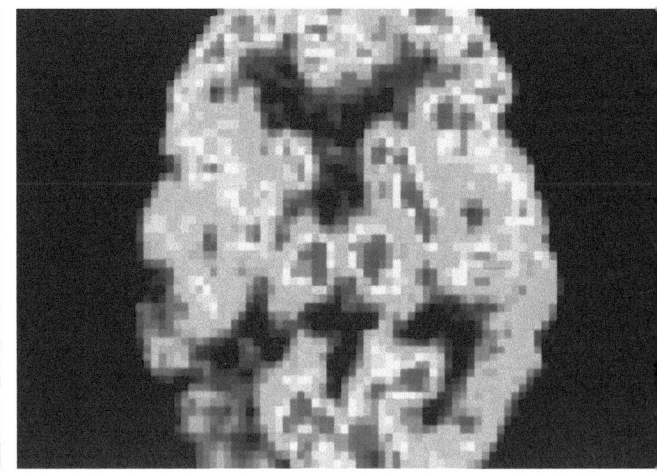

Learning Outcomes

1. Distinguish between analog and digital information, and briefly discuss analog-to-digital conversion.
2. Define and use the terms *bit*, *byte*, and *word* as they are applied to computers in general (i.e., not specific to nuclear medicine).
3. Identify the parts of a computer's central processing unit, and discuss the function of each.
4. Discuss issues related to connecting computers in a network.
5. Discuss the functions and benefits of a radiology information system (RIS) and a picture archiving and communications system (PACS).

Introduction

Computers have revolutionized nuclear medicine, as they have so many other aspects of modern life. This appendix considers the essential nature of digital information and the process of conversion of analog information to digital form. It reviews basic computer composition and operation and computer networks, so that the reader can become familiar with the computer technology associated with modern gamma cameras. Finally, it touches briefly on computer systems specific to nuclear medicine and radiology. It does not purport to be comprehensive on any of these topics; it is rather intended to provide the technologist with a working knowledge of basic concepts and terminology. Nor does it cover computer analysis of nuclear medicine images, which is a textbook topic unto itself. The reader interested in greater depth is referred to "Additional Resources" at the end of this Appendix.

Analog vs Digital

One of the major trends of the modern age is the movement from analog to digital systems in many aspects of life. The difference between the two can most easily be described by thinking of wristwatches. An analog wristwatch has an hour hand, a minute hand, and (sometimes) a second hand. Each hand has an infinite number of possible positions around the face of the watch. If we needed to, we could, with an analog wristwatch, tell time down to the microsecond or even the nanosecond. But because our scale (the watch face markings) is limited, we must infer the exact time by estimating the position of the hands.

We can make this information more accessible by *digitizing* it into discrete values. On a digital wristwatch, the number of possible values for the seconds might be 60 (i.e., 1 increment = 1 sec), or 600 (i.e., 1 increment = 0.1 sec). The digital value of the current time is displayed down to this increment. If we need greater accuracy (e.g., for race timing), we can increase the number of increments even further. Digital timepieces can report times

(a) Analog energy spectrum

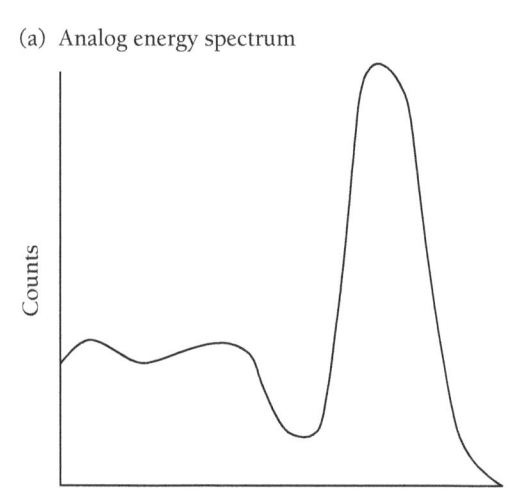

(b) Digital energy spectrum

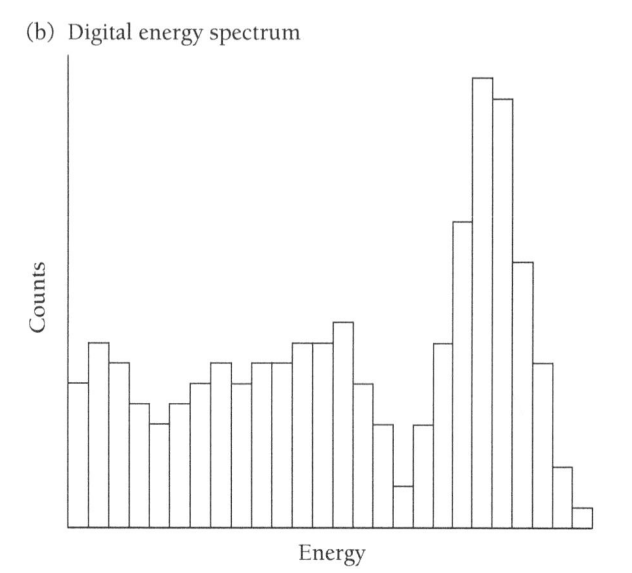

Figure D-1 Analog and digital energy spectra. The analog spectrum has an infinite number of points. The digital spectrum has a finite number of points, each of which has a discrete height. The chief advantage of the digital spectrum is that the X and Y values of each bar are easily accessed.

with high precision, without requiring any estimation on the part of the user. In addition, the digital format lends itself to additional functions, such as a timer and an alarm. Further, a digital watch is driven by reliable microprocessor technology, rather than the gear-and-spring mechanics of an analog wristwatch.

Figure D-1 illustrates another example of the distinction between analog and digital data, using an energy spectrum. The analog graph in Figure D-1a is smooth and continuous, and an infinite number of points can be identified on it; one definition of *analog* is "continuously variable." However, we cannot determine the exact X and Y values of the individual points that create the smooth line. The information contained in the analog energy spectrum is not readily available to us. The energy spectrum in Figure D-1b, on the other hand, has a limited number of data points, but because they are discrete we can easily determine and manipulate their values. For example, we can add the Y values of a series of columns to determine total counts in a particular energy window.

Thus, digitization offers the benefits of defined data, more applications, and the use of microprocessor technology. Digital data are easily stored and transmitted, and algorithms using digital data are reproducible. It is for the most part immune to signal distortion and the resultant errors that can occur when analog data are transmitted electronically. These benefits have proved extremely useful to modern society, and they similarly have been applied with great success to nuclear medicine in the form of digital images and computers.

Computer Fundamentals

A *computer* is a "programmable electronic machine that performs high-speed operations and assembles, stores, correlates, or otherwise processes information" (*American Heritage High School Dictionary*, 3rd ed., 1993). We can think of it as a symbol-manipulating and information-processing machine. How does it accomplish this electronically? The essential element of any computer is an electrical device called a *transistor* (described in Appendix B), which acts as a switch in that it can have two possible states: ON or OFF. A computer consists of many, many transistors and connecting circuits, and functions using *Boolean algebra* and a base-2 numbering system called *binary*.

Boolean Algebra

This field of mathematics was developed in the 1850s by George Boole as an exploration of logical thought processes. It became highly useful in the twentieth century, because it has direct applicability to the transistors and switching circuits that perform the essential functions of a computer. Boolean algebra employs the numbers 0 and 1, and translates them as "false" and "true" or "absent" and "present," respectively. It uses 3 operators, usually described as AND, OR, and NOT. The operators perform operations on 1 or 2 input signals. The AND operator requires two inputs, and produces a "true" output only if both input signals are present. The OR operator produces a "true" output if either input signal is present. The NOT operator negates a single input signal, that is, it turns a "true" (present) input signal into a "false" (absent), and vice versa. Another way of describing this is that it exchanges a "1" input for a "0" output or a "0" input for a "1" output. These possibilities are shown in the form of truth tables and Venn diagrams (**Figure D-2**).

As precursors to modern computers were developed, the principles of Boolean algebra were directly applicable to the aggregation of switching circuits that those precursors contained. The development of the transistor, with its binary nature, further strengthened this connection. Today's computers consist of millions of transistors and logic gates. A logic gate is an electric switch that performs a logical operation on one or more input signals and produces a single output signal. Through the use of logic gates in large numbers and various combinations,

(a) Truth tables

Input #1	Input #2	AND output	OR output
0	0	0	0
1	0	0	1
0	1	0	1
1	1	1	1

Input #1	NOT output
1	0
0	1

(b) Venn diagrams

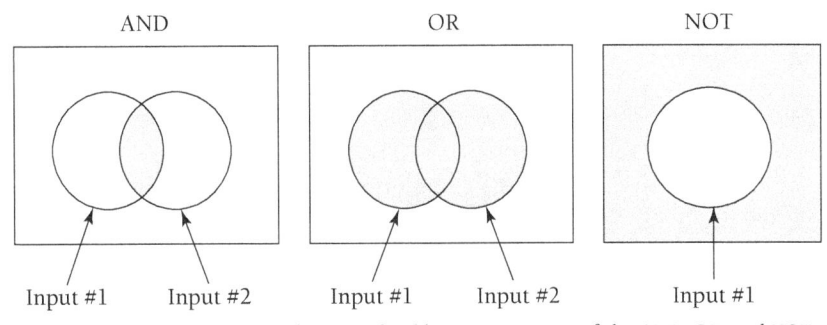

Figure D-2 Operations in Boolean algebra. Figure D-2a shows truth table representations of the AND, OR, and NOT operators. A "1" in the tables represents a signal that is present, and "0" a signal that is not present. These operators can be represented pictorially in Venn diagrams (Fig. D-2b). In each diagram, the shaded area represents the combination of signal inputs that produce a "1" or "true" output. The NOT Venn diagram shows that the output signal is the opposite of the input signal.

a computer can perform a multitude of mathematical manipulations and decision-making functions.

Binary Numbers

The *binary number system* (**Figure D-3**) is a system of counting that utilizes only the values 0 and 1. We can understand binary by comparing it to a base-10 system, such as our familiar numbering system. We count up to 9 in the rightmost column, and when we get to 10, we add 1 to the next column to the left and return the right column to 0. When that second column has accumulated 10, we add 1 to the third column and return the second column to 0. Binary works the same way, but with only two possibilities, not 10. Mathematically, the base-10 number 120 can be written as $(1 \times 10^2) + (2 \times 10^1) + (0 \times 10^0)$. Similarly in base 2, the number 101 is $(1 \times 2^2) + (0 \times 2^1) + (1 \times 2^0)$. Just as the positions of the numbers in a decimal representation are important (for example, 120 is different from 210), so the positions in a binary number are important (101 is different from 110). A computer does its arithmetic and logic calculations in binary and then converts the results to base-10 form so that we can understand them.

Bits, Bytes, and Words

The Information Age has evolved an entire terminology to describe units of digital information. These are used frequently and should be a part of the vocabulary of a nuclear medicine technologist. A *bit* (*binary digit*) is a single position of a binary number representation or a digital array. A bit can be ON or OFF; it can have values of 1 or 0. It is the fundamental information unit of the computer. A *byte* is a unit of 8 bits. A byte can represent a large number of binary codes, up to 256 possibilities, as shown in Figure D-3.

Note that the number of available bits in a digital array limits the range of possibilities that the array can represent. An array with n bits can represent up to 2^n different numbers, or letters, or colors, or whatever the array is being used for. (One often sees this written as $2^n - 1$, counting only nonzero possibilities, but in the world of computers, zero is a significant number.) Consider the example of a computer displaying nuclear medicine images. The computer uses a single digital array to define a lookup table (LUT) consisting of shades of gray, ranging from zero (white) to its highest value (black); this LUT is then used to correlate image density to counts per pixel. If the LUT array has 3 bits, the maximum number of

Computer Fundamentals 331

Decimal Value:	Binary Representation:	bit 7	bit 6	bit 5	bit 4	bit 3	bit 2	bit 1	bit 0
0		0	0	0	0	0	0	0	0
1		0	0	0	0	0	0	0	1
2		0	0	0	0	0	0	1	0
3		0	0	0	0	0	0	1	1
4		0	0	0	0	0	1	0	0
5		0	0	0	0	0	1	0	1
6		0	0	0	0	0	1	1	0
7		0	0	0	0	0	1	1	1
8		0	0	0	0	1	0	0	0
9		0	0	0	0	1	0	0	1
//									
16		0	0	0	1	0	0	0	0
32		0	0	1	0	0	0	0	0
64		0	1	0	0	0	0	0	0
128		1	0	0	0	0	0	0	0
255		1	1	1	1	1	1	1	1

(Bits of an array representing numbers)

Figure D-3 The binary numbering system. Each bit is encoded by a single transistor, which can be either ON or OFF. The 8-bit (or 1-byte) array shown here can represent any integer value between 0 and 255.

shades of gray the computer can display is 2^3, or 8. If the array is allotted 6 bits, the maximum number of shades of gray increases to 64 (2^6). If 8 bits are used, the available shades of gray increase to 256 (2^8).

The small size of the bit requires the use of large multiples, utilizing the prefixes of the metric system, but with a slight twist. The prefix *kilo-*, which means "× 1,000" in most scientific notations, means "× 2^{10}" in computerese. Fortunately, 2^{10} = 1,024, which is only slightly larger than 1,000. Similarly, the prefix *mega-* is 2^{20} and *giga-* is 2^{30}, which are, respectively, a little bigger than 1 million and 1 billion (the meaning of these prefixes in the metric system). The rough equivalency between the scientific and digital meanings allows the prefixes to be understood in much the same way.

A *word* is a group of bits that a computer can process at one time. This must be matched to the design of the computer, specifically to the size of the arithmetic-logic unit (see "Central Processing Unit"). The more bytes included in a word, the more information can be processed in each operation. Thus we can speak of computers that work 2 bytes at a time (16-bit computers), 4 bytes at a time (32-bit computers), or 8 bytes at a time (64-bit computers). Longer word length allows for greater precision, increased speed, and better memory management. The variability from one generation of computers to the next has created some confusion, however, leading to a redefinition of the term *word* to mean 16 bits. In nuclear medicine, the terms *byte mode* and *word mode* have specific meanings related to acquisition of data into an image matrix.

Analog-to-Digital Conversion

An analog signal has an infinite number of positions to the right of the decimal point. Of that infinitely long number, only the first few numbers after the decimal are meaningful; the rest do not change the signal's overall meaning. In daily life, we round numbers to the desired number of decimal places, according to rules we learned in elementary school. Within the confines of an electrical machine, an *analog-to-digital converter* (ADC) performs a similar process. There are several types of ADCs in common use; three are described here.

- A *ramp* ADC uses the incoming voltage signal to charge a capacitor. The capacitor discharges, and the time required for this discharge is measured by a clock. Larger pulses take longer to discharge. The digital value of the signal is the number of clock ticks required for the signal to reach baseline (**Figure D-4**).
- The *successive-approximation* ADC compares the voltage size of the signal to sizes that it guesses

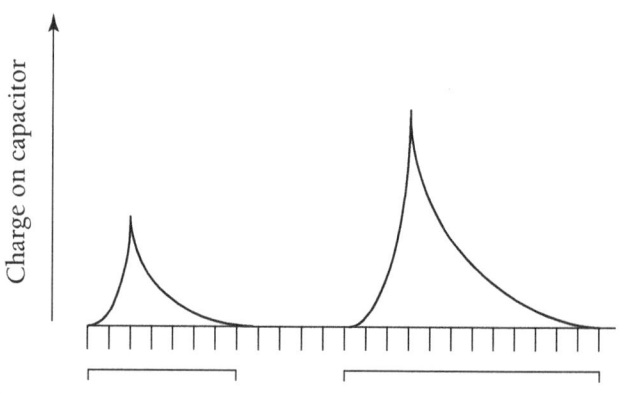

Figure D-4 Ramp ADC. The input signal is used to charge a capacitor; the vertical direction represents the capacitor charge. The time required for the capacitor to discharge determines the digital value of the signal.

(a) ADC array

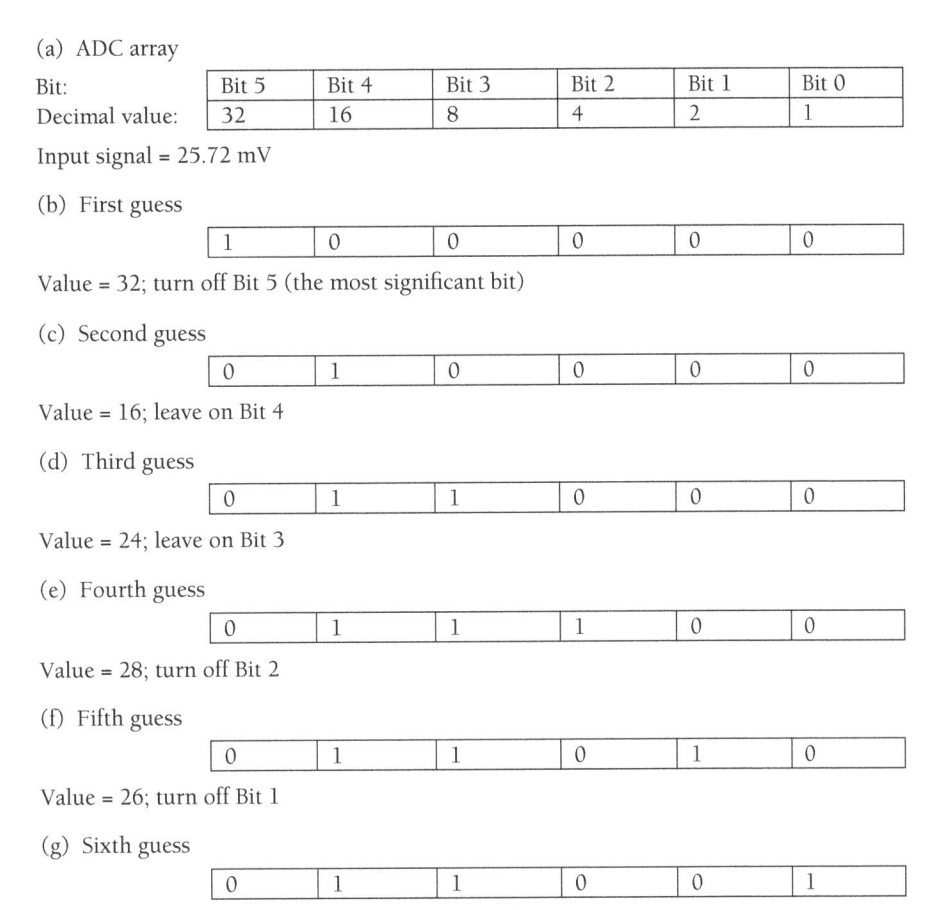

Bit:	Bit 5	Bit 4	Bit 3	Bit 2	Bit 1	Bit 0
Decimal value:	32	16	8	4	2	1

Input signal = 25.72 mV

(b) First guess

1	0	0	0	0	0

Value = 32; turn off Bit 5 (the most significant bit)

(c) Second guess

0	1	0	0	0	0

Value = 16; leave on Bit 4

(d) Third guess

0	1	1	0	0	0

Value = 24; leave on Bit 3

(e) Fourth guess

0	1	1	1	0	0

Value = 28; turn off Bit 2

(f) Fifth guess

0	1	1	0	1	0

Value = 26; turn off Bit 1

(g) Sixth guess

0	1	1	0	0	1

Value = 25; leave on Bit 0 (the least significant bit)

Figure D-5 Successive-approximation ADC. A 6-bit ADC is shown for illustration purposes. The process starts with the leftmost bit, called the most significant bit. Each bit is turned on in succession, and the resulting ADC value is compared to the input signal. If the ADC value is larger than the input signal, the bit is turned off; if it is smaller, the bit is left on. Adapted from: Lee, KH. *Computers in Nuclear Medicine: A Practical Approach.* 2nd ed. Reston, VA: Society of Nuclear Medicine; 2005: Appendix B. With permission of the Society of Nuclear Medicine.

(**Figure D-5**). Each bit in turn, starting with the leftmost (most significant) bit, is turned on. The ADC total is then compared to the analog voltage signal, and the bit is turned off if the ADC total is too high or is kept on if it is too low. This process continues through the remaining bits of the ADC, until the final ADC total approximates the analog voltage signal.

- The *flash ADC* contains a number of comparators, each with a discrete threshold. The analog signal is simultaneously compared to each one, and all comparators with thresholds below the signal turn their values to "true." A digital encoder then translates this to a digital number. This kind of ADC is very fast and quite inexpensive.

Recent-generation computers utilize flash ADCs for most purposes.

Most ADCs work by sampling the analog signal and creating a digital signal based on its samples. The rate at which the ADC samples thus determines the quality of the digital signal (**Figure D-6**). A faster sampling rate produces a more exact reproduction of the analog signal but requires faster electronics and more storage space, while a slower sampling rate causes a loss of information in the analog-to-digital conversion process. Most radiologic applications require a high sampling rate.

ADCs are the key to the digital world and are generally trouble-free, but we must remember two important things about them. First, the accuracy of the converted number depends on the number of bits in the ADC, which determines the maximum number of positions that can be demarcated. Second, the analog-to-digital conversion process takes time, and the greater the ADC size, the more time it takes. Analog-to-digital conversion should never be a limiting factor in terms of system performance, in respect to either time or accuracy.

Computer Architecture

Although computers have a wide variety of physical appearances, for the most part they rely on the same underlying hardware components. (The term *hardware* is used to refer to the tangible components of the computer, while *software* refers to the programs that direct the actions of the hardware.) **Figure D-7a** shows a generic block diagram illustrating the connections among these units. The "heart" of the computer is its *central processing unit*, or CPU, which performs all operations and directs the other functional units. It may also be referred to as the

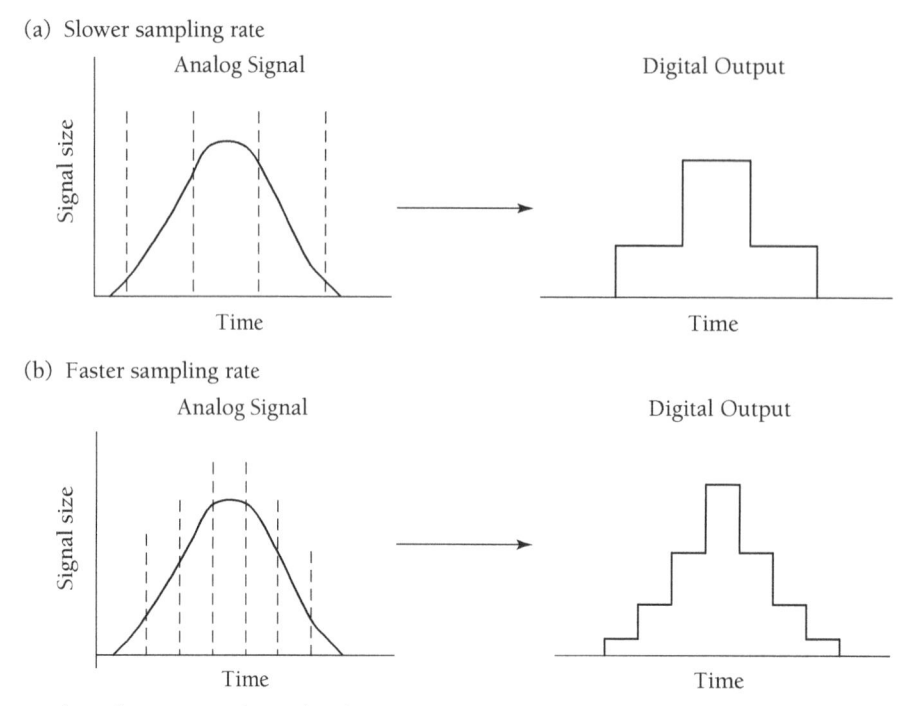

Figure D-6 The importance of sampling rate in analog-to-digital conversion. When a changing signal (shown here on a time axis) is to be converted from analog to digital, the ADC must sample the signal and convert the sampled values to digital ones. The dashed lines represent two different sampling rates. The faster sampling rate more accurately reproduces the analog signal than the slower sampling rate.

microprocessor. Software programs and data in current or recent use are stored in the memory unit. Bulk storage provides long-term storage of images, data, and other information. Input devices include the keyboard and mouse as well as gamma camera signals; output devices may include video display terminals (VDTs), printers, and multiformatters.

The CPU communicates with the other devices through either a serial or a parallel connection. A *serial* connection sends each bit of information in succession, while a *parallel* connection has multiple connecting wires, so that many bits are sent as a group. The *bus* is a high-capacity connecting cable that allows the functional units to communicate and share data with one another; its bandwidth determines the speed at which data are transferred between units. The bus interface unit, a part of the CPU, controls data transfers on the bus. The bus uses a *communications protocol* that allows information from one device to be properly interpreted by another device. The computer can thus be created using components from different manufacturers, rather than requiring the purchase of a complete system. The modular approach also simplifies hardware upgrades and repairs.

Central Processing Unit

A schematic diagram of the internal components of a CPU is shown in Figure D-7b. Its major functional subunits are the *control unit* and the *arithmetic-logic unit* (ALU). As the name implies, the control unit directs the actions of the computer, based on the instructions it receives from the software. The ALU performs mathematical and logical operations on specific data as directed by the control unit.

The registers hold the data being worked on, and the decode unit translates software instructions into language that the ALU understands. A CPU can perform only one instruction per clock cycle, so the CPU's internal clock rate is an important parameter of computer functionality. Speed in turn is dependent on the time required for a pulse to travel the longest path within the CPU. Speed is usually quoted in units of gigahertz (GHz; 1 GHz = 1 billion instructions per second). The increase in speed has been a major aspect of computer evolution, for both nuclear medicine systems and those sold for home and office use.

But computers can perform even faster by breaking up tasks into smaller chunks and putting multiple microprocessors to work on them. This can be accomplished by including more than one ALU in the CPU, by incorporating multiple CPUs into one computer, or by utilizing multiple computers. These options all fall into the category of *parallel processing*. Whichever scheme is utilized, parallel processing requires additional engineering and programming, with the ultimate reward of a faster computer. The ability to perform parallel processing was important in the implementation of iterative reconstruction techniques.

Software

The instructions that direct basic computer operation, and the basis for interaction with the user, are found in the computer's *operating system*, or OS. The OS receives instructions, interprets them, and invokes software and hardware to act on them. The OS includes the boot program that starts the computer, the instructions for communication with input and output devices, file

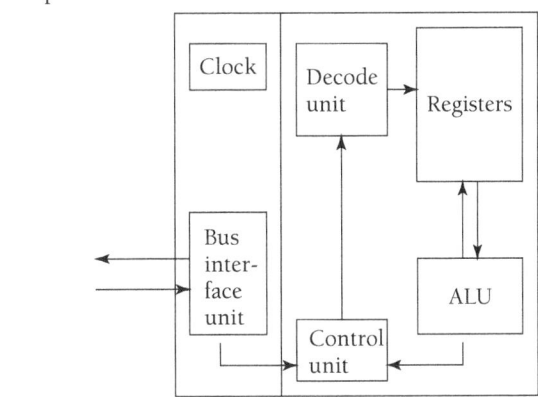

Figure D-7 Generalized schematic of computer architecture. John von Neumann, considered by many to be the father of modern computers, originally proposed this architecture. Within the CPU (Fig. D-7b), the arithmetic-logic unit (ALU) performs the actual operations, the control unit directs those operations, the decode unit translates the instructions, and the bus interface unit communicates with other devices. The registers hold data for use by the ALU. The clock unit controls the rate of interactions within the CPU.

management and utility programs, and the *graphical-user interface* (GUI). The GUI allows the user to direct the computer via "point and click" operations on the computer screen. Application software includes programs for nuclear medicine image acquisition, display, and analysis, as well as programs that perform word processing, number manipulation, and so on. These programs are written in higher-level computer languages, such as Fortran, BASIC, C++, and Java. The OS translates these higher-level languages into machine language or assembly language, which is directly understandable by the CPU. The particular language used by a specific CPU is called the *instructional set architecture*, and it defines how the software and hardware interact.

A peripheral device such as a printer or VDT requires a *driver*, which is a program that allows the operating system to communicate with the device. Many peripheral devices have their own memory, allowing the CPU to send data to a slow peripheral device and then move on to other tasks. Good design of the interfaces between computer components, with special attention to the bus and the memory architecture, increases both the flexibility and the speed of the computer.

Memory

Information storage is another aspect of computers that has improved significantly, much to the benefit of nuclear medicine. Computers need to store information for both the short term and the long term; the parts of the computer that do the former are called *memory*, while those that maintain data for long periods are referred to as *mass storage devices*. Short-term memory generally consists of solid-state devices, which use transistors to encode bit values. They are *volatile*, in that the data are lost when the power is turned off. Memory can be described operationally with such terms as *RAM* (random access memory), *ROM* (read-only memory), and *PROM* (programmable read-only memory). Long-term mass storage devices such as disks and tapes may employ either magnetic or optical methods for recording data; these are nonvolatile. A special memory bank called *cache memory* stores data and programs that have recently been used, for rapid access by the CPU. Buffers provide a memory space to temporarily store data in current use by various devices.

Computer Networks

One way to increase the efficiency of computers is by linking them together in a *network*. For example, individual nuclear medicine computers may be specialized for acquisition, processing, or display, but all are connected to allow their images and data to be shared among the various computers. The terminology used for networked systems is common enough that nuclear medicine personnel need to be conversant in it.

Networked computers can be connected by cables in a *local-area network* (LAN). Several common kinds of cables exist. The use of cable connections limits the physical size

(a) Token-ring network

Nodes (computer workstations)

Token for signaling data transfer

Ring for data transfer

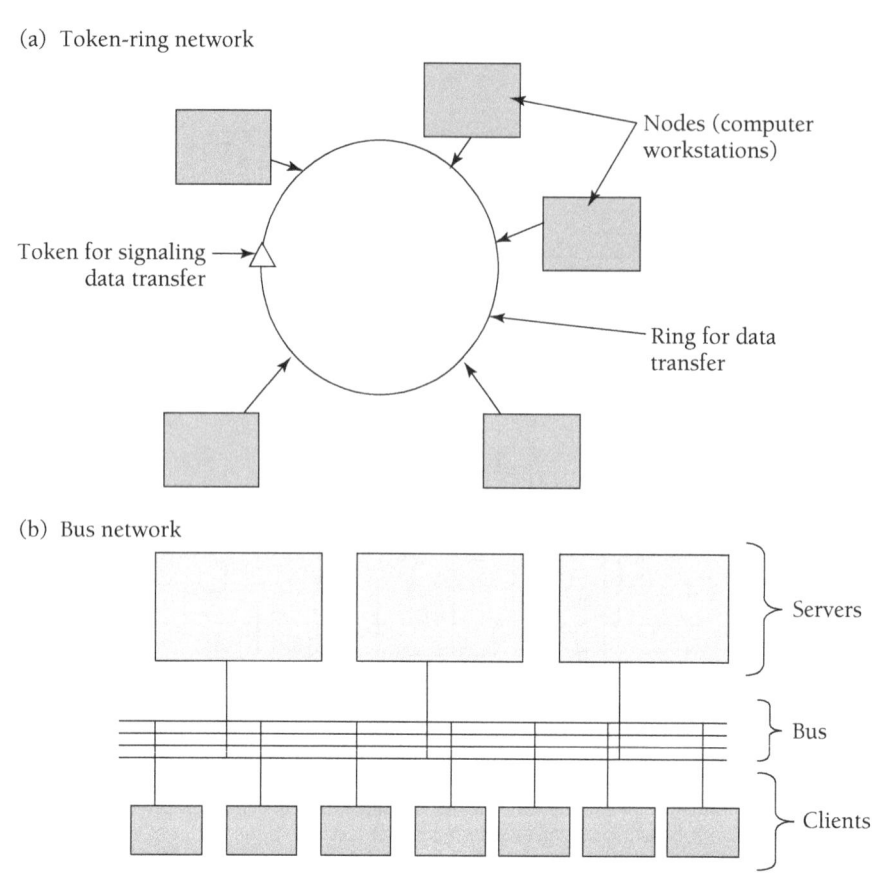

(b) Bus network

Servers

Bus

Clients

Figure D-8 Two common types of computer networks. The name *token-ring network* refers to the use of a token ring that continuously circles the ring. When a computer wishes to send information to another computer, it grabs the token ring as it goes by and attaches to it the information to be sent. The token-ring network is generally slower in data transfer than the bus network, which also has greater flexibility in terms of its ability to add both servers and clients.

of the network, usually to a single building or complex of closely spaced buildings (hence the "local-area" designation). If computers in widely separated buildings are to be networked, a *wide-area network* (WAN) is used instead. In a WAN, computers communicate via telephone lines or other types of connections.

Within a LAN or WAN, computers may have equal control and computing power (a *peer-to-peer network*) or may be divided into specialized types. Computers called *servers* provide services to computers called *clients*; this arrangement, called a *client–server network*, is the most common one in use today. A network may have multiple servers, each specialized to a particular aspect of network function. Client computers (or *workstations*) may then have reduced functionality themselves, because they can rely on the servers for specialized programs. Client–server networks require an investment in hardware and technical expertise, but are able to support a large number of users in an efficient fashion.

Another aspect of a LAN is its architecture, that is, how the computers are physically connected, which in turn determines the efficiency of data transfer. Network topologies include the star network, the ring network, and the bus network. The latter two are diagrammed in **Figure D-8**. Each has advantages and drawbacks; the bus network seems to offer the greatest flexibility for adding workstations and is often used for complex situations. Whichever network topology is used, there must also be a communications protocol that governs data transmission across the network. The communications protocol specifies network addresses, how data are packaged, and what to do in the case of a collision of two data packets.

As networks are developed, it often becomes advantageous to network the networks together. For example, in a hospital, the *radiology information system* (RIS), which holds information about radiology exams, may be networked to the *hospital information system* (HIS), which contains information about patients, doctors, insurance coverage, and so on. The RIS (see the following section) may also be networked to the nuclear medicine computer network and the hot lab computer, allowing patient data to be entered automatically rather than by hand. Networking of networks has great benefits in terms of information sharing, but also requires careful attention so that a problem in one system does not cause problems in other networks.

The biggest network of all is the Internet. It is essentially a peer-to-peer network of networks, in that no one entity controls or has priority over it. The Internet can be accessed by any computer, for both finding and sharing information. The Internet has indeed been revolutionary, in that it has made information widely available at very low cost. In terms of nuclear medicine usage, it allows for the sharing of images on a much wider scale than is possible for LANs and WANs. Important considerations for sending images on the Internet include security, reliability, and confidentiality of patient data. A suite of communications protocols controls the movement of information across the Internet.

Radiology-Specific Computer Systems

Just as computers were applied to nuclear medicine imaging starting soon after their development, so they have also been widely utilized in the larger radiology department. Many imaging systems, such as CT and MRI, use computers for acquisition and/or reconstruction. Other computer systems maintain ancillary functions such as radiopharmaceutical dose administration records. The next two sections address two department-wide computer systems, one for tracking patients and studies and the other for managing images from a variety of modalities.

Radiology Information Systems

One obvious use of a computer is for scheduling and tracking the completion of imaging procedures. This is carried out by a radiology information system. The main functions of a RIS include:

- Registration and patient information
- Scheduling of examinations
- Workflow and resource management
- Patient and study tracking
- Reporting
- Billing

Most of these systems consist of large linked databases, using an *accession number* as the primary linking field. Each patient interaction with the radiology department is given a unique accession number. In a multistep procedure, such as a bone scan, each part (e.g., injection and imaging) has its own accession number. This system also allows a single patient to have multiple exams of the same type over time, because each visit is individually identifiable.

Hospitals and outpatient clinics have similar systems (hospital information systems) for tracking their patient visits, hospital admissions, procedures performed, test results, and so on. A fairly recent development is to incorporate the RIS into the HIS. This has the advantage of putting all aspects of hospital/clinic operation into a single computer entity. Disadvantages include an increased need for training and (potentially) less flexibility for radiology-specific functions. Whichever system houses radiology department operations, technologists should expect to use these systems and their successors for their entire working lives.

Picture Archiving and Communications Systems

Most radiology departments have moved toward a completely digital environment in regard to images. The computer system is called a *picture archiving and communications system*, or PACS. When fully implemented, a single display station connected to a PACS is able to display images from all imaging modalities. Images are stored digitally rather than on film, and they can be transmitted rapidly to any display station. Rather than a film library and film librarians, the radiology department employs large-capacity computer storage devices and computer specialists to maintain its PACS and its library of past patient studies. Considerable benefits in terms of accessibility, productivity, and economics are gained by the conversion to a PACS.

For a PACS to work, all of the image data must share a common format. The format that has become the standard is called *DICOM*, for Digital Imaging and Communications in Medicine. The DICOM format specifies how image data and nonimage information (patient name, acquisition date, acquisition time, etc.) are to be recognized in various computer systems. Nuclear medicine has been the last of the radiologic modalities to settle on a DICOM format, because nuclear medicine has some unique needs, including the storage of raw data, regions of interest, and time–activity curves. All imaging system manufacturers produce "DICOM-compatible" images, although the phrase may not mean the same thing in all cases.

The issue of storage space is an important one in PACS. Even in digital form, a nuclear medicine image requires a finite amount of space on a hard disk. A complex study, such as a gated myocardial perfusion image set, may require several megabytes of memory. Radiology images, with their greater level of detail, require even more space. Considerable effort has been devoted to finding ways to compress images so that they take up less space. Nuclear medicine images are generally compressed in a *lossless* manner, meaning that none of the image detail is lost. Some compression techniques are *lossy*, because the image is corrupted to some extent in the compression process. If lossy compression algorithms are employed, the user needs to verify that image quality is maintained.

Keep in mind that a PACS is not a replacement for the nuclear medicine computer network. While it might be possible to put nuclear-medicine-specific programs into the PACS, that may not be a wise idea. A better choice may be to maintain the nuclear medicine network for image acquisition and processing and to transfer "finished" images (e.g., screen-capture displays) and data to the PACS. This prevents individuals who don't know the ins and outs of nuclear medicine from obtaining incorrect results due to incorrect processing techniques.

The implementation of a PACS requires considerable expense. Image workstations require high-quality VDTs or liquid crystal display (LCD) monitors, storage systems need both large capacity and high-speed access, and a network must be constructed to allow for rapid communication and data transfer. Staff members, from technologists to radiologists to clinical physicians, must be instructed in the system's capabilities and functions.

Ultimately, a radiology PACS may be tied into a complete electronic system for hospital records. Imagine a clinician at a workstation on a medical ward, able to view his or her patient's lung scan and chest x-ray, check the pharmacy record for incompatibilities between the patient's current medications and heparin, compare today's electrocardiogram with yesterday's, and retrieve an office note from the patient's last visit, all without leaving his or her seat. While this scenario is still some time from being a reality in most hospitals, it may soon become commonplace, thanks to computers.

Summary

Computers are so commonplace these days that their operation is for the most part taken for granted. But an understanding of how they work, from analog-to-digital conversion to performance of basic operations, to network and PACS architecture, allows the technologist to utilize them more efficiently. Moreover, the ever-advancing nature of computer development will continue to affect medical computer systems, including those found in nuclear medicine departments. So it is well worth the effort to have a greater understanding of computers, rather than to treat them as "black boxes" and interact with them on only a superficial basis.

As computer technology continues to advance, so the complexities of the nuclear medicine computer system and its connections to other computer networks will continue to change. The significant progress made in the last 20 years is astounding, but the pace of developments relating to computers will remain steady or even increase. It is therefore important that the nuclear medicine technologist understand the underlying basics of computer technology, in order to make intelligent choices in the future.

Additional Resources

Bushberg JT, Seibert JA, Leidholdt EM, Boone JM. *The Essential Physics of Medical Imaging*. 2nd ed. Philadelphia, PA: Lippincott Williams and Wilkins; 2002: Chapters 4, 17.

Henkin RE, Boles MA, Dillehay GL, et al., eds. *Nuclear Medicine*. St. Louis, MO: Mosby-Year Book; 1996: Chapters 14, 15.

Kuni CC. *Introduction to Computers and Digital Processing in Medical Imaging*. Chicago, IL: Year Book Medical Publishers; 1988: Chapters 1, 2.

Lee KH. *Computers in Nuclear Medicine: A Practical Approach*. 2nd ed. Reston, VA: Society of Nuclear Medicine; 2005: Chapters 1–6, Appendices. A, B, and p. 2.

APPENDIX E Collimator Mathematics

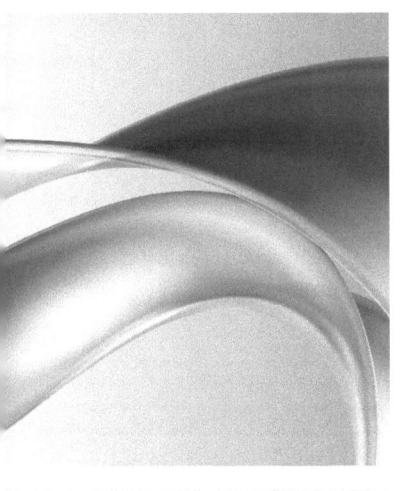

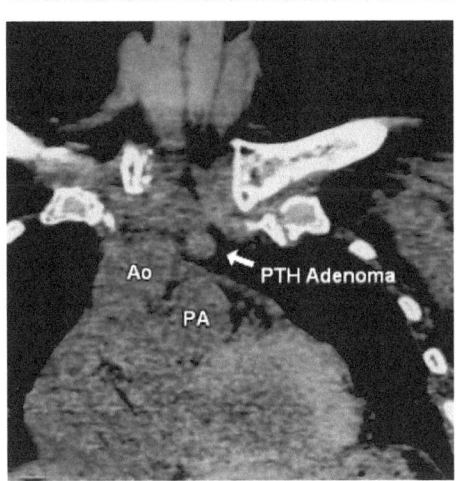

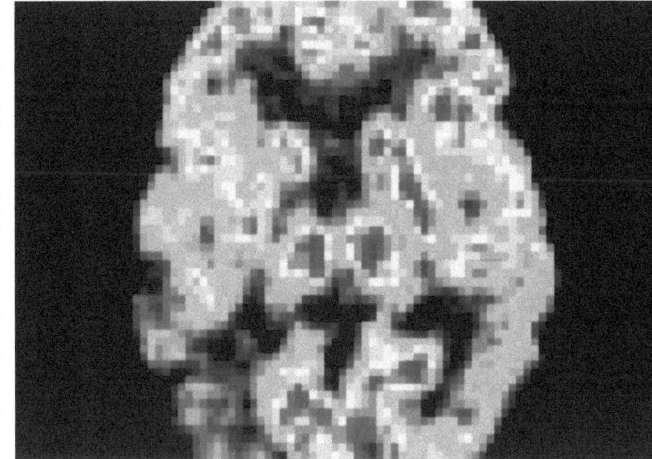

Learning Outcomes

1. Given the desired field of view (FOV) size, calculate the distance from the scintillation crystal for an organ-probe measurement.
2. For a parallel-hole collimator, given the hole length, hole diameter, and object–collimator distance, calculate the effective length and collimator resolution.
3. Given the intrinsic resolution and collimator resolution, calculate the system resolution for a parallel-hole collimator.
4. Explain why the sensitivity does not change with object–collimator distance for a multihole collimator.
5. Given the hole diameter and linear attenuation coefficient, calculate the septal thickness required to achieve 5% septal penetration.
6. For a pinhole collimator, given the aperture diameter, cone length, and object–aperture distance, calculate the collimator resolution; given the intrinsic resolution, calculate the magnification factor and the system resolution.

Introduction

The science of collimator design is based on the physics of gamma ray interactions and on basic geometry. Technologists generally do not design collimators, so the text itself concentrates on the effects of design characteristics on resolution and sensitivity, the uses of collimators, and the advantages and disadvantages of different types. This appendix reviews some of the mathematical formulas relating to collimators, and it is intended for those who desire to understand the underlying science in greater detail. The equations do not constitute an exhaustive source of such formulas. Rather, they are intended to introduce the reader to the most important collimator parameters and show mathematically the effects that those parameters have on resolution and sensitivity.

Flat-Field Collimator

The simplest kind of collimator, found in nuclear medicine on single-photomultiplier-tube (PMT) scintillation detectors such as thyroid probes, is called a *flat-field collimator*. This collimator is designed to limit the FOV to a circular area, but not to create a geometric mapping as is done with multihole collimators. **Figure E-1** shows a scintillation crystal equipped with a flat-field collimator. The FOV increases in radius as the distance between the crystal and the object increases. We can calculate the appropriate distance for a desired FOV radius according to the formula (1)

$$b = L\left(\frac{0.2R + r}{r}\right) \qquad \text{(E-1)}$$

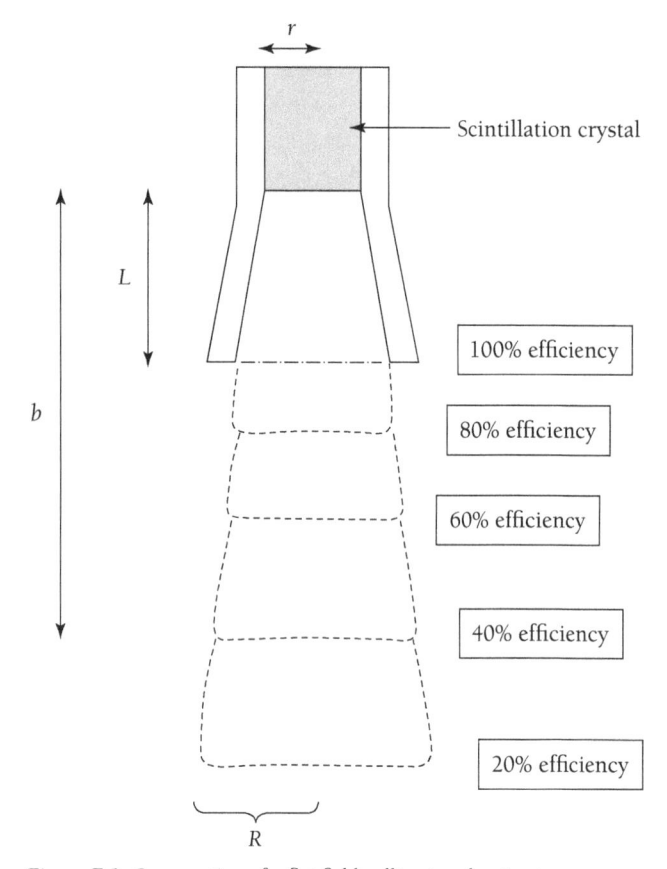

Figure E-1 Cross section of a flat-field collimator, showing isoresponse lines. At any given distance b from the crystal, the response to a uniform source is equal across the FOV (R represents the radius of the isoresponse circle). As b increases, the proportion of the total counts interacting in the crystal declines, but the area of isoresponse increases as more angled gamma rays are allowed through the collimator. Note that b in this situation is not from the end of the collimator, as in multihole collimator calculations, but rather from the face of the crystal.

where r is the scintillation crystal radius, L is the collimator length beyond the front face of the crystal, R is the radius of the desired FOV, and b is the distance between the crystal face and the object. The size of the FOV is therefore directly proportional to b and inversely proportional to L. Equation E-1 can be used to calculate b for a given probe and desired FOV (i.e., the size of the organ to be counted). Flat-field collimators demonstrate uniform efficiency at a given distance; the dashed lines shown in Figure E-1 are isoresponse lines, such that a point source will yield the same count rate at any location within the circular radius R. Thus a small side-to-side variation in position of the source within the FOV will not change the measured count rate.

Sample Calculation E-1 Flat-Field Collimator Distance

A thyroid probe is to be used for external counting of the spleen, which has a length of about 11 cm. The thyroid probe has a collimator length of 12 cm and a crystal radius of 2.5 cm. What distance should the probe be from the skin surface?

Converting the spleen size from 11 cm (desired diameter of the isoresponse area) to a radius of 5.5 cm, and adding in a fudge factor for individual variability, we will use 6 cm in Equation E-1:

$$b = 12 \text{ cm} \left[\frac{(0.2)(6 \text{ cm}) + 2.5 \text{ cm}}{2.5 \text{ cm}} \right]$$
$$= (12 \text{ cm})(1.48) = 17.8 \text{ cm}.$$

Most labs would round up to 20 cm for the sake of simplicity. But the calculation confirms that a counting distance of at least 18 cm is needed.

Multihole Collimator

The mathematics of multihole collimators is considerably more complex than that of flat-field collimators. First, there is an additional design parameter, namely, the septal thickness. Second, we need to consider not only FOV size but also sensitivity and spatial resolution. In addition, a number of different types of collimators are used in nuclear medicine, including slant-hole, converging and diverging, cone-beam, and fan-beam varieties as well as the standard parallel-hole collimator. The reader is referred to "Additional Resources" at the end of this appendix for the intricate details. The purpose here is to show how collimator design parameters affect image size, magnification, resolution, and sensitivity, using some basic mathematical formulas.

Resolution

Figure E-2 diagrams the geometric calculation of collimator resolution for a parallel-hole collimator. The collimator resolution R_{coll} (the radius of the circle of counts created by a point source of radioactivity) provides an estimate of the full width at half-maximum (FWHM) of the point-spread function. We can use the geometric principle of similar triangles to obtain

$$\frac{d}{L} = \frac{R_{coll}}{L+b} \tag{E-2}$$

where the parameters are as defined in Figure E-2b. Solving for R_{coll}, we get

$$R_{coll} = \frac{d(L+b)}{L}. \tag{E-3}$$

More correctly, however, L must be decreased slightly to account for the fact that some septal penetration will occur. The effective length L_e of the collimator holes takes septal penetration near the ends of the septa into account:

$$L_e = L - 2/\mu_\ell \tag{E-4}$$

where μ_ℓ is the linear attenuation coefficient of the collimator material at the specified gamma ray energy. This

(a) Collimator resolution geometry

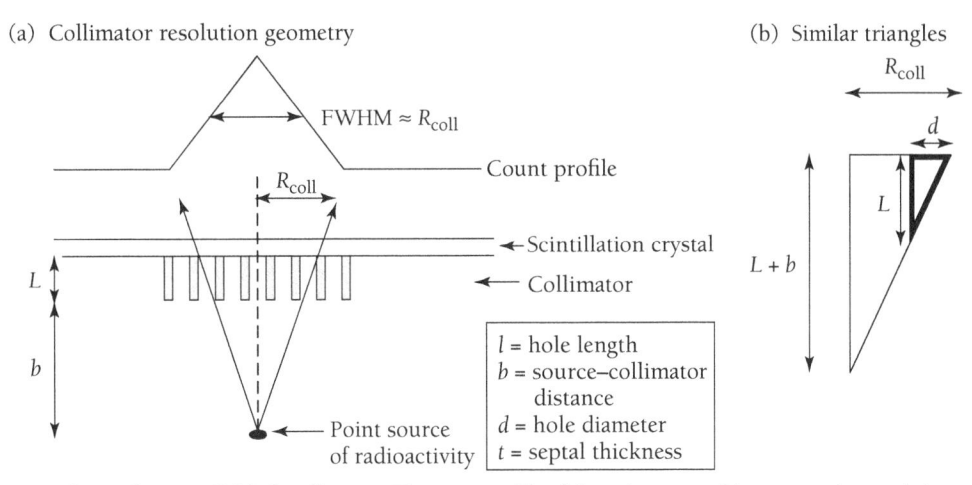

(b) Similar triangles

Figure E-2 Collimator resolution for a parallel-hole collimator. The count profile of the point source (shown superimposed above the crystal) represents the point-spread function of the source. The two single-headed arrows represent the widest angle that gamma rays can travel without crossing a septum. Collimator resolution R_{coll} is defined as the radius of the circle formed by taking this widest angle in all directions. It serves as an approximation of the width of the count profile at one-half the maximum height. Figure E-2b shows how R_{coll} is calculated geometrically. In the actual equation, L_e is substituted for L to account for septal penetration.

increases the calculated value for collimator resolution slightly:

$$R_{coll} \approx \frac{d(L_e + b)}{L_e}. \quad (E\text{-}5)$$

The difference between L and L_e is about 1 mm for low-energy collimators and about 8 mm for medium-energy collimators (2).

Sample Calculation E-2   Effective Hole Length and Collimator Resolution

A collimator is to be specially made to image 200-keV gamma rays. It will be manufactured from lead. Calculate the effective length of the collimator and the collimator resolution at 2-cm distance, given that the holes are to be 2.5 mm in diameter and 30 mm in length.

The μ_m (mass attenuation coefficient) value for 200-keV photons in lead is 0.936 cm^2/g, and the density of lead is 11.34 g/cm^3. The value for μ_l is

$$\mu_\ell = \frac{0.936 \text{ cm}^2}{\text{g}} \times \frac{11.34 \text{ g}}{\text{cm}^3} = \frac{10.6}{\text{cm}} = \frac{1.06}{\text{mm}}.$$

From Equation E-4, the effective hole length is then

$$L_e = 30 \text{ mm} - \frac{2}{1.06/\text{mm}} = 30 \text{ mm} - 1.9 \text{ mm} \approx 28 \text{ mm}$$

and the collimator resolution (Eq. E-5) is

$$R_{coll} = \frac{(2.5 \text{ mm})(28 \text{ mm} + 20 \text{ mm})}{28 \text{ mm}} = 4.3 \text{ mm}.$$

The most important thing to notice about Equation E-5 is that it includes the object–collimator distance b as well as the hole length and diameter. Resolution degrades (R_{coll} gets larger) as this distance increases. For example, resolution deteriorates by a factor of about 2 for an object–collimator distance of 4 to 6 cm, compared to an object–collimator distance of 0 cm. Degradation of resolution with increasing distance is less for long-bore collimators (larger L_e) than for short-bore collimators, a fact that has been used in the design of collimators for single-photon emission computed tomography (SPECT).

The spatial resolution of the gamma camera as a whole is a function of both the intrinsic resolution R_{int} and the collimator resolution:

$$R_{system} = \sqrt{R_{int}^2 + R_{coll}^2}. \quad (E\text{-}6)$$

(When combining multiple functions that can be represented by Gaussian-shaped curves, the resulting function is also Gaussian, and its width is given by adding the individual widths in quadrature [3].) For most gamma cameras, collimator resolution is larger than intrinsic resolution and therefore is the main determinant of system resolution. Further improvements in system resolution can come only through improvements in collimator resolution, which in turn decrease sensitivity. It is to this subject that we turn next.

Sample Calculation E-3   Collimator and System Resolution for Long-Bore vs Short-Bore Collimators

A SPECT study is to be acquired with an average distance between patient and collimator of 12 cm. Given a 2-mm hole diameter, how much difference will there be in the collimator resolution if the effective hole length is increased from 30 to 45 mm? Given intrinsic resolution of 4 mm, how much difference would this change make in the system resolution?

Multihole Collimator

Use Equations E-5 and E-6 to calculate R_{coll} and R_{sys} for each situation.

For a 30-mm bore length:

$$R_{coll} = \frac{(2\text{ mm})(30\text{ mm} + 120\text{ mm})}{30\text{ mm}} = 10\text{ mm}$$

$$R_{sys} = \sqrt{(4\text{ mm})^2 + (10\text{ mm})^2} = 10.8\text{ mm}.$$

For the 45-mm bore length:

$$R_{coll} = \frac{(2\text{ mm})(45\text{ mm} + 120\text{ mm})}{45\text{ mm}}$$
$$= 7.3\text{ mm}$$

$$R_{sys} = \sqrt{(4\text{ mm})^2 + (7.3\text{ mm})^2} = 8.3\text{ mm}.$$

Resolution R_{sys} is improved by almost 25% with the longer-bore collimator.

Sensitivity

In the discussion of flat-field collimators, we referred to the count rate response as *efficiency*, which is the term usually employed for nonimaging radiation detectors. When the same concept is used in relationship to imaging systems, the term *sensitivity* is used. The sensitivity of a multihole collimator is indicated by the symbol g, and it is defined as the ratio of the number of gamma rays passing through the collimator holes to the number emitted from the source. Once again, the formulas describing sensitivity are derived from geometry, and they depend on collimator design parameters such as hole shape and septal thickness as well as hole diameter and length.

The determination of collimator sensitivity is most easily understood using a point source. First, let us consider the value of g for a single hole of the collimator. Using the notation of Figure E-2, a hole with diameter d has an area of $\pi(d/2)^2$. The gamma rays from the point source are emitted isotropically (in all directions), so that the total gamma ray flux at the crystal, a distance L from the source (i.e., the point source at the collimator surface), is proportional to the area of a sphere with radius L, which equals $4\pi L^2$. The sensitivity g of a single hole is the ratio of the area of the crystal seen through the hole to the total area of the isotropic sphere of gamma ray flux:

$$g = \frac{\pi(d/2)^2}{4\pi L^2} = \frac{d^2}{16L^2}. \quad \text{(E-7)}$$

If the point source is moved away from the collimator, the denominator in this equation becomes $4\pi(L_e + b)^2$. Thus in the single-hole situation, sensitivity decreases as the source–collimator distance increases.

For a multihole collimator, we can calculate the number of holes exposed by the point source as the area of exposed crystal divided by the area of a single hole:

$$\text{Number of holes exposed} = \frac{\pi R_{coll}^2}{\pi(d/2)^2}. \quad \text{(E-8)}$$

We must also take into account that a portion of the crystal face is covered by lead septa. The uncovered crystal surface is calculated as

Fraction of crystal surface that is uncovered

$$= \frac{\pi(d/2)^2}{\pi[(d+t)/2]^2}. \quad \text{(E-9)}$$

We then combine all of these factors into an equation for sensitivity:

Sensitivity = (sensitivity of a single hole) × (number of holes exposed) × (fraction of crystal surface not covered by septa) × (correction factor for hole shape)

$$g = \frac{\pi(d/2)^2}{4\pi(L_e + b)^2} \times \frac{\pi R_{coll}^2}{\pi(d/2)^2} \times \frac{\pi(d/2)^2}{\pi[(d+t)/2]^2} \times K^2. \quad \text{(E-10)}$$

But we can substitute $d(L_e + b)/L_e$ for R_{coll} (Eq. E-5) in this formula:

$$g = \frac{\pi(d/2)^2}{4\pi(L_e + b)^2} \times \frac{\pi(d(L_e + b)/L_e)^2}{\pi(d/2)^2} \times \frac{\pi(d/2)^2}{\pi[(d+t)/2]^2} \times K^2.$$

(E-11)

Note the implication of this substitution. As the source moves away from the face of the collimator, its radiation intensity as measured through a single hole of the collimator decreases according to the inverse square law ($[L_e + b]^2$ in the denominator of the leftmost term). But at the same time, with a multihole collimator, the area of the crystal that "sees" the source increases by exactly the same amount ($[L_e + b]^2$ in the numerator of the middle term). These two effects cancel each other out, leaving us after simplification with

$$\text{Point-source sensitivity} = \frac{d^2}{4L_e^2} \times \frac{d^2}{(d+t)^2} \times K^2. \quad \text{(E-12)}$$

The hole length variable used in this equation is L_e, accounting for the septal penetration that we know will occur with the thin lead septa of a multihole collimator. The second quantity, $d^2/(d+t)^2$, is reasonably close to 1, so sensitivity varies approximately as d^2. This analysis assumes that the collimator holes are round. In fact, collimators are made more efficient by using other hole shapes, such as squares, hexagons, triangles, and more elaborate arrangements; the value for the correction factor K and the exact form of the mathematical equations will differ for the different shapes.

The most important aspect of these calculations from the point of view of the technologist is their implications. We can see from Equation E-5 that resolution will improve (R_{coll} gets smaller) if the hole diameter d is decreased or the hole length L is increased. A change in hole diameter that improves resolution slightly will at the same time greatly decrease sensitivity, as sensitivity is proportional to d^2 and thus to R_{coll}^2. In addition, resolution is degraded (R_{coll} gets larger) if the source–collimator distance b increases, but sensitivity does not depend on distance. We can conclude first that sensitivity is a function of hole diameter and hole length, but not of the source–collimator distance, and second that a small improvement in resolution will have a significantly negative effect on sensitivity.

Septal Thickness

The final design feature that must be considered for multihole collimators is the septal thickness, which depends on the gamma ray energy or energies being imaged. We know from nuclear physics that the absorption of gamma rays is a probability function, such that no thickness of material can stop all gamma rays. We will instead be happy with a reasonably small amount of septal penetration. Table 7-1 shows 1 to 2% septal penetration for lower-energy collimators and greater than 5% for high-energy collimators; we will use 5% as an "acceptable" value in the following calculations.

Figure E-3 shows the geometry of septal penetration through a single septum (expanded in Fig. E-3b for visual clarity). For 5% septal penetration, we need to solve for w in the equation

$$e^{-\mu_\ell w} \leq 0.05 \quad \text{(E-13)}$$

where μ_l is the linear attenuation coefficient of the collimator material and w is the minimum path length for a gamma ray crossing a septum (Fig. E-3b). Because ln 0.05 = −3, we can reduce this equation to

$$w \geq 3/\mu_\ell. \quad \text{(E-14)}$$

Keep in mind that μ_ℓ is determined by the composition of the collimator material and the gamma ray energy of the radionuclide being imaged.

In most collimators, the hole length L is much greater than the hole diameter d and septal thickness t, so the hypotenuse of the large triangle in Figure E-3c is taken to be equal to the hole length. Using this approximation, we can relate the septal thickness t to the shortest path w by the geometric law of similar triangles:

$$\frac{2d+t}{t} = \frac{L}{w}. \quad \text{(E-15)}$$

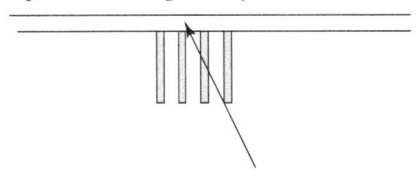

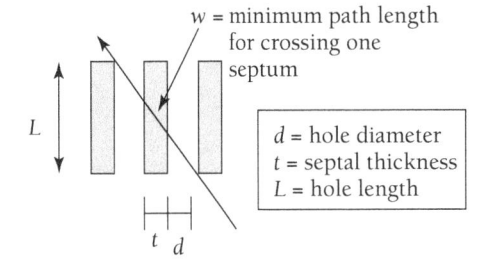

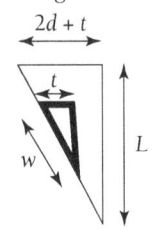

Figure E-3 Geometry of septal thickness. The gamma ray path (arrow) shown in Figures E-3a and E-3b is the shallowest possible angle for a gamma ray that penetrates a single septum; w is the length of this path through the septum only. Figure E-3c shows the similar triangles; because collimator holes are always much longer than they are wide, L is used as an approximation of the hypotenuse of the larger triangle.

By rearranging, we can get

$$t = \frac{2dw}{L-w}. \quad \text{(E-16)}$$

Substituting $w > 3/\mu_\ell$, we can solve for t:

$$t \geq \frac{6d}{L\mu_\ell - 3}. \quad \text{(E-17)}$$

The equation shows that septal thickness depends on hole diameter and length as well as the attenuation coefficient of the collimator material. Smaller and/or longer holes provide greater surface area for absorption of the gamma rays, and thus require less septal thickness.

If one is designing a collimator, one needs to consider not only the energy of the gamma ray(s) being imaged, but also the energies of other emissions of the radionuclide. For example, Ga-67 has imageable gamma ray emissions at 93, 185, and 300 keV. But 4.3% of Ga-67 decays produce a 393-keV gamma ray. If a collimator is to be designed specifically for Ga-67, these photons should be considered when deciding on septal thickness. Another example is I-124, which is sometimes present as a contaminant in I-123 preparations. Iodine-124 decay yields both annihilation photons and 600-keV gamma rays, which will fly through a collimator designed to stop the 159-keV gamma rays of I-123.

> **Sample Calculation E-4 Septal Thickness**
>
> Calculate the minimal septal thickness for the collimator described in Sample Calculation E-2.
>
> The collimator hole length is 30 mm, the diameter is 2.5 mm, and μ_ℓ is 1.06/mm. Using Equation E-17, the septal thickness is
>
> $$t = \frac{(6)(2.5 \text{ mm})}{(30 \text{ mm})(1.06/\text{mm}) - 3} = \frac{15 \text{ mm}}{28.8} = 0.52 \text{ mm}.$$

Pinhole Collimator

Finally, let us examine the pinhole collimator as an example of a focused collimator. The pinhole collimator magnifies the object being imaged, with the degree of magnification dependent on the distance between the object and the collimator. The magnification factor, in turn, affects the system resolution. As with parallel-hole collimators, the size of the pinhole aperture is a major determinant of both resolution and sensitivity. But in the case of the pinhole collimator, sensitivity and resolution both vary with the object–collimator distance.

Magnification and Field of View

The pinhole collimator's magnification (the ratio of image size to object size) is a function of the length L of the collimator relative to the object–collimator distance b (**Figure E-4**):

$$\text{Magnification factor} = \frac{\text{image size}}{\text{object size}} = \frac{L}{b}. \quad \text{(E-18)}$$

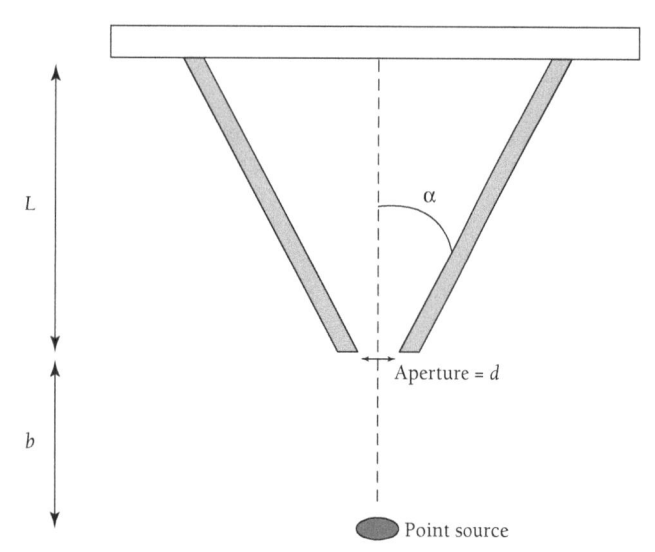

Figure E-4 Geometry of a pinhole collimator. The ratio of cone length (L) to aperture–object distance (b) determines the amount of magnification; a smaller value of b produces greater magnification.

Note that the amount of magnification changes as b changes. Normally, we image with b much less than L. When b equals L, the image size is equal to the object size (i.e., no magnification). If b is larger than L, the image is smaller than the object (i.e., minification). The implication is that magnification varies with depth in the object, which is important because we are generally imaging a three-dimensional object.

The FOV also varies with b, in a direct relationship. The closer the object is to the pinhole, the smaller the FOV, because a steeper angle is required for gamma rays to pass through the aperture. As the object–aperture distance increases, the FOV diameter likewise increases. The FOV size can thus be changed simply by moving the camera up or down relative to the object.

Aperture Penetration

As with parallel-hole collimators, we must consider the issue of septal or aperture penetration. The cone of the collimator is made of lead, but the aperture itself is often made of tungsten. In many systems the aperture is removable or interchangeable with apertures of different hole diameters. **Figure E-5a** shows a detailed view of the pinhole

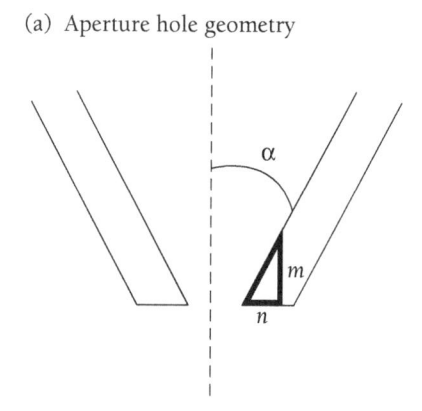

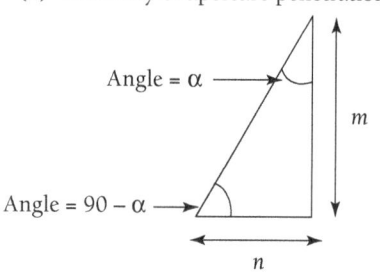

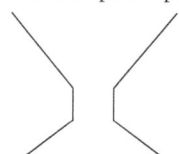

Figure E-5 Detail of pinhole collimator, showing the geometry of aperture penetration. The line labeled m represents one mean free path length ($1/\mu_\ell$) through the aperture material. The assumption of the analysis in the text is that photons will be likely to penetrate the triangle with the heavy outline in Figure E-5a. Figure E-5b shows the geometry of that triangle, and Figure E-5c shows the actual aperture configuration that is commonly used.

aperture, using a simple geometric shape. Figure E-5b shows the triangle that will be penetrated by the gamma rays. The effective diameter of the aperture opening d_e is greater than the measured opening, because the thin corners of the aperture allow for significant penetration. We will use the mean free path ($1/\mu_\ell$) as a measure of m, corresponding to 36.7% of gamma rays passing through the aperture without interacting, according to the shielding equation. The distance n is then equal to $m \tan \alpha$, where α is the cone angle (measured from the vertical).

Given this analysis, the effective hole diameter should be $(d + 2n)$, or $[d + (2/\mu)(\tan \alpha)]$. But the actual shape of the aperture (Fig. E-5c) and its construction from tungsten alter the formula slightly to

$$d_e = \left[d\left(d + \frac{2}{\mu} \tan \alpha\right) \right]^{1/2}. \tag{E-19}$$

It is this value that will be used to calculate resolution and sensitivity.

Resolution

Collimator resolution is calculated much as in the parallel-hole collimator case:

$$R_{coll} = \frac{d_e(L+b)}{L}. \tag{E-20}$$

When the collimator resolution is put into the system resolution equation, however, we must also take the magnification into account:

$$R_{system} = \sqrt{\left(\frac{b}{L}\right)^2 R_{int}^2 + R_{coll}^2}. \tag{E-21}$$

The inclusion of the inverse of the magnification factor causes the first term under the square root to get smaller (because b is usually less than L, b/L is less than 1). The magnification thus effectively reduces the intrinsic spatial resolution. The system resolution is dominated by the collimator resolution even more so than in the parallel-hole situation. Collimator resolution, in turn, is determined primarily by aperture size.

Sensitivity

The sensitivity of the pinhole collimator is much lower than that of any multihole collimator. But with this collimator, sensitivity depends on the depth and position of the object in the FOV. We again start with the definition of sensitivity—the number of gamma rays from a point source passing through the pinhole relative to the number emitted (Fig. E-4):

$$\text{Sensitivity} = \frac{\text{area of aperture}}{\text{surface area of sphere}}$$
$$= \frac{\pi(d_e/2)^2}{4\pi b^2} = \frac{d_e^2}{16 b^2}. \tag{E-22}$$

Sample Calculation E-5 Pinhole Collimator Calculations

A pinhole collimator has a 20-cm cone and is used to image I-131 in the thyroid at about 8-cm distance from the aperture. The aperture is 3 mm in diameter. Calculate the magnification factor, collimator resolution, and system resolution, assuming an intrinsic resolution of 5 mm.

$$\text{Magnification factor} = \frac{20 \text{ cm}}{8 \text{ cm}} = 2.5$$

$$d_e = \left[(3 \text{ mm})\left(3 \text{ mm} + \frac{2}{\mu_\ell} \tan \alpha\right) \right]^{1/2}.$$

Assume $\alpha = 30°$, $\tan \alpha = 0.577$, and μ_ℓ for 364 keV = 4.27/cm = 0.427/mm.

$$d_e = \left[(3 \text{ mm})\left(3 \text{ mm} + \frac{2}{0.427/\text{mm}} \times 0.577\right) \right]^{1/2}$$
$$= 4.14 \text{ mm}$$

$$R_{coll} = \frac{(4.14 \text{ mm})(20 \text{ cm} + 8 \text{ cm})}{20 \text{ cm}}$$
$$= \frac{(4.14 \text{ mm})(28 \text{ cm})}{20 \text{ cm}} = 5.8 \text{ mm}$$

$$R_{sys} = \sqrt{\left(\frac{8}{20}\right)^2 (5 \text{ mm})^2 + (5.8 \text{ mm})^2}$$
$$= \sqrt{4 \text{ mm} + 33.6 \text{ mm}} = 6.13 \text{ mm}.$$

This assumes that the point source lies along the line passing perpendicularly through the center of the aperture. If the point source is not centered (**Figure E-6**), the aperture has the shape of an ellipse, so the aperture area changes to

$$\text{Aperture area} = \pi \left(\frac{d_e}{2}\right)^2 \cos \theta. \tag{E-23}$$

In addition, the denominator must reflect the location of the point source relative to the center of the aperture. The radius of the isotropic sphere of equal gamma ray flux is the short side of the right triangle in Figure E-6, marked x. But the distance to the aperture is equal to the distance b divided by the cosine of the angle θ, so the sensitivity is

$$\text{Sensitivity} = \frac{\pi(d_e/2)^2 \cos \theta}{4\pi (b/\cos \theta)^2} = \frac{d_e^2 \cos^3 \theta}{16 b^2}. \tag{E-24}$$

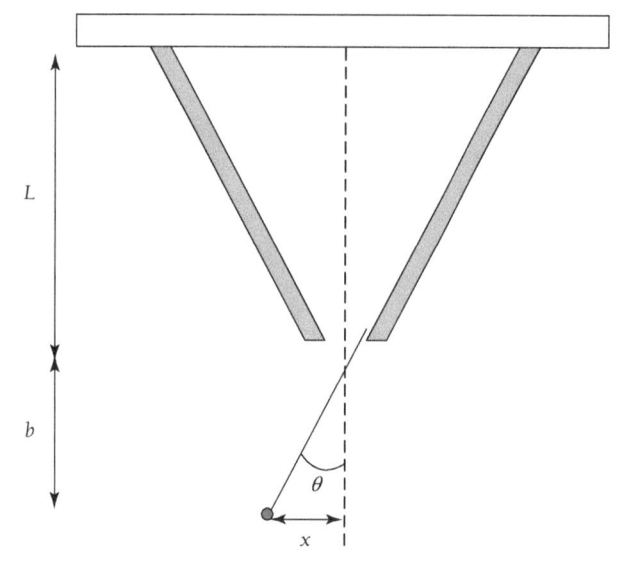

Figure E-6 Geometry of pinhole collimator sensitivity. A point source at a distance x from the perpendicular is seen at an angle θ. The length of the line connecting the point source to the center of the aperture is $b/\cos\theta$. At an angle, the aperture takes on an elliptical shape, with an area of $\pi(d_e/2)^2 \cos\theta$. The resulting sensitivity is given in Equation E-24.

When $\theta = 0°$, this formula reduces to Equation E-22. Thus the sensitivity is degraded as we move away from the centerline of the aperture (i.e., as θ increases from 0°). When coupled with the change in magnification factor with depth, the variation in sensitivity may lead to distortion near the edges of the FOV.

Summary

Gamma ray energy and object–collimator distance are the two main factors that determine the appearance of an image from a gamma camera. Sensitivity and resolution depend on hole length, hole diameter, and septal thickness. These factors affect collimator performance in logical ways, as described in this appendix. The technologist needs to be aware of the impact that these factors have on image resolution. Understanding and using the equations that describe resolution and sensitivity can help one to make good choices in clinical imaging.

References

1. Christian PE. Radiation measurement systems. In: Fahey F, Harkness B. *Basic Science of Nuclear Medicine* [CD-ROM]. Reston, VA: Society of Nuclear Medicine; 2001.
2. Cherry SR, Sorenson JA, Phelps ME. *Physics in Nuclear Medicine*. 3rd ed. Philadelphia, PA: W.B. Saunders; 2003:239–245.
3. Phelps ME, ed. *PET: Physics, Instrumentation and Scanners*. New York, NY: Springer; 2006:42.

Additional Resources

Cherry SR, Sorenson JA, Phelps ME. *Physics in Nuclear Medicine*. 3rd ed. Philadelphia, PA: Saunders; 2003:Chapter 14.
Henkin RE, Boles MA, Dillehay GL, et al., eds. *Nuclear Medicine*. St. Louis, MO: Mosby-Year Book; 1996:Chapter 8.
Moore SC, Kouros K, Cullum I. Collimator design for single photon emission tomography. *Eur J Nucl Med*. 1992;19:138–150.
Rollo FD. *Nuclear Medicine Physics, Instrumentation, and Agents*. St. Louis, MO: Mosby-Year Book; 1977:Chapter 10.
Simmons GH. *The Scintillation Camera*. New York, NY: Society of Nuclear Medicine; 1988:Chapter 4.

APPENDIX F: Laboratory Accreditation

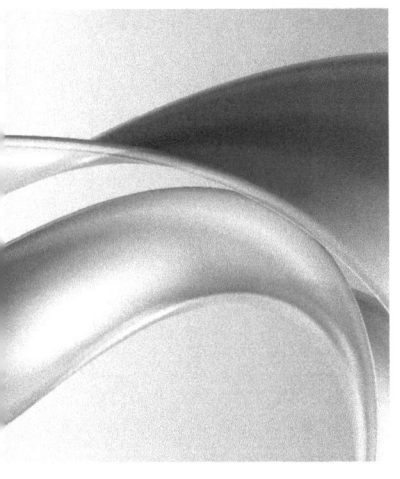

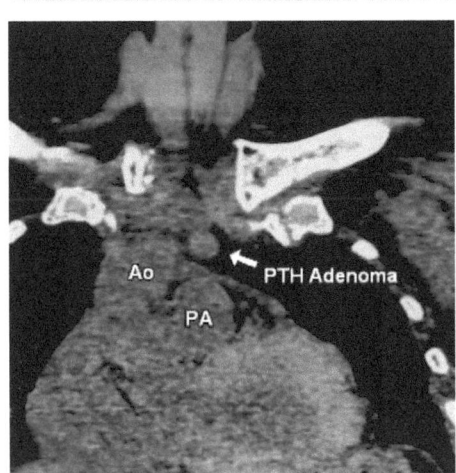

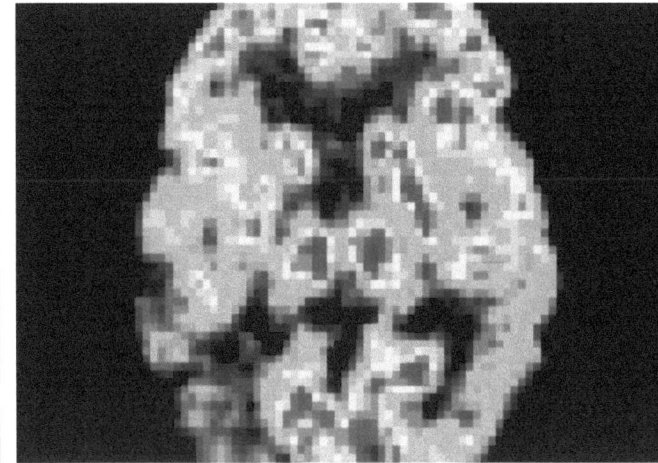

Learning Objectives

1. State the requirements of the Medicare Improvements for Patients and Providers Act (MIPPA) legislation on the need for accreditation of nuclear medicine laboratories, and identify the agencies that accredit nuclear laboratories.
2. Identify at least five areas of departmental operation that are assessed in the accreditation process.
3. State the roles of the physicians, technologists, and medical physicists in the accreditation process.
4. Discuss strategies to make the accreditation process easier and more meaningful to the department.

Introduction

For many years, accreditation of nuclear medicine laboratories was part of the hospital accreditation process performed by The Joint Commission (TJC; formerly known as the Joint Commission on Accreditation of Healthcare Organizations). Starting in the 1980s, changes in reimbursement made the hospital in some ways a less attractive location for doing business. Physicians and entrepreneurs began to locate imaging equipment in offices and imaging centers, which in turn removed the oversight of TJC.

In 2008, the U.S. Congress passed the Medicare Improvements for Patients and Providers Act (MIPPA). This legislation addressed a number of inconsistencies and other adjustments related to Medicare reimbursement. One section specifically addressed advanced diagnostic imaging (defined as magnetic resonance and computed tomography as well as nuclear medicine and PET; x-ray, fluoroscopy, and ultrasound are not included). This section requires that providers of the technical component of advanced imaging procedures be accredited in order to receive payment for services rendered to patients covered by Medicare. Three accrediting agencies are identified: TJC, the American College of Radiology (ACR), and the Intersocietal Accreditation Commission (IAC).

While the pros and cons of government regulation can be argued, one should recall that these procedures are reimbursed at high levels, and Medicare is within its rights to require high quality in return. There has certainly been anecdotal evidence of improperly performed procedures, poor-quality equipment, and incomplete reporting. Regardless, the requirement for laboratory accreditation began in 2012 and will continue for the foreseeable future. In addition, private insurers are starting to require laboratory accreditation. Hospitals are not included in the advanced imaging section of MIPPA because they are not reimbursed under the Medicare Physician Fee Schedule, but many hospital radiology departments are pursuing ACR or IAC accreditation, both as proof of image quality and for reimbursement by private insurers. So nuclear medicine technologists should expect to participate in accreditation activities, no matter what their employment location.

Accrediting Organizations

The three agencies that accredit advanced imaging departments have different approaches and emphasize different aspects of department function. All consider the quality standards included in the MIPPA law, which include

- Credentials of physicians, technologists, and other staff
- Continuing education
- Performance of imaging and ancillary equipment
- Protocols for imaging studies
- Reporting
- Safety of patients and personnel
- Quality assurance and quality control

Accreditation is granted for up to three years and may require routine (e.g., annual) reporting as well as triennial reapplication for accreditation. Each organization reviews and updates its standards on a regular cycle.

American College of Radiology

The ACR accreditation process concentrates on the quality of images produced by the imaging device. In its process, each gamma camera or PET tomograph is individually considered. Oversight and equipment testing by a medical physicist with specialty certification in nuclear medicine are required. A separate Technical Standard on the use of radiopharmaceuticals provides the qualifications for physicians and technologists, expectations regarding the handling of radioactive materials, quality control of nonimaging equipment, and the expectations for reporting. Required documentation includes the most recent report of inspection by the Nuclear Regulatory Commission or state radiation protection inspector. Submission of specific phantom images and patient studies is a requirement of ACR accreditation. Phantom images must be assessed qualitatively and quantitatively according to specific instructions provided by the ACR. Patient studies and diagnostic interpretations must also be submitted as part of the application, and physicians must participate in an ongoing peer review process.

Intersocietal Commission on Accreditation of Nuclear Laboratories (ICANL)

This organization originally concentrated on accreditation of the performance of nuclear medicine studies in cardiology offices; it currently accredits in the areas of nuclear cardiology, general nuclear medicine, and PET. The ICANL standards relate to overall laboratory function, including credentials of medical, technical, and ancillary personnel; physical space, equipment, and instrumentation (this includes mobile sites); procedure protocols; radiation safety; and study interpretation and reporting. Camera performance is only one aspect of the larger picture in the ICANL process.

The Joint Commission

Accreditation of advanced diagnostic imaging by TJC is a part of its ambulatory care program, and is more holistic in that it takes a comprehensive look at the entire facility. Its standards include safety and functionality, infection control and prevention, management of medications, performance improvement, and patient rights (in addition to the standards of the MIPPA law). Significant effort is expected on policy and procedure manuals.

One aspect of TJC accreditation will sound familiar to nuclear medicine professionals. "Tracer methodology" is used to track individual patients as they move from one department to the next. This allows TJC to see how services are provided in a way similar to that experienced by a patient, and it may uncover quality issues that are not apparent when a department has prepared itself for an inspection.

The Accreditation Process

Verification that imaging equipment is performing according to high standards is one of the chief aims of the accreditation process. The standards specify the tests needed to demonstrate the quality of images and information obtained, and their frequency (**Table F-1**). The methodology used to perform these tests is specified by the National Electrical Manufacturers Association (NEMA), which publishes recommended procedures for gamma cameras, SPECT tomographs, and PET tomographs. Many of these tests are difficult to perform correctly, and many departments contract this aspect of the accreditation process to a medical physicist.

In addition to performance standards, the laboratory is expected to maintain a quality control program, in order to spot problems before they affect clinical images. This part of the accreditation process belongs to the technologists. A well-designed quality control program includes

- Protocols that are understood and followed by all technologists
- Limits for test results that prompt corrective action if exceeded
- A recordkeeping system that demonstrates any changes in instrument function

A regular cycle of preventive maintenance, along with the quality control program, will maintain the camera's or tomograph's performance so that clinical images are always of highest quality. For example, both the ACR and ICANL require at least annual camera or tomograph system evaluation using a phantom. The ICANL accreditation also requires semiannual preventive maintenance. Acceptance testing of new cameras is required by all accreditation standards.

Some of the regularly performed quality control tests, such as extrinsic floods or Jaszczak phantom studies, are time-consuming. They are easily put aside when the schedule gets busy. It may be necessary to close a camera for an afternoon, or put in some weekend hours, in order to maintain the schedule of testing required for accreditation. Planning ahead and scheduling both the camera time and necessary radionuclide sources greatly increase the likelihood that the required testing will be performed in

Table F-1

Characteristics to Be Monitored Annually or at Other Intervals as Stated

1. Planar image quality
   a. System uniformity and intrinsic uniformity, if possible
   b. Spatial resolution (intrinsic or system)
   c. Spatial linearity
   d. Energy resolution
   e. Sensitivity
   f. Multiple-window spatial registration
   g. Count rate capability
   h. Collimator integrity
2. Tomographic image quality
   a. Uniformity and noise
   b. Spatial resolution
   c. Contrast
3. PET tomograph image quality
   a. Spatial resolution (radial, tangential, and axial)
   b. Count rate performance, including count loss correction, may include:
      i. Total coincidences
      ii. Random coincidences
      iii. Scatter coincidences
      iv. Net true coincidences
      v. Noise-equivalent count rate
   c. Sensitivity in 2D and 3D modes, if applicable
   d. Image quality, accuracy of attenuation and scatter corrections
   e. Correct scaling for activity measurements and SUV scaling
4. SPECT/CT and PET/CT systems
   a. Accuracy of image registration
   b. Accuracy of CT-based attenuation correction
5. CT systems
   a. Bed position/gantry/positioning laser alignment
   b. Slice localization from scanned projection radiograph
   c. Slice thickness
   d. CT number accuracy and linearity
   e. Image quality
      i. High-contrast resolution
      ii. Low-contrast sensitivity and resolution
      iii. Image uniformity
      iv. Noise
   f. CT dose index and patient radiation dose for representative examinations
   g. Review of dose reduction protocols
   h. Safety evaluation, to include stray radiation measurements, audio and visual signals, and posting requirements
6. Dose calibrator
   a. Constancy (daily)
   b. Linearity (quarterly)
   c. Accuracy
   d. Geometry (at installation and after repair)
7. Radiation detectors and survey instruments
   a. Calibration (before first use and following repair)
   b. Battery operation and constancy (daily)
   c. Accuracy check and recalibration, if needed
8. Well counter and thyroid probe
   a. Calibration/peaking (daily)
   b. Constancy (daily)
   c. Reproducibility (chi-square test) (quarterly)
   d. Efficiency
9. Intraoperative probe
   a. Battery operation and constancy (daily)
   b. Efficiency (if probe is used to perform wipe tests)

American College of Radiology-Society of Nuclear Medicine Technical Standard for Diagnostic Procedures Using Radiopharmaceuticals, revised 2011.
American College of Radiology Technical Standard for Medical Nuclear Physics Performance Monitoring of Gamma Cameras, revised 2008.
American College of Radiology Technical Standard for Medical Nuclear Physics Performance Monitoring of SPECT-CT Imaging Equipment, revised 2009.
American College of Radiology Technical Standard for Medical Nuclear Physics Performance Monitoring of PET Imaging Equipment, revised 2011.
American College of Radiology Technical Standard for Medical Nuclear Physics Performance Monitoring of PET-CT Imaging Equipment, revised 2008.
Intersocietal Commission on Accreditation of Nuclear Laboratories, ICANL Standards for Nuclear Cardiology, Nuclear Medicine, and PET Accreditation, revised 2010.

the required time frame. Assigning the responsibility for the quality control program to a particular technologist similarly means that at least one person is paying close attention to the testing required for accreditation. The ACR standard asks the department to assign the responsibility for the quality control program to an individual technologist.

Study Protocols and Patient Care Policies

Another important aspect of the accreditation process is the department protocol manual for patient studies. Study protocols should reflect both the department's procedure methods and the community's standard of practice. A good source for the latter is the Society of Nuclear Medicine (SNM) Practice Guidelines, available at the SNM website (www.snm.org). Each study protocol should have its own description, the date of most recent modification or review, and the approval of the department chair or medical director. The protocols must be reviewed annually as a requirement of accreditation.

However, directions and protocols are valuable only if they are followed. The protocol manual needs to be readily available to the technologists performing the patient procedures. Further, the technologists must perform those procedures according to the protocol and not according to their own whims. A new protocol suggested by a world-renowned expert should not be put into effect until it is approved by the department head. Only when imaging procedures are performed consistently will the results of those procedures be truly valid.

Clearly, appropriate care for patients is paramount to the quality of any healthcare organization. But good patient care does not happen on its own. It requires both establishment of policy and daily enactment of that policy. In nuclear medicine, patient care is addressed in policies that cover

- Handling of radioactive materials and other medications
- Infection control and sanitation
- Radiation safety
- Use of ancillary equipment
- Patient transportation and mounting/dismounting from imaging tables
- Electrical safety, functionality of emergency stops, and so on.
- Disaster procedures (including radiation emergency response)

In addition to routine review of patient care policies, every problematic incident should be used as a tool to identify how policies and practices can be improved. Situations indicating poor patient care should be reviewed with all staff so that the level of care is consistent throughout the department.

Customer satisfaction is an important aspect of high-quality care. Accredited labs are required to post a notice addressing consumer complaints. These are forwarded to the accrediting agency, which in turn must report then to the Centers for Medicare and Medicaid Services (CMS).

Tips for Successful Accreditation

A laboratory can view the accreditation process in one of two ways: as a very large task to be undertaken every three years, under a looming deadline; or as an ongoing process of quality assurance including protocol improvement, image quality, equipment testing, maintainance of staff competency, and documentation. Hopefully, most can see the wisdom of the latter approach. A key way to lighten the burden is to set up data collection points at regular intervals. For example, all accreditation processes require documentation of continuing-education hours by physicians and technologists. The department can set an internal annual deadline to collect this information, which is then safely maintained in the department. While it may be the responsibility of each individual to keep track of his or her own continuing-education hours, assigning one person to keep track of the accumulated papers again means that someone is paying attention. This approach prevents the mad scramble to find old records and documents in advance of the due date for submission of reaccreditation documents.

Many nuclear medicine departments only employ a medical physicist on a consulting basis, but there are definite benefits to an ongoing relationship. A contract that includes annual visits from the medical physicist would allow the medical physicist to review all camera and equipment quality control processes and results, and to make recommendations on how to be prepared for the reaccreditation cycle. Again, early attention to reaccreditation avoids the "crunch time" that often crops up at the last minute. Similarly, regular attention to the department's radiation safety records will keep them in order, removing another possible area of concern at reaccreditation time. As a final incentive, note that CMS intends to make unannounced site visits.

Summary

A high level of camera and department operational quality should be a goal of every nuclear medicine department. Accreditation ideally only documents what the department is already doing. The need for the MIPPA law indicates that this has not been true for all nuclear medicine laboratories. The tie to Medicare reimbursement provides an enforcement mechanism to ensure that advanced diagnostic imaging is routinely done at a level of excellence.

A department should view lab accreditation as a necessary expenditure of time and effort to verify the quality of its cameras, images, reporting, and patient care. The allowance of camera and technologist time and effort to complete the required tests is (ideally) repaid with improved image quality and decreased downtime. Regular review of study protocols and patient satisfaction surveys will help the department to be more consistent in its day-to-day operation. The credential and continuing-education requirements help to ensure that all personnel have appropriate education and are keeping up with changes in the field. Lab accreditation is a net positive for the field of nuclear medicine.

Additional Resources

Technical standards are available online from ACR and ICANL (6/24/2012):
http://www.acr.org/Quality-Safety/Standards-Guidelines
http://www.icanl.org/nuclear/main/standards.htm
Practice guidelines for nuclear medicine imaging are found at the SNM website (11/20/2011): http://interactive.snm.org/index.cfm?PageID=772

GLOSSARY

Absolute efficiency—the intrinsic ability of a radiation-detecting material, such as a scintillation crystal, to convert gamma rays into detector output signals.

Absorptive collimation—the removal of gamma rays by absorption in a dense material such as lead, usually based on the gamma ray's angle in space. Compare to *electronic collimation*.

Acceptance testing—the evaluation of a newly purchased imaging device, to compare its actual abilities to the vendor's or supplier's specifications.

Accuracy—a quality control check in which an instrument's reading is compared to the true value for the measurement, allowing the correctness of the instrument's output or reading to be evaluated.

Action level—a numeric value for a test result that triggers a corrective action of some kind.

Aliasing—an artifact in which higher-frequency components of an image or signal are incorrectly interpreted at lower frequencies, causing a distortion of the overall image or signal. This occurs in nuclear medicine when high spatial frequencies (those beyond the Nyquist frequency) are incorporated into the reconstruction process in 3D imaging.

Amplifier—a device that increases the strength of an electrical signal, usually in a linear fashion.

Analog—descriptive of a signal that is allowed to vary continuously or take on any value to an infinite degree of precision. Compare to *digital*.

Analog-to-digital converter—a device that converts analog data into a digital format.

Analytic reconstruction—a method of reconstructing a 3D image matrix that uses mathematical formulas applied to the measured values for each ray-sum (e.g., count/pixel values in each 2D projection or LORs in a PET reconstruction). Compare to *iterative reconstruction*.

Annihilation photon—either of two 511-keV photons emitted in opposite directions following the annihilation interaction of a positron and an electron.

Anode—in a radiation detection device, a positively charged electrode, whose function is to attract free electrons. Compare to *cathode*.

Artifact—an error in the representation of information (such as an image) that is due to the equipment or technique, rather than an actual difference in the underlying object.

Attenuation—the loss of a photon from a photon beam due to a photoelectric or Compton interaction.

Attenuation map—a (usually 3D) representation of the body in which the intensity of each voxel represents the degree of attenuation in that part of the body.

Axial—in the direction of the imaging system's axis; for SPECT the direction of the axis of rotation and for PET the direction of the gantry bore. Compare to *transaxial*.

Axis of rotation—the line in space around which a gamma camera rotates. Compare to *center of rotation*.

Background—detected counts that do not come from the radiation source being measured or, in an image, from the organ of interest.

Backprojection—an image reconstruction technique in which each pixel value in a 2D projection is projected into all voxels of the 3D image matrix at the corresponding angle (i.e., the "paint roller" technique).

Baseline shift—a situation in which the output of an electronic device, viewed in graphical form, shows deviation from its usual unactivated (i.e., baseline) output level.

Beam hardening—the energy shift that occurs when a polychromatic x-ray beam passes through a material and more lower-energy photons are absorbed than higher-energy photons, such that the exiting beam is "harder" (of higher energy) than the entering beam.

Bed position—a single location of the gantry relative to the longitudinal axis of the patient in a PET acquisition.

Bias voltage—a predetermined applied voltage (the operating point) in an electrical device that causes electrons to move in a particular direction. The bias voltage in a radiation detector causes it to operate in the expected, predictable way.

Blank scan—a scan obtained using the transmission source with nothing in the gantry or field of view (also called a *reference scan*).

Bolus—an injectate (such as a radiopharmaceutical or IV contrast medium) introduced into the body in a very short time, such that the material travels as a unit through the first part of the circulatory or gastrointestinal system.

Bucket—a group of PET detector blocks that are treated similarly in regard to allowed coincidences.

Buffer—a short-term memory location in a computer.

Byte mode—acquisition mode in which 1 byte (8 bits) of computer memory is allotted per pixel, thereby limiting the maximum number of counts in a pixel to 255. Compare to *word mode*.

Calibration—the adjustment of the readout of a radiation-detecting instrument in order to match some known value; for example, the activity or radiation field strength of a NIST-traceable source.

Calibration factor—a number that provides some kind of calibration or correlation from measured units to a different set of units. Examples include the isotope-specific calibration factors in a dose calibrator and the well counter calibration factor in PET.

Cathode—in a radiation detection device, a negatively charged electrode, whose function is to attract positively charged entities and/or to release electrons. Compare to *anode*.

Center of rotation—the center of the 3D image matrix being used for reconstruction of a SPECT study. Compare to *axis of rotation*.

Centroid—the midpoint between two sources or locations of radioactivity, such as those in the 180°-opposed images of a center-of-rotation QC test.

Cine display—a method of viewing radiologic images one after another, in a continuous-loop "movie" format; *cine* is short for *cinematic*.

Circumferential—in a circular direction, usually around the gantry of a tomograph. Compare to *longitudinal*.

Coefficient of variation—an expression of the standard deviation of a set of measurements as a percentage of the mean, thus allowing the standard deviations of measurement sets with different means to be compared.

Coil—a loop of wire carrying a current and therefore able to create and/or register a magnetic field (e.g., in an MRI tomograph).

Coincidence—two events that happen simultaneously or nearly simultaneously; specifically in PET, two photons registered in a PET tomograph within the coincidence timing window.

Coincidence imaging—any imaging technique that relies on coincident detection of annihilation photons.

Colinear—aligned with each other, such as two annihilation photons emitted from an annihilation interaction.

Collimator—a part of an imaging system that restricts and/or directs gamma rays.

Collimator resolution—the component of spatial resolution of a gamma camera that can be attributed to the collimator.

Constancy—a quality control check in which the instrument's response to a long-lived radionuclide or other unchanging or slowly changing source of radiation is measured; the reading of the source should be constant from one day to the next.

Contrast—the relative difference in counts per pixel or intensity between two points in an image.

Contrast resolution—the ability to distinguish between areas in an image (such as different tissues) due to the difference in count densities of the two areas.

Convolution—a mathematical operation that combines two mathematical functions, producing a third function that represents one of the two original functions as modified by the other. Compare to *deconvolution*.

Co-registration—the alignment of two objects, such as a PET study and a CT data set, so that the two can be viewed and analyzed on a point-by-point basis.

Correction matrix—a matrix in which each pixel stores a correction factor to be applied to the corresponding pixel in an image matrix, often as the image is being acquired.

Count—a radiation entity (such as a photon) that has been detected by a radiation-detecting instrument and meets the criteria of the instrument (such as being within the energy window set by the pulse height analyzer). Compare to *event*.

Cross plane—in PET, the set of coincidences registered in pairs of crystals that are in two different rings of the PET tomograph; these are assigned to a sinogram that is positioned halfway between the two rings. Compare to *direct plane*.

Current mode—a method of radiation detector operation in which the current (i.e., the number of electrons per second) is measured, resulting in an inherently time-averaged signal. Compare to *pulse mode*.

Cyclotron—a particle accelerator used to create neutron-deficient radionuclides; it is called a cyclotron because the path of the accelerated particles is circular.

Data acquisition system—in CT and MR tomographs, the part of the system that transmits data from the gantry to the computer system.

Dead time—the minimum time separation required for two radiation events to be correctly recorded as two separate events; the processing time per event.

Decay time—in a scintillator, the time required for all scintillation photons to be released after absorption of a gamma ray.

Deconvolution—the inverse of convolution; a mathematical operation that recovers a primary input function after it has been convolved with another function. Compare to *convolution*.

Delay events (or delays)—all coincidence events counted in a delayed coincidence timing window that is set up to count potential random events. Compare to *prompt events*.

Dephasing—the loss of phase coherence (e.g., of precessing hydrogen nuclei).

Depletion layer—in a semiconductor detector made from *n*-type and *p*-type materials, the volume in which holes and electrons combine.

Detector block—a group of PET scintillation crystals that register photons via a small number of photomultiplier tubes; the detector block is treated as a unit in terms of electronics and repair.

Digital—descriptive of a signal that is allowed to take on only specified, discrete values. Compare to *analog*.

Diode—an electrical device that passes current through a circuit in only one direction.

Direct plane—in PET, the set of coincidences registered by pairs of crystals that are both in the same ring of the PET tomograph. Compare to *cross plane*.

Discriminator—an electronic circuit that identifies a signal as being above a threshold value; its output is often a logic (true or false) pulse.

Doping—the practice of adding an impurity to a material such as a semiconductor, usually to improve some aspect of the material's behavior.

Dynamic triangulation—a display technique that allows the viewer to choose an area of interest on one slice of a 3D image set, after which the display program identifies the same area in the other orthogonal projections.

Echo time—the time between the excitation pulse and the measurement of the signal in an MRI pulse sequence.

Efficiency—the ability of a radiation-detecting instrument to convert measurable events into measured counts, usually stated as the ratio of detected count rate to actual activity.

Electron volt (eV)—the amount of potential energy gained by an electron when it is placed in an electric field of 1 V.

Electronic collimation—the selection of gamma rays based on their arrival time or some other detection characteristic, rather than by absorption of gamma rays that are not acceptable. Compare to *absorptive collimation*.

Emission tomography—a tomographic imaging technique in which the imaging photons are being emitted from inside the body; for example, SPECT or PET. Compare to *transmission tomography*.

Energy resolution—the ability of an energy-sensitive radiation detector to distinguish between gamma rays (or other radiation entities) with closely spaced energies.

Energy window—the range of acceptable gamma ray energies for a given radiation detection task, allowing unacceptable energies to be excluded.

Event—a radiation entity (such as a photon) that has interacted in a radiation-detecting instrument but has not been evaluated for meeting the instrument's criteria (such as being within the energy window set by the pulse height analyzer). Compare to *count*.

Excited state—a condition of an atom or an atomic nucleus in which not all electrons or nucleons are in the lowest possible energy state. Compare to *ground state*.

Extrinsic—for gamma cameras, with a collimator installed between the radiation source and the scintillation crystal. Compare to *intrinsic*.

Field of view—the useful imaging area of an imaging device, usually measured in cm or inches along one or two axes.

Filter—(1) A mathematical modifying function applied to an image; nuclear medicine examples include smoothing filters and the filter applied to the 2D projections in filtered backprojection. (2) A shield that absorbs low-energy x-rays created in an x-ray tube, leaving only x-rays energetic enough to pass through the body.

Flip angle—the angle (relative to the longitudinal plane) through which an RF pulse causes the net magnetic moment of hydrogen atoms to rotate.

Flood image—an image of a uniform distribution of radioactivity.

Fourier transformation—a mathematical process whereby data are converted from the spatial domain to the spatial frequency domain; it expresses a signal or image as a series of sine waves with varying amplitudes and frequencies.

Frame mode—an acquisition method in which accepted counts are stored in the appropriate pixels of an image matrix that was created before the acquisition commenced. Compare to *list mode*.

Free induction decay—the basic signal in an MR tomograph, caused by the loss of magnetization in the transverse plane.

Frequency distribution—a graph showing the measurement values on the X-axis and the number of times (or frequency) that each value was obtained on the Y-axis.

Frequency domain—a way of expressing information based on its frequency (cycles per second or cycles per cm; the latter is known as the spatial frequency domain). Compare to *spatial domain*.

Full width at half-maximum (FWHM)—a technique for describing the width of a peak seen on a graph; the width measurement is made at the half-height point of the peak.

Gain—the ratio of output to input electrical power in an electrical device such as an amplifier; the term is generically used in reference to electronic multiplication of signal size, such as occurs in a PMT.

Gantry—the superstructure of a circular imaging device such as a PET or CT tomograph.

Gated imaging—an acquisition method in which imaging is synchronized with a repeating physiologic process such as respirations or cardiac contractions; a physiologic signal such as the ECG R wave is the gate used to synchronize the acquisition process.

Gaussian—see *normal distribution*.

Geometric efficiency—the fraction of total emissions from a radiation source that intersect with the active area of a radiation detector.

Geometry—a collection of factors that may affect a radiation measurement, such as the volume of the source being measured or the type of container it is in, as well as the physical location of the source relative to the detector.

Gradient—in MRI, a magnetic field that is changing (getting larger) in a linear fashion over a designated space; a magnetic field with a slope.

Ground state—a condition of an atom or an atomic nucleus in which all electrons or all nucleons are in the lowest possible energy state. Compare to *excited state*.

High voltage—the electromotive force (such as a battery) providing the electric field that causes the movement of electrons in a radiation-detecting instrument.

Histogram mode—the PET acquisition mode in which the computer memory locations for each sinogram are set up prior to acquisition. Compare to *frame mode* and *list mode*.

Hounsfield units—the units of attenuation that are assigned to voxels in a CT study; they are expressed relative to the attenuation of water (0 Hounsfield units) and range from −1,000 (air) to +3,000 (metal; dense bone is about +1,000).

Hygroscopic—able to absorb and hold water molecules from the environment; this is a detrimental characteristic of some scintillation materials.

Image matrix—a 2D grid of squares known as pixels, into which image information (e.g., accepted counts) is placed to create a digital image.

In phase—the condition of a group of entities moving or rotating in synchrony with one another. Two classic examples are sine waves with the aligned peaks and troughs and hydrogen atoms precessing together in response to a magnetic field.

Information carrier—an entity that is "carrying" information about the detection of radiation. Examples include electrons in a gas-filled detector, scintillation photons in a scintillation crystal, and the X, Y, and Z output signals from a gamma camera head.

Information density—in gamma camera imaging, the average counts per unit area in a defined region of an image, usually expressed as cts/cm^2 or cts/pixel.

Interference pattern—a pattern of light and dark produced when light waves intersect. A notable occasion of this in nuclear medicine is Moiré patterns, which appear when the bar widths of a bar phantom are approximately the same size as collimator holes.

Intrinsic—for gamma cameras, without a collimator. Compare to *extrinsic*.

Ion pair—an electron that has been freed from its atomic orbital as a result of an interaction (e.g., with a radiation entity) and the positively charged ion it leaves behind.

Ionization—(1) Generally, any interaction that separates an electron from its parent atom. (2) Specifically for charged particles, an interaction of the electric field of the charged particle with the electric field of an orbital electron of an atom such that the orbital electron is ejected from the atom's orbital structure.

Isotropic—uniform in all directions, such as the radiation flux from a point source of radioactivity.

Iterative reconstruction—a method of reconstructing a 3D image matrix that makes multiple attempts (iterations) to find the right 3D image matrix to account for the measured projections. Compare to *analytic reconstruction*.

k-space—the data matrix in which MRI signal information is stored.

Kernel—a mathematical formula that is applied to each of a set of entities (e.g., to each pixel in an image or to each 2D projection in filtered backprojection).

Level—in CT imaging, the CT number that is the midpoint of the image display window, in Hounsfield units. It is used in conjunction with a specified window width.

Light pipe—a transparent material that provides a high-quality optical connection between two reflective surfaces, such as a scintillation crystal and a photomultiplier tube.

Line of response—the line connecting two scintillation crystals that have detected coincident annihilation photons; each line of response has its own memory location on a sinogram.

Line-spread function—a method to determine a gamma camera's spatial resolution by measuring the full width at half-maximum of the count profile drawn perpendicular to a thin line source.

Linearity—(1) The ability of a radiation detection instrument to respond to variable quantities in a linear fashion, usually over several orders of magnitude (e.g., activity linearity of a dose calibrator or energy linearity of a scintillation detector). (2) In a gamma camera, the ability to reproduce a radiation distribution consisting of straight lines, such as a bar phantom.

List mode—an acquisition method in which each data point is stored as an (X, Y) coordinate, rather than in a pixel of an image matrix; time markers (e.g., every msec) and physiologic markers (e.g., ECG R waves) are stored as well, in time sequence. Compare to *frame mode*.

Logic pulse—an electrical pulse that can only take on one of two values, usually described as ON and OFF or TRUE and FALSE. In binary notation, these are treated as 1 and 0, respectively.

Longitudinal—(1) In the direction of the long axis (of an organ or of the patient's body). (2) In an MR tomograph, the direction of the external magnetic field. Compare to *circumferential*.

Lookup table—a computer array that facilitates the exchange of one type of data for another in an orderly fashion. For nuclear medicine image display, the counts/pixel values in an image matrix are converted via a lookup table into intensities of a gray scale or to colors of a color scale.

Low-pass filter—see *roll-off filter*.

Magnetic moment (properly the magnetic dipole moment)—the magnetic field created by an object that has magnetic properties (such as a hydrogen nucleus spinning on its axis). It is best described by a vector quantity, as it has both magnitude and direction.

Matrix dimension—the number of pixels in each direction of an image matrix; common matrix dimensions in nuclear medicine include 64 × 64 (coarse), 128 × 128, and 256 × 256 (fine).

Maximum intensity projection—a representation of a 3D image matrix in which each projection shows the highest-count voxel in the row of the 3D image matrix perpendicular to the projection angle. It can be displayed as a 3D rotating image, or as a single 2D coronal image in which each pixel displays the highest-count voxel in the corresponding row of the 3D image matrix.

Mean attenuation length or mean free path—the average distance traveled by a gamma ray of specific energy in a particular absorbing material; its value is equal to the inverse of the material's linear attenuation coefficient.

Misregistration—absence of correct co-registration.

Modulation transfer function—a method of expressing a gamma camera's ability to image an object as a function of the frequencies contained within the object.

Monoenergetic—having only a single energy, such as a gamma ray or an alpha particle. Compare to *polychromatic*.

Mu-metal—a nickel-iron alloy with high magnetic permeability, making it effective at screening low-frequency magnetic fields.

Multichannel analyzer—an electronic device that reports outputs from a number of channels, such as a scintillation detector with numeric outputs from a large number of small energy windows. Compare to *single-channel analyzer*.

Noise—any undesired fluctuation that appears superimposed on a signal; in nuclear medicine, this can be due to electrical variations, the random nature of radioactive decay, variability in detection efficiency, and/or variability associated with assigning counts to pixels in an image matrix.

Noise-equivalent count rate—the effective signal-to-noise ratio in a PET tomograph, taking randoms and scatters into account.

Normal/Gaussian/bell-shaped distribution—a symmetric curve with a defined "bell" shape that is often used to approximate the frequency distribution of complex phenomena.

Normalization—(1) The act of putting two images or other types of data on equal footing. (2) In PET, the correction that accounts for the different efficiencies of the individual lines of response for detection of annihilation photon coincidences.

Nucleon—either of the constituent particles (proton or neutron) normally found in the nucleus of an atom.

Null—the point in a magnetic field gradient at which the actual magnetic field is equal to the nominal field.

Nyquist frequency—the highest frequency that can be accurately represented by an imaging system, based on its pixel dimension.

Offset—for a SPECT study, the amount of correction needed to align the image matrix's center of rotation with the physical axis of rotation.

Orbit—the manner in which a gamma camera rotates in a SPECT acquisition, including the mode of rotation (continuous vs step-and-shoot), the shape of the orbit, the total angle of rotation, and the number of projections acquired.

Order of magnitude—a power of 10. For example, a PMT amplifies the scintillation crystal output by 6 orders of magnitude, which is a factor of 10^6, or 1 million.

Parallax—an apparent change in location of an object due to one's point of observation.

Paramagnetic—descriptive of a material that is able to align with a magnetic field (but is not intrinsically magnetic).

Partial volume effect—the within-voxel averaging that occurs in any 3D imaging technique, due to the finite size of the voxels.

Particulate—consisting of particles (such as beta and alpha particles as opposed to photons).

Peaking—in a gamma camera, the process of matching the energy window to the observed energy peak of the gamma ray being imaged.

Phantom—a QC tool used mainly with gamma cameras, often providing some kind of test pattern that is evaluated on the resulting image.

Phase coherence—the alignment of precessing hydrogen nuclei so that they are all in phase with one another.

Photodiode—an electronic device that converts visible-light photons into an electrical signal, such that the signal is proportional to the amount of light received.

Photoemissive—descriptive of a material that releases electrons when it interacts with visible-light photons.

Photopeak—the peak in the energy spectrum of a radionuclide that corresponds to a specific gamma ray emission.

Photopenic—descriptive of an area of an image showing fewer counts than other areas, or fewer counts than it should show.

Pitch—in helical CT imaging, the ratio of the table speed to the gantry rotation speed.

Pixel—a single unit or picture element of a 2D image matrix.

Pixelated—descriptive of an imaging system employing many small scintillation crystals rather than a single large crystal as in the Anger camera design; in most pixelated systems, each count is localized only to the crystal registering the gamma ray interaction and not to an exact location.

Planar—two-dimensional, not tomographic. In gamma camera imaging, information in the third dimension is included in the planar image.

Polychromatic—having a range of possible energies, such as a Bremsstrahlung x-ray or a $\beta-$ particle. Compare to *monoenergetic*.

Potential—(1) Potential energy possessed by a charged particle due to its location in an electrical field. (2) Electrical energy available to drive radiation detection.

Power spectrum—a graphical representation of an image in the spatial-frequency domain (amplitude vs frequency), showing the contribution of information at various frequencies.

Precession—the wobble motion (a combination of spinning and falling or tipping) of the central axis of a spinning object, such as a hydrogen nucleus or a child's top.

Precision—in a situation of multiple measurements, the degree to which measured values are close to one another, indicating that the measurement is reproducible.

Primary radiation—photons and charged particles resulting from radioactive decay, compare to *secondary radiation* and *tertiary electrons*.

Projection—an external view of the body from a particular angle that is used to reconstruct a 3D representation of radioactivity in the body.

Prompt events (or prompts)—all coincidence events counted in the initial coincidence timing window. Compare to *delay events*.

Pulse mode—a method of radiation detector operation in which each radiation entity is measured as a single event, such that the resulting measurement is the number of pulses counted (e.g., in a given length of time, such that the time averaging is explicit in the units of measurement). Compare to *current mode*.

Quality assurance—the processes by which an organization determines whether it is accomplishing its intended functions in an acceptable manner.

Quality control—the procedures by which a measuring instrument of some kind is tested to ensure its appropriate function.

Quantum mottle—the noise that results from the fact that only a finite number of x-rays or gamma rays are used to acquire an image.

Radial—on a line radiating from the center (e.g., of a gantry). Compare to *tangential*.

Random event (or a random)—a coincidence of two photons that are from two separate annihilation interactions and just happen to be registered as a coincidence. Compare to *true event* and *scatter event*.

Raster—the line-by-line scanning pattern used to create an image on a screen, such as occurs in a video display terminal.

Ray-sum—the total radioactivity (in an emission image) or attenuation (in a transmission image) of a column of tissue that is perpendicular to the camera face; its value is represented by the total counts/pixel (in an emission image) or the total attenuation along the column (in a transmission image).

Rebinning—the process of reformatting 3D PET LORs into one or more sets of 2D projections.

Recovery coefficient—a multiplier that increases the count density in a given region based on the small size (area or, more commonly, volume) of that region; the smaller the region, the higher the correction factor.

Reference scan—an acquisition utilizing the transmission radionuclide used for attenuation correction in a SPECT or a PET study, acquired with nothing in the tomograph gantry; may also be called a *blank scan* or an air scan.

Registered collimator—a collimator often used with a pixelated camera system, in which the collimator holes are the same size as the scintillation crystal faces; this effectively allows each crystal–collimator pair to act as a single-component radiation detector, removing the collimator resolution from determination of the system resolution.

Regularization—a mathematical methodology that adds known constraints into the 3D image reconstruction process, thus causing the reconstruction to be faster and/or more correct.

Relaxation—in MRI, the process by which the hydrogen nuclei, having been given excess energy by a radiofrequency pulse, lose their excess energy.

Repetition time—the time between successive excitation pulses in an MRI pulse sequence.

Resolution—see *spatial resolution* (specific use in this text) or *energy resolution*.

Resonance—the phenomenon in which, under certain circumstances, energy can be transferred from one entity to another with high efficiency.

Reverse bias voltage—an applied voltage that causes electrons to move in a direction that is opposed to their natural or expected direction of movement.

Rod source—a radioactive material shaped in the form of a rod and used for transmission-based attenuation correction in SPECT or PET.

Roentgen (R)—a measure of radiation field strength; radiation field strength of 1 roentgen is an amount of radiation that creates 1 electrostatic unit of either positive or negative charge in 1 cubic centimeter of air.

Roll-off filter—a mathematical function that is used to modify the ramp filter in filtered backprojection; the roll-off filter starts with an amplitude of 1 at low frequencies and rolls off to 0 amplitude at higher frequencies. Also called a *low-pass filter*.

Sampling theorem—the idea that if one wishes to measure a signal with a particular frequency, the sampling rate used to measure the signal must be at least twice that frequency. For nuclear medicine, the sampling theorem implies that the pixels used to image a small object should be no larger than one-half the size of the object.

Scatter—the redirection of a gamma ray following a Compton interaction.

Scatter event (or a scatter)—a true coincidence in which one or both of the annihilation photons experienced a Compton scattering event before being detected. Compare to *true event* and *random event*.

Scatter fraction—the percentage of total counts in a study that are scattered photons.

Scintillation light output—the amount of scintillation light produced by the interaction of a gamma ray in a specific scintillator, usually expressed relative to the output of sodium iodide.

Scintillator—any material that can release visible-light or ultraviolet photons when an electron moves from a higher-energy orbital to a lower-energy orbital; the resulting photons are called scintillation photons.

Scout scan—see *topogram*.

Secondary radiation—photons and free electrons resulting from the interaction of primary radiation entities. In particular, secondary electrons are those ejected (via primary radiation interactions) that have more than 10 eV kinetic energy and thus can have ionization interactions themselves. Compare to *primary radiation* and *tertiary electrons*.

Segmentation—the process of partitioning a complex image into a few segments. In nuclear medicine, segmentation occurs when a patient-specific attenuation map is used to identify tissue types (bone, soft tissue, air) to which standard attenuation coefficients are then applied.

Semiquantitative—providing a numeric estimate or range for a value such as a QC measure, but not a single number.

Sensitivity—in a gamma camera, the ratio of measured count rate to activity available.

Septa—(1) The lead found between holes in a gamma camera collimator. (2) Thin tungsten slats that are found between rings of scintillation crystals in 2D PET imaging.

Septal penetration—the penetration of a gamma ray through a septum of a collimator. Septa are designed to be sufficient to cause the absorption of the gamma ray, but because attenuation obeys laws of probability, there is always some likelihood of septal penetration.

Shimming—a set of engineering techniques used to maintain the homogeneity of magnetic fields in an MR tomograph.

Signal-to-noise ratio—the relative amounts of (desired) signal and (unwanted) noise in a situation in which both are present; in general this ratio needs to be greater than at least 3 to reliably distinguish the signal above the noise.

Sinegram—a graph showing the location of the source or the offset vs the view number in a SPECT center-of-rotation test.

Single-channel analyzer—an electronic module that reports out a single value, such as a scintillation detector in which the output is the number of counts registered within the energy window (the single channel). Compare to *multichannel analyzer*.

Single event (or a single)—a photon in a PET study that is determined to be not in coincidence with any other photon.

Sinogram—(1) In SPECT, an "image" created by taking the same row of image data from each projection and concatenating these into an image matrix, which is then used to evaluate the acquired projections for patient motion. (2) The raw image data matrix in a PET study.

Smoothing—a computer processing technique that changes count/pixel values of an image (or a series of dynamic images) to be more similar to one another.

Solid state—descriptive of an electronic device that is made out of solid material, thus confining the electrons to the solid material itself. When used as a reference to a radiation detector, it is in contrast to a gas-filled detector.

Spatial domain—the representation of an object in space, in one, two, or three dimensions. Compare to *frequency domain*.

Spatial resolution—the ability of an imaging instrument to visualize small objects; for gamma cameras, the ability to reproduce the details of a nonuniform source of gamma rays.

Spectroscopy—the analysis of spectra, specifically energy spectra generated from radionuclide sources.

Spectrum—a display of the output of a radiation detection instrument over a range of values of some quantity, such as energy.

Spin—in MRI, a hydrogen nucleus, so called because it precesses or spins in response to a magnetic field.

Standard deviation—a measure of the spread of a set of measurements (i.e., of the frequency distribution).

Standardized uptake value—an expression of a radiopharmaceutical's uptake relative to a completely even distribution of the radiopharmaceutical throughout the body.

Star artifact—an image artifact that looks like a star, with arms in several directions. The cause is either septal penetration or reconstruction via the backprojection process.

Stop—in a SPECT study, a single projection in step-and-shoot mode (so named because the camera is not moving while it is acquiring a projection).

Structured background—background that arises from something other than the object being imaged. Examples include rays created by the backprojection process in analytic reconstruction and the featureless background of random and scatter events in PET.

System resolution—spatial resolution of a gamma camera, combining the intrinsic and collimator resolution.

Tangential—on a line perpendicular to a line radiating from the center (e.g., of a gantry). Compare to *radial*.

Tertiary electrons—electrons freed by interaction with primary or secondary radiation that have less than 10 eV kinetic energy. These do not cause additional ionizations but may be detected in an electronic circuit. Compare to *primary radiation* and *secondary radiation*.

Time constant—the characteristic response time of a radiation-detecting instrument to changing radiation fields.

Time-of-flight—a PET acquisition technique that uses the time difference between the detection of two annihilation photons to more exactly place the location of the annihilation interaction along the LOR.

Tomograph—one of several imaging devices (PET, SPECT, CT, MRI) used to acquire images for tomography.

Tomography—an imaging process that provides images in multiple slices of the body; from the Greek *tomo* (to cut) and *graphein* (to write or display).

Topogram—a planar x-ray acquired by moving a CT gantry, with the x-ray beam on, from the top to the bottom of the desired FOV without rotating the gantry; this is used to identify the range of the gantry excursion for the CT acquisition. It is also called a *scout scan*.

Transaxial—perpendicular to the longitudinal axis of an object being imaged, or to the axial direction of an imaging system. Compare to *axial*.

Transmission tomography—a tomographic imaging technique in which the source of the imaging photons is outside of the body, such that the transmission of the photons through the body is measured. Compare to *emission tomography*.

True event (or a true)—a coincidence that results from the annihilation photons from a single annihilation interaction. Compare to *random event* and *scatter event*.

Truncation—incompleteness, specifically not including the entire body when acquiring a transmission image set that is to be used for attenuation correction.

Unblank pulse—the output signal from the pulse height analyzer in a gamma camera, which turns on (unblanks) the electron gun of a cathode ray tube so that a dot will be placed on a phosphor screen. In modern gamma cameras, it is a logic pulse that allows an event to go forward or be dropped.

Uniformity—the ability of a gamma camera to produce a uniform image in response to a uniform source of gamma rays.

Virtual plane—a plane found between direct planes of a PET tomograph, into which are placed cross-plane events between rings on either side of the virtual plane.

Voxel—a volume element of a 3D image matrix.

Well counter calibration—a calibration factor that converts counts/sec measured in a PET tomograph to activity concentration.

Window width (or just window)—in CT imaging, the range of CT numbers used for a particular display. It is used in conjunction with a specified level.

Windowing—the technique of using only part of the available count/pixel range to display a nuclear medicine image.

Word mode—acquisition in which 2 bytes (16 bits) of computer memory is allotted per pixel, therefore allowing up to 65,535 counts to be stored in each pixel. Compare to *byte mode*.

Zoom—an acquisition or display modification that magnifies the object relative to the field of view.

INDEX

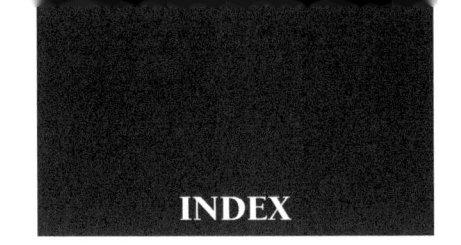

Figures and tables are indicated by f and t following the page number.

A

AAPM. *See* American Association of Physicists in Medicine
Absolute efficiency, 48
Absorption fraction, 85
Absorptive collimation, 83
AC. *See* Attenuation correction
Acceptance testing
   and accreditation, 348
   gamma camera, 122, 123t
   NEMA and, 180
   PET, 243–244
   SPECT, 180, 180f
Acceptor impurity, 30
Accession number, 337
Accreditation, laboratory, 347–350
Accrediting organizations, 348
Accuracy testing, 11–12
ACF (attenuation correction factor), 166, 222
Acoustic noise, MRI and, 293
Acquisition
   CT, 260–261, 262t, 263f, 268–269
   digital images, 76–77
   parameters, 106–108, 109t
   PET, 210–215, 215f, 223–226, 224–225f
   planar imaging, 106–108, 109t
   SPECT, 132–133, 133f, 155–161, 156t
   time-of-flight, 225, 238
   2D vs. 3D, 238
ACR (American College of Radiology), 112, 185, 247
Action levels, 113, 117
Activation centers, 18
Activity linearity, 12–14
Activity nonlinearity, 14, 15f
Adaptive filters, 172
ADC (analog-to-digital converter), 72, 332–333, 332f, 333f
Add in quadrature, 42
Administered activity, PET, 237–238
Air-core resistive magnets, 289
Air scan, 245–246, 246f
Aliasing, artifact, 160–161, 161f
American Association of Physicists in Medicine (AAPM)
   camera uniformity, 180
   sensitivity measurement, 188
   spatial resolution measurement, 187
   tomographic slice uniformity, 188
American College of Radiology (ACR), 112, 185, 247, 348
   Imaging Network, 240
American Registry of Radiologic Technologists, 294
Amplifiers, 22, 314, 316–317, 316f
Analog, 330
Analog images, 71–72
Analog-to-digital converter (ADC), 72, 332–333, 332f, 333f
Analytic reconstruction, 133, 134–135, 134f, 142
Anger, Hal, 55, 56, 198. *See also* Gamma camera
Angular sampling, 158
Annihilation photons, 198f, 199–200
Annihilation photon detection, 200–201, 200t
Anode, 3, 20, 308
Antibonding orbital, 307–308
Anticoincidence logic circuit, 22, 314–316, 316t
AOR (axis of rotation), 181
Arc correction, 236, 236f
Artifacts. *See also specific artifacts*
   collimators, 125, 127f
   CT, 265, 271–272, 273f
   PET, 249–251, 249t, 250–251f
   SPECT, 160–161, 160–161f, 190–194, 191–193f
   star, 88, 88f
Attenuation
   defined, 164, 303, 303f
   equation, 164, 303
   PET, 229–230, 229f
   planar imaging, 97, 97t, 98f
   radionuclide, 219
   SPECT, 152, 164–166, 164–166f
   tissue, 256, 257f
   x-rays, 256
Attenuation coefficient, 200t, 303
Attenuation correction (AC)
   Chang, 166, 167–168t
   defined, 163
   PET, 204–205, 205f, 218, 222, 229–230, 229f, 247
Attenuation correction factor (ACF), 166, 222
Attenuation length, 200t
Attenuation maps
   CT-generated, 171–172, 219–220
   patient-specific, 163, 166–172, 170–171f
Automated corrections, 124, 126f
Autopeaking, 113
Autotuning of PMTs, 65–66
Avalanche photodiodes, 68, 216, 317, 317f
Axial direction, 213f
Axial sensitivity, 223, 224f
Axial shields, 210
Axis of rotation (AOR), 181

B

Background
   defined, 39, 96
   PET, 228
   planar imaging, 96
   radiation measurement, 39–40
   SPECT, 152
   structured, 152
Backprojection, unfiltered, 134–135, 135f
Backprojection step in iterative reconstruction, 143
Backscatter peak, 47
Band-pass filters, 140, 141
Band structure, 18, 19f, 29–30, 30f
Bar phantoms, 103, 105–106, 117–119, 118–119f
Baseline shift, 23, 47–48, 49f, 101
Bayesian inference method, 173
Beam hardening, 165, 265
Beam pitch, 260
Beat rejection, 77
Bed overlap artifacts, 250f, 251
Bed positions, 212
Benchmark testing, 122
Binary number system, 331, 331f
Binding energy, 298
Bioeffects of static magnetic fields, 292
Biomarkers, 240
Bismuth germanate (BGO), 200–201
Bit, 331
Blank scan, 222, 245–246, 246f

361

Bloch, Felix, 277
Body coils, 290
Body contour orbit, 158
Bohr, Niels, 298
Bonding orbital, 307–308
Boolean algebra, 314, 330, 331f
Bore (collimator hole length), 86, 155
Bow-tie filters, 259, 259f, 265
Breakup phenomenon (noise), 144
Breast-specific gamma imaging, 69–70, 69f
Bremsstrahlung
　interaction, 300, 300f
　radiation, 8, 16
　x-rays, 254, 255, 256, 256f
Broad-beam geometry, 164f, 165, 219, 219f
Buckets (detector blocks), 215f, 216
Budinger, Thomas, 228
Bull's-eye artifacts, 192
Butterworth filter, 141, 141f, 160
Byte, 331
Byte mode, 73

C

Cache memory, 335
Calibration
　defined, 12, 23, 46
　　Geiger counter and ionization survey meter, 12
　　scintillation detectors, 23–24
CardiArc, 175–176f, 176
Cassen, Benedict, 56
Cassettes (detector blocks), 216
Cast collimators, 84
Cathode, defined, 3, 308
Cathode ray tubes (CRTs), 61, 319, 319f
Center of rotation (COR), 181–185, 182–184f
Central field of view (CFOV), 116
Central processing unit, 333–334, 335f
Certifications, 274, 294
Chang attenuation correction, 166, 167f, 168f
Characteristic survey, 325f, 326–327, 326f
Characteristic x-ray, 46–47, 255, 298, 300
Charge trapping, 31–32, 32f
Chi-square test, 27, 43, 43t
Cine display, 145, 148
Circumferential direction, 257
Claustrophobia, MRIs and, 293
Clinical Trials Network, 240
CNR (contrast-to-noise ratio), 99
Coded-aperture tomography, 132
Coefficient of variation, 41
Coils, for MRI, 284, 289–290

Coincidence circuit, 217–218, 217f
Coincidence imaging, 197–198, 229
Coincidences. *See also* Random coincidences
　crossplane, 210
　detection of, 201, 202f
　multiple, 228
　PET, 217–218, 217f
　scatter, 204
　sum peaks and, 47, 48–49f
Coincidence timing calibration, 247
Coincidence timing window (CTW), 197, 210, 217–218
Cold-spot imaging, 228
Collimation
　absorptive, 83
　electronic, 200
　semiconductor detectors, 33, 33f
Collimator-hole angulation, 186
Collimator pitch, 259
Collimator resolution, 86, 86f, 88, 89t, 340–341, 341f
Collimators, 83–94. *See also specific collimators*
　artifacts, 125, 127f
　choice of, 155–156
　concepts, 84–85, 85f
　cone-beam, 92, 93, 156
　converging, 92–93, 92–93f
　design parameters, 85–88, 86f, 340–341, 341f
　distance factor, 87, 341
　diverging, 92–93, 92–93f
　energy choices, 89, 107
　fan-beam, 93, 93f, 156
　flat-field, 25, 339–340, 340f
　focused, 156
　gamma camera (Anger's), 56–58, 60, 69
　hole diameter and length, 86, 155, 340–341, 341f
　integrity, 119–120, 120f
　manufacturing, 84, 85f
　non-Anger cameras, 69
　overview, 83–84
　parallel-hole, 88–89, 89t
　performance, 88
　pinhole, 89–92, 90–91f, 344–346, 344f, 346f
　planar imaging, 106–107
　prepatient and postpatient, 259
　resolution/sensitivity choices, 89
　septal thickness, 87–88, 343–344
　slant-hole, 92, 92f, 155–156, 157f
　SPECT, 155–156, 157f
　x-ray tube, 255
Color scales, 79–80
Comparison step, iterative construction, 143
Compton edge, 46

Compton interactions, 97, 97t, 300–301
Compton region, 46
Compton scatter, 45–46, 97
Computed tomography (CT), 253–275
　acquisition, reconstruction, and display, 257–264
　artifacts, 265, 271–272, 273f
　attenuation map for PET, 220
　attenuation map for SPECT, 171–172
　contrast, 264, 271, 273f
　data management, 264
　development of, 132, 253–254, 257
　diagnostic vs. low-dose, 270
　gantry, 257–259, 258–259f
　Hounsfield units, 262, 263t, 270–271, 272f
　image acquisition, 260–261, 262t, 263f, 268–269
　image display, 262–264, 263f, 264t, 268–269, 272f
　image preprocessing and reconstruction, 256–257, 261–262
　noise, 264–265
　PET/CT systems, 268–273, 271–273f
　pitch, 259–260, 260f
　quality control, 264–265
　radiation dosimetry, 265–267, 265f, 267f
　regulatory issues, 273–274
　spatial resolution, 264
　SPECT/CT systems, 267–268, 267–270f
　technical issues, 269–273
　techniques, 132
　x-rays and, 254–257, 254–257f
Conduction band, 18, 19f, 307–308
Conduction electron, 30
Conductor, 308
Cone-beam collimators, 92, 93, 156
Cone-beam geometry, 259
Confidence interval, 40
Confidence-weighted backprojection, 225
Conjugate pair, 183
Constancy check, 11, 12t, 27, 35
Continuing education, 112, 348, 350
Continuous discharge region, 5
Contrast
　CT, 264
　digital image, 80
　PET, 231
　planar images, 98–99, 99f
　resolution and, 154, 155f
　SPECT, 153–154
Contrast agents, 271, 273f, 293

Contrast-to-noise ratio (CNR), 99
Converging collimators, 92–93, 92–93f
Convolution, 135, 136f
COR (center of rotation), 181–185, 182–184f
Coronal plane, 144
Correction map, 65, 124, 126f
Coulomb force, 15, 298, 305–306
Coulomb's law, 306
Council of Radiation Control Program Directors, 274
Count
 adding, 63–64
 gamma camera, 58
 per minute (CPM), 25
 skimming, 63–64
 time and, 106
 tracking, 23
Count profiles, 117, 118f
Count rate
 capabilities of gamma cameras, 120–122, 121f
 noise-equivalent, 219, 233–235, 234f, 234t, 237–238, 248
 PET, 233–235, 234f, 234t, 237–238
 sensitivity and, 100–101, 100–102f
Covalent bond, 307
CPM (counts per minute), 25
Critical frequency, 141
Critical temperature, 289
Cross calibration, 238–239, 245
Crossplane coincidences, 210
Cross planes, 202, 212
CRTs (cathode ray tubes), 61, 319, 319f
Crystals
 for annihilation photon detection, 200–201, 200t
 coupling to PMTs, 124–125
 defects, 124, 125f
 gamma camera, 60, 68
 thickness, 100, 100f
CT. See Computed tomography
CT-generated attenuation map, 219–220
CTW (coincidence timing window), 197
Current, 310, 311f
Current mode, 4, 5–6
Cutie Pie detectors, 8–9, 8f, 11–12
Cutoff frequency, 141
CZT-based systems, 31, 32f, 68, 69, 176

D

Damadian, Raymond, 278
Data acquisition system (DAS), 259
Data set, precision of, 40
Data storage in MRI, 285
Data transmission in CT, 259
Dead time
 correction, 221, 247, 247f
 nonparalyzable vs. paralyzable, 44, 44f
 PET, 228–229, 237
 planar images and, 101
 pulse mode and, 6, 16
Decay correction in PET, 222
Decay time of scintillators, 18, 200, 200t, 217–218
Deconvolution, 135, 136f
Delayed-coincidence method, 218
Delay sinogram, 211f, 213, 218
Delocalized bonding, 18, 19f, 307–308
Departmental quality assurance, 112
Dephasing, 281
Depletion layer, 31, 312–314, 314f
Depth of interaction effect, 236, 237f
Detection efficiency, 48–51
Detector block failure, 246, 246f
Detector blocks, 215–216
Detector identification maps, 215, 246–247
Detector orbit, 157–158, 158–159f
Differential uniformity, 115–116
Digirad Cardius 3 XPO, 175–176, 175f
Digital, 71–72, 329–330
Digital images
 acquisition of, 76–77
 contrast and, 80
 display and storage, 61, 77–80
 image matrices and, 72–76
Digital Imaging and Communications in Medicine (DICOM), 337
Digital zoom, 76
Diode, 317, 318f
Dipole, 306, 306f
Dipper, 6
Direct planes, 201, 212
Diverging collimators, 92–93, 92–93f
Division circuit, 61
Donor impurity, 30
Doping, 18, 312
Dose calibrators, 6–7f, 6–8, 11t, 12–15
 calibration curve, 7
 dipper, 6
 isotope selector buttons, 7
 isotope-specific conversion factors, 7
 molyshield, 8
Dose-length product (DLP), 266
Dosing (quality assurance procedure), 112
Driver, 335
Dynamic imaging, 67, 77, 225
Dynamic triangulation, 144–145, 148f
Dynodes, 19–20

E

Echo, 284
Echo time (TE), 284
Edge packing, 59
Effective energy, 255
Effective sensitivity, 248–249
Efficiency
 components, 48–49
 definition, 48, 302
 factor determination, 49–51
 of gas-filled detectors, 15
 of scintillation detectors, 17
Electric circuit, 308–309, 310–312
Electric field, 306, 306f
Electromagnetism, 278–281
Electron orbitals, 298, 299f
Electronic collimation, 200
Electronics
 gamma camera, 62
 malfunctions in PET, 249
 scintillation detector, 21–23
 semiconductor detector, 32–33
EM (expectation maximization), 143
Emission tomography, 132
Energy correction in gamma cameras, 64, 64f
Energy discrimination in PET, 216–217
Energy linearity, 24, 25f
Energy resolution, 26–27, 26f, 34–35, 36f
Energy spectra, 44–47, 45–46f, 64, 64f
Energy window
 acquisition parameters, 108
 calibration in PET, 246–247
 detection efficiency, 49
 incorrect, 122, 124f
 PET, 216
 photopeak energy percentage, 26
 planar imaging, 108
 sliding energy window, 64
 SPECT, 156
Error 3D image matrix, 143
Estimated 2D projections, 142
Estimated 3D image matrix, 133–134, 143
Estimated projections, 133
Estimation-from-singles method, 218
Events
 absorbed gamma rays, 58
 misposition, 64
 in PET, 203–204, 205f, 218, 228
 prompt, 213
 scatter, 204
 single, 203, 204, 218, 228
 true (trues), 203
Excitation interaction, 299

Excitation pulse, 281
Excited-state orbitals, 300
Expectation maximization (EM), 143
Exponential gray scale, 80
Exposure rate meters, 8–9
Extrinsic flood uniformity, 114, 115, 117
Extrinsic resolution, 88

F
Fan-beam collimators, 93, 93f, 156
Faraday cage, 289
FBP. *See* Filtered backprojection
FDA (Food and Drug Administration), 198
FDG (fluorodeoxyglucose), 228, 249, 250f
FID (free induction decay) signal, 281–282
Field of view (FOV), 59
Fillable flood phantom, 125, 127f, 180–181
Filling bladder artifact, 193, 193f
Film composition, 323
Film development, 324
Film exposure, 324, 324f
Filtered backprojection (FBP), 139–142, 140–142f
  PET, 225
  SPECT, 159–160, 160f
Filters and filtering. *See also specific filters*
  resolution recovery, 172, 173f
  SPECT, 139–142, 140–142f, 172, 173f
  x-ray tube, 255
Flashing artifact, 190
Flat-field collimator, 25, 339–340, 340f
Flat-field flood source, 115, 181
Flood histogram, 215
Flood image, 62
Flood phantom artifact, 125, 127f
Floods, intrinsic vs. extrinsic, 114–117, 115–117f
Flow void, 291
Fluorodeoxyglucose (FDG), 228, 239, 249, 250f
Focal-plane tomography, 132
Focal spot, 254
Focused collimators, 156
Focusing grid, 19
Foil collimators, 84
Forward bias, 31, 314
Forward projection step, iterative reconstruction, 142
Fourier rebinning (FORE), 224
Fourier transformation, 137, 138f, 285
Four-quadrant bar phantoms, 103
FOV (field of view), 59

Frame mode, 76–77
Free induction decay (FID) signal, 281–282
Frequency distribution, 40, 41f
Frequency domain, 136–137, 137–139f
Frequency encoding gradient, 284, 285–287
Frequency space, 136
Full width at half-maximum (FWHM), 26, 103, 105f, 119, 187
Full width at tenth-maximum (FWTM), 103, 105f, 187

G
Gadolinium oxyorthosilicate (GSO), 201
Gamma camera, 55–70
  acceptance testing, 122, 123t
  Anger's camera components, 60–61
  Anger's camera development and concepts, 56–59
  autotuning, 65–66
  breast-specific gamma imaging, 69–70, 69f
  care of, 68
  cathode ray tubes (CRTs), 61
  collimators, 56–58, 60, 69
  construction of, 66–67
  count skimming or adding, 63–64
  detector material, 68–69
  development of, 56
  diagram of, 58f
  digital image display and storage, 61
  division circuit, 61
  electronics, 62
  energy corrections, 64–65, 64–66f
  guidelines for use, 66–68
  imaging modes, 67–68
  installation, 67
  light pipe, 61
  linearity corrections, 64–65, 64–66f
  modern cameras, 61–62
  monitoring, 66, 66f
  non-Anger types, 68–70, 69f, 175–177, 175f
  nonuniformity, 62–63, 63f
  overview of operation, 56–57
  patient positioning, 67
  photomultiplier tubes (PMTs), 61–62, 65–66
  physical size, 69
  pixelated architecture, 69
  position circuits, 59, 61
  positioning logic, 56, 58–59, 59–60f

  pulse height analyzer, 48, 61
  purchase considerations, 122
  scintillation crystal, 60
  spatial resolution and, 101–106, 102f, 104f
  sum circuit, 61
  troubleshooting, 123–125, 124–127f
  uniformity corrections, 62–65
Gamma constant, 11
Gamma curves, 80
Gas amplification, 5
Gas-filled detectors, 3–16
  basic operation, 3–6, 4f
  current vs. pulse mode, 5–6
  dose calibrators, 6–7f, 6–8, 11t, 12–15
  Geiger-Müller survey meters, 9–11, 10f
  ionization survey meters, 8–9, 8f, 11–12
  limitations of, 15–16
  overview, 3
  quality control, 11–14t, 11–15
  voltage response curve, 4–5, 4f
Gated frame mode, 77
Gated imaging, 67, 225
GE Discovery NM 530c, 175f, 176
Geiger counters, 5, 9, 11–12
Geiger discharge, 5, 5f, 9
Geiger-Müller region, 5, 5f, 9
Geiger-Müller survey meters, 9–11, 10f
General purpose collimators, 89
Geometric efficiency, 49
Geometric fraction, 85
Geometries used for SPECT TBAC, 169, 170f
Geometry
  broad-beam, 164f, 165
  cone-beam, 259
  detector, 49
  factors for dose calibrators, 15
  narrow-beam, 164, 164f
  ring, 235–237, 236–237f
  source, 169
Gibbs phenomenon, 160, 160f
Gradient coil, 284
Gradients, defined, 289
Gray scale, 78–79, 79f
GSO (gadolinium oxyorthosilicate), 201
Gyromagnetic ratio, 279

H
Hamming filters, 189, 261
Hann filters, 141
Head coils, 290
Health Physics Society, 267
Helical CT, 259
High-pass filters, 140
High-resolution collimators, 89

Histogram mode, 212
Hofstadter, Robert, 18, 56
Hole diameter and length, 86, 155
Hot-body scale, 79
Hot-spot artifacts, 250, 251f
Hot-spot imaging, 228
Hounsfield units, 262, 263t, 270–271, 272f
Howler, 32
Hygroscopic, 18, 60

I
ICANL (Intersocietal Commission on Accreditation of Nuclear Laboratories), 112, 348
IEC (International Electrotechnical Commission), 243
Image buffer, 76
Image characteristics
   MRI, 284–288
   PET, 227–231
   SPECT, 151–154
Image contrast. See Contrast
Image digitization and display, 71–81
   acquisition of, 76–77, 210–215, 215f
   analog images, 71–72
   color scales, 79–80
   contrast, 80
   devices, 80, 175–176f, 175–177, 318–321, 319–320f
   digital images, 72–80
   digital zoom, 76
   display of images, 77–80
   frame mode, 76–77
   frequency, 105, 136–137
   gated frame mode, 77
   gray scale, 78–79, 79f
   image matrix choices, 72–73, 72–73f
   image matrix trade-offs, 74–76, 75f
   limitations of, 80–81
   list mode, 77
   lookup table, 78–79
   pixel saturation, 73–74, 75f
   screen capture, 80
   smoothing, 77–78, 78f
Image display
   CT, 262–264, 263f, 264t, 268–269, 272f
   PET, 210–215, 215f, 223–226, 224–225f
   SPECT, 144–149
Image formation MRI, 288
Image matrix
   choices, 72–73, 72–73f
   defined, 61
   digital images and, 72–76
   PET, 214
   planar images and, 107
   size and noise trade-off, 74–76, 75f
   3D, 133–134, 143
Image noise. See Noise
Image quality
   CT, 264–265
   planar images, 109t
   SPECT, 156t, 159–161, 160–161f
Image segmentation, 169, 230–231
Image weighting in MRI, 290–291, 291f
Imaging modes, 67–68, 223, 224
Imaging planes
   coronal, 144
   cross, 202, 212
   direct, 202, 212
   PET, 213f
   sagittal, 144
   tomographic, 145f
   transverse, 281
   virtual, 212
IMRT (intensity-modulated radiation therapy), 254
"India ink" images, 229
Information density, 68
In phase precessing, 281
Insulator, 4, 308, 309
Integral flood uniformity, 115, 117
Integrate mode, 8
Intensity-modulated radiation therapy (IMRT), 254
Interleaving, 213
International Electrotechnical Commission (IEC), 243
Interobserver, 81
Interpretation of results, 112
Intersocietal Commission on Accreditation of Nuclear Laboratories (ICANL), 112
Intraobserver, 81
Intrinsic efficiency, 48
Intrinsic resolution, 88
Intrinsic sensitivity, 88
Intrinsic uniformity flood, 114–115, 115f
Iodine escape peak, 47
Ion chambers, 8–9
Ionization, 3, 297
Ionization interaction, 298
Ionization region, 4–5
Ionization survey meters, 8–9, 8f, 11–12
Ion pair, defined, 3, 297
Iron-core electromagnets, 289
Isotope selector buttons, 7
Isotope-specific conversion factors, 7
Iterations, 133
Iterative cycle, 142–143, 143f
Iterative reconstruction, 133, 142–144, 161

J
Jaszczak, Ronald, 189
Jaszczak phantom, 189–190, 189–190f
The Joint Commission (TJC), 111–112, 347, 348

K
Kernel, 78f, 140f
Kilovolt peak (kVp), 255, 256f, 261
K-space, 285

L
Larmor equation, 279–281
Lauterbur, Paul, 278
Lead x-rays, 47
LEAP (low-energy all-purpose) collimators, 89
LED monitoring, 66, 66f
Levy–Jennings plot, 42, 42f, 116f, 117, 326f, 327
Light pipe, 61
Likelihood (ML process), 143
Linear gray scale, 78
Linearity, 12–14, 24, 25f, 117
Linearity corrections in gamma cameras, 64–65, 64–66f
Linear sampling, 157
Line of response (LOR), 201, 228
Line-spread function (LSF), 103, 105–106, 106f, 118
Liquid crystal display (LCD), 320–321
List mode, 77
LLD (lower-level discriminator), 22, 316, 316t
Logarithmic gray scale, 80
Logical notation, 285, 285t, 286f
Logic circuits or gates, 314–316, 316t, 330
Longitudinal direction, 133f
Lookup table (LUT), 78–79, 331
LOR (line of response), 201, 228
Low-dose vs. diagnostic CT, 270
Low-energy all-purpose (LEAP) collimators, 89
Lower-level discriminator (LLD), 22, 316, 316t
Low-pass filters, 140–141, 140f
LSF. See Line-spread function
Lutetium oxyorthosilicate (LSO), 201
Lutetium yttrium oxyorthosilicate (LYSO), 201
LUT (lookup table), 78–79

M
Mach band phenomenon, 81, 81f
Magnetic gradients, 284–285, 284f
Magnetic moment, 278

Magnetic resonance imaging (MRI), 277–295
  acoustic noise, 293
  advantages of, 278
  bioeffects of static magnetic fields, 292
  claustrophobia, 293
  computer systems, 290
  contrast agents, 293
  data storage, 285
  electromagnetism, 278–281
  forming of, 284–288
  free induction decay signal, 281–282
  frequency encoding gradient, 284, 285–287
  gradients, 289
  image characteristics, 284–288
  image formation, 288
  instrumentation, 288–290
  logical notation, 285, 285t, 286f
  magnetic gradients, 284–285, 284f
  magnets, 289, 292–293
  moving fluids, 291
  net magnetization, 279, 279–280f
  noise, 293
  overview, 277–278
  PET/MRI combined, 293–294f, 293–295
  phase encoding gradient, 284, 285, 287–288, 288f
  precession and the Larmor equation, 279–281
  proton density weighting, 291
  pulse sequence, 283–284, 283f
  receiver coils, 290
  relaxation, 282, 283f
  relaxation characteristics, 290, 291–292f, 291t
  RF coils, 289
  RF flip angle, 281, 282f
  RF pulse characteristics, 289
  safety issues, 291–293
  slice selection gradient, 284, 285, 287
  tissue characteristics and image appearance, 290–291
  tissue disturbance and differentiation, 281–283
  T1 relaxation, 282–283, 290
  transmit coils, 289–290
  T2 relaxation, 283, 290–291
Magnets, 289, 292–293
Mansfield, Peter, 278
Matrix size and dimensions, 72, 156–157, 214
Maximum a posteriori (MAP), 173
Maximum-intensity projection (MIP) image, 147–148
Maximum-likelihood expectation maximization (MLEM), 143–144

Maximum-likelihood (ML), 143–144
MCA (multichannel analyzer), 22, 23–24
Mean free path, 302
Mean value, 40
Measles effect, 124, 125f
Measured 2D projections, 133, 142
Memory (computer), 73–74, 335
Metz filter, 172
Microcast collimators, 84
Microlinear collimators, 84
MIP (maximum-intensity projection) image, 147–148, 215
Mispositioning events, 64
Misregistration artifacts, 249–251, 271–272, 273f
ML (maximum-likelihood), 143–144
MLEM (maximum-likelihood expectation maximization), 143–144
Mock standards, 50
Modulation, 105
Modulation transfer function (MTF), 103–106, 107–108f
Moiré patterns, 118, 119f
Moly shield, 8
Motion artifacts, 190, 192f, 193, 249, 250f
Moving fluids, 291
MPI (myocardial perfusion imaging), 164
MR computer systems, 290
MRI. See Magnetic resonance imagining
MR spectroscopy, 278
MTF (modulation transfer function), 103–106, 107–108f
Multichannel analyzer (MCA), 22, 23–24
Multidetector CT tomograph, 259
Multiformatter, 319–320
Multiple coincidences, 228
Multiple-window spatial registration (MWSR), 120, 121f
Myocardial perfusion imaging (MPI), 164

N
NaI(Tl), thallium-activated sodium iodide, 18–19, 19f, 29, 200
Narrow-beam geometry, 164, 164f
National Electrical Manufacturers Association (NEMA)
  acceptance testing, 180
  quality control tests, 35, 243–244
  scatter fraction protocol, 247–248
  sensitivity protocol, 248–249
  spatial resolution protocol, 248
  standards, 122
  tomography, 132
  volume sensitivity, 188–189

National Institute of Standards and Testing (NIST), 7, 12
Naviscan high-resolution organ-specific PET scanner, 225
NECR. See Noise-equivalent count rate
NEMA. See National Electrical Manufacturers Association
NEX (number of excitations), 287
NIST (National Institute of Standards and Testing), 7, 12
NMR (nuclear magnetic resonance) spectrometer, 278
Noise
  acoustic, 293
  breakup phenomenon, 144
  CT, 264–265
  defined, 40
  image matrix size and, 74–76, 75f
  MRI, 293
  PET, 228
  planar images, 96
  ratios, 96, 99
  SPECT, 142, 152, 169, 173
Noise-equivalent count rate (NECR), 219, 233–235, 234f, 234t, 237–238, 248
Noise regularization (NR), 164, 173
Non-Anger gamma cameras, 68–70, 68f, 175–177, 175f
Nonparalyzable system, 44, 44f
Nonpenetrating radiation, 302
Nonuniformity of PMTs, 62–63, 63f
Normalization, 220, 220f
Normalization scan, 220, 244–245
Normalized images, 78
NR (noise regularization), 164, 173
NSA (number of signal averages), 287
n-type semiconductor, 30, 314
Nuclear counting statistics, 40–44, 41f, 43f, 43t
Nuclear magnetic resonance (NMR) spectrometer, 278
Null, 284
Number of excitations (NEX), 287
Number of signal averages (NSA), 287
Nyquist frequency, 137–139, 139f, 160–161

O
Object–collimator distance, 87, 108, 341, 343
Object space, 136
Oblique reorientation, 144
Off-peak windows, 124
Offset, 181
1/r blurring, 135, 136f
Operator-determined parameters in PET, 235
Optical density, 326

Optoelectronic data transmission, 259
Ordered-subsets expectation maximization (OSEM), 143–144, 144f, 161
Organ-specific PET systems, 225–226

P

Parallax of pinhole collimation, 91, 91f
Parallax effect in PET tomographs, 236, 237f
Parallel-hole collimators, 88–89, 89t
Parallel-line equal-spacing (PLES) bar phantoms, 103
Paralyzable system, 44, 44f
Parathyroid adenoma localization, 34
Partial volume effect (PVE), 153, 154f, 230–231, 231f, 251
Particulate radiation, 15–16
Patient interview, 112
Patient motion, effects of
  PET, 230
  planar images, 97
  SPECT, 152–153, 153f
Patient positioning, 67
Patient radiation doses in CT, 266
Patient-specific attenuation maps, 163, 166–172, 170–171f
Peak broadening, 21, 26
Peaking, 46, 113, 114f
Penetrating radiation, 302
Penetration fraction, 85
Performance Measurements of Positron Emission Tomographs (NEMA), 243
Performance measures
  PET, 231–234, 232t, 235–238
  planar images, 99–100, 100t
  SPECT, 154–155, 155f
Performance phantom, 189
Permanent magnets, 289
PET. *See* Positron emission tomography
PET/CT systems, 268–273, 271–273f
PET/MRI systems, 293–294f, 293–295
PHA. *See* Pulse height analyzer
Phase coherence, 281
Phase encoding gradient, 284, 285, 287–288, 288f
Phoswich, 237
Photocathodes, 19
Photodiodes, 69, 256, 317–318, 317f
Photoelectric interaction, 97, 97t, 300
Photoemissive materials, 19
Photographic system, troubleshooting of, 125, 127f

Photomultiplier tubes (PMTs)
  autotuning, 65–66
  coupling to scintillation crystal, 124–125
  description of, 19–21, 20–21f, 21t
  nonuniformity of, 62–63, 63f
  scintillation detectors, 19–21, 20–21f, 21t
  thresholding, 61–62
  troubleshooting, 124, 124f
Photons, 300
Photopeak
  defined, 22
  energy percentage, 26
  energy spectra, 45
  monitoring, 66
Picture Archiving and Communications System (PACS), 337–338
Pig (moly shield), 8
Pinhole collimators, 89–92, 90–91f, 344–346, 344f, 346f
Pitch, in helical CT, 259–260, 260f
Pixelated architecture, 69
Pixels, 61, 72
Pixel saturation, 73–74, 75f
Pixel size determination, 119, 186
Planar imaging, 95–109
  acquisition parameters, 106–108, 109t
  attenuation, 97, 97t, 98f
  background, 96
  bar phantoms, 103, 105–106
  characteristics, 95–98
  collimators, 106–107
  contrast, 98–99, 99f
  counts and time, 106
  energy window, 108
  image matrix, 107
  line-spread function, 103, 105–106, 106f, 118
  modulation transfer function, 103–106, 107–108f
  noise, 96
  object-collimator distance, 87, 108
  patient motion, 97
  patient positioning, 67
  performance measures, 99–100, 100t
  quality control, 112–119, 113t
  resolution loss with distance, 96–97
  scatter, 97, 97t, 98f
  sensitivity and count rate, 100–101, 100–102f
  spatial resolution, 101–106, 102f, 104f
  third-dimension superposition, 96, 96f
  uniformity, 100
PLES (parallel-line equal-spacing) bar phantoms, 103

PMTs. *See* Photomultiplier tubes
p-n junction, 30–32, 314, 314f
Point-source sensitivity, 63
Point-spread function (PSF), 103, 105f
Poisson fluctuations in delayed-coincidence method, 218
Poisson statistical model, 40–41
Polychromatic, x-ray beam, 255
Position circuits, 59, 61
Positioning logic, 56, 58–59, 59–60f
Position-sensitive PMT (PSPMT), 69
Positron Attrius, cardiac PET scanner, 225–226
Positron emission tomography (PET), 197–252
  acceptance testing, 243–244
  acquisition, 210–215, 215f, 223–226, 224–225f
  administered activity, 237–238
  annihilation photons, 198f, 199–200
  annihilation photon detection, 200–201, 200t
  artifacts, 249–251, 249t, 250–251f
  attenuation, 219, 229–230, 229f
  attenuation correction, 204–205, 205f, 222, 229–230, 229f, 247
  avalanche photodiodes, 68, 216
  axial sensitivity, 223, 224f
  background, 228
  blank scan, 222, 245–246, 246f
  coincidence circuit, 217–218, 217f
  coincidences, detection of, 201, 202f, 217–218, 217f
  coincidence timing calibration, 247, 273f
  contrast, 231
  corrections, 220–222
  count rate, 233–235, 234f, 234t
  cross calibration, 238–239, 245
  CT-generated attenuation map, 219–220
  data collection, 201–203
  dead time, 228–229, 237
  dead time correction, 221, 247, 247f
  decay correction, 222
  delayed-coincidence window, 218
  detector blocks, 215–216
  detector identification maps, 215, 246–247
  dynamic imaging, 225
  energy discrimination, 216–217
  energy window calibration, 246–247
  events, types of, 203–204, 205f, 217–218, 228, 234t
  gated imaging, 225
  history of, 198–199
  image characteristics, 227–231

Positron emission tomography (PET) (*Contd.*)
  image display, 210–215, 215*f*, 223–226, 224–225*f*
  instrumentation, 209–226
  noise, 228
  noise-equivalent count rate, 219, 233–235, 234*f*, 234*t*, 237–238, 248
  normalization, 220, 220*f*
  normalization scan, 220, 244–245
  operator-determined parameters, 235
  organ-specific systems, 225–226
  overview, 197–198, 209–210
  partial volume effect, 230–231, 231*f*
  patient motion, 230
  performance measures, 231–238, 232*t*
  physics of, 199–200
  quality control, 243–249, 244*t*
  quantitative abilities, 206–207
  radionuclides, positron-emitting, 199, 199*t*, 219, 219*f*
  radionuclides, single-photon-emitting, 219
  random coincidences, 203–204, 217*f*, 217–218, 224, 225*f*, 228
  reconstruction, 210–215, 224–225, 247
  resolution, limits on, 235
  ring geometry, 235–237, 236–237*f*
  scatter, 228, 230, 247
  scatter coincidences, 204
  scatter correction, 221–222, 221*f*, 224
  scatter fraction, 232–233, 247–248
  scintillation crystal, 17, 199–200
  sensitivity, 231–232, 248–249
  singles, estimation of randoms from, 218
  sinograms, 201–203, 202–203*f*, 213
  spatial resolution, 231, 248
  standardized uptake value, 238–240
  time-of-flight (TOF), 201, 205–206, 206–207*f*, 225, 238
  tomograph composition, overview, 210
  transmission sources and geometries, 218–220
  2D vs. 3D imaging modes, 223–224, 224*f*, 238
  uniformity, 246
Positron-emitting radionuclides, 199, 199*t*
Posterior probability, 173
Postfiltering, 144
Postpatient collimators, 259
Postzoom, 76

Potential, 310
Power spectrum, 137, 138–139*f*
Power supply, 66
PP (pulse programmer), 290
Preamplifier, 22
Precession, 279–281
Precessional frequency, 280
Precision of data set, 40
Prepatient collimators, 259
Preprocessing of CT images, 261–262
Primary charged particle, 298
Printers, 321
Prior probability, 173
Procedural quality assurance, 112
Processor (film), 324–325, 324*f*
Projection
  PET, 202, 203*f*
  SPECT, 132, 133, 134*f*, 142–143, 143*f*
Prompt events, 213
Prompt sinogram, 211*f*, 213
Proportional counters, 5
Proportionality of radiation detection, 18–19
Proportional region, 5
Proton density, 284
Proton density weighting, 291
PSF (point-spread function), 103, 105*f*
PSPMT (position-sensitive PMT), 69
p-type semiconductors, 30, 314
Public health concerns about radiation, 266–267
Pulse clipping, 101, 101*f*
Pulse height analyzer (PHA)
  defined, 22
  gamma cameras, 48, 61
  PET, 216
  scintillation detectors, 22
  semiconductor detectors, 32
Pulse height spectrum, 22, 22*f*
Pulse mode, 4, 5–6, 16
Pulse pileup, 23, 47–48, 49*f*, 101, 229
Pulse programmer (PP), 290
Pulse sequence in MRI, 283–284, 283*f*
Pulse shapes, 23, 312, 313*f*
Purcell, Edward, 277
Pure beta-emitting radiopharmaceutical, detection of, 8, 8*t*
PVE. *See* Partial volume effect

Q

Quadrant sharing, 216
Quality assurance, 111–112
Quality control (QC). *See also* Testing
  and accreditation, 348–349, 349*t*
  CT, 264–265

film processor, 325–326
gas-filled detectors, 11–14*t*, 11–15
NEMA and, 35, 243–244
PET, 243, 244–249, 244*t*
planar gamma cameras, 112–119, 113*t*
scintillation detectors, 27, 27–28*t*
semiconductor detectors, 35–36, 35*t*
spatial resolution, 248
SPECT, 180–186, 181*t*
troubleshooting, 123–125, 124–127*f*
uniformity, PET, 246
uniformity, SPECT, 180–181
Quantitation in PET, 206–207
Quantum mottle, 96, 264
Quench gas, 11

R

R (Roentgen), 8–9
Radial direction, 187, 188*f*
Radiation dosimetry in CT, 265–267, 265*f*, 267*f*
Radiation measurement, 39–51
  background, 39–40
  baseline shift, 23, 47–48, 49*f*, 101
  dead time, 44, 44*f*
  detection efficiency, 48–51
  energy spectra, 44–47, 45–46*f*, 64, 64*f*
  nuclear counting statistics, 40–44, 41*f*, 43*f*, 43*t*
  overview, 39
  pulse pileup, 23, 47–48, 49*f*, 101, 229
  statistical testing, 42–44
Radiation safety of SPECT TBAC sources, 169–171
Radio-frequency (RF), 281
Radionuclides
  for PET AC, 219, 219*f*
  positron-emitting, 199, 199*t*, 219, 219*f*
  for SPECT AC, 167–169, 170*f*
Radon transform, 132
RAMLA (row action maximum likelihood algorithm), 213
Ramp filters, 139, 140*f*
Random coincidences, 203–204, 217–218, 217*f*, 224, 225*f*, 228
Range, 302
Rate meter, 8–9, 23, 32, 318
Rate mode, 8
Ray artifacts, 190–192, 191*f*, 249, 250*f*
Ray-sum, 134, 134*f*
RC (resistor and capacitor) circuit, 6, 310–312, 311*f*, 313*f*
Readout gradient, 285
Rebinning, 224–225

368 Index

Receiver coils, 290
Recombination region, 4
Reconstruction
    analytic, 133–135, 135f, 139–142
    CT, 256–257, 261–262
    iterative, 133, 142–144, 143f, 161, 172
    PET, 210–215, 224–225, 247
    SPECT and, 133
    x-rays, 256–257
Recovery coefficient, 230–231, 231f
Rectilinear scanner, 56, 57f
Reference beam, 257
Reference scan, 169, 171f, 185–186, 185f, 245–246, 246f
Region of limited proportionality, 5
Registered collimators, 69
Regularization, defined, 173
Regulatory issues
    PET, 198
    PET/CT, 273–274
    PET/MRI, 294
Relaxation
    characteristics of tissues, 290, 291–292f, 291t
    in MRI, 282, 283f, 290, 291–292f, 291t
Repetition time (TR), 284
Resistance, 310
Resistivity, 309
Resistor, 309–310
Resistor and capacitor (RC) circuit, 6, 310–312, 311f, 313f
Resolution
    defined, 55
    limits in PET, 235
Resolution loss with distance
    planar images, 96–97
    SPECT, 152, 172–173, 173f
Resolution recovery (RR), 164, 172–173, 173f
    filters, 172, 173f
Resolution/sensitivity collimator choices, 89
Resonance, 277
Restorative filters, 172
Reverse bias, 31, 314
RF (radio-frequency), 281
RF coils, 289
RF flip angle, 281, 282f
RF pulse characteristics, 289
Ring artifacts, 190, 192–193, 192f
Ring difference, 223
Ring geometry, 235–237, 236–237f
Ringing artifact, 160, 160f
Rod sources for attenuation correction, 169, 170f, 210, 219, 219f
Rod windowing, 219
Roentgen (R), 8–9
Roll-off filters, 140, 140f, 159–160
Rose criterion, 99

Rotation, center of, 181–185, 182–184f
Rotational stability, 186, 186f
Rotation angle in SPECT acquisition, 158
Row action maximum likelihood algorithm (RAMLA), 213
R-R interval, 77
RR (resolution recovery), 164, 172–173, 173f

S
Safety of MRI, 291–293
Sagittal plane, 144
Saturation voltage, 4–5
SC (scatter compensation), 164, 172
SCA (single-channel analyzer), 22, 23, 24f
Scaler, 23, 318
Scatter
    Compton, 45–46, 97, 300–301
    and detection efficiency, 49
    PET, 230
    planar imaging, 97, 97t
    SPECT, 152, 164–166, 164–166f, 172
Scatter coincidences, 204
Scatter compensation (SC), 164, 172
Scatter correction, 221–222, 221f, 224, 247–248
Scatter fraction, 85, 172, 232–233, 247–248
Scatter subtraction, 97
Scintigraphy, 18
Scintillation, basic principles of, 17–21
Scintillation camera. See Gamma camera
Scintillation crystal
    for annihilation photon detection, 200–201, 200t
    coupling to PMTs, 124–125
    gamma camera component, 60, 68
Scintillation detectors, 17–28
    applications, 24–26
    calibration, 23–24
    configurations, 25–26, 25f
    decay time, 18
    diagram of, 21, 22f
    electronics, 21–23
    energy linearity, 24, 25f
    energy resolution, 26–27, 26f
    overview, 17
    peak broadening, 21, 26
    PET, 200–201, 200t
    photomultiplier tubes, 19–21, 20–21f, 21t
    pulse height analyzer, 22
    pulse height spectrum, 22, 22f
    pulse shapes, 23
    quality control, 27, 27–28t
    signal amplification, 22

thallium-activated sodium iodide, 18–19, 19f, 29, 200
    tracking counts, 23
Scintillation light yield, 18
Scintillation photons, 17
Scintiscans, 18
Scout scan, 261
Screen capture, 80
Semiconductor detectors, 29–37
    applications, 33–34
    band structure, 18, 29–30, 30f, 308, 308f
    characteristics, 31–32, 31t, 32f
    collimation and shielding, 33, 33f
    depletion layer, 30–31, 31f, 314, 314f
    diagram of, 32, 32f
    electronics, 32–33
    energy resolution, 34–35, 36f
    handling, 36
    operation of, 32–33
    performance measures, 34–35
    properties of, 29–32
    quality control, 35–36, 35t
    radiation detection, 30–32, 31f
    sensitivity measures, 34
    spatial resolution, 35
Semiconductor materials in non-Anger cameras, 68–69
Sensitivity
    collimator choices, 89
    count rate and, 100–101, 100–101f
    defined, 55
    effective in PET, 248–249
    intrinsic, 88
    of multihole collimator, 342–343
    of pinhole collimator, 345–346, 346f
    point-source, 63
Sensitivity check, 119
Sensitivity maps, 65
Sensitivity measures
    AAPM and SPECT, 188
    NEMA protocol for PET, 248–249
    PET, 231–232, 248–249
    semiconductor detectors, 34
    SPECT, 154–155
    system volume, 188–189
Sentinel lymph node localization, 33–34
Septa, 83, 87, 87f, 210, 210f, 223
Septal penetration, 87–88, 87–88f, 87t
Septal thickness, 87–88, 87f, 87t, 343–344, 343f
Seven-pinhole tomography, 132
Shepp–Logan filter, 261
Shimming, 289
Signal amplification, 22, 316–317
Signal-to-noise ratio (SNR), 96
Signal-to-noise ratio in PET, 233

Index   369

Sineogram graph, 183
Sine waves, 137, 138f
Single-channel analyzer (SCA), 22, 23, 24f
Single events (singles), 203, 204, 218, 228, 237
Single-photon emission computed tomography (SPECT), 131–194
  acceptance testing, 180, 180f
  acquisition parameters, 132–133, 133f, 155–161, 156t
  analytic reconstruction, 134–142, 134f, 134f, 136f
  artifacts, 160–161, 160–161f, 190–194, 191–193f
  attenuation, 152, 164–166, 164–166f
  background, 152
  center of rotation, 181–185, 182–184f
  Chang attenuation correction, 166, 167–168f
  cine modes, 148
  clinical benefits of improvements, 177, 177f
  collimator choices, 155–156, 157f
  collimator-hole angulation, 186
  computed tomography techniques, 132
  continuous mode, 157
  contrast, 153–154
  detector orbit, 157–158, 158–159f
  development of computed tomography techniques, 132
  energy window, 156
  filtered backprojection, 139–142, 159–160, 160f
  filters, 139–142, 140–142f, 172, 173f
  frequency domain, 136–137, 137–139f
  image characteristics, 151–154
  image display, 144–149
  implementation of correction methods, 174–177
  improving image quality, 155–161, 156t, 163–178
  iterative reconstruction, 133, 142–144, 143f, 161, 172
  Jaszczak phantom, 189–190, 189–190f
  matrix size, 156–157
  MLEM process, 143–144
  noise, 142, 152, 169
  noise regularization, 173
  Nyquist frequency, 137–139, 139f, 160–161
  OSEM process, 143–144, 144f
  overview, 132–133
  partial volume effect, 153, 154f
  patient motion, 152–153, 153f, 192f, 193
  patient-specific attenuation maps, 166–172, 170–171f
  performance measures, 154–155, 155f
  pixel size determination, 119, 186
  quality control, 179–190, 181t
  radiation safety of TBAC sources, 169–171
  radionuclide choice for TBAC, 167–169
  reference scan, 169, 171f, 185–186, 185f
  resolution loss with distance, 152
  resolution recovery, 172–173, 173f
  rotational stability, 186, 186f
  scatter, 152, 164–166, 164–166f
  scatter compensation, 164, 172
  source geometry, 169
  spatial resolution, 154–155, 155f
  spatial resolution measurement, 35, 187, 188f
  step-and-shoot mode, 133, 157
  surface rendering, 145, 147
  system volume sensitivity, 188–189
  3D image matrix, 133–134, 143
  three-dimensional display techniques, 145–148
  time per stop, 158–159
  tomographic measures of performance, 187–190
  two-dimensional display techniques, 144–145, 145–148f
  unfiltered backprojection, 134–135, 135f
  uniformity, 180–181
  viewing recommendations, 148–149
  volume rendering, 145, 147
  zoom, 157
Single-photon-emitting radionuclide for PETAC, 219
Singles-by-estimation technique, 218
Sinograms
  CT, 257, 258f
  delay, 211f, 213
  PET, 201–203, 202–204f
  prompt, 211f, 213
  SPECT, 152, 153f
Slant-hole collimators, 92, 92f, 155–156, 157f
Sleeve method (activity linearity testing), 14
Slew rate, 289
Slice selection gradient, 284, 285, 287
Sliding energy window, 64
Smoothing, 77–78, 78f
Smoothing filter, 77
SNR (signal-to-noise ratio), 96
  in PET, 233
Society of Motion Picture and Television Engineers (SMPTE), 122
Society of Nuclear Medicine (SNM), 92, 198, 240
  Technologist Section (SNMTS), 274
Sodium iodide
  disadvantages, 29
  gamma camera, 60
  PET and, 200
  scintillation in, 19–20
Software methods, SPECT, 174–175, 174f
Source geometry for TBAC, 169
Spans, 223
Spatial domain, 136
Spatial frequency domain, 136
Spatial resolution
  bar phantoms, 117–119, 118–119f
  CT, 264
  defined, 26
  gamma cameras and, 101–106, 102f, 104f
  measures of, 35, 187, 188f
  PET, 231, 248
  PET protocol, 248
  planar imaging, 101–106, 102f, 104f
  semiconductor detectors, 35
  SPECT, 154–155, 155f
SPECT. See Single-photon emission computed tomography
SPECT/CT systems, 267–268, 267–270f
Spectroscopy, 44
Spectrum Dynamics D-SPECT system, 175–176f, 176–177
Spillover of counts, 153
Spin (net magnetization), 279
Spin density, 291
Spin echo sequence, 284
Spin lattice, 290
Spin-lattice relaxation, 283
Spin-spin interactions, 283, 290
Spiral CT, 259
Split-photopeak monitoring, 66
Square waves, 137, 138f
Squelch feature, 32
Standard deviation, 40–42
Standardized uptake value (SUV), 238–240
Star artifact, 88, 88f
Static imaging, 67
Static magnetic fields, 292
Statistical degrees of freedom, 43
Statistical precision, 41
Statistical testing, 42–43
Statistics, nuclear counting, 40–44, 41f, 43f
Structured background, 152
Sum circuit, 61

Sum of sine waves, 137, 138f
Sum peaks, 47, 48–49f
Superconducting magnets, 289
Surface rendering, 145, 147
SUV (standardized uptake value), 238–240
System performance, 88

T

Tangential directions, 187, 188f
TBAC (transmission-based AC), 166–172
TE (echo time), 284
Technologist, radiation protection in CT, 267, 267f
Tertiary electrons, 4, 298, 301
Tesla (units of measure), 280
Testing. *See also* Quality control (QC)
   acceptance, 122, 123t, 180, 180f, 243–244
   accuracy, 11–12
   activity linearity, 14
   benchmark, 122
   Chi-square, 27, 42–43
   geometry factors for dose calibrator, 15
   infrequent PET, 246–249
   nonroutine gamma camera, 119–122
   routine PET, 244–246
Test patterns, 122, 123f
Thallium-activated sodium iodide, NaI(Tl), 18–19, 19f, 29, 200
Thin entrance window, 9, 10
Third-dimension superposition, 96, 96f
3D display techniques, 145–148
3D image matrix, 133–134, 143
3D vs. 2D. *See* 2D vs. 3D imaging modes
Thresholding, 61, 62f
Time. *See also* Dead time
   counts and, 106
     decay, 18
     echo, 284
     relaxation, 283
     repetition, 284
     rotation, 257
Time constant, 10, 10f, 311–312, 318
Time-of-flight (TOF-PET), 201, 205–206, 206–207f, 225, 238
Time per stop in SPECT, 158–159
Tissue attenuation, 256, 257f
Tissue characteristics and image appearance in MRI, 290–291
Tissue disturbance and differentiation in MRI, 281–283
Tomographic measures of performance in SPECT, 187–190
Tomographic slice uniformity, 188
Tomography overview, 131, 132
T1 relaxation, 282–283, 290
T1 relaxation time, 283
Topogram, 261
Townsend avalanche, 5, 9
TR (repetition time), 284
Transceiver, 289
Transistor, 314, 315f, 330
Transmission-based AC (TBAC), 166–172
Transmission tomography, 132
Transmit coils, 289–290
Transverse plane, 281
Transverse slices, 144
Troubleshooting gamma cameras, 122–125, 124–127f. *See also* Quality control (QC)
True events (trues), 203
Truncation artifacts, 193–194, 193f, 272
T2 relaxation, 283, 290–291
T2 relaxation time, 283
Tumor localization, 34
Tuning, 63
2D display techniques, 144–145, 145–148f
2D projections, 132–134, 135f, 142, 143
2D vs. 3D imaging modes, 210, 223–224, 224f, 238

U

Ultra-SPECT, 174
Unblank pulse, 61
Unfiltered backprojection (UBP), 134–135, 135f
Uniformity
   correction map, 65, 124, 126f
   correction techniques, 63–65
   defined, 55, 62
   differential, 115–116
   planar imaging, 100
   quality control for, 180–181, 246
   in SPECT, 117, 180–181
   tomographic slice, 188
Uniformity flood, 114–117, 115–117f
Uniformity measurement in SPECT, 187–188
Update step, 2D projection, 143
Upper-level discriminator (ULD), 22, 316, 316t
Useful field of view (UFOV), 116

V

Valence band, 18, 307–308, 308f
Video display terminal (VDT), 79, 122, 123f, 320, 320f
Viewing recommendations (SPECT images), 148–149
Virtual plane, 212, 215f
Voltage response curve, 4–5, 4f
Volume rendering, 145, 147
Volume sensitivity, 188–189
Voxel (volume element), 134, 153

W

Warm-metal scale, 79
Weighting, image in MRI, 290–291, 291f
Whole-body image, 67
Wiener filter, 172
Windowing, 80, 263, 263f
Windows, filters, 140. *See also* Energy window
Word, 331
Word mode, 73
Work function, defined, 9

X

X-axis gradient, 284
X-axis offset, 181–183, 182–183f
X-ray energy spectrum, 255–256, 256f
X-rays
   attenuation, 256
   Bremsstrahlung, 254, 255, 256, 256f, 300, 300t
   characteristic, 46–47, 255, 298
   energy spectrum, 255–256, 256f
   lead, 47
   polychromatic beam, 255
   production of, 254–255, 255f
X-ray tube, 254, 255, 255f

Y

Y-axis gradient, 284
Yellowing of the crystal, 124

Z

Zoom factor, 76, 157